Disease Management

Disease Management
A guide to clinical pharmacology

Michael D Randall MA, PhD, FBPhS
Professor of Pharmacology
University of Nottingham Medical School
Nottingham, UK

Karen E Neil BPharm (Hons), PhD, MRPharmS
Pharmacist
Nottingham, UK

Pharmaceutical Press

Published by the Pharmaceutical Press

66-68 East Smithfield, London E1W 1AW, UK

© The Royal Pharmaceutical Society 2016

(**PhP**) is a trade mark of RPS Publishing

RPS Publishing is the publishing organisation of the Royal Pharmaceutical Society

First edition published 2003
Second edition published 2009
Third edition published 2016

Printed in Great Britain by TJ International, Padstow, Cornwall

ISBN 978 0 85711 209 5 (print)
ISBN 978 0 85711 210 1 (ePDF)
ISBN 978 0 85711 211 8 (ePub)
ISBN 978 0 85711 212 5 (mobi)

A catalogue record for this book is available from the British Library

Contents

Part J Dermatology 385

Preface

Our aim is to put pharmacology, which is being learnt or was learnt some time ago, into the context of clinical practice. We believe that this book will be of use to later-year pharmacy students who are encountering clinical pharmacy and pharmacology for the first time, and to pre-registration pharmacists who are putting their training into practice, and will be of general interest to pharmacists in practice. However, the prescribing role of other healthcare professions is likely to expand and we believe that *Disease Management* will also prove a useful resource for introducing and dealing with important issues associated with medicines management.

Disease Management has grown from a course in clinical pharmacy and pharmacology (Disease and the Goals of Treatment), with which we have been involved in the Master of Pharmacy course at the University of Nottingham. In that course, we have used a case-study based approach, coupled to summary lectures, to introduce important therapeutic areas. In doing this we have become aware of the value of a disease-based approach to learning. In *Disease Management* we have sought to build on the course by taking common diseases such as diabetes, hypertension, asthma, depression and peptic ulceration, and dealing with the therapeutic issues. The structure that we have adopted is to provide a brief outline of the disease characteristics and clinical features. We have generally worked on the basis that diagnosis is beyond the scope of this book but have provided clinical features, particularly in the context of alerting symptoms for referral. These are followed by brief accounts of the pharmacology of the agents used to manage the conditions. Where guidelines exist and are in widespread use, we have incorporated brief summaries. The reader is of course referred to the more detailed guidance available and should also recognise that there is currently a wealth of resources that provide clinical guidance, such as the National Institute for Health and Care Excellence (NICE).

We have focused on drug choice and taken a holistic approach to recognise that a patient may have several related or unrelated conditions, e.g. rational drug choice in hypertension should be based on managing the hypertension without affecting other concurrent conditions such as asthma. Similarly, drug interactions represent an important therapeutic challenge and here we have attempted to highlight important examples of interactions and how they may be dealt with. Given the plethora of information on drug interactions we have largely drawn on *Stockley's Drug Interactions* (Baxter 2013) for information, because this provides an evidence-based approach with considered advice.

The topics of drug choice are intended to enable the reader to appreciate the rationale behind logical prescribing and advice in medicines management. We have also considered the patient rather than the disease, and here we have produced some points in which patients should be counselled about their disease and their drug treatment.

Our initial concept was to produce a short textbook focused on primary care but we now believe that we have produced an introduction to the management of diseases that are commonly encountered in, but not exclusive to, primary care. As such, we believe that *Disease Management* will provide a useful generalist introduction to medicines management.

Since the first edition of *Disease Management* there have been many changes in therapeutics and this is reflected in the third edition. In this new edition the revisions to clinical guidelines have been incorporated to reflect some substantial changes, notably in the management of hypertension, the use of statins and chronic heart failure. Key to therapeutics is the rational choice of medicines, and this is reflected in a new chapter focused on the considerations of drug choice in prescribing, taking account of prescribing in special cases. Although *Disease Management* is a generalist introduction, a new chapter on anticancer chemotherapy has been included, and this also deals with some of the newer, more targeted therapies introduced recently.

Michael D Randall, Karen E Neil

Reference

Baxter K, ed. (2013). *Stockley's Drug Interactions,* 10th edn. London: Pharmaceutical Press.

General reading

In producing this book we have used an extensive range of excellent standard textbooks and reference sources. These are listed here both as acknowledgement and to enable the reader to carry out further reading. More specific references, further reading and resources are provided in each chapter.

General medicine

Davey P (2014). *Medicine at a Glance*, 4th edn. Oxford, Wiley Blackwell.

Longmore M, Wilkinson I, Davidson EH *et al.* (2012). *Oxford Handbook of Clinical Medicine*, 7th edn. Oxford: Oxford University Press.

Kumar P, Clark M (2012). *Kumar and Clark's Clinical Medicine*, 6th edn. Edinburgh: WB Saunders.

Basic and clinical pharmacology

Bennett PN, Brown MJ (2012). *Clinical Pharmacology*, 11th edn. Edinburgh: Churchill Livingstone.

Brunton L, Chabneer BA, eds (2011). *Goodman & Gilman's The Pharmacological Basis of Therapeutics*, 12th edn. New York: McGraw-Hill.

Grahame-Smith DG, Aronson JK (2002). *Oxford Textbook of Clinical Pharmacology and Drug Therapy*, 3rd edn. Oxford: Oxford University Press.

Rang HP, Ritter JM, Flower RJ, Henderson G (2015). *Rang and Dale's Pharmacology*, 8th edn. London: Elsevier Churchill Livingstone.

Waller DG, Renwick AG, Hillier K (2005). *Medical Pharmacology and Therapeutics*, 2nd edn. Edinburgh: WB Saunders.

Clinical pharmacy

Addison B, Brown A, Edwards R, Gray G (2016). *Minor Illness or Major Disease. The clinical pharmacist in the community*, 6th edn. London: Pharmaceutical Press.

Baxter K, ed. (2013). *Stockley's Drug Interactions*, 10th edn. London: Pharmaceutical Press.

Blenkinsopp A, Paxton P, Blenkinsopp J (2014). *Symptoms in the Pharmacy: a guide to the management of common illnesses*, 7th edn. Oxford: Wiley Blackwell.

Greene RJ, Harris ND (2008). *Pathology and Therapeutics for Pharmacists*, 3rd edn. London: Pharmaceutical Press.

Lee A, ed. (2005). *Adverse Drug Reactions*, 2nd edn. London: Pharmaceutical Press.

Rutter P (2013). *Community Pharmacy*, 3rd edn. Edinburgh: Churchill Livingstone.

Walker R, Whittlesea C (2011). *Clinical Pharmacy and Therapeutics*, 5th edn. Edinburgh: Churchill Livingstone.

Wills S (2005). *Drugs of Abuse*, 2nd edn. London: Pharmaceutical Press.

Dietary supplements and clinical nutrition

Barnes J, Anderson LA, Phillipson JD (2007). *Herbal Medicines*, 3rd edn. London: Pharmaceutical Press.

Mason P (2000). *Nutrition and Dietary Advice in the Pharmacy*, 2nd edn. Oxford: Blackwell Science.

Mason P (2011). *Dietary Supplements*, 4th edn. London: Pharmaceutical Press.

Webster-Gandy J, Madden A (2011). *Oxford Handbook of Nutrition and Dietetics*, 2nd edn. Oxford: Oxford University Press.

Online resources

Bandolier is an excellent site with extensive summaries of recent clinical trials and experiments: www.medicine.ox.ac.uk/bandolier (accessed October 2015).

British National Formulary may be accessed and interacted with: www.bnf.org.uk (accessed October 2015).

Cochrane Collaboration for access to systematic reviews of healthcare interventions: www.cochrane.org (accessed October 2015).

Medicines and Healthcare products Regulatory Agency (MHRA) provides information on drug safety: www.mhra.gov.uk (accessed October 2015).

NHS Choices provides patient information on a range of conditions and treatments: www.nhs.uk (accessed October 2015)

The National Institute for Health and Care Excellence (NICE) provides guidance on prescribing policies: www.nice.org.uk (accessed October 2015).

Note to the reader

In producing this book we have attempted to provide a logical background to disease management. Although we have summarised some key guidelines, this book is not intended to provide definitive guidance, and the reader should of course consult appropriate national and local guidelines. The examples of drug interactions, adverse drug reactions and counselling points are not exhaustive and are included to illustrate common or important examples. Similarly, *Disease Management* is not intended to replace professional experience and the reader is reminded of the need to consult the latest information presented in the latest *British National Formulary,* summary of product characteristics and evidence-based resources for the latest drug information.

The case studies may deliberately contain less than ideal regimens and are intended to illustrate important therapeutic issues. Once again, the reader is reminded of the importance of consulting the *British National Formulary.*

Acknowledgements

In producing *Disease Management* we are grateful to a number of colleagues who have provided comments on our drafts for the first edition. In particular, we are indebted to Professor Tony Avery, University of Nottingham Medical School and a general practitioner, who commented on much of the clinical content. We are also extremely grateful to Dr Guy Mansford, a Nottinghamshire GP, and to Mrs Katie Grundy, a community pharmacist, for the much appreciated comments on many of the chapters. We are grateful to Naresh Chauhan, a community pharmacist in Nottingham, who provided detailed feedback on the first edition of *Disease Management*.

We would like to thank Professor Dave Kendall and Dr Ivan Stockley for their encouragement and shared enthusiasm for pharmacology. We should also like to thank Dr Tony Short for introducing us to the value of case study-based teaching.

In addition we would like to thank the many colleagues within the University of Nottingham Medical and Pharmacy Schools who have also provided detailed comments and criticisms on individual chapters in the first edition: Professor Claire Anderson, Professor of Social Pharmacy; Sandra Beatty, Hospital Pharmacist; Dr Sue Chan, Lecturer in Cell Signalling; Professor Vicky Chapman, Professor of Neuropharmacology; Dr Dick Churchill, general practitioner and Associate Professor in General Practice; Dr Jeff Fry, Associate Professor and Reader in Molecular Toxicology; Dr Katie Hewitt, Research Fellow; Dr Roger Knaggs; Professor Charles Marsden, Professor of Neuropharmacology; Dr Rob Mason, Senior Lecturer in Neuroscience; Dr Kishor Patel; Dr Nick Pierce, Consultant; Dr Gary Whitlock. We are also indebted to: Dr Anna Cadogan; Anne Lee, Principal Pharmacist, Glasgow Royal Infirmary; Dr Swaran P Singh, Senior Lecturer in Community Psychiatry, St George's Hospital, London; and Mrs Louise Walmsley, Health Visitor, Nottingham, for their most helpful comments and advice. We would also like to thank Karen's sister, Alison Devine, Professional Services Manager, Alliance Boots and brother, Paul Wallace, a final year pharmacy student, Liverpool John Moores University for their helpful and honest comments.

Karen would like to thank Ju-hee Kim (affectionately known as Sylvia), Rose Hindle, and both the Wallace and the Neil families for their support and encouragement.

We are indebted to the staff of the Pharmaceutical Press, and especially Paul Weller, Tamsin Cousins, Louise McIndoe, Linda Paulus, Mildred Davis, Christina Karaviotis, and Erasmis Kidd for their invaluable assistance and advice in the production of the first, second and third editions.

Despite the extensive help that we have received, any of the errors and omissions within *Disease Management* are the sole responsibility of the authors and we would very much appreciate any constructive comments directed to michael.randall@nottingham. ac.uk

About the authors

Michael D Randall read natural sciences at the University of Cambridge and specialised in pharmacology. After his first degree, he remained at Cambridge, carrying out research into the vascular actions of the endothelial factors, nitric oxide and the endothelins, and obtained a PhD in cardiovascular pharmacology. He was then a postdoctoral research fellow at the University of Wales College of Medicine (now Cardiff University's Medical School), continuing research into vascular pharmacology. In 1993 he was appointed to a lectureship, and is now a professor of pharmacology and Director of Teaching in the School of Life Sciences at the University of Nottingham Medical School, teaching pharmacology to both medical and pharmacy students.

Karen E Neil studied pharmacy at the University of Nottingham, before completing pre-registration training based at Broadgreen Hospital in Liverpool. She then returned to Nottingham to develop an interest in pharmacology gained during her final year as an undergraduate. She researched a variety of mechanisms involved in mediating second-messenger cross-talk, with particular interest in pathways associated with β-adrenoceptors, nitric oxide and phosphodiesterases, and achieved a PhD in molecular pharmacology. The application of pharmacology to clinical pharmacy beckoned and this developed from experience gained as a community pharmacist and researcher investigating adverse drug events and particularly drug interactions. She has been involved in teaching clinical pharmacy to pharmacy undergraduates, using problem-based learning, for a number of years. She has been a special lecturer in clinical pharmacology at the University of Nottingham Medical School.

Abbreviations

5ASA	5-aminosalicylate	CAPP	Captopril Prevention Project
5HT	5-hydroxytryptamine (serotonin)	CBT	cognitive-behavioural therapy
ACE	angiotensin-converting enzyme	CCK	cholecystokinin
ACEI	angiotensin-converting enzyme inhibitor	CDH	chronic daily headache
		CFC	chlorofluorocarbon
ADH	antidiuretic hormone	cGMP	guanosine cyclic 3':5'-monophosphate
ADME	absorption, distribution, metabolism, or excretion		
		CGRP	calcitonin gene-related peptide
ADP	adenosine diphosphate	CHAOS	Cambridge Heart Antioxidant Study
ADR	adverse drug reaction	CHD	coronary heart disease
AED	antiepileptic drug	CHF	chronic heart failure
AF	atrial fibrillation	CHM	Commission on Human Medicines
AIDS	acquired immune deficiency syndrome	CK	creatine kinase
		CKD	chronic renal disease
AIN	acute interstitial nephritis	CL	clearance
ALP	alkaline phosphatase	CL_{cr}	creatinine clearance
ALT	alanine transaminase	C_{max}	maximum concentration
AMP	adenosine monophosphate	C_{min}	minimum concentration
ANP	atrial natriuretic peptide	CNS	central nervous system
APTT	activated partial thromboplastin time	CO_2	carbon dioxide
ARDS	adult respiratory distress syndrome	CoA	coenzyme A
AST	aspartate transferase	COC	combined oral contraceptive
AT	angiotensin	COMA	Committee on Medical Aspects of Food and Nutrition Policy
ATP	adenine triphosphate		
AUC	area under the curve	COMT	catechol-O-methyltransferase
AV	atrioventricular	CONSENSUS	Cooperative North Scandinavian Enalapril Survival Study
BCG	bacille Calmette-Guérin		
BHF	British Heart Foundation	COPD	chronic obstructive pulmonary disease
BMI	body mass index		
BNF	*British National Formulary*	COX	cyclo-oxygenase
BP	blood pressure	CPK	creatine phosphokinase
BTS	British Thoracic Society	CRF	corticotrophin-releasing factor
CABG	coronary artery bypass grafting	CRP	C-reactive protein
CAD	coronary artery disease	CSM	Committee on Safety of Medicines
CAI	cholesterol absorption inhibitors	C_{ss}	steady-state concentration
cAMP	adenosine cyclic 3':5'-monophosphate	CTZ	chemoreceptor trigger zone
		CVA	cerebrovascular accident
CAPD	continuous ambulatory peritoneal dialysis	DCCT	Diabetes Control and Complications Trial

DCT	distal convoluted tubule	HMG	hydroxymethylglutaryl
DDT	dichlorodiphenyltrichloroethane	HOPE	Heart Outcomes Prevention Evaluation
DEET	diethyltoluamide (diethylmethylbenzamide)	HOT	Hypertension Optimal Treatment
DEXA	dual-energy X-ray absorptiometry	HPA	hypothalamic–pituitary–adrenal
DHA	docosahexanoic acid	HRT	hormone replacement therapy
DHEA	dehydroepiandrosterone	IARC	International Agency for Research on Cancer
DHP	dihydropyridine		
DIG	Digitalis Intervention Group	IBS	irritable bowel syndrome
DMARD	disease-modifying antirheumatoid drug	IBW	ideal body weight
		ICD-10	*International Statistical Classification of Diseases and Related Health Problems*, 10th edn
DNA	deoxyribonucleic acid		
DPP-4	dipeptidyl peptidase-4		
DSM-IV	*Diagnostic and Statistical Manual of Mental Disorders*	Ig	immunoglobulin
		IHD	ischaemic heart disease
DVLA	Driver and Vehicle Licensing Agency	INR	international normalised ratio
		IONA	Impact Of Nicorandil in Angina
DVT	deep vein thrombosis	IP_3	inositol triphosphate
ECG	electrocardiogram	JVP	jugular venous pressure
ECT	electroconvulsive therapy	K_{ATP}	ATP-sensitive K^+ channels
EEG	electroencephalogram	K_m	Michaelis–Menten constant
eGFR	estimated glomerular filtration rate	LDH	lactate dehydrogenase
EPA	eicosapentaenoic acid	LDL	low-density lipoprotein
EPO	erythropoietin; evening primrose oil	LFT	liver function test
ESR	erythrocyte sedimentation rate	LH	luteinising hormone
ET	endothelin	LIFE	Losartan Intervention For Endpoint reduction in hypertension
FBC	full blood count		
FDA	(US) Food and Drug Administration	LMWH	low-molecular-weight heparin
FEV_1	forced expiratory volume in the first second	LVH	left ventricular hypertrophy
		MAOI	monoamine oxidase inhibitor
FSH	follicle-stimulating hormone	MCH	mean corpuscular haemoglobin
FVC	forced vital capacity	MCV	mean corpuscular (cell) volume
GABA	γ-aminobutyric acid	MDI	metered dose inhaler
GAD	general anxiety disorder	MDMA	3,4-methylenedioxymethamfetamine or ecstasy
GFR	glomerular filtration rate		
GGT	γ-glutamyl transferase (transpeptidase)	MDRD	modification of diet in renal disease
G6PD	glucose-6-phosphate dehydrogenase	MHRA	Medicines and Healthcare products Regulatory Agency
GI	gastrointestinal		
GLP-1	glycogen-like peptide-1	MI	myocardial infarction
GLUT	glucose transporter	MMR	measles, mumps and rubella
GORD	gastro-oesophageal reflux disease	MODY	maturity-onset diabetes of the young
GP	general practitioner		
GTN	glyceryl trinitrate	MOH	medication overuse headache
Hb	haemoglobin	MRSA	meticillin-resistant *Staphylococcus aureus*
HbA_{1c}	glycated haemoglobin		
Hct	haematocrit	MS	multiple sclerosis
HDL	high-density lipoprotein	NACC	National Association for Colitis and Crohn's Disease
HIV	human immunodeficiency virus		

NANC	non-adrenergic non-cholinergic	RA	rheumatoid arthritis
NARI	noradrenaline (norepinephrine) reuptake inhibitors	RAAS	renin–angiotensin–aldosterone system
NaSSA	noradrenergic and specific serotonergic antidepressant	RAS	renin–angiotensin system
		RBC	red blood cell
NHS	National Health Service	REIN	Ramipril Efficacy In Nephropathy
NICE	National Institute for Health and Care Excellence	REM	rapid eye movement
		RICE	rest, ice, compression and elevation
NK	neurokinin	RIMA	reversible inhibitor of MAO-A
NMDA	N-methyl-D-aspartate	RPSGB	Royal Pharmaceutical Society of Great Britain
NO	nitric oxide		
NPA	National Pharmaceutical Association	4S	Scandinavian Simvastatin Survival Study
NPC	National Prescribing Centre	SACN	Scientific Advisory Committee on Nutrition
NPY	neuropeptide		
NRT	nicotine replacement therapy	SAD	seasonal affective disorder
NSAIDs	non-steroidal anti-inflammatory drugs	SERM	selective oestrogen receptor modulator
NSF	National Service Framework	SIADH	syndrome of inappropriate secretion of antidiuretic hormone
NSP	non-starch polysaccharide		
OA	osteoarthritis	SIGN	Scottish Intercollegiate Guidelines Network
OCD	obsessive compulsive disorder		
ORT	oral rehydration therapy	SLE	systemic lupus erythematosus
OTC	over-the-counter	SM	smooth muscle
PAF	platelet-activating factor	SMAC	Standing Medical Advisory Committee
PCV	packed cell volume		
PDEI	phosphodiesterase inhibitor	SNRI	serotonin–noradrenaline (norepinephrine) reuptake inhibitors
PE	pulmonary embolism		
PEF	peak expiratory flow	SPC	summary of product characteristics
PG	prostaglandin	SRM	serotonin receptor modulator
PGRs	prandial glucose regulators	SSRI	selective serotonin reuptake inhibitor
PI	phosphatidyl inositol		
PLA$_2$	phospholipase A$_2$	T$_3$	triiodothyronine
PMR	patient medication record	T$_4$	thyroxine
POM	prescription-only medicine	TB	tuberculosis
POP	progestogen-only pill	TCA	tricyclic antidepressant
PPAR	peroxisome proliferator-activated receptors	TDM	therapeutic drug monitoring
		TEN	toxic epidermal necrolysis
PPI	proton pump inhibitor	TENS	transcutaneous electrical stimulation
PRISM	Platelet Receptor Inhibition in Ischemic Syndrome Management		
		TFT	thyroid function test
PROGRESS	Perindopril Protection Against Recurrent Stroke Study	THC	Δ^9-tetrahydrocannabinol
		THR	traditional herbal registration
PSA	prostate-specific antigen	TIA	transient ischaemic attack
PTCA	percutaneous transluminal coronary angioplasty	TNFα	tumour necrosis factor-α
		TPN	total parenteral nutrition
PTH	parathyroid hormone	tRNA	transfer ribonucleic acid
PUFA	polyunsaturated fatty acid	TrT	troponin T

TSH	thyroid-stimulating hormone	V_{max}	maximum rate of reaction
TxA$_2$	thromboxane	VLDL	very-low-density lipoprotein
U&Es	urea and electrolytes	VSM	vascular smooth muscle
UKPDS	UK Prospective Diabetes Study	VTE	venous thromboembolism
UT	urinary tract	WBC	white blood cell
UTI	urinary tract infection	WFSBP	World Federation of Societies of Biological Psychiatry
UV	ultraviolet		
V_d	volume of distribution	WHO	World Health Organization

PART **A**

The patient

1

Signs and symptoms

Symptoms and patient histories in the pharmacy

Role

The pharmacist has a central role in assessing a patient's complaint or condition, with a view to providing information, recommending appropriate treatment or referring the patient to a general practitioner (GP). Indeed the pharmacist may be the first health professional consulted by many patients, especially as an appointment is not required.

The consultation

Unlike the hospital doctor or GP, the pharmacist is unlikely to have the luxury of carrying out a full medical history and may not have access to the patient's medical records or test results. Indeed, the consultation may well be happening in a busy shop. Hence, the pharmacist has to establish the relevant facts, to differentiate between minor complaints and potentially serious conditions, and make a judgement or even diagnosis 'on the spot'. First, the patient must be identified and once this is established the pharmacist might then ask the person to explain what he or she believes the problem to be; this should then prompt more specific questions related to the condition. Throughout the interview the pharmacist should take the opportunity to assess the patient to make a judgement about how ill he or she looks and also to examine the patient for

any signs that may point to disease, e.g. the following might be revealed:

- Skin colour: signs of jaundice or changes in skin coloration.
- Coloration of the sclera (may reveal jaundice).
- Marks on the skin: e.g. a change in a mole, a rodent ulcer or spider naevi (see Chapter 36).
- Breathing: is the patient short of breath or having trouble completing a sentence?
- Digital clubbing: the fingers take on a 'drumstick' appearance and this can indicate chronic pulmonary, cardiac or liver diseases.
- Does the patient *appear* to have a fever?
- Does the patient appear anxious? Signs of anxiety might indicate how serious the patient feels that the problem is or reveal a hidden concern.

The pharmacist should also attempt to make a judgement about the educational background or medical knowledge of the person, so that the questioning and any subsequent counselling may be appropriately phrased. A patient volunteering specific facts or requesting a specific medicine may reveal their medical knowledge or lack of it.

Establishing the facts

The questioning should be directed towards aiding a diagnosis or making a judgement as to the need for referral or over-the-counter (OTC) treatment.

Relevant lines of questioning might be related to the following:

- What the problem appears to be.
- How bad the symptoms are.
- How long the patient has been aware of the problem.
- The main presenting symptoms.
- Any accompanying symptoms.
- What makes the condition worse?
- What provides relief?
- Any relevant social factors.
- Does the patient have a previously diagnosed medical condition?
- A drug history with particular attention to the use of OTC treatments.

The above may be summarised by the popular mnemonic, WWHAM (Blenkinsopp *et al.*, 2014):

Who is the patient?
What are the symptoms?
How long have the symptoms been present?
Action taken, medicines tried?
Medicines taken for other conditions?

The drug history may be relevant to the current symptoms or influence the recommendation for OTC medicines or referral. Patients may regard non-prescription medicines and herbal remedies as being less important and so they should be directly questioned about their usage. In addition, it is clearly important for the pharmacist to establish if the patient is suffering from a previously diagnosed chronic condition, such as diabetes mellitus, asthma, chronic obstructive pulmonary disease (COPD), epilepsy, liver disease, renal disease and cardiovascular disease, or receiving long-term treatment, e.g. corticosteroids. It may be that the presenting complaint is associated with this condition or its treatment but this may not be obvious to the patient. Chronic conditions will also influence the use of OTC medicines and the importance of referral.

Patients may also make direct requests for named OTC medicines. In such cases this may suggest that a patient has a previously diagnosed condition, for which an OTC medicine may be appropriate within the limitations of its licence, e.g. a patient may be requesting sumatriptan for previously diagnosed migraine (see Chapter 23). A request for simvastatin to reduce cholesterol (and cardiovascular risk) would prompt a full history to check that the patient fulfils the criteria to receive it as an OTC medicine (see Chapter 13), and also provides an opportunity to explore any health concerns and provide appropriate lifestyle advice

In the case of women of childbearing age it is important to establish if the patient *could be* pregnant and it may be sensible to assume that the patient is pregnant until proven otherwise. This level of caution is essential because many drugs may damage the fetus, especially in the early stages of pregnancy when the patient may not herself be aware that she is pregnant.

Once the presenting complaint has been established, the pharmacist should use his or her professional skills to select relevant searching questions, e.g. if a patient complains of a cough, an open and open-ended question may be:

'Tell me about the cough'

and, depending on the response, detailed questioning may enable the pharmacist to determine the underlying nature of the complaint (and thus course of action), e.g. the questioning might proceed as follows.

What are the symptoms?

'Is there any sputum?'
'What colour is the sputum?'
'Have you noticed any blood in the sputum?'
Alternatively, ask the patient to describe the sputum.

Indeed the last question is a more indirect approach than the question 'Have you coughed up any blood?' Using appropriate questions is important because patients may wish to deny to themselves sinister symptoms such as haemoptysis (coughing up blood) or by contrast they may not appreciate their importance.

How long?

'How long have you had the cough?'

Action taken, medicines tried?

'Are you taking any medicines prescribed by a doctor or bought from a pharmacy?'

This essential question enables the identification of iatrogenic problems such as drug-induced blood dyscrasias in patients prescribed immunosuppressants or a cough induced by an angiotensin-converting enzyme (ACE) inhibitor. It may also identify problems where a drug has already been prescribed but the treatment has failed. Medicines taken for other conditions should also be considered. A drug history is imperative when OTC medication is recommended, allowing the exclusion of contraindications and avoidance of drug interactions. Additional relevant questions might be:

'Have you ever smoked?'

This is a more searching question than 'Do you smoke?' because the person may have given up yesterday (perhaps in response to the symptom) and the answer would be no! Alcohol consumption is also likely to be under-reported by patients.

'Are you having any difficulty in breathing?'
'Have you noticed a wheezing noise or rattle?'

The outcome

The interview should enable the pharmacist to make a reasonable attempt at identifying the condition and then to decide on the appropriate course of action, whether advice, treatment or referral. If the outcome is that the pharmacist believes that it is in the patient's best interests to consult a GP, the importance of this should be emphasised without unduly worrying the patient. It is, however, important to give an indication of the urgency of referral, e.g. a patient presenting with cystitis and systemic symptoms such as fever should be seen urgently rather than wait for the next available appointment. In all cases the pharmacist should ensure that the patient understands fully the course of action that you recommend.

Signs and symptoms

In dealing with responding to symptoms the reader is referred to *Minor Illness or Major Disease* by Addison *et al.* (2016), *Symptoms in the Pharmacy* by Blenkinsopp *et al.* (2014) and *Community Pharmacy* by Rutter (2013), which deal with responding to a range of common symptoms (see end of chapter).

Symptoms

A symptom is a perceived change in well-being by the patient that may or may not be associated with significant illness. The patient complains of a symptom and it is different from 'normal'. Several symptoms may present together to suggest or exclude a disease; this forms part of differential diagnosis, e.g. a patient may report breathlessness and also notice swollen ankles, which may appear unrelated but to the pharmacist may point to chronic heart failure (see Chapter 16). The following are some examples of symptoms:

- cough
- tiredness
- aches
- chest pains
- breathlessness
- indigestion.

Signs

A sign is a clinical change in a person, which may be observed by a clinician and indicates a disease. The following are some common examples of signs:

- changes in skin (colour, markings)
- digital clubbing (fingers clubbed in lung and hepatic diseases)
- heart murmurs
- sounds on listening to the lungs (wheezes [rhonchi], crackles [crepitations])
- dullness to percussion of thorax (changes in sound on tapping)
- changes to the retina
- enlarged lymph nodes.

There is obviously some overlap between signs and symptoms as a patient might notice ankle oedema but not realise that it is a significant sign of heart failure.

Important examples of signs and symptoms

Cough

A cough may be a trivial symptom, either reflecting a minor ailment or possibly pointing to a serious underlying disease (Table 1.1).

Chest pains

Once again, chest pains represent an important symptom, which might be due to a minor illness or a serious condition and some common causes are detailed in Table 1.2.

Given the above (Table 1.2) presentations and diverse conditions, questioning should be directed towards establishing the following:

- The location and nature of the pain and additional symptoms.
- What provokes the pain?
- What relieves the pain (including the use of OTC medicines and rest)?
- Recent activity? For example, exertion that may have strained a muscle.
- Past medical history.
- If GTN (glyceryl trinitrate) failed to control the symptoms, is it actually in date?

Breathlessness

Similarly, breathlessness may be due to a whole range of conditions and the possible aetiologies include:

- congenital: cystic fibrosis
- infection: chest infection, tuberculosis
- inflammatory: asthma, anaphylaxis
- neoplastic: carcinoma
- haematological: secondary to anaemia
- psychogenic: panic attacks

Table 1.1 Some causes of a cough	
Underlying condition	**Comments**
Coryza (cold) (Chapter 20)	Associated with cold symptoms
Acute bronchitis (Chapter 20)	Often following a cold: there may be production of sputum, with wheezing and a temperature
Tracheitis	A dry, rasping and painful cough which is often associated with a viral infection
Pneumonia (Chapter 20)	Infection of the alveoli which leads to sputum (which may be bloodstained and is often rusty in appearance), breathlessness, pleuritic chest pains and fever
COPD (Chapter 22)	- COPD - Associated with exacerbations - The 'smoker's cough' may herald the onset of COPD
Asthma (Chapter 22)	- May be associated with wheezing and breathlessness - Often a nocturnal cough and this may be the only symptom in a child
Drug-induced (Chapters 12 and 16)	For example, with ACE inhibitors
Anxiety	A long-term 'nervous cough'
Foreign body	Associated with recent inhalation of an object
Tuberculosis (Chapter 34)	Associated with tiredness, malaise, weight loss, fever and haemoptysis
Bronchiectasis	- Dilated bronchioles with persistent infections and mucus - Copious amounts of sputum which may be bloodstained
Congestive heart failure (Chapter 16)	Associated with breathlessness and oedema
Lung cancer	A history of smoking associated with haemoptysis. A change in a 'smoker's cough' is a serious alerting symptom

ACE, angiotensin-converting enzyme; COPD, chronic obstructive pulmonary disease.

Table 1.2 Some causes of chest pains	
Underlying condition	**Comments**
Musculoskeletal in origin (Chapter 31)	Pain may be worse on moving an arm or follows strenuous or unusual exercise. This is a common explanation and is often the default diagnosis
Respiratory (Chapter 22)	The pain is likely to be associated with breathing and to be due to an underlying respiratory disease, e.g. asthma
Pleuritic pains	This may be due to some form of respiratory disease but, if associated with calf swelling, haemoptysis or risk factors for thromboembolism, it may point to pulmonary embolism
Gastric origin: peptic ulceration, reflux	Here there may be a relationship to food, being either brought on by a meal (gastro-oesophageal reflux disease) or temporarily relieved by food (peptic ulceration) (Chapter 8). It should be relieved rapidly by antacids. In patients >55 years of age, if this symptom is of recent onset it raises the suspicion of carcinoma, which should be excluded
Angina (Chapter 15)	Angina has the following characteristics, which often allow it to be diagnosed by a history: • A crushing feeling in the chest • Often accompanied by pains down the arm (often left) • Pains may radiate to the jaw • Stable angina is induced by exercise, emotional stress, cold weather or a meal • Unstable angina may occur at rest • It should be relieved by rest (unless unstable) or GTN • Characteristic ECG changes
Myocardial infarction (Chapter 15)	• This must be differentiated from angina and is characteristically severe chest pains, which are not relieved by rest or GTN • May be accompanied by nausea, breathlessness, pallor, sweating and pains down the arms and/or jaw • Often diagnosed by ECG changes and so-called 'cardiac enzymes' • Some patients may experience a silent myocardial infarction, which does not cause chest pains

ECG, electrocardiogram; GTN, glyceryl trinitrate.

- degenerative: COPD
- cardiac: chronic heart failure, acute left ventricular failure, myocardial infarction
- thromboembolic: pulmonary embolism
- functional: in pregnancy, ascent to altitude, obesity
- iatrogenic: bronchospasm secondary to drug treatment (e.g. (β blockers, non-steroidal anti-inflammatory drugs [NSAIDs]); chronic pulmonary damage (e.g. amiodarone). (See Chapter 6.)
- traumatic: physical damage to the chest.

In all cases, the serious nature of the potential conditions should lead to a referral, and the key question is the degree of urgency required.

Pain

Pain affects many parts of the body and represents an interesting complaint as it may point to a range of trivial or serious conditions, e.g. an uncomplicated tension headache would be treated by simple analgesia but a severe headache typical of migraine (see Chapter 23) with accompanying symptoms such as nausea and photophobia would require referral. A headache that is severe and explosive (the patient might describe it as feeling like being 'hit on the back of the head with a brick') might point to a subarachnoid haemorrhage, which is a medical emergency. In taking a history of pain it may help to ask the patient to describe the severity on a scale of 1–10, with 10 representing 'the worst ever'.

Pain affecting other systems in the body requires close questioning of the relevant system, e.g. musculoskeletal pain may be the response to a recent injury or due to a chronic condition such as arthritis – in which case a diagnosis might be suggested by the time course of onset and provoking factors.

Gastrointestinal pain similarly represents a challenge. The first issue is one of location, e.g. heartburn is an obvious indication of upper gastrointestinal problems such as gastro-oesophageal reflux disease and would be exacerbated by eating. Lower gastrointestinal pain, which is colicky in nature, might point to a visceral cause, whereas pain with bloating, which is relieved by defecation, would be consistent with irritable bowel syndrome.

A 'funny turn'

This symptom encompasses a range of events from dizziness to total loss of consciousness that may involve fitting. As one might imagine, the range of events has a wide number of possible causes including the following.

Cardiovascular

Cardiovascular events such as a stroke (including a transient ischaemic attack), arrhythmias and postural hypotension, which is particularly prevalent in elderly people and those taking vasodilators or diuretics. Vaso-vagal syncope (fainting) may involve bradycardia with vasodilatation as a response to fear, pain, emotion or standing for a prolonged period and result in a faint.

Neurological

Neurological causes include epilepsy, strokes, migraine and infections including meningitis.

Endocrine

Endocrine causes include postural hypotension due to Addison's disease, thyrotoxicosis and diabetes with hypoglycaemia or hyperglycaemia.

Psychological

Psychological causes include panic attacks.

Iatrogenic

Iatrogenic causes include postural hypotension, in those taking vasodilators or diuretics as mentioned above or confusion with benzodiazepines. In response to a funny turn, the following questions may help to implicate or exclude certain causes:

- What provokes an attack? For example, flashing lights in certain forms of epilepsy.
- Were there any prodromal symptoms? For example, an aura in epilepsy.
- Was there loss of consciousness?

- Was there injury? Tongue biting would be consistent with epilepsy.
- Were there any unusual movements? This might implicate epilepsy.
- Was there incontinence? Incontinence of urine is common in epilepsy.
- What colour did the patient go? Extreme pallor during the episode and flushing after the attack might suggest a cardiac cause.
- How did the patient recover? With neurological causes there may be confusion.
- How long did it last?
- Does the patient have a current illness or is he or she receiving any drugs?

Given the potential seriousness of the above causes of a 'funny turn', it is likely that a referral would be made.

Referral

The pharmacist has a major role in responding to symptoms. Initially, the pharmacist should respond with advice and where necessary prescribe OTC medicines for 'minor' conditions that would respond. Compliance problems with prescribed medicines can often be rectified by the pharmacist. Equally, the pharmacist should be able to recognise potentially serious symptoms and refer patients to their GP, NHS drop-in centres or, in an emergency, a hospital accident and emergency department. Consultation via telephone, publications or online resources with NHS Choices is also a valuable source of referral information, triage and algorithms for patients.

In general, referral should be made for patients with potentially serious symptoms, for persistent symptoms and high-risk patients such as:

- babies
- children
- elderly people
- patients with diabetes
- pregnant or breastfeeding mothers
- immunocompromised patients.

In addition, many other disease states representing high risk (e.g. ischaemic heart disease, epilepsy, COPD, asthma) and then deterioration in the condition might warrant referral.

One should also be mindful of patients who frequently request OTC medicines for symptomatic relief, because they may be used to hide symptoms, e.g. the use of OTC H_2-receptor antagonists in peptic ulceration. Another reason to refer would be due to the failure of OTC medicines to control or relieve a condition or requests for OTC medicines that are not covered by their licence. In addition, the following examples of alerting symptoms should also prompt a referral.

Gastrointestinal

Some important gastrointestinal referral points are shown in Table 1.3.

Cardiorespiratory

Some important cardiorespiratory referral points are shown in Table 1.4.

Neurological and psychiatric

Some important neurological and psychiatric referral points are shown in Table 1.5.

Others

Some other important referral points are shown in Table 1.6.

This list of referrals is intended as a list of common examples that should prompt referral to the patient's GP or urgent referral to hospital. Obviously, if there is any doubt the patient should be referred and, as emphasised in Chapter 6, the pharmacist should be alert to the possibility of patients presenting with an adverse drug reaction (ADR). The list is clearly not exhaustive and local referral protocols may already be established with GPs.

Table 1.3 Some important gastrointestinal referral points	
Leading feature	**Features and comments**
Mouth ulcers	• Recurrent and/or failure of OTC therapy • Possible ADR • Associated with agents that may cause neutropenia such as carbimazole, carbamazepine and clozapine (Chapter 6)
Swallowing	• Dysphagia (difficulty in swallowing) • Odynophagia (painful swallowing) that is not simply due to a sore throat
Vomiting (Chapters 9 and 10)	• Haematemesis (vomiting blood) – any and urgent referral if profuse. Bleeding may be profuse or present as 'ground coffee' in appearance (Chapter 8) • Symptoms of dehydration such as decreased output of urine, headache and confusion – care in special groups; taking laxatives or diuretics (advise to omit doses) • Nausea of more than 3–4 days
Dyspepsia/'indigestion' (Chapter 8)	• Indigestion persisting after 2 weeks of OTC histamine H_2-receptor antagonists or 4 weeks of OTC omeprazole • Pain consistent with peptic ulceration • Following use of NSAIDs • Prolonged indigestion, also new or changed symptoms in patients >45 years of age, or alerting symptoms including anorexia, weight loss, anaemia and upper abdominal masses
Bowel habits (Chapter 10)	• Sustained (>2 weeks) alteration in bowel habits (particularly in those over 45 years of age) • Passing blood (frank or melaena, black 'tarry' stools) – this may be due to gastrointestinal bleeding • Severe diarrhoea while taking antibiotics, especially clindamycin – antibiotics may lead to colitis • Steatorrhoea – significant if not explained by concomitant orlistat • Pale stools
Weight loss	Weight loss or wasting that is unexplained
Liver problems (Chapter 11)	Jaundice

ADR, adverse drug reaction; NSAIDs, non-steroidal anti-inflammatory drugs; OTC, over-the-counter.

Table 1.4 Some important cardiorespiratory referral points

Leading feature	Features and comments
Chest pain (Chapter 15)	• Chest pain at rest or on exertion • Chest pain suggesting a myocardial infarction and that is not relieved by nitrates should prompt emergency hospital referral. Consider administering aspirin (150–300 mg)
Breathlessness	• Any of new onset or deterioration • Including breathlessness at night while lying down (Chapter 16) • Breathlessness (often wheezy) with signs of anaphylaxis such as urticaria, angio-oedema with swollen lips or eyelids, should lead to urgent hospital referral (Chapter 21)
Wheezing	Any
Cough	• Persistent cough of >2–3 weeks, or with a history of bronchitis or green sputum (Chapter 20) • A change in smoker's cough • Persistent dry nocturnal cough in a child, which may indicate asthma (Chapter 22) • Haemoptysis (coughing up blood) • Cough with ACE inhibitors (Chapters 12 and 16), if the cough is intolerable
Symptoms consistent with anaemia	Any (Chapter 18) – identify possible cause, including use of NSAIDs and associated gastrointestinal bleeding
Dizziness on standing (postural hypotension)	Especially in patients taking ACE inhibitors, diuretics, α blockers and antipsychotics
Painful unilateral calf swelling	Especially if accompanied by breathlessness and/or pleuritic pain, this should lead to urgent referral to hospital (Chapter 17)
Ankle swelling	Any – new or deterioration
Xanthomas	Yellowish lipid deposits, especially on eyelids (xanthelasmas), cornea and tendons (Chapter 13)
Sore throat	• Persistent sore throat (Chapter 20) • Sore throat with rash, fever, enlarged lymph nodes or infected tonsils (Chapter 20) • Sore throat or rashes, especially in patients taking drugs known to cause neutropenia such as carbimazole, clozapine and carbamazepine (Chapter 6)
Sinusitis	Sinus pain or discharge that does not resolve after 7 days (Chapter 20)

ACE, angiotensin-converting enzyme; NSAIDs, non-steroidal anti-inflammatory drugs.

Table 1.5 Some important neurological and psychiatric referral points

Leading feature	Features and comments
Headache (Chapter 23)	• Headache that is severe, follows injury or accompanied by other alerting signs • Recurrent or persistent migraine not relieved by OTC medicines
Seizures or loss of consciousness	Any, including absences (Chapter 24)
Signs or behaviour pointing to psychiatric disorders	Any (Chapters 25–28)
Insomnia	With repeat requests (>2 weeks) for OTC sleeping remedies (Chapter 27)
Problems with movement or tremor	Refer for specialist opinion (Chapter 29)

OTC, over-the-counter.

Table 1.6 Some other important referral points

Leading feature	Features and comments
Symptoms suggestive of diabetes mellitus (Chapter 37)	Including polydipsia (increased drinking), polyuria, recurrent thrush, frequent skin infections, ketone breath
Symptoms suggestive of hyperthyroidism (Chapter 38)	Including tachycardia, palpitations, fine tremor, warm peripheries, bulging eyes
Symptoms suggestive of hypothyroidism (Chapter 38)	Including tiredness, weight gain, cold intolerance, dry skin and hair, goitre, puffiness around the eyes
Cushingoid symptoms	• Features include moon face, thinning of the skin, easy bruising and central weight gain • Including patients taking corticosteroids
Problems with urination	• Difficulty in passing urine • Blood in urine • Recurrent thrush or cystitis • Urinary dysfunction suggestive of prostatic hypertrophy
Urogenital problems	• Vaginal bleeding; in pregnancy this should lead to urgent referral • Recurrent infections • Urinary dysfunction, including haematuria (passing blood) and prostate problems • Any renal problems
Somatosensory problems	• Eye problems • Eye infections where OTC treatment is not appropriate or is ineffective. One should be mindful of the risk of serious eye conditions that require urgent referral • Hearing problems • Otitis media not responding to simple analgesia • Disturbances of balance
Dermatological problems (Chapter 36)	• Eczema for the first time • Infected eczema (bacterial infection, eczema herpeticum) • Impetigo • Use of OTC topical steroids for >1 week • Secondary infection of bites • Psoriasis • Rosacea • Acne after 2 months of OTC treatment or risk of scarring • Jaundice • Spider naevi • Changes in moles • Rodent ulcers • Chickenpox in patients taking steroids • Shingles • Rashes: especially after taking a drug. Non-blanching rashes where there is suspicion of meningitis should lead to immediate hospital referral • Burns larger than a thumbnail in size • Purpura (easy bruising), especially in patients taking either drugs associated with thrombocytopenia or warfarin
Lumps	Especially in: • breast • testicles • neck • armpit

(continued)

Table 1.6 *(continued)*	
Leading feature	**Features and comments**
Musculoskeletal	• Pain on weight bearing • Significant pain not relieved by simple analgesia • Any significant trauma at high speed or significant load • Any significant limb or motor dysfunction • Muscle pains with statins and/or fibrates (Chapter 13) • Tendon pain with certain drugs, including quinolones
Drugs	• Overdose of drugs (especially paracetamol) requires urgent referral to hospital, even in the absence of any symptoms
Travel	Ill after foreign travel

OTC, over-the-counter

CASE STUDIES

Case studies on coughs

A cough may be trivial symptom, either reflecting a minor ailment or possibly associated with serious underlying disease. The following cases are intended to illustrate the possible causes.

Case 1

A 4 year old with a cough as the presenting symptom was taken to their pharmacist. The pharmacist asked the following questions:

- 'Is it nocturnal?' – this might point to asthma.
- 'How long has the child had a cough?' – this would identity chronic conditions such as asthma, whereas a shorter duration would be consistent with an infection.
- 'Is there a family history of asthma?' – a family history of asthma and/or atopy might suggest asthma.
- 'Is it productive?' – this might point to a bacterial chest infection.
- 'Is it productive of vast quantities of sputum?' – large amounts of sputum that may contain blood might point to bronchiectasis.
- 'Is it a dry cough?' – this might point to a simple upper respiratory tract infection.
- 'Is it associated with wheezing?' – this may point to bronchiolitis or asthma.
- 'Is he eating and drinking normally?' – this may give an indication as to how ill he is.

It was found that the cough was non-productive and of recent onset, and a diagnosis of a viral infection was made. Reassurance was given and paracetamol was recommended for any fever and the mother was advised to take the toddler to the GP if it was no better after 2 weeks or it worsened in that time.

Case 2

In the course of a morning, a number of 60-year-olds present to their GP with coughs and additional questioning went along the lines of:

- 'Have you ever smoked?'
- 'Is it a dry or productive cough?'
- 'How long have you had it?'

Patient A: A productive cough of recent onset with green sputum.

- This is consistent with bacterial infection and a chest infection was diagnosed.

Patient B: A smoker with a productive cough over many years, which is worse in winter and the sputum is grey or sometimes green.

- Smoking is a major risk factor for respiratory diseases and a 'smoker's cough' is an early sign of COPD. His present condition is consistent with severe COPD with an infection. Haemoptysis (coughing up blood) may occur in other serious conditions such as tumour, which should be excluded. An exacerbation of COPD was diagnosed.

Patient C: Smoker with changes in cough characteristics or persistent dry cough and coughing up blood.

- This may be a presenting symptom of carcinoma and other signs (which may include: haemoptysis, digital clubbing, pleural pain, weight loss, signs of metastasis, central nervous system changes including fits) are all ominous symptoms of carcinoma. The suspicion of carcinoma was raised.

Patient D: Non-smoker with productive cough, haemoptysis, weight loss, night sweats and risk factor for tuberculosis (TB) (homeless).

- A productive cough is a major respiratory symptom and night sweats are consistent with TB and Hodgkin's disease. The suspicion of TB was raised.

Patient E: Cough and breathlessness on mild exertion and lying down in bed at night.

- The suspicion of chronic heart failure was raised.

Patient F: Cough while taking an ACE inhibitor for chronic heart failure.

- These might point to inadequate treatment or an ACE inhibitor-induced cough.

References

Addison B, Brown A, Edwards R, Gray G (2016). *Minor Illness or Major Disease. The clinical pharmacist in the community*, 6th edn. London: Pharmaceutical Press.

Blenkinsopp A, Paxton P, Blenkinsopp J (2014). *Symptoms in the Pharmacy: a guide to the management of common illnesses*, 7th edn. Oxford: Wiley Blackwell.

Rutter P (2013). *Community Pharmacy*. Edinburgh: Churchill Livingstone.

Online resources

www.nhs.uk
The website of NHS Choices, with advice available on how patients should respond to symptoms.

Clinical laboratory tests

The following sections are intended as a guide to the most commonly used laboratory tests. Reference values are included as a guide and represent average population values. It should be noted that these values may alter according to the assay procedure, particularly when measuring enzymes, and local values should be sought when interpreting clinical data.

Clinical biochemistry

The monitoring of clinical biochemistry is used alongside clinical symptoms to diagnose disease, regulate drug therapy and identify adverse drug reactions. Biochemical blood tests include:

- urea and electrolytes (U&Es): a standard request may provide sodium, potassium, urea and creatinine levels
- liver function tests (LFTs)
- lipid profiles
- glucose and glycated haemoglobin (HbA$_{1c}$)
- thyroid function tests (TFTs).

Urea and electrolytes

The plasma concentration of urea and the electrolytes sodium, potassium, calcium and magnesium in blood plasma is used to indicate renal function, dehydration and electrolyte disturbances caused by drugs or disease, e.g. the retention of electrolytes may indicate impaired renal function or electrolyte loss may occur due to diarrhoea and vomiting, or the overuse of diuretics.

Drugs and the monitoring of U&Es

The requirement for electrolyte monitoring is discussed in individual chapters. A summary of some important drug-related electrolyte disturbances is given in Table 2.1.

Renal function tests

Renal function is often predicted from the results obtained from U&E monitoring. The main indicators are urea and creatinine. Urea is produced by protein metabolism and levels are raised following high protein intake, renal impairment, tissue damage and/or catabolism. So, although levels may be elevated in renal disease, they do not provide a reliable estimate of renal function.

Creatinine is produced from creatine in the skeletal muscle at a fairly constant rate and in normal individuals is renally cleared, so plasma levels are an index of renal function. A more precise predictor of renal function is therefore calculated as an estimate of the glomerular filtration rate (GFR) calculated from the

Table 2.1 Examples of drugs causing electrolyte disturbance

Electrolyte disturbance	Symptoms	Drugs implicated
Hypokalaemia (reduced potassium)	Hypokalaemia due to fluid loss (consider diuretics, vomiting, diarrhoea): may occur in hepatic failure due to aldosterone release; may lead to neuromuscular disturbances, cramps, muscle weakness, and tetany leading to paralysis and respiratory failure. Arrhythmias may also occur, especially in patients at increased risk, e.g. taking digoxin	Especially thiazide and loop diuretics; β_2-adrenoceptor agonists, corticosteroids, lithium and theophylline
Hyperkalaemia (increased potassium)	Hyperkalaemia may lead to a limp paralysis, arrhythmias and sudden death, but is initially asymptomatic	ACE inhibitors, aldosterone receptor antagonists, analgesics, angiotensin II receptor antagonists, potassium salts (salt substitute, effervescent preparations, e.g. low-sodium cystitis products and potassium citrate mixture), potassium-sparing diuretics and heparin
Hyponatraemia (reduced sodium)	Symptoms of hyponatraemia include orthostatic hypotension, reduced skin turgidity, confusion and ultimately convulsions. Hyponatraemia due to excess water may present as anorexia, heart failure, muscle weakness and oedema	ACE inhibitors, aldosterone inhibitors, analgesics, antidepressants, carbamazepine, loop diuretics, omeprazole, potassium-sparing diuretics, thiazide diuretics and tolbutamide
Hypernatraemia (increased sodium)	Hypernatraemia occurs in renal failure, producing symptoms of confusion, drowsiness, lethargy, dry skin, hypotension, muscle twitching, peripheral vasoconstriction and ultimately coma	Corticosteroids, NSAIDs, lithium
Hypomagnesaemia (reduced magnesium)	Hypomagnesaemia increases the risk of arrhythmias	Aminoglycosides, bisphosphonates, immunosuppressants, loop diuretics and thiazide diuretics
Hypercalcaemia (increased calcium)	Symptoms of hypercalcaemia include abdominal pain, anorexia, constipation, fatigue, nausea and vomiting, polyuria with nocturia and thirst. Progression to confusion, delirium, psychosis, gallstones, renal impairment (due to calculi or stones), stupor and coma may occur	Androgens, antacids, calcium salts, fat-soluble vitamins, sex hormones, thiazide diuretics, vitamin A derivatives and vitamin D derivatives
Hypocalcaemia (decreased calcium)	Hypocalcaemia tends to be asymptomatic. Worsening hypocalcaemia may produce paraesthesia of the face, fingers and toes, tetany or prolonged tonic muscle spasms and ultimately convulsions and psychosis	Loop diuretics, bisphosphonates

ACE, angiotensin-converting enzyme; NSAIDs, non-steroidal anti-inflammatory drugs.

plasma creatinine levels (see Chapter 19) and adjusted for age, weight and sex. The ideal body weight should be used if the patient's weight is more than 20% in excess of it. A more accurate GFR may be calculated by comparing the amount of creatinine collected in a 24-hour urine sample to the blood plasma measurement, using the Cockcroft–Gault equation:

$$\text{Creatinine clearance (mL/minute)} = \frac{1.23\,(\text{males})\text{ or }1.04\,(\text{females}) \times 140 - \text{age (years)} \times \text{weight (kg)}}{\text{Serum creatinine (}\mu\text{mol/L)}}$$

Although creatinine levels and clearance have been used for many years as a measure of renal function, it is now recommended (by a National Service Framework) that it be assessed by estimated GFR (eGFR). This is based on a study by Levey and colleagues (1999) which indicated that the so-called modification of diet in renal disease (MDRD) formula gives a more reliable measure. The MDRD formula takes account of serum creatinine levels, gender, age, ethnic origin, serum nitrogen urea and albumin, and takes the form:

$$eGFR = 170 \times [\text{Serum creatinine}]^{-0.999} \times (\text{Age})^{-0.176} \times (0.762 \text{ if female}) \times (1.180 \text{ if patient black}) \times [\text{Serum urea nitrogen}]^{-0.170} \times [\text{Albumin}]^{0.318}$$

and is reported in mL/minute per 1.73 m² (where m² refers to body surface area).

This equation should not be used for children, malnourished patients, or in pregnancy, in acute renal failure or oedema. From the eGFR values, renal function is expressed as:

- eGFR >90 mL/minute per 1.73 m²: normal renal function (Stage 1)
- eGFR 89–60 mL/minute per 1.73 m²: mild renal impairment (Stage 2)
- eGFR 30–59 mL/minute per 1.73 m²: moderate renal impairment (Stage 3)
- eGFR 15–29 mL/minute per 1.73 m²: severe renal impairment (Stage 4)
- eGFR <15 mL/minute per 1.73 m²: established renal failure (Stage 5).

The use of drugs in renal impairment may involve the avoidance or reduction of doses, according to the extent to which the kidneys are involved in the elimination of drugs. Individual chapters should be consulted for more detail. Important examples of drugs to be used with caution, often at reduced doses and with regular monitoring, or avoided in renal failure include:

- non-steroidal anti-inflammatory drugs (NSAIDs)
- angiotensin-converting enzyme (ACE) inhibitors
- tetracycline
- metformin
- digoxin
- gold salts
- penicillamine
- ciclosporin
- lithium.

Liver function tests

Impaired liver function may be detected from alterations in the levels of bilirubin, the enzymes transaminase, alkaline phosphatase and/or γ-glutamyl transferase (transpeptidase; GGT), and albumin and coagulation factors (see Appendix 2). An assessment of the LFT can be used to identify liver disease. For further discussion of liver disease see Chapter 11 and for drug-related liver disease see Chapter 6.

Acute cellular damage

Damage to hepatocytes leads to hepatic enzymes leaking out of the liver cells and passing into the hepatic circulation. Therefore, blood plasma levels of the enzymes alanine transaminase (ALT) and aspartate transaminase (AST) are increased in patients with acute hepatocyte damage. However, they are somewhat non-specific and AST is also found in cardiac muscle and skeletal muscle and therefore blood levels may be raised following either damage to cardiac cells after a myocardial infarction or non-specific muscle damage.

The damaged liver also fails to clear bilirubin, a breakdown product from the haem component of red blood cells. The unconjugated form of bilirubin, termed 'free bilirubin', therefore builds up in the blood, causing a yellowing of the skin, together with pruritus (see Chapter 11).

Chronic cellular damage

Chronic cellular damage, such as alcohol-induced cirrhosis, results in the deposition of fibrous tissue in place of dysfunctional hepatocytes. Transaminase levels are often normal but synthetic activity of the liver may be impaired and this impacts on albumin and clotting factors, which are normally produced by the liver. Therefore patients may have hypoalbuminaemia and an increased prothrombin time (or international normalised ratio or INR: see Chapter 17) due to reduced clotting ability.

Cholestasis

In cholestasis, substances that are normally secreted by the liver build up due to impaired metabolism or excretion, e.g. in obstructive cholestasis the liver can no longer excrete bilirubin and alkaline phosphatase (ALP) also accumulates. The enzyme GGT is also elevated but is not a reliable indicator of cholestasis because it may be induced by drugs such as alcohol and anticonvulsants, thereby increasing levels in the absence of cholestasis. A drug history is useful in determining alternative causes of raised GGT levels.

Summary of LFT interpretation

In general, LFTs are considered abnormal when a value is more than double the maximum value of the normal reference range.

Acute hepatitis

- Large elevations of ALT and AST.
- Possible slight increases in ALP and GGT.
- Possible large elevation of bilirubin.
- Prothrombin time may occasionally be increased.
- No change in albumin levels.

Chronic cellular damage

- ALP, ALT and AST tend to be normal or only slightly increased.
- GGT levels may show an elevation.
- Albumin levels are low.
- Bilirubin levels may show marginal to large increases.
- Prothrombin time is prolonged.

Cholestasis

- ALP levels show a large increase.
- GGT is usually elevated.
- ALT and AST tend to be only marginally raised or normal.
- Bilirubin levels may show marginal to large increases.

- Albumin levels are normal.
- Prothrombin time may occasionally be increased.

Drugs requiring regular LFTs

(See also individual chapters.)

The requirement for monitoring LFTs when prescribing is indicated in individual chapters. Examples of drugs for which monitoring is appropriate include:

- statins
- fibrates
- amiodarone
- isotretinoin
- isoniazid
- methyldopa
- rifampicin
- pioglitazone
- sodium valproate
- sulfasalazine.

Herbal preparations should also be considered when patients present with signs of hepatic disease (see Chapters 4, 6 and 11).

Lipids

A full screen of lipids (see Chapter 13) from patients when fasting includes the measurement of:

- total cholesterol (ideal target <5mmol/L)
- high-density-lipoprotein (HDL)-cholesterol (ideal: >0.9 mmol/L male, >1.2 mmol/L females and >20% of total cholesterol)
- low-density-lipoprotein (LDL)-cholesterol (<3.35–4.0 mmol/L)
- triglyceride (<2.1 mmol/L)
- ratio total cholesterol:HDL-cholesterol (<4.5)

Isotretinoin treatment may alter serum lipids and monitoring is recommended 1 month after treatment is initiated and again at the end of treatment (Chapter 6).

Glucose

See Chapter 37.

Thyroid function tests

Thyroid function is determined by comparing clinical features, as discussed in Chapter 38, with biochemical values of thyroid-stimulating hormone (TSH), free thyroxine (fT_4) and free triiodothyronine (fT_3). Drug treatments requiring regular monitoring of thyroid function include lithium and amiodarone (see Chapters 6 and 38).

Summary

Monitoring requirements are also considered within individual chapters. Further information can be found in the summary of product characteristics (SPCs), in the latest *British National Formulary* or direct from the drug manufacturer. It should be noted that requirements for monitoring change according to the clinical presentation of the patient, together with risk factors. For monitoring of drug levels in blood plasma, see Chapter 7 and Appendix 2.

Haematology

Haematological monitoring is used as a general screening test to aid the diagnosis of inflammatory conditions or drug-related blood dyscrasias, identify anaemias and monitor coagulation such as during warfarin therapy. Tests include (see Appendix 2):

- full blood count (FBC): standard request provides haemoglobin, white blood cell count (WBC), platelets, mean cell volume (MCV), mean corpuscular haemoglobin (MCH), red blood cell count (RBC), haematocrit (Hct) and estimates of differentiated types of white blood cells
- erythrocyte sedimentation rate (ESR)
- blood coagulation
- vitamin B_{12} and folate.

Full blood count

Appendix 2 summarises some of the main haematological parameters measured. Drugs requiring a regular FBC include immunosuppressants, clozapine and methyldopa.

Monitoring of oral anticoagulants

See Chapter 17.

Immunological tests

These tests generally involve the detection of antibodies that may point to autoimmune disease or may indicate general immune status. The following tests are used:

- Autoantibody or autoimmune screening includes the detection of antibodies to preparations of thyroid cytoplasm, parietal cells, mitochondria, smooth muscle, and liver or kidney microsomes.
- Rheumatoid factor: a positive test confirms a diagnosis of rheumatoid arthritis/autoimmune rheumatoid disorders.
- C-reactive protein (CRP) is elevated during infection and/or severe inflammation and may be repeated to monitor the outcome of treatment. CRP is more specific for inflammation, necrosis or infection and changes more rapidly than ESR.
- Thyroid antibodies (Graves' disease: see Chapter 38).
- Immunoglobulins: patients presenting with epigastric pain may be tested for the presence of serum immunoglobulin G (IgG) against *Helicobacter pylori* infection (see Chapter 8).
- Paul-Bunnell test (infectious mononucleosis or glandular fever) in response to persistent sore throat, lethargy, fever, headache and cervical adenopathy.
- Prostate-specific antigen (PSA): a positive test provides an early indication of prostate cancer even when the patient is asymptomatic. This is, however, a relatively non-specific test, because only a proportion of patients who have a high value have malignancy.

Microbiology

Microbiology tests are performed on samples such as urine, sputum, cerebrospinal fluid, faeces, or swabs from the vagina or cervix, nose or eyes. These tests tend to be requested when treatment has failed, or sinister causes are suspected, e.g. in symptoms suggestive of meningitis or if there is a risk of sexually transmitted infections such as chlamydia, gonorrhoea or syphilis.

References

British National Formulary, latest edition. London: British Medical Association and Royal Pharmaceutical Society of Great Britain.

Levey AS, Bosch JP, Lewis JB *et al.* (1999). A more accurate method to estimate glomerular filtration rate from serum creatinine: A new prediction equation. *Ann Intern Med*, 130: 461–470. pmid: 10075613.

Further reading

Hoffbrand AV, Moss PAH (2001). *Hoffbrand's Essential Haematology,* 7th edn. Oxford: Blackwell Science.

3

Lifestyle

Lifestyle interventions are essential to the prevention and treatment of almost all diseases. There is therefore a move towards greater emphasis on promoting healthy lifestyle in the management of disease. This is not an easy task as the harm caused by an unhealthy lifestyle may not be experienced for a number of years; conversely some benefits of improving lifestyle are not always observed immediately, thereby reducing motivation of patients to make these changes. Added to this, people do not respond well to being told to change their lifestyle and even those willing to change may find it difficult to change lifelong habits.

A useful approach is to provide education as to the benefits of pursuing a healthy lifestyle and regular support in implementing changes. This can take the form of poster campaigns, the provision of verbal and written advice, health clinics, and signposting to useful internet sites and health clubs.

The aim of this chapter is to emphasise the importance of providing lifestyle advice alongside drug treatment and highlight current recommendations. The effects of diet on drug treatment are also considered.

Clinical features

Typically an unhealthy lifestyle includes excessive calorific intake, particularly from saturated fat, sugar and alcohol. A vicious circle of weight gain, fatigue, low self-esteem and lack of motivation to exercise then develops and poor health will inevitably follow. The following are just some conditions caused or exacerbated by an unhealthy lifestyle:

- anxiety
- arthritis
- cancer
- depression
- diabetes mellitus
- dyspepsia
- ischaemic heart disease
- hypertension
- stroke
- liver disease
- osteoporosis.

A healthy diet

A healthy diet comprises an intake of calories appropriate for energy expenditure and from a variety of food groups, to include a balance of carbohydrate, non-starch polysaccharides (NSPs), protein, fats, water, and vitamins and minerals.

A useful way to explain the balance of food for a healthy diet is to display a picture of 'the wheel of good health', which shows a plate divided into segments with proportions relevant to a healthy intake of each food type. Fruit and vegetables and bread, cereals and potatoes therefore dominate the picture. Changes often required are a reduction in fat, particularly saturated fat, sugar and salt intake. Another important recommendation is the intake of five portions of a variety of fruit and vegetables daily (Williams 1995). Although this is an arbitrary value, it reinforces the health benefits of a diet rich in fruit and vegetables. A diet rich in fruit and vegetables has been estimated to reduce heart disease, stroke and cancer by up to 20% (Department of Health 2000). The World Health Organization (WHO) estimates that up to 2.7 million lives worldwide could be saved each year with increased fruit and vegetable consumption (WHO 2003). The health benefits are due to complex interactions of vitamins, minerals and phytochemicals including flavonoids, glucosinilates and phyto-oestrogens, some of which have protective antioxidant properties. Fruit and vegetables are also an important source of NSPs.

A portion of fruit and vegetables including canned, frozen and dried products is defined as 80 g for adults and children over 5 years of age. A common misconception is that fruit and vegetables count only if they are fresh. Consuming five portions or more a day is therefore easier than many people think. Fruit juice (150 mL) may be counted once a day and baked beans also count. Potatoes are excluded because these represent a 'starchy staple'. It should be noted that intake should be appropriate to age, sex and activity. An approximate guide (Food Standards Agency or FSA 2001) is:

1 dessert bowlful of salad
1 banana, apple or orange
1 cupful or handful of grapes, cherries or similar
½–1 tablespoonful of dried fruit.

Recommendations for a healthy diet:

- The dominance of starchy food in a meal – low glycaemic index (GI) foods especially.
- A diet rich in fruit and vegetables.
- Increased consumption of oily fish (at least one portion per week, see Chapter 13).
- Reducing saturated fat and sugar (the daily intake of sugar is currently too high and should be reduced to ~30 g/day).
- Reducing salt (maximum 6 g/day, see Chapter 12).
- Maintaining a healthy weight.
- Increasing water intake.
- The importance of breakfast for controlling weight.

Drug–food interactions

A number of clinically significant interactions including food have been reported and the reader should consult *Stockley's Drug Interactions* (Baxter 2013). Food interactions may predictably involve absorption interactions but also effects on cytochrome P450 isoenzymes, leading to metabolic interactions. An important example is that constituents of grapefruit juice are inhibitors of CYP3A4 and so may inhibit drug metabolism by this isoenzyme, leading to increased plasma concentrations and the risk of adverse events. Examples of drugs that may be affected by consumption of grapefruit juice include amiodarone, felodipine, nisoldipine, verapamil (and possibly other calcium-channel blockers), sildenafil, vardenafil and simvastatin. Table 3.1 includes other examples of clinically significant food–drug interactions.

Alcohol

The consumption of excess alcohol is associated with acute health risks (e.g. poisoning, accidents), and chronic disease such as cardiovascular disease, cancer, hepatic disease and mental health problems. The high calories associated with alcohol also contribute towards the risk of obesity and associated morbidity. Alcohol misuse continues to be a major health concern

Table 3.1 Drug interactions with food

Interaction	Consequences	Comments
Aspirin with vitamin C	Reduced absorption of vitamin C	Aspirin reduces the absorption of vitamin C by approximately a third
Bisphosphonates with food, iron or zinc	Reduced absorption by polyvalent cations	• Alendronate, ibandronic acid and risedronate should be taken at least 30 minutes before the first food of the day • Clodronate should be taken at least 1 hour before or after food • Etidronate and tiludronate should be given at least 2 hours before or after food • Timing should be similar for polyvalent cations, which are also present in antacids
Ciprofloxaxin and norfloxacin with dairy products, zinc or iron	Reduced bioavailability	• Avoid dairy products within 1–2 hours of these antibiotics • Note that enteral feeds may also reduce absorption significantly • Quinolones should also be taken 2 hours before zinc and iron
Colestyramine or orlistat with fat-soluble vitamins (A, D, E, K)	Reduced absorption of vitamins	• Supplements may be required with long-term treatment • Supplements should be taken at least 2 hours after orlistat or at bedtime and 1 hours before or 4–6 hours after colestyramine
Diuretics or lithium with sodium chloride (salt)	• Excess salt increases excretion of lithium, reducing levels. Conversely, reducing salt intake increases lithium levels • Sodium chloride opposes beneficial effects of diuretics by increasing water retention by kidney	• Patients prescribed lithium should be counselled about maintaining salt and fluid intake • Patients prescribed diuretics should avoid excess salt in their diet
Isoniazid with fish or cheese	• Reduced absorption • Histamine poisoning reaction may occur with mature cheese and some fish (e.g. salmon, tuna, mackerel)	• Advise patients to take at least 30 minutes before or 2 hours after food • Check diet if patients report chills, diarrhoea, flushing, itching, headache, tachycardia and/or wheeze
Isotretinoin with vitamin A (retinol) Lansoprazole	• A condition similar to vitamin A overdose may result from concurrent administration • Bioavailability reduced by up to 50%	• High doses of vitamin A (>4000–5000 units) should be avoided with isotretinoin • Lansoprazole should be taken at least an hour before food
MAOIs	Risk of life-threatening hypertensive crisis with tyramine-rich foods such as cheese, salami, yeast extracts, pickled herrings and some beers and wines	• Patients prescribed irreversible MAOIs such as phenelzine should avoid these foods • Large amounts of these foods may affect some patients taking the reversible MAOI moclobemide
Methotrexate, phenobarbital, phenytoin primidone with folates, vitamin D	• Methotrexate acts as a folate antagonist, the latter therefore affecting toxic and therapeutic effects • Folate deficiency may occur with long-term phenobarbital, phenytoin or primidone treatment but supplements should be introduced with monitoring because serum levels of antiepileptics may fall • Long-term phenytoin use can lead to osteomalacia, large doses of vitamin D supplementation may be required	Folic acid is given with methotrexate to reduce adverse effects

Table 3.1 *(continued)*

Interaction	Consequences	Comments
Tetracyclines with dairy products, iron and zinc	Milk and other dairy products and dietary calcium reduce the absorption of most tetracyclines significantly. Zinc reduces absorption by up to 50%	• Take 1 hour before food or 2 hours after • Doxycycline and minocycline less affected by food • 3 hours separation between drug and iron or zinc may be required (see *Stockley's Drug Interactions* (2013))
Warfarin (and other coumarins)	• Cranberry juice can produce potentially life-threatening increases in INR • Vitamin K reduces the effects of warfarin, a vitamin K antagonist	• Patients limit or avoid drinking cranberry juice or taking other cranberry products • Large changes in consumption of vitamin K-containing foods, e.g. green vegetables, green tea and vitamin K supplements, should be avoided • Less significant interactions may occur with supplements, e.g. fish oils, glucosamine, coenzyme Q10, vitamin E, though patients should have their INR checked when starting these preparations

INR, international normalised ratio; MAOI, monoamine oxidase inhibitor.

with binge drinking a particular problem that impacts on society and health service resources. Pharmacists should be alert for patients presenting with effects of alcohol misuse and provide information of local services providing specialist help (Mason 2003). Symptoms include irritability, anxiety, insomnia, smelling of alcohol, self-neglect and unsteady gait. Signs of chronic alcohol abuse may include reddening of the palms and signs of alcoholic liver disease such as spider naevi (see Chapter 36) and jaundice (see Chapter 11).

Pharmacological activity

Alcohol has central nervous system (CNS)-depressant and disinhibitory effects through non-specific actions similar to those of general anaesthetics. Peripheral effects of alcohol include increased gastric acid secretions, resulting in chronic gastritis. Hormonal effects can include reduced synthesis of testosterone (which may lead to impotence), reduced release of antidiuretic hormone (which causes diuresis and may lead to dehydration, which contributes to a 'hangover') and increased levels of corticosteroids.

Long-term effects

Long-term alcohol abuse is in some, but not all, patients associated with liver damage. Initial changes involve reversible fatty infiltration of the liver and may proceed to cirrhosis of the liver (see Chapter 11). Alcoholism is also associated with thiamine (vitamin B_1) deficiency, due to malnutrition and impaired metabolism, and this may lead to neurological problems such as Wernicke's encephalopathy. Excessive alcohol consumption is also associated with cancer of the mouth, larynx and oesophagus.

Current guidelines in the UK recommend that the safe limits of weekly alcohol consumption are 14 units for women and men, where a unit is defined as one small glass of wine, a 'shot' of spirit or a half-pint of weak beer. However, there is confusion as to what constitutes a unit and, for example, generous self-measures of wine in large glasses may yield several units. For guidance, on average a bottle of wine contains approximately 10 units and one pint of strong lager contains 3 or more units. The recommendations also suggest that women and men should not consume more than 2–3 units per day to avoid binge drinking. It is also recommended to have 2–3 days a week without consuming alcohol. Despite these guidelines for safe drinking, consumption of alcohol in excess of these limits is widespread and some authorities regard consumption of more than 35 units per week as hazardous.

The recommendations for drinking in pregnancy have varied over the years but the most recent evidence suggests that there is no safe limit and current guidelines recommend that alcohol should not be consumed during pregnancy. Alcohol can also affect conception and so those wishing to conceive should limit alcohol consumption or stop drinking.

Drug interactions

The main interaction occurring between drugs and alcohol is with other drugs with CNS-depressant activity. This includes analgesics, anticonvulsants, antidepressants, sedating antihistamines, benzodiazepines and antipsychotics (also risk of postural hypotension), increasing side effects and the ability to perform skilled tasks such as driving. Other examples of drug interactions with alcohol are detailed in Table 3.2.

Caffeine

Caffeine consumption has become increasingly fashionable and caffeine dependence, together with

patients increasing their intake due to the development of tolerance, is more common although not easily defined. The effect of caffeine on health may be minimal compared with alcohol. However, it can be a neglected cause of symptoms that may be confused with other conditions. Patients presenting with the following symptoms should therefore be asked about their caffeine intake: anxiety and/or panic, increased blood pressure, tremor, dyspepsia, dizziness, headaches, insomnia, palpitations, vertigo and tinnitus. Excess caffeine intake is also associated with withdrawal effects including headache, fatigue, anxiety, depression and poor concentration.

Pharmacology

Caffeine is a methylxanthine compound, therefore exhibiting similar pharmacology to other methylxanthines such as theophylline. These act as adenosine receptor antagonists, opposing the inhibitory effect of adenosine pathways in the CNS, and this may affect

Table 3.2 Drug interactions with alcohol		
Drug	**Consequences**	**Comments**
Antihypertensives	• Reduced effect of antihypertensives • Risk of additive effect of hypotension	Alcohol increases blood pressure (see text) so patients should be advised to reduce alcohol intake
Central nervous system depressants	See text	
Isoniazid	• Increased effect on driving and risk of hepatitis • Effects of isoniazid possibly reduced	Alcohol intake should be limited
Lithium	Impaired performance of skilled tasks such as driving	Patients should be advised accordingly
Methotrexate	Increased risk of hepatic cirrhosis and fibrosis	Manufacturers recommend that patients taking methotrexate avoid drugs, including alcohol, associated with hepatotoxicity
Metoclopramide	Increased absorption of alcohol	Patients should be advised of this and the possible effect on driving and other skilled tasks
Metronidazole	Disulfiram (flushing)-type reaction	Patients should be warned because this reaction is unpleasant and potentially frightening
Paracetamol	Increased risk of hepatotoxicity with heavy drinking	Close monitoring is recommended for heavy drinkers prescribed regular paracetamol
Phenytoin	Increased serum phenytoin levels	• Dose increase may be required for heavy drinkers • Note that dose may need to be reduced in hepatic impairment
Verapamil	Increased blood alcohol levels and prolonged effects	Patients should be warned

sleep. Methylxanthines also inhibit phosphodiesterases and so augment the actions of catecholamines, leading to an increase in heart rate and bronchodilation. Diuresis is thought to occur following renal vasodilatation, leading to an increase in glomerular filtration rate. Caffeine also stimulates gastrin production and may therefore exacerbate gastrointestinal disease.

Drug interactions

There appear to be few clinically significant interactions with caffeine, with the exception of reduced clearance in the presence of disulfiram. Increased levels of caffeine may produce symptoms similar to those of alcohol withdrawal and patients should therefore be advised to limit caffeine consumption. As caffeine stimulates the release of catecholamines, resulting in increased heart rate and blood pressure, caffeine intake should be limited by patients prescribed medication for cardiovascular disease and anxiety. Additional drug–disease interactions may include excessive intake of caffeine in patients taking medication for gastrointestinal disease.

Food supplements

Patients may request food supplements and advice given should be evidence based. In general, supplements such as vitamins and minerals should not replace a healthy balanced diet and high doses of single vitamins or minerals should be avoided. Indeed, a major conclusion from the Heart Protection Study (2002) was that antioxidant supplementation with vitamins A, C and E was not associated with an improvement in mortality of high-risk patients and that a balanced diet was more appropriate. Furthermore, some studies have now revealed harmful effects of these antioxidant supplements as highlighted by a Cochrane review (Bjelakovic et al. 2008).

Despite concerns over indiscriminate use of certain vitamins, it is clear that special groups (such as pregnant and breastfeeding women, infants, children, adolescents, vegans, elderly people and those who are convalescing) benefit from and indeed require vitamin and mineral supplementation. Some examples of appropriate recommendations of supplements are summarised in Table 3.3. It should also be noted that vitamin and mineral supplements supplied within the

Table 3.3 Recommendation of food supplements		
Special considerations for use of vitamins and minerals	**Supplement**	**Comments**
Alcohol misuse	Thiamine (vitamin B_1) and multivitamins	Risk of Wernicke's encephalopathy and Korsakoff's psychosis necessitates thiamine supplementation in chronic alcoholism. Multivitamins may also be recommended because diet is likely to be poor
Individuals who are elderly, housebound or have low exposure to sunlight	Vitamin D	Consider additional risk factors for osteoporosis and long-term treatment with drugs such as phenytoin
Preconception to first 12 weeks of pregnancy	Folic acid 400 micrograms	• For the prevention of neural tube defects • Patients prescribed proguanil or antiepileptic drugs, e.g. carbamazepine require 5 mg on prescription
Ante- or postnatally, following surgery, menorrhagia, vegetarians, symptoms of deficiency, e.g. breathlessness on exertion	Iron	Patients may request iron supplements over-the-counter and it is important that appropriate questions are asked to assess the risk of anaemia. Some preparations do not contain adequate levels of iron salts and patients should be referred to their general practitioner for a blood test and an appropriate dose prescribed
Vegetarians	Calcium, vitamin D, iron and vitamin B_{12}	Vegan vegetarians are particularly at risk of nutrient deficiency due to the absence of meat and dairy products in the diet (the Food Standards Agency and Vegan Society at www.vegansociety.com provide useful information)

EU are currently regulated by the Food Supplements Directive, which came into effect in the UK in 2005.

Exercise

It has long been known that physical activity is important for good health. However, scientific evidence is increasingly quantifying the contribution of physical activity to health and disease. A report commissioned by the British government found that physical activity reduces the risk of coronary heart disease, stroke and type 2 diabetes by 50% and premature death by 20–30% (Wanless 2004). There is also evidence for the therapeutic benefits for these diseases and also musculoskeletal disorders such as osteoarthritis. Communication of this information to patients can be an important motivator for increasing physical activity. Indeed, in 2004 the UK's Chief Medical Officer recommended that adults should exercise for at least 30 minutes each day for at least 5 days a week for health benefits. The 30 minutes may consist of an accumulation of 10-minute sessions, which may include simple changes such as walking for a bus instead of driving. This level of activity has been shown to reduce the risks highlighted above, together with improving mental health and reducing the risk of many cancers. Prolonged activity up to 45–60 minutes a day is recommended to prevent obesity and 60 minutes for young people and children, including exercise for bone health, muscle strength and flexibility.

Stress

Prolonged excessive stress is known to be detrimental to health, being associated with mental health problems, reduced immunity and cardiovascular disease, e.g. a study of over 10 000 civil servants found that stress at work increases the risk of the metabolic syndrome, a predictor for the development of cardiovascular disease and type 2 diabetes (Chandola *et al.* 2006). Patients presenting with insomnia, changes in appetite, panic attacks, muscle pain, headaches, hypercholesterolaemia, gastrointestinal problems and low mood would particularly benefit from advice regarding stress reduction, such as taking regular exercise.

Tobacco smoke

Tobacco smoking is the single most harmful lifestyle activity and is clearly linked to cancers, respiratory disorders and cardiovascular disease. Smoking cessation may therefore be considered to be the most important intervention by health professionals in the treatment and prevention of disease. The powerful addictive nature of nicotine, however, makes this an extremely difficult task, although the availability of nicotine replacement therapy (NRT) has improved quit rates in combination with support and willpower.

Pharmacological activity

Tobacco smoke contains nicotine, carcinogenic tars (polycyclic hydrocarbons) and carbon monoxide. Nicotine stimulates subtypes of nicotinic receptors leading to neuronal excitation. These receptors are distributed on neurons in the brain and on autonomic ganglia and neuromuscular synapses (mainly in the heart and lungs) in the periphery. Carbon monoxide reduces the oxygen-carrying capacity of haemoglobin, contributing further to the adverse cardiovascular effects outlined above. Irritant, carcinogenic and other toxic substances found in cigarette smoke include arsenic, benzene, lead, DDT (dichlorodiphenyltrichloroethane, an insecticide), nitric acid and toluene (methylbenzene). Carcinogenic tars may lead to chronic obstructive pulmonary disease (COPD) and cancer of the lungs, upper respiratory tract, oesophagus, pancreas and bladder.

Treatment of nicotine addiction

Patients who smoke more than ten cigarettes a day may benefit from nicotine replacement, counselling and support. All preparations of NRT have been shown to be effective in smoking cessation, with cessation rates increased by 50–70% (Cochrane review by Stead *et al.,* 2007). The National Institute for Health and Care Excellence guidance recommends that NRT or bupropion should be prescribed only after the agreement of a target stop date with the smoker. Initial treatment is for 2 weeks for NRT or 3–4 weeks of bupropion. The dosage form is selected according to patient preference. Bupropion may also be used but current NICE (2002) guidelines do not recommend concurrent use with NRT.

Withdrawal symptoms include:

- dysphoric or depressed mood
- insomnia
- irritability, frustration or anger
- anxiety
- difficulty concentrating
- restlessness
- decreased heart rate
- increased appetite and weight gain.

Varenicline, a partial nicotinic receptor agonist, is a recent introduction to aid smoking cessation and is recommended for patients wanting to stop smoking and preferably in addition to behavioural support (NICE 2007). As a partial agonist, it will provide weak stimulation to reduce withdrawal reactions but oppose the actions of nicotine itself.

Electronic cigarettes (e-cigarettes) are now available and widely used as a way of delivering nicotine as a vapour without smoke. Their use is controversial as there is no long-term evidence as to their safety or harmful effects. They certainly reduce the exposure of the lungs to carcinogenic tars, although the effects of the vapours have yet to be determined. The use of e-cigarettes could also present a gateway to nicotine addiction and encourage smoking as an alternative. Given these issues their benefits or otherwise have yet to be established.

Concurrent disease

Some considerations of prescribing or recommending therapy for smoking cessation in concurrent diseases are detailed in Table 3.4.

Drug interactions and adverse effects

Tobacco smoke

Components of tobacco smoke, thought to be polycyclic hydrocarbons, induce cytochrome P450 enzymes in the liver, thereby increasing the metabolism of some drugs, e.g. the metabolism of theophylline is accelerated in smokers and so higher dosages are required. However, on cessation the induction of enzyme activity will be reduced and so the dosage should be decreased.

Increased insulin-opposing hormones caused by smoking necessitate greater insulin doses in people with diabetes who smoke and a reduced dosage on cessation of smoking (*Stockley's Drug Interactions –* Baxter 2013). Smoking also adds to the already increased cardiovascular risk of patients with diabetes mellitus. A further increased risk of thromboembolic disease occurs in women taking oral contraceptives if they also smoke.

Bupropion

The increased risk of seizures should be considered when co-prescribing drugs known to lower the seizure threshold (see Chapters 6 and 24). A maximum dose of 150 mg daily of bupropion is recommended when prescribed with other drugs that lower the convulsive threshold.

Bupropion also exhibits a number of metabolic interactions including with antipsychotics such as haloperidol and risperidone, antiepileptics (note that bupropion is contraindicated in epilepsy), selective serotonin reuptake inhibitors (SSRIs) and tricyclic antidepressants. The effects of these interactions should be monitored carefully. Adverse effects of bupropion may also occur in combination with drugs competing for the same metabolic enzymes, e.g. valproate, ritonavir, clopidogrel, paroxetine and fluoxetine. Note that the long half-life of drugs such as fluoxetine may also increase the risk of interactions after the cessation of treatment.

Drug–disease interactions are detailed in Table 3.4.

General counselling

For smoking cessation to be successful, patients must make the decision to stop. Health professionals therefore need to recognise the different stages involved in arriving at this decision. This ranges from the patient who has never considered stopping smoking to the patient who is ready to stop. Information leaflets may be given to patients who smoke and encouragement to stop smoking given at every opportunity. A successful attempt to quit is more likely when the patient has actually made the decision and is ready to stop. The patient should be advised to set a date to stop smoking

Table 3.4 Concurrent disease and prescribing of smoking cessation aids (derived from the *British National Formulary* (BNF))

Disease	Cautions and contraindications	Comments

Cardiovascular disease, including peripheral vascular disease	• Nicotine products are used with caution in severe cardiovascular disease such as:
	  – severe arrhythmias
	  – recent myocardial infarction, TIA or CVA
	• Monitoring is appropriate for other conditions
		• These patients should be encouraged to stop smoking due to the adverse effects outlined in the text
		• Monitoring for signs of deterioration is required. The harmful effects produced by toxic components of smoke are obviously removed but unwanted effects due to nicotine remain. This information may be useful for patients reluctant to stop using NRT

Depression, bipolar disorder	• The use of bupropion is contraindicated • Varenicline has been associated with depression and should be used with caution in patients with a history of psychiatric disease	Increased risk of precipitating or exacerbating the manic phase
Diabetes mellitus	NRT and bupropion should be used only with caution	• See risk of seizures with bupropion use in diabetes mellitus • The effects of nicotine may mask the signs of hypoglycaemia and increase the risk of damage to the microvascular circulation • Smoking cessation is imperative in these patients due to the increased risk of diabetic complications (Chapter 37) and NRT may be useful in the short term with monitoring
Epilepsy, risk of seizures	Bupropion is contraindicated when there is a risk of seizures as follows: • a history of seizures or eating disorders • a CNS tumour • during acute withdrawal from alcohol or benzodiazepines	Bupropion may be used with caution and close monitoring when benefit exceeds risk in the following situations: • alcohol abuse • history of head trauma • diabetes • concurrent use of stimulants or anorectic drugs, which may lower the seizure threshold (e.g. antidepressants, antimalarials, sedating antihistamines, corticosteroids, theophylline, tramadol)
Hyperthyroidism	NRT should be used only with caution	Nicotine may exacerbate symptoms of hyperthyroidism and complicate its management
History of gastritis and peptic ulcer	NRT should be used with caution	Nicotine may worsen gastritis and peptic ulcer disease and patients should be monitored accordingly. Smoking cessation is, however, particularly important for these patients
Pregnancy and breastfeeding	• Bupropion is contraindicated • NRT should be used only when attempts to quit without it have failed	• Smoking cessation should be strongly encouraged in pregnant women and those with young children • Intermittent use of NRT is preferred and avoiding liquorice-flavoured products
Chronic generalised skin disease	Nicotine patches are contraindicated	NRT patches should not be used on broken skin
Renal and hepatic impairment	NRT, bupropion and varenicline should be used with caution	• Dose adjustment may be required • Avoid bupropion in severe hepatic cirrhosis

CNS, central nervous system; CVA, cerebrovascular accident; NRT, nicotine replacement therapy; TIA, transient ischaemic attack.

completely and discard all remaining cigarettes. The importance of willpower and the use of NRT to alleviate the symptoms of withdrawal should be stressed.

The following points may help the patient to be successful:

- Explain that chest symptoms such as increased secretions may occur initially on cessation but these should abate within 2–3 weeks.
- Try to avoid situations associated with smoking, e.g. take up a hobby in the evening if this is when most cigarettes are smoked.
- Encourage the patient to return with questions or difficulties.
- Avoid excess intake of caffeine because this may worsen the withdrawal effect of nicotine.
- A list of the benefits of smoking cessation may particularly help patients who are long-term smokers. Rapid improvements in taste and sense of smell, circulation and lung function are experienced. The risk of a heart attack decreases rapidly on smoking cessation (Kenfield *et al.* 2008).
- Other benefits include increased exercise capacity, reduced odour, avoiding premature ageing of the skin and tooth loss.

NRT (patches, gum, inhalator, lozenges, sublingual, nasal spray)

- The nasal spray should not be used when driving due to the risk of sneezing or watery eyes.
- Side effects include nausea, dizziness, headache, cold and influenza-like symptoms, palpitations, dyspepsia, insomnia and vivid dreams (particularly with the 24-hour patch). The 24-hour patch should be removed if these symptoms are troublesome: a 16-hour patch may be more suitable.
- Patches should not be applied to broken skin.
- Patches are not appropriate for occasional smokers.

Bupropion

- Side effects include dry mouth, gastrointestinal disturbances, insomnia, tremor, tachycardia and hypertension.
- Blood pressure should be monitored weekly if bupropion is used with NRT. Patients who

relapse should be encouraged to self-refer due to the risk of increased blood pressure.
- Bupropion should be used with caution when driving or performing skilled tasks.
- Bupropion increases the risk of side effects with over-the-counter (OTC) cough preparations containing dextromethorphan.

Varenicline

- Start 1–2 weeks before target stop date.
- Avoid abrupt withdrawal.
- Side effects include gastrointestinal disturbances, changes to appetite, dry mouth, taste disturbance, headache, dizziness and sleep disorders.
- Report changes in mood to their general practitioner.
- May affect driving, so patients should not drive until they know they are not affected.

Over-the-counter medicines

OTC medicines are also prone to misuse and this may complicate diagnosis and use of prescribed medication that may interact. Examples of OTC drugs associated with abuse include the following:

- Sedative antihistamines, including those contained in cough medicines, may be used chronically for insomnia, leading to dependence (see Chapter 27).
- Laxatives may be misused for weight loss, particularly by female patients and those suffering from anorexia nervosa.
- Patients addicted to opioids may misuse codeine and other opioid-containing preparations, such as kaolin and morphine. The antihistamine cyclizine is also subject to misuse by these patients as it is thought to increase the effects of opioids.
- Sympathomimetics such as ephedrine and pseudoephedrine are used for their alerting and euphoric effects, for fatigue, improving athletic performance (see banned substances in the *British National Formulary*), for weight loss, to reduce craving for amphetamines and for the manufacture of amphetamines.
- Caffeine-containing products include some analgesics and preparations marketed for increased energy, e.g. Pro Plus and drinks such as Red Bull (see Caffeine above).

Contraception

The choice of contraception is an important lifestyle decision for sexually active people and this is a critical area for health promotion. The transmission of sexually transmitted infections such as chlamydia is on the increase and some pharmacies are providing screening, treatment and sexual health promotion services as part of the National Chlamydia Screening programme. The prescribing of hormonal contraception is considered below in relation to the presence of concurrent disease and drug interactions.

Pharmacology

Hormonal contraception comprises a combination of oestrogen and a progestogen (combined oral contraceptive, COC) or a progestogen alone (POP). These agents modify the hormonal control of the menstrual cycle and in particular the oestrogens inhibit the release of follicle-stimulating hormone (FSH) from the anterior pituitary, preventing the development of ovarian follicles. Progestogens inhibit the release of luteinising hormone (LH), preventing ovulation, and also alter the cervical mucus to prevent insemination. Both hormones affect the endometrium and oppose implantation.

Hormonal contraception may be administered as an oral tablet, dermal implant or injection. COCs are also prescribed to reduce symptoms of menstrual disorders such as dysmenorrhoea and reduce the risk of ovarian and endometrial cancers. Adverse effects, however, include an increased risk of venous thromboembolism, mood changes and mineralocorticoid effects that can lead to increases in blood pressure. Prescribing of COC therefore requires an initial risk assessment of concurrent diseases.

COCs pose a risk for cardiovascular disease and the *British National Formulary* specifies risk factors that either preclude the use of COCs or mean that they should be used with caution. These include:

- a family history of cardiovascular disease
- diabetes mellitus
- hypertension
- smoking
- age >35 years
- obesity
- migraine (Table 3.5).

COCs also pose a risk for venous thrombosis due to an increase in the levels of coagulation factors. Indeed, in the 1990s a new generation of COCs

Table 3.5 Prescribing of oral contraceptives in the presence of concurrent disease		
Condition	**Effect on drug choice**	**Comments**
Cardiovascular disease and venous thrombosis risk	See text	
Depression Inflammatory bowel disease	• COC used with caution in severe depression • COC used with caution	• Patients should report worsening mood associated with COC • Increased risk of contraceptive failure due to reduced absorption
Migraine	• COC contraindicated if: • typical focal aura – severe migraine >72 hours despite treatment – treatment with ergot derivatives • Cautious use of COC if treated with $5HT_1$-receptor agonists and for migraine without focal aura	Increased frequency and/or worsening symptoms should be reported by patients
Sex-steroid-dependent cancer	Use with caution	

COC, combined oral contraceptive.

was withdrawn due to the increased risk. Current recommendations suggest that the presence of two or more risk factors should preclude the use of COCs, and cautious use is advised if any of the following risk factors are present:

- family history, e.g. first-degree relative <45 years (gestodene and desogestrel should be avoided)
- obesity
- immobility (e.g. after surgery)
- varicose veins

Other considerations are summarised in Table 3.5.

Choice of drugs

COCs are the most effective form of reversible contraception and are appropriate for patients who are sufficiently motivated to remember to take a dose within 12 hours every day. COCs have many advantages such as reducing dysmenorrhoea, symptoms of fibroids and ovarian cysts, benign breast disease, anaemia, premenstrual syndrome, and the risk of ovarian and endometrial cancer. Disadvantages, however, include an increased risk of thrombosis (see above), adverse effects such as nausea, weight gain and mood changes, and mineralocorticoid effect, which can increase blood pressure. There is also a small increase in risk of breast cancer and the MHRA (Medicines and Healthcare products Regulatory Agency) recently highlighted an increase in the risk of cervical cancer with long-term use of hormonal contraceptives. These risks need to be considered alongside the benefits and the availability of screening services.

POPs are often regarded as being more suitable for patients who cannot take COCs due to age, smoking status, cardiovascular risks or migraine. However, for most POPs they must be taken within 3 hours of the same time each day to maintain efficacy. POPs are considered the pill of choice in breastfeeding mothers as COCs may suppress lactation.

Drug interactions

The interaction of drugs with hormonal contraception involves increased metabolism in the presence of enzyme inducers such as carbamazepine, phenobarbital, phenytoin, rifampicin, rifabutin and St John's wort (see Chapter 6).

Patients prescribed potent enzyme inducers such as rifampicin and rifabutin are advised to use an intrauterine device or barrier methods. High doses of oestrogen or 'tricycling' whereby three cycles of pill are taken without the usual 7-day breaks are alternatives for less potent inducers but are not without risk.

Self-assessment

Consider whether the following statements are true or false concerning advice to patients about their lifestyle:

1 Thirty minutes of moderate intensity exercise are recommended each day on five or more days a week to reduce obesity.
2 Grapefruit juice inhibits the metabolism of calcium-channel blockers.
3 Vitamin K-containing foods may alter the actions of warfarin.
4 Varenicline tablets should be used with caution in patients with a history of depression.

Practice points

- Pharmacists should participate in health promotion campaigns; provide leaflets with information on healthy lifestyle and signpost to information sources, e.g. resources promoting healthy eating and the consumption of five portions of fruit and vegetables.
- *At Least Five a Week* (Department of Health 2004) should be consulted for a useful summary of evidence of the benefits of physical activity in health and disease.
- The pharmacist has a major role in educating patients in relation to safe alcohol consumption and smoking cessation.

CASE STUDY

A 36-year-old woman requests a blood pressure test in the pharmacy and you notice that her breath smells of tobacco smoke. Her patient medication record (PMR) reveals that she takes Microgynon tablets. You measure her blood pressure as 160/85 mmHg. You ask her if she smokes and she admits that she has recently increased to 40 cigarettes a day due to a period of stress.

What course of action do you take?

- This patient has potentially three risk factors for cardiovascular disease and she should therefore be advised to see her general practitioner for a review of her oral contraceptive. Her systolic blood pressure is elevated, though this would need to be repeated on a further two occasions and taking into consideration any recent caffeine consumption, smoking and anxiety. In addition she is aged over 35 years and a smoker. Combined hormonal contraception is not recommended if a patient has two or more risk factors for arterial disease. A referral for smoking cessation support and information about stress management would also benefit this patient. You should explain the risks, without causing alarm, to ensure that she does speak to her GP.

References

Baxter K, ed. (2013). *Stockley's Drug Interactions,* 10th edn. London: Pharmaceutical Press.

Bjelakovic G, Nikolova D, Gluud LL *et al.* (2008). Antioxidant supplements for prevention of mortality in healthy participants and patients with various diseases. *Cochrane Database System Rev* issue 2: CD007176.

Chandola T, Brunner E, Marmot M (2006). Chronic stress at work and the metabolic syndrome: prospective study. *BMJ,* 332: 521–525.

Department of Health (2000). *The NHS Plan.* London: DH.

Department of Health (2004). *Physical Activity, Health Improvement and Prevention. At least five a week. Evidence on the impact of physical activity and its relationship to health.* London: DH.

Food Standards Agency (2001) *The Balance of Good Health.* Information for educators and communicators. London: FSA in consultation with the Department of Health.

Food Standards Agency (2005). *Eatwell. Your guide to healthy eating* London: FSA.

Heart Protection Study (2002). MRC/BHF Heart Protection Study of antioxidant vitamin supplementation in 20 536 high risk individuals: a randomised placebo controlled trial. *Lancet* 360: 23–33.

Kenfield SA, Stampfer MJ, Rosner BA *et al.* (2008). Smoking and smoking cessation in relation to mortality in women. *JAMA,* 299: 2037–2047. pmid: 18460664.

Mason P (2003). Alcohol misuse – a case study. *Pharm J,* 271: 777–779.

National Institute for Health and Care Excellence (2002). *Guidance on the use of nicotine replacement therapy (NRT) and bupropion for smoking cessation.* Technology appraisal guidance, No. 39. London: NICE.

National Institute for Health and Care Excellence (2007). *Varenicline for smoking cessation.* Technology appraisal guidance, No. 123. London: NICE.

Stead LF, Perera R, Bullen C *et al.* (2007). Nicotine replacement therapy for smoking cessation (Cochrane review). *Cochrane Database System Rev* issue 3: CD000146.

Wanless D (2004). *Securing Good Health for the Whole Population.* Final report. London: Department of Health.

Williams C (1995). Healthy eating: clarifying advice about fruit and vegetables. *BMJ,* 310: 1453–1455. pmid: 7613282.

World Health Organization (2003). *Fruit, Vegetables and NCD Disease Prevention. Global strategy on diet, physical activity and health.* Geneva: WHO.

Online resources

www.foodstandards.gov.uk
The website of the Food Standards Agency; provides evidence-based advice and nutrition leaflets with advice for different age groups (accessed September 2015).

www.nutrition.org.uk
The website of the British Nutrition Foundation, a charity providing useful information and resources promoting healthy eating (accessed September 2015).

www.fpa.org.uk
The website of the Family Planning Association; provides information for both patients and health professionals (accessed September 2015).

4

Herbal medicine and alternative remedies

Herbal remedies are natural products largely of plant origin and may contain pharmacologically active compounds, which may be beneficial or have adverse effects. The use of certain natural products is established in medicine, e.g. by the use of digoxin from foxglove, but many remedies are poorly characterised in terms of efficacy and side-effect profile.

The use of herbal remedies is widespread, being particularly attractive due to the publicity of adverse effects associated with conventional medicine. Indeed the public perception that herbal medicines are safe has probably led to an under-reporting of adverse events and patients failing to report the use of herbal medicines alongside prescribed and over-the-counter (OTC) medicines. This problem is highlighted by the use of St John's wort, which has pharmacological actions similar to selective serotonin reuptake inhibitors (SSRIs) but has a range of significant interactions with conventional medicines (Table 4.1). Another issue is the lack of quality control, in that the composition of active ingredients may vary considerably between preparations.

Drug history-taking and responding to symptoms should involve active enquiry about herbal medicines. Any change in clinical outcome should be assessed for possible drug interactions or adverse drug reactions (ADRs) thought to result from concurrent use of conventional and herbal drugs. Suspected problems should be reported using the Yellow Card system.

Evidence

It is difficult for health professionals to recommend the use of many herbal preparations in the absence of sound evidence of safe efficacious use, particularly in combination with conventional medicines. Added to this, an extensive variety of preparations is available and doses and purity may vary. Some herbal preparations have a product licence or marketing authorisation whereby safety, quality and efficacy, together with evidence for safe use, are provided. These products are identifiable by a PL number on the label. Most herbal preparations are, however, unlicensed products under the Medicines Act 1968. They are not therefore assessed for safety and quality and lack the rigorous testing of conventional drugs. The introduction of the Traditional Herbal Registration (THR) scheme

Table 4.1 Examples of interactions between herbal and conventional medicines for which clinical evidence exists or potential interactions based on *in vivo* or *in vitro* pharmacological activity

Physiological effects	Implicated herbs and interactions with conventional drugs	Comments
Anticoagulant or antiplatelet activity	Danshen (Chinese herb), dong quai (Chinese), garlic, feverfew, ginkgo, ginger, ginseng (*Panax*), kangen-karyu (Chinese) and liquorice with warfarin or antiplatelet drugs (aspirin, dipyridamole, clopidogrel and ticlopidine)	• An isolated report of spontaneous bleeding from the iris in a patient taking low-dose aspirin and ginkgo biloba • Possible ADRs with ginkgo, most relating to bleeding abnormalities and including a fatal haemorrhage in a patient taking ginkgo with ticlopidine (*Stockley's Drug Interactions –* Baxter 2013). It may be sensible for patients prescribed antiplatelet treatment to avoid these herbal preparations • Case reports of significantly increased effects of warfarin with dansheen or dong quai • Patients reporting increased bleeding, e.g. bruising, should be asked about their use of herbal preparations • These products should also be avoided or discontinued at least 24–48 hours before surgery and considered alongside an increased risk of bleeding with drugs such as NSAIDs and SSRIs
Cardioactive activity, e.g. antiarrhythmic, inotropic or calcium channel effects	Cola, coltsfoot, fenugreek, ginger, ginseng (*Panax*), motherwort, shepherd's purse and wild carrot with antiarrhythmics (amiodarone), digoxin and other cardioactive agents	Patients at increased risk include those with cardiovascular disease and/or taking drugs with cardiovascular activity
Diuresis	Dandelion, elder, Java tea, nettle, saw palmetto, shepherd's purse and squill	• Potential to interact with concurrent diuretic and other antihypertensive treatment (Chapter 12) • Particular caution may be required with drugs associated with significant hypotensive effects such as ACE inhibitors, α-adrenoceptor antagonists and antipsychotics
Hormone activity	Dong quai (Chinese), vitex berry (*Agnus castus*), hops flower, ginseng root, black cohosh, saw palmetto with tamoxifen	There is little evidence of a problem but these products demonstrate binding to oestrogen receptors and some physiological oestrogenic activity. The action of tamoxifen, and other drugs that reduce stimulation of oestrogen receptors, may therefore be opposed by these herbs. They may also stimulate the growth of oestrogen-sensitive tumours of the breast
	Saw palmetto with antiandrogens (finasteride)	Saw palmetto has been reported to possess antiandrogen activity and this should be considered when prescribing antiandrogens for prostatic hyperplasia
Hyperglycaemic	Ginseng (*Panax*), hydrocotyl, rosemary	Increased risk for patients with diabetes mellitus and also concurrent treatment with corticosteroids (Chapters 22 and 37)
Hypoglycaemic	Aloe vera, burdock, celery, corn silk, dandelion, garlic, ginger, ginseng, ispaghula, juniper, marshmallow, nettle, sage	Increased risk of hypoglycaemia in patients with diabetes due to possible additive effects
Immunomodulation	Cat's claw, camomile (German), echinacea, ephedra, ginseng (*Eleutherococcus*), mistletoe, saw palmetto with immunosuppressants (corticosteroids, azathioprine)	Risk of potentiation or antagonism of immunosuppressants

Table 4.1 *(continued)*

Physiological effects	Implicated herbs and interactions with conventional drugs	Comments
Increased levels of digoxin	Ginseng (Siberian) with digoxin	Siberian ginseng contains glycosides related to digoxin
Increased effects	Ginseng with MAOIs (phenelzine)	Increased side effects such as headache, insomnia and psychoactive effects
	St John's wort with triptans, SSRIs	An increased risk of serotonergic effects, so should be avoided
Decreased effects	St John's wort with anticonvulsants (phenytoin, phenobarbital), warfarin, digoxin, theophylline, ciclosporin, hormonal contraceptives, antiHIV drugs	• St John's wort induces cytochrome P450 isoenzymes • Avoid concurrent use • Dose adjustment is not appropriate due to varying doses of St John's wort according to preparation
Laxative effects	Aloes, cascara, ispaghula, rhubarb and senna	• Risk of abuse by patients with anorexia nervosa • Increased risk of dehydration and electrolyte disturbances in patients taking drugs such as diuretics (Chapters 12 and 16)
Sedation	Celery, kava, camomile (German), ginseng, hops, nettle, sage, and valerian with opioids, antihistamines, alcohol, antidepressants, benzodiazepines	• Possibility of severe sedation with concurrent use of St John's wort with SSRIs (paroxetine) and other antidepressants; avoid concomitant use (see above) • It may be a sensible precaution to avoid concurrent use of St John's wort with all antidepressants due to the risk of additive pharmacological effects • Increased effects of CNS depressants • Patients requesting herbal products for insomnia should be advised as for conventional hypnotics (Chapter 27) • As a precaution, patients should not take herbs such as valerian up to 2 hours before driving or performing other skilled tasks
Sympathomimetic activity	Aniseed, arnica, borage, capsicum, cohosh (black, blue), cola, ephedra, gentian, ginseng (*Panax*), nettle, parsley, valerian and vervain	• Reduced effect of antihypertensives
Thyroid effects	Kelp with amiodarone, thyroxine, lithium and antithyroid drugs	Iodine content of kelp may alter thyroid function (caution also with warfarin due to vitamin K content)

Urinary effects (see diuresis and hormone activity above)	Saw palmetto	• Patients at risk include those with concurrent prostatic hyperplasia, incontinence or taking drugs such as diuretics
		• If possible, patients requesting herbs for bladder problems should be asked about symptoms, which may indicate prostatic hyperplasia requiring referral to their general practitioner, including:
		  – a sensation of incomplete bladder emptying on urination
		  – needing to urinate within 2 hours of previous urination
		  – frequent urination during the night
		  – non-continuous urine flow
		  – a weak urinary stream
		  – difficulty starting urinating
		  – difficulty postponing urination

Information obtained from *Stockley's Drug Interactions* (Baxter 2013), and *Herbal Medicines* by Barnes *et al.* (2007).

ACE, angiotensin-converting enzyme; ADRs, adverse drug reactions; CHF, chronic heart failure; CNS, central nervous system; MAOIs, monoamine oxidase inhibitors; NSAIDs, non-steroidal anti-inflammatory drugs; SSRIs, selective serotonin reuptake inhibitors.

by the MHRA (Medicines and Healthcare products Regulatory Agency) should help to improve patient safety when using these products. Those registered with the scheme are assessed by the MHRA for safety, quality and the provision of patient information. It should be noted, however, that indications are based on traditional uses rather than evidence of efficacy. Products are identifiable by a THR number on the label and those with marketing authorisation will continue to display a PL number. *Professional Standards and Guidance for the Sale and Supply of Medicines by Pharmacists* (Royal Pharmaceutical Society of Great Britain 2007) recommends that pharmacists competent to supply complementary therapies, including herbal medicines are required to: 'assist patients in making informed decisions by providing them with necessary and relevant information; ensure any stock is from a reputable source; recommend a remedy only where you can be satisfied of its safety and quality, taking into account the MHRA registration schemes for homeopathic and herbal remedies'.

The most important role of health professionals in the use of herbal preparations is to advise patients of potential problems, particularly associated with concurrent use of conventional medicine (Table 4.1) and to help identify adverse effects, which should be reported as discussed above. When available, the evidence of efficacy and safety may be communicated to patients and this information is increasingly available in systematic reviews of current trials, e.g. Cochrane and Bandolier reviews.

Safety issues

In 2002, the Medicines Control Agency or MCA (now part of the MHRA) produced a report on the *Safety of Herbal Medicinal Products,* concluding overall that these medicines did not pose a major threat to human health. A number of safety issues were, however, highlighted:

- licensing issues and particularly risks associated with unlicensed products
- addition of prescription medicines (sildenafil, glibenclamide, warfarin, alprazolam) and toxic heavy metals to herbal products; other examples are corticosteroids in herbal eczema creams for children and fenfluramine in a slimming product
- interactions with conventional medicines
- hepatotoxicity with comfrey and coltsfoot
- hypersensitivity to herbs with allergenic potential, e.g. chamomile, feverfew
- contamination by microbes, pesticides, fumigants and toxic metals.

Attention was given to patient groups at risk of adverse reactions such as pregnant or breastfeeding mothers, elderly people, children, or with cardiovascular disease and those undergoing surgery, e.g. some herbs such as blue cohosh, burdock, fenugreek, hawthorn, nettle and raspberry were found to exert a stimulant effect on uterine smooth muscle, making them unsuitable for pregnant women. Herbal teas were also identified as a source of pharmacologically active herbal ingredients. A case was described in which hepatotoxicity occurred in a newborn baby after the consumption of a herbal tea by the mother during pregnancy. The tea contained pyrrolizidine alkaloids associated with hepatotoxicity.

Current safety issues are reported in regular Drug Safety Updates by the MHRA and the Herbal Safety News section of the MHRA website. Examples of reports include:

- interactions between conventional drugs and St John's wort (see Table 4.1)
- hepatotoxicity with kava-kava and black cohosh
- renal failure with certain Chinese herbs
- severe skin reactions with *Psoralea corylifolia* fruit in Chinese herbal remedies
- the substitution of plantain by digitalis, leading to serious cardiac arrhythmias.

Interactions between herbal and conventional medicines

Examples of interactions between herbal and conventional medicines, for which clinical evidence exists, are given in Table 4.1. The possibility of drug interactions extrapolated from *in vitro* and *in vivo* pharmacological activity is also considered. For further information the reader is referred to *Stockley's Drug Interactions* (Baxter 2013) and *Herbal Medicines* by Barnes *et al.* (2007).

Homeopathy

There is no proven scientific evidence for efficacy of homeopathy. However, these remedies continue to be available on the National Health Service and many patients choose homeopathy. Healthcare professionals should be alert for a possible delay in consulting advice for serious symptoms (see Chapter 1) by patients choosing homeopathy. Advice should be provided only after adequate training. It should be noted that adverse effects involving an exacerbation of symptoms may be reported. Patients should discontinue treatment and consult a healthcare professional. There are no known interactions with conventional medicines.

The main principle of homeopathy is the treatment of 'like with like', as implied by the prefix 'homeo-', e.g. insomnia is treated with an extract from the green coffee bean *(Coffea)*. Extremely small quantities of the homeopathic preparation are administered following serial dilution, agitation and formulation. A product is recommended according to the presenting complaint but also the individual, providing a holistic approach.

Nomenclature used to express potency uses centesimal and decimal systems. For the centesimal system, mother tincture is prepared from an extract of the source material, which may be plant, animal, insect, biological or chemical material, in a mixture of alcohol and water. One drop of mother tincture is then added to 99 drops of diluent (20–60% triple-distilled alcohol and water). The resulting solution is shaken vigorously (a process known as succussion) and then serial dilutions are made, indicated by a multiple of 'c' representing the number of successive dilutions of 1 in 100, e.g. a potency of 6c gives a concentration of 10^{-12}. It is the process of serial dilution and claims of increased therapeutic potency (potentisation) with each dilution that many people find difficult to accept.

The decimal system involves the addition of one drop of mother tincture to nine drops of diluent and is represented as a multiple of 'x'. The letters M and CM are used to represent greater dilution levels of 1000 and 10 000, respectively. If one compares the two systems for denoting potency, therefore, 6c is equivalent to 12x.

The following points of advice may be given to patients taking homeopathic preparations. The active ingredient is placed on the surface of the dosage form and absorbed through the oral mucosa. Inappropriate handling is therefore thought to inactivate the product. Patients should be counselled as follows:

- The product should be kept in its original container.
- Homeopathic medicines should not be handled but transferred to the mouth via the container cap.
- Take at least 30 minutes before or after food.
- Suck or chew tablet before swallowing.
- Mother tincture should be diluted in a mouthful of water, gargled and then swallowed.
- Highly flavoured or aromatic foods should be avoided, e.g. peppermints.
- Avoid the inhalation of aromatic products containing eucalyptus and camphor, as well as smoking and coffee or tea.
- Stop the treatment when the condition improves.

Homeopathy and pregnancy

Highly diluted homeopathic remedies are considered safe for use during pregnancy but should not delay referral to exclude serious conditions.

> **Practice points**
> - Health professionals should enquire routinely about the use of herbal remedies by patients.
> - Herbal remedies should be avoided in pregnancy and lactation, due to the absence of safety data.
> - The risk of ADRs caused by herbal preparations is increased, as for conventional drugs, with polypharmacy, long-term use, high doses, history of allergy, patients at extremes of age and impaired renal and hepatic function.
> - Safety information produced by the MHRA should be communicated to patients.

Self-assessment

Consider whether the following statements are true or false concerning herbal medicines:

1 These are natural products and therefore unlikely to be associated with side effects.
2 All herbal preparations should have a THR number.
3 Suspected adverse events should not be reported on a Yellow Card as these are not drugs.
4 They are unlikely to cause a problem for people undergoing surgery.
5 St John's wort should not be taken with hormonal contraceptives, antidepressants, anticonvulsants (phenytoin, phenobarbital), warfarin, digoxin, theophylline, antiHIV drugs or ciclosporin.

CASE STUDIES

Case 1

A 25-year-old woman has recently been diagnosed with Crohn's disease. She has been given dietary advice and her symptoms have improved. Her symptoms have, however, worsened in the last 24 hours and she does not understand why. She says that she feels very low and is tearful. She has started taking St John's wort. She is also complaining of a sore throat and chest infection. Should she take echinacea? She is very keen on taking herbal remedies, as they are natural. She gives you her prescription:

venlafaxine 75 mg twice daily
azathioprine 50 mg three times daily
prednisolone 5 mg enteric coated tablets as directed
mesalazine 400 mg enteric coated tablets two three times daily.

While you dispense her medication, she starts to tell you about a party that she went to the previous night.

Is it appropriate for this patient to take St John's wort with echinacea? What general advice would you give to this patient about herbal medicines?

There were a number of issues to consider from this case:

- Was she taking a calcium supplement to reduce the risk of osteoporosis due to her prednisolone treatment, particularly in view of malabsorption as a result of her Crohn's disease (see Chapter 10)?
- How much alcohol was she consuming? Alcohol is a central nervous system depressant and may therefore worsen her depression (assumption that patient has depression because of prescription for venlafaxine) and could also exacerbate her Crohn's disease. The corticosteroid may also contribute to her low mood (see Chapter 6).
- St John's wort should not be given with antidepressant therapy. She should be referred back to her general practitioner if her antidepressant treatment is not effective. Perhaps check first how long she has been taking the venlafaxine, because there may be a delay in efficacy at the start of treatment.
- Hopefully her sore throat is the result of too much singing the night before. However, in view of her immunosuppressant therapy, she should be referred to her GP for a full blood count.
- Echinacea may interfere with immunosuppressive therapy because it is thought to have immunomodulatory activity.
- It may be wise to advise this patient to avoid herbal medicine in view of her drug treatment.

Case 2

A 21-year-old woman asks what you think about kelp tablets for weight loss. Her gym instructor recommended them.

What further questions would you ask?

- It is important to establish if the patient is overweight and to consider her lifestyle and diet (see Chapter 3). Her medical history and any current medication should also be considered.
- Further questioning reveals a history of thyroid dysfunction and excessive calorie intake from lager.

Are kelp tablets suitable for this patient?

- No. Kelp tablets contain iodine, which could exacerbate her thyroid problem (see Chapter 38). There is also a risk of the presence of toxic heavy metals. Possible mechanisms for the weight-loss effect of kelp tablets include increased thyroid activity and/or laxative effects and are not, therefore, a healthy option for weight loss. General lifestyle factors should be considered and the patient advised that the best way to lose weight is to increase exercise and reduce her calorie intake (see Chapter 3). This patient was only marginally overweight and this was corrected by avoiding lager and continuing her exercise routine.

Case 3

A 56-year-old woman informs you that she has been taking a herbal remedy containing ginseng root to relieve her menopausal symptoms. She has found that her symptoms have improved and thought that you would like to know so that you could recommend them to other patients. You notice from her computer records that she is currently taking tamoxifen 20 mg/day for breast cancer.

Are you happy for the patient to continue with the herbal remedy?

- No. In view of her tamoxifen treatment and the absence of sufficient safety data, the ginseng root is not recommended because it has been shown to possess oestrogen receptor-binding activity. There is a risk that the herbal preparation could interfere with her tamoxifen treatment. This case illustrates the importance of asking patients about their use of herbal preparations, as the information is not always volunteered.

Case 4

A patient asks your advice on the use of karela (*Momordica charantia*) for diabetes. She says that she has found good evidence on the internet for its blood sugar lowering effect and is worried she is at risk of diabetes.

How do you respond?

- Initially, the patient's risk factors should be assessed and blood glucose measured. Referral to her GP may be required or to a local pharmacy providing this service. On inspection of the internet site that she found it reveals claims such as 'lower blood sugar naturally' and advertising to buy on-line. The next place to look might be the MHRA website to check for any current safety warnings. This reveals a warning in 2005 regarding the presence of heavy metals in some preparations of karela. The patient should be advised to avoid these products. Diabetes UK has also provided a warning (www.diabetes.org.uk) regarding concerns over the advertising of karela to lower blood sugar and the absence of good evidence for safe use in diabetes. Karela cannot therefore be recommended. As karela is widely available it is important to be aware that patients may take it alongside other medicines for diabetes. *Stockley's Drug Interactions* (Baxter 2013) warns of the potentiation of antidiabetic drugs and that unexplained changes in blood sugars may be attributed to the use of karela, including as a cooking ingredient added to curries.

References

Barnes J, Anderson LA, Phillipson JD (2007). *Herbal Medicines,* 3rd edn. London: Pharmaceutical Press.

Baxter K, ed. (2013). *Stockley's Drug Interactions*, 11th edn. London: Pharmaceutical Press.

Medicines Control Agency or MCA (2002). *Safety of Herbal Medicinal Products*. London: Department of Health. Available at: http://webarchive. nationalarchives.gov.uk/20141205150130/http:// www.mhra.gov.uk/home/groups/es-herbal/documents/ websiteresources/con009293.pdf (accessed June 2016).

Royal Pharmaceutical Society of Great Britain (2007). *Professional Standards and Guidance for the Sale and Supply of Medicines*. London: Royal Pharmaceutical Society of Great Britain.

Further reading

Barnes J (2002). Herbal therapeutics (1). An introduction to herbal medicinal products. *Pharm J*, 268: 804–806.

Barnes J (2002). Herbal therapeutics (2). Depression. *Pharm J*, 268: 908–910.

Barnes J (2002). Herbal therapeutics (3). Cognitive deficiency and dementia. *Pharm J*, 269: 160–162.

Barnes J (2002). Herbal therapeutics (4). Hyperlipidaemia. *Pharm J*, 269: 193–195.

Barnes J (2002). Herbal therapeutics (5). Insomnia. *Pharm J*, 269: 219–221.

Barnes J (2002). Benign prostatic hyperplasia. *Pharm J*, 269: 250–252.

Fugh-Berman A (2000). Herbdrug interactions. *Lancet*, 355: 134–138. pmid: 10675182.

Kayne SB (2008). *Complementary and Alternative Medicine,* 2nd edn. London: Pharmaceutical Press.

Online resources

https://www.gov.uk/government/organisations/medicines-and-healthcare-products-regulatory-agency
The website of the MHRA with policy information for the use and licensing of herbal medicines and the latest safety information (accessed June 2016).

www.nimh.org.uk
The National Institute of Medical Herbalists provides information and research relating to herbal medicines and access to suitably trained herbalists (accessed June 2016).

Treatment

5

Drug choice and prescribing

At the centre of clinical pharmacology and therapeutics is the skill of drug choice and prescribing. These are complex processes which build on a thorough knowledge of drug action and pathophysiology. One of the fundamental principles of medicine is *primum non nocere,* the Latin phrase which means 'First, do no harm'. This is exemplified by drug choice and prescribing, in which the benefits of treatment should always outweigh the disadvantages.

Drug choice and prescribing are increasingly based on guidelines which are evidence-based and the aim should be to become familiar with and apply current guidelines. In the United Kingdom the National Institute for Health and Care Excellence (NICE) has developed a range of guidelines based on evidence for efficacy, safety and economic considerations. Complementary to these, a number of professional organisations have also developed clear guidelines – for example, the British Thoracic Society guidelines concerning asthma. In addition to these there is the concept of 'P-drugs' and this refers to the practitioner having their own 'preferred' drug from a particular class. For example, a practitioner might chose atorvastatin as their preferred statin, becoming familiar with the dosages, interactions, relevant pharmacokinetics and other prescribing issues.

In terms of drug choice and prescribing, the World Health Organization (WHO) have produced their steps to good prescribing (de Vries *et al.* 1994):

Step 1: Define the patient's problem. This requires a thorough understanding of pathophysiology.
Step 2: Specify the therapeutic objective.

- What do you want to achieve with the treatment?
- What are the specific goals of treatment?

There should be precise objectives in mind; for example, in treating hypertension there are specific targets to control blood pressure, with the overall aim of reducing cardiovascular events and reducing mortality.

Step 3: Verify the suitability of your P-treatment. This requires the practitioner to be confident in the safety and efficacy of their preferred drug.
Step 4: Start the treatment. This involves the prescription of a drug.
Step 5: Give information, instructions and warnings.

- This is an essential part of the process and requires communication to the patient about what is prescribed (and why), when to take the drug, how to take the drug and the dosage.
- A key skill is to communicate to the patient the common and important side effects.

The *British National Formulary* and Patient Information leaflets contain exhaustive lists of the possible side effects and adverse reactions; the challenge for the practitioner is to identify the key events to caution the patient about. One approach for each P-drug is to identify a small number of key possible events and communicate these to the patient and, by choosing the key events, this should increase the likelihood of the patient remembering them!

Step 6: Monitor (and stop?) treatment.

- Many treatments require that the patient is monitored in terms of response and changes in physiology and so it is important that appropriate monitoring is carried out, e.g. measuring blood pressure, plasma electrolytes and renal function while taking angiotensin-converting enzyme (ACE) inhibitors.
- For some drugs with a narrow therapeutic window there may be requirements to carry out therapeutic drug monitoring (Chapter 7).
- In planning therapy there should always be a timeframe, whether a week's treatment on an antibiotic, long-term treatment with an antidepressant or lifelong treatment with an antihypertensive.

Considerations in drug choice

Lifestyle changes and advice

Pharmacological therapy should not be viewed as the only solution to medical conditions and should be used alongside lifestyle modifications and advice. One of the best examples of this is in the treatment of hypertension (see Chapter 12), where weight loss, reduction in alcohol consumption, increased exercise, salt reduction and a healthy diet should all be considered prior to, and then alongside, drug treatment.

Concurrent diseases

A holistic approach to the patient should take account of co-morbidities and this should guide drug choice. Drug choice should be designed so as not to exacerbate concurrent diseases, and in some cases co-morbidities may make a compelling reason to choose one drug to manage both conditions. Examples of concurrent diseases are covered in the subsequent chapters, but a couple of examples are the avoidance of β blockers in a patient with ischaemic heart disease who also has asthma (see Chapter 22), and the compelling reason to use ACE inhibitors in a patient who has hypertension but also has diabetes (see Chapter 12).

Allergies

Before a drug is prescribed, the patient and their medical records should be checked for any known drug allergy. Hospital drug charts all have a prominent box for drug allergies to be documented or alert steps in electronic prescribing. As covered in Chapter 6, drug allergies represent an important Type B adverse drug reaction, and affected drugs or classes of drugs should be avoided accordingly.

Age

The age of the patient is an important consideration, with the extremes of age posing a particular challenge. Neonates and babies have developing metabolic pathways and so drug metabolism may be impaired and drug action prolonged. More elderly patients may exhibit impaired drug metabolism and once again the effects and side effects of drugs may be enhanced. In the case of children their body weight should also be accounted for in determining dosages. Paediatric prescribing is a specialist area of therapeutics and children's formularies (e.g. the *British National Formulary for Children*) exist to support the prescriber. Given the complexities of prescribing for children, some drugs have specific minimum ages for prescribing or for availability over-the-counter (OTC). Guidelines also take account of age – for example, because of increased risks, antidepressant therapy is now avoided where possible in children under 18 years of age.

Liver function

The effects of hepatic function on drug choice are considered in more detail in Chapter 11. In general, hepatically cleared drugs are potentially affected by hepatic dysfunction. Liver function tests can provide some insight but are poorly predictive. The *British National Formulary* provides guidance for most drugs, and this typically involves avoidance or dose reduction of affected drugs. Liver disease can also pose challenges of sodium retention, impaired coagulation and enhanced actions on the central nervous system (see Chapter 11).

Renal function

About a quarter of drugs available are renally excreted, and so renal impairment may reduce elimination of these drugs leading to accumulation and toxicity, such as with digoxin. Renal function should be assessed by creatinine clearance and/or estimated glomerular filtration rate (eGFR). Once again the *British National Formulary* provides guidance (and dosages for most drugs in relation to the patient's eGFR). Strategies for prescribing in renal impairment include:

- Dose reduction.
- Choosing shorter acting agents as the plasma half-life may be increased, e.g. in diabetes, gliclazide and tolbutamide have shorter half-lives and are the preferred sulphonylureas.
- Increase the dosage interval, e.g. aminoglycosides are high-risk drugs and their dosage interval is increased in renal impairment to reduce toxicity.
- Choose non-renally excreted alternatives, e.g. amlodipine is principally cleared via hepatic metabolism and may be chosen in hypertension with concurrent renal impairment.
- Some drugs should be avoided in renal impairment, e.g. metformin.
- Some drugs require renal excretion to act and may become ineffective in renal impairment, e.g. thiazide diuretics, nitrofurantoin.

Females of childbearing age

The risk of teratogenesis or harm to the fetus is a key issue as first established by the use of thalidomide in the early 1960s. Prescribing in pregnancy exemplifies the concept of balancing the advantages of therapy versus the risks, and the aim is to avoid drug treatment where possible. This is compounded by the fact that almost all drugs cross the placenta and so the fetus will be exposed to the drug, its metabolites and their effects. The risk of harm to the developing fetus is generally accepted to be greatest in the first trimester, during which time there is considerable organogenesis, although drug exposure later in pregnancy can also lead to complications. The greatest risk being during the first trimester poses a challenge as many pregnancies are unplanned and the patient may not be aware of their pregnancy at this stage. In treating females of childbearing age, one should ask the question: *Could the patient be pregnant?* Some drug treatments require a negative pregnancy test prior to therapy; for example, the retinoids used in dermatology.

Although limiting drug treatment during pregnancy is achievable in some areas, there are a number of long-term medical conditions in which drug therapy is required. For example, challenges are posed by conditions such as diabetes, epilepsy, hypertension, depression and where anticoagulation is required. Although these specific issues are dealt with in the relevant chapters, the underlying principle is to choose the drugs with the greatest safety profile in pregnancy and avoid drugs associated with teratogenesis. For example, in patients with epilepsy, a number of the older agents are associated with birth defects, and evidence-based guidelines advocate the use of drugs such as lamotrigine and carbamazepine (see Chapter 24) which have good safety profiles.

Once again the *British National Formulary* drug monographs contain advice about the safety of drugs in pregnancy and should be consulted. However, in some cases, owing to a lack of evidence or experience with a drug, for the sake of caution it is not recommended.

Pregnancy itself can alter drug action and pharmacokinetics. The increased volume of distribution and enhanced metabolism of some drugs may mean that dosages have to be altered. For example, pregnancy reduces the plasma concentration of lamotrigine and so control of epilepsy may be impaired and may require an increase in dosage.

Adverse drug reactions and interactions

These are core drug safety issues and are covered in detail in Chapters 6 and 7. In terms of drug choice these should always be taken into account to mini-mise patient harm.

Pharmacokinetics

The pharmacokinetic properties of a drug will impact on both drug choice and the regimen. Firstly, the ideal regimen for a drug is usually once daily and this may be achieved with drugs with relatively long half-lives so that plasma concentrations stay within the therapeutic range over 24 hours. Once-daily dos-ing has the advantage of improving compliance over regimens requiring multiple doses per day. Given this advantage, some drugs with a short half-life are for-mulated as sustained release preparations to allow once-daily dosing.

Route of administration

Where possible the oral route is preferred for ease of administration and overcomes the need for par-enteral administration and the associated compli-cations (e.g. setting up an intravenous infusion). However, this is not always possible for labile drugs such as insulin (which is degraded in the stomach), when a rapid response is required (e.g. in severe infections where intravenous antibiotics may speed up treatment) or when the patient cannot swal-low due to disease or debilitation (including severe infections).

Generic versus proprietary preparations

The general guidance to the prescriber is where pos-sible to prescribe generically, as this invariably has an economic advantage, and the generic version is also more likely to be available. For OTC medicines there is often a cheaper generic version, which is equally effective, and it is in the patient's best interests to be directed to them. In some cases there are phar-macokinetic differences between different pharma-ceutical preparations and for these drugs the *British National Formulary* will recommend that the patient is prescribed the particular pharmaceutical form they are stable on. Examples of this include prepa-rations of lithium, carbamazepine, theophylline and ciclosporin.

Prescribing

The act of prescribing is a legally recognised action in which the practitioner produces a prescription for a patient, whether it be in the community on an FP10 or on a hospital drug chart. In both cases the patient must be identified with their name and address, and age if under 12 years of age. The prescribed drugs should be identified with the appropriate dosage route, frequency and length of treatment.

Dosages

Dosage errors can lead to serious consequences and so should be unambiguous, e.g. mg or microgram are acceptable but, in the case of microgram, neither μg nor mcg are acceptable as they could be misread and lead to error. Similarly nanogram should be written in full and not as ng. Some drugs, e.g. insulin and heparins, are prescribed as 'units', where a unit is a measure of biological activity and should not be abbreviated to u.

Hospital drug charts

Many hospitals still retain paper-based drug charts and somewhat surprisingly they can differ from hospital to hospital, and this can potentially lead to errors as practitioners move between hospitals. Drugs charts commonly have patient demographics, a 'Medicines Communication Section', a section for allergies to be stated, which must always be com-pleted, and a section to indicate other special drug charts (e.g. insulin) (Figure 5.1).

Once-only drugs

Drugs for immediate management are stated on the front page. These are likely to include drugs for emergency treatment, e.g. intravenous furosemide in the immediate management of pulmonary oedema (Figure 5.2).

Regular drugs

This section is populated as a prescription and record of drug administration. Prescribed drugs are stated with dosage, route, frequency, and start and stop dates with a section for instructions (e.g. when to monitor) and indications (why the drug has been

MEDICINE PRESCRIPTION AND ADMINISTRATION RECORD	NAME ....
Hospital number...……..…. WARD...........................…..CONSULTANT......................…..….….…	Address
DATE OF ADMISSION..…..….........	DATE OF BIRTH ....
MEDICINES COMMUNICATION SECTION	Height cm Weight kg Surface area m²
	ALLERGY SECTION If none known tick ☐ Medicine/Other Effect Signature .... Date ....
TTO Pharmacy comments : Ready / Will be ready Lunchtime / Mid-afternoon / Evening / Next day circle Date .... Sig .... Bleep	
Other cards in use (please tick) Chart ... of ... Anticoagulant Blood Cytotoxics Enteral Epidural Insulin TDM antimicrobial Nerve sheath PCA SC TPN Other specify	

Figure 5.1   Typical patient details section on the front of a drug chart. Note the box for documentation of allergies or confirmation of no known allergies.

ONCE-ONLY, PRE-OPERATIVE MEDICINES AND PGDS									
Date	Medicine	Dose	Route	Instructions	Time Req	Prescribers sig and print name and bleep	Time given	Nurse sig	Pharm

Figure 5.2   Once-only drugs section of a drug chart.

prescribed). Drug charts commonly contain a section for a low molecular heparin against deep vein thrombosis, and all patients should be assessed for their risk (Figure 5.3).

As-required medication

For drugs given as required (p.r.n.), a separate section contains a prescription for the drug with an indication of the maximum daily dose and minimal

NON-ADMINISTRATION

If a dose is omitted for any reason, the nurse should enter on the administration record below his/her initials and the code number shown. Remember Pre-op fasting is NOT a contraindication to giving the majority of medicines. 50ml of water should be offered with the Medicine for adults. For exclusions please refer to the Pre-operative Medicine Drug Administration Policy.

1   Unable to administer – Inform Doctor in case alternative route required
2   Patient refused
3   Medicine unavailable – Inform Doctor or Pharmacist
4   Strict NBM [*nil by mouth*] on Doctor's instructions only
5   Other – please state in nursing notes, including action taken

ALLERGY SECTION

If none known tick ☐

Medicine/Other Effect

Signature .... Date ....

Administration record

REGULAR PRESCRIPTION Date												
Drug				06								
Dose	Route	Start date	Stop/ Review date	08								
				12								
Additional instructions/ indication			Pharm	14								
				18								
Signature		Print name & bleep		22								
Drug				06								
Dose	Route	Start date	Stop/ Review date	08								
				12								
Additional instructions/ indication			Pharm	14								
				18								
Signature		Print name & bleep		22								
Drug				06								
Dose	Route	Start date	Stop/ Review date	08								
				12								
Additional instructions/ indication			Pharm	14								
				18								
Signature		Print name & bleep		22								

Figure 5.3   Regular drugs section for regimens. Many drug charts now have a low-molecular-weight heparin for prescription following assessment of the need for thromboembolic prophylaxis.

AS-REQUIRED DRUGS ADMINISTRATION RECORD											
Drug				Date							
Dose	Route	Min interval	Max dose in 24hrs	Time							
Additional instructions		Start date	Pharm	Dose							
				Route							
Prescriber signature		Print name & bleep		Given by							

Figure 5.4 As-required medication section of a drug chart.

interval between dosing, e.g. paracetamol might be prescribed for analgesia as required as 1 g, with a minimum dosage interval of 4 hours and a maximum daily dose of 4 g (Figure 5.4).

Variable dosages

Some drugs are prescribed as variable dosages in relation to response, and examples would include analgesia in relation to pain relief obtained.

Prescribing errors

Drug safety is a major issue that has received widespread interest. In the UK the landmark 2009 EQUIP study identified that the level of prescription errors was 8.9% based on a large sample of hospital prescriptions (Dornan *et al.* 2009). In many cases these were considered as minor errors and almost all were intercepted by the pharmacists. However, of the errors identified, 1.74% were potentially fatal. The commonest error involved dosage. The study reported that it was the application of knowledge that contributed to prescription errors, and that basic knowledge was not a key issue.

Safeguards

For the prevention of prescribing errors, there is the established system: prescriber followed by pharmacist checking and final checking on drug administration. The World Health Organization has produced a video *Learning from Error* (WHO 2008), which should be viewed by all those involved in the medication process as it follows a medication error and its cause.

Practice points

- Prescribing errors are alarmingly frequent, with dosage errors being the most common.
- Look out for key drug interactions.
- Be familiar with key adverse drug reactions (ADRs).
- Is the patient renally impaired?
- How should the patient be monitored? Electrolytes? Renal and hepatic function? Is therapeutic drug monitoring required?
- Females of childbearing age: could they be pregnant or breastfeeding?
- Key counselling points: what to tell the patient, including important key side effects.
- Be alert for the occurrence of adverse events.

References

de Vries TPGM, Henning RH, Hogerzeil HV *et al.* (1994). *Guide to Good Prescribing: A practical manual.* Geneva: World Health Organization (www.who.org).

Dornan T, Ashcroft D, Heathfield H *et al.* (2009). *An In-depth Investigation Into Causes of Prescribing Errors by Foundation Trainees in Relation to Their Medical Education. EQUIP Study.* London: General Medical Council.

Video

World Health Organization (2008). *Learning from Error.* Geneva: WHO. http://www.who.int/patientsafety/education/vincristine_download/en/
This is essential viewing for all of those involved in prescribing, dispensing and drug administration.

Further reading

Freyer AM (2008). Drug-prescribing challenges during pregnancy, practice points, additional resources. *Obstet Gynaecol Reprod Med* 18: 180–186.
Ross S, Bond C, Rothnie H *et al.* (2009). What is the scale of prescribing errors committed by junior doctors? A systematic review. *Br J Clin Pharmacol* 67(6): 629–640.

Adverse drug reactions and interactions

Adverse drug reactions (ADRs) and drug interactions are related topics, e.g. a drug interaction results in a change to the expected treatment outcome and occurs as a result of concurrent exposure to another drug, food or chemical. The result may be an adverse event but this is not always the case. In either event ADRs and drug interactions tend to be more important for drugs that exhibit a narrow therapeutic window, which is the margin between a therapeutic dose and a toxic dose. However, this is not always the case and some drugs may cause severe adverse reactions at low or therapeutic doses. A thorough knowledge of these topics is essential for safe prescribing and drug safety, in both prevention of events and recognition of adverse outcomes. A key element of prescribing is that the benefits of a drug treatment must always outweigh its drawbacks, of which ADRs are the major component.

The purpose of this chapter is to explore the nature and mechanisms, when known, resulting in ADRs and interactions. For a more comprehensive coverage of these topics the reader is referred to Lee's *Adverse Drug Reactions* (2006), the *British National Formulary* and *Stockley's Drug Interactions* (Baxter 2013).

Adverse drug reactions and side effects

These terms are difficult to distinguish and in practice are often used interchangeably. It may be helpful to consider side effects of a medicine as predictable secondary effects that may be beneficial (e.g. sedation with antihistamines when used as an over-the-counter [OTC] sleep medicine) or undesirable (e.g. sedation with antihistamines used for allergy relief). By contrast, ADRs are side effects that are always deleterious.

The magnitude of ADRs with significant morbidity and mortality is substantial, with 6.5% of hospital admissions being ADR related, leading to a mortality rate of 0.15% (Pirmohamed *et al.* 2004). Of these, non-steroidal anti-inflammatory drugs (NSAIDs) were associated with the greatest proportion of admissions (29.6%) and the causes included peptic ulceration, renal impairment, cerebrovascular accident and wheezing. Based on this study and other work the following are associated with the greatest burden of ADRs and their use should always ring alarm bells:

- NSAIDs (e.g. peptic ulceration, asthma, renal dysfunction)
- diuretics (e.g. electrolyte disturbances, postural hypotension)
- warfarin (e.g. bleeding)
- angiotensin-converting enzyme (ACE) inhibitors and angiotensin receptor antagonists (e.g. electrolyte disturbances, renal dysfunction)
- antidepressants (e.g. cardiac toxicity with tricyclic antidepressants)

- lithium (e.g. renal impairment)
- β blockers (e.g. bronchospasm)
- opioids (e.g. constipation)
- digoxin (e.g. toxicity)
- oral steroids (e.g. adrenal suppression)
- oral hypoglycaemic agents (e.g. hypoglycaemia).

ADRs are often divided into type A (augmented response) and type B (bizarre or idiosyncratic reactions).

Type A: augmented response

This type of ADR can be explained or predicted on the basis of the drug's pharmacology. Type A reactions are often dose dependent and may often be managed by dose reduction. If they are anticipated, measures may be taken to ameliorate or prevent the problem, e.g. the use of antiemetics in patients receiving chemotherapy, or laxatives with opioid analgesics.

Type B: bizarre or idiosyncratic reactions

These ADRs are unrelated to the known pharmacology of the drug, which makes them less common and unpredictable; they may also be severe. This group of ADRs is often related to genetics or immunology, which means that certain individuals may be at a higher risk than others.

Risk factors for developing ADRs

When considering ADRs there are a number of risk factors that may predispose a patient to adverse responses:

- extremes of age
- gender
- concurrent drug usage
- concurrent disease, e.g. respiratory disease and β blockers
- pharmacokinetic variables, e.g. renal or hepatic function
- pharmaceutical factors, e.g. nature of dosage form or excipients
- genetics, e.g. glucose-6-phosphate dehydrogenase (G6PD) deficiency.

Mechanisms of adverse reactions

The effects of a drug may be enhanced by various pharmacodynamic or pharmacokinetic factors, leading to enhanced side effects or adverse reactions.

Pharmacological mechanisms

These represent the most straightforward examples that may be predicted from a sound knowledge of a drug's pharmacology. The best example is β-adrenoceptor antagonists which, to varying degrees, will block β_2-adrenoceptors on the bronchial smooth muscle, opposing the actions of circulating adrenaline (epinephrine), which may lead to bronchoconstriction, and it is for this reason that they are contraindicated in asthma. Other examples are given in Table 6.1. These predictable responses are dose dependent and so increases in plasma concentration, which may occur as a consequence of pharmacokinetic mechanism (as outlined below) or drug interactions (see later), necessarily increase their likelihood and impact.

Pharmacokinetic mechanisms

Pharmacokinetic ADRs result from impaired absorption, distribution, metabolism or excretion (ADME). The first potential site is absorption and this might be delayed if, for example, gastric emptying is slowed and the consequences might be retarded absorption, leading to failure of therapy, which is itself an ADR. Metabolism and elimination are far more important, e.g. a reduced rate of elimination, often due to impaired renal function, is likely to increase plasma concentrations, leading to augmented effects. These are common causes of ADRs and may often be prevented by careful prescribing and patient monitoring. Impaired renal function is common in elderly people and neonates, and should be measured so that drug doses or dosage intervals are adjusted as appropriate to prevent an ADR. An important example of this is digoxin, which is predominantly (about two-thirds) cleared by the kidneys, and in renally impaired patients the plasma concentration may reach toxic levels (Figure 6.1). Accordingly, when using digoxin the dose should be determined in relation to renal function.

The alternative strategy that is used with aminoglycosides such as gentamicin is to increase the dosage interval in renally impaired patients.

Table 6.1 Examples of adverse drug reactions that may be predicted from the pharmacology of the drug class; further information is given in the relevant chapters

Drug class	Side effect	Pharmacological mechanism	Possible solutions
β blockers	Cold extremities	Antagonism of peripheral β_2-adrenoceptors	• Choose a more cardioselective agent such as atenolol, which has less affinity for β_2-adrenoceptors • Choose a β blocker with vasodilator actions, e.g. nebivolol
β blockers	Bradycardia	Antagonism of chronotropic cardiac β_1-adrenoceptors	Withdraw β blockers gradually to prevent rebound tachycardia
β blockers	Bronchospasm	Antagonism of bronchial β_2-adrenoceptors	All β blockers are contraindicated in asthma. A cardioselective one may be used with extreme caution under specialist supervision. Cardioselective β blockers should be used with caution in COPD
α blockers, diuretics, ACE inhibitors	Postural hypotension	Impairment of blood pressure regulation	• Caution on standing • Take first dose of α blocker or ACE inhibitor on retiring to bed
Thiazide and loop diuretics	Hypokalaemia	Activation of the renin–angiotensin–aldosterone system (Chapter 16)	Potassium levels should be monitored
Nitrates	Flushing, headache	Vasodilatation	• Headache relieved by paracetamol • Sublingual tablets may be discarded by spitting them out
Oral anticoagulants	Increased bleeding	Plasma concentration too high or increased bleeding tendency	Monitoring of INR required and dose adjustment may be required
Opioids	Constipation	Inhibition of lower GI tract motility	Use a laxative such as lactulose or senna
Tricyclic antidepressants; certain older antihistamines (e.g. promethazine)	Antimuscarinic effects such as dry mouth, blurred vision, constipation and urinary retention	Antagonism of muscarinic receptors	• Consider an SSRI for depression • Choose a newer antihistamine with less muscarinic binding, e.g. loratadine
Sulphonylureas	Hypoglycaemia	Augmented pharmacological effect	• Careful monitoring with dose adjustment • Use short-acting agents
Broad-spectrum antibiotics	Diarrhoea	Alterations of lower gastrointestinal flora	Caution: severe diarrhoea should alert one to the risk of pseudomembranous colitis. Otherwise a short course of loperamide may be used with caution
NSAIDs	Gastric damage	Inhibition of the production of cytoprotective prostaglandins	• Use a less irritant NSAID such as ibuprofen • Consider a COX-2 inhibitor. • Combine NSAID with misoprostol or a PPI

(continued)

Table 6.1 *(continued)*			
Drug class	**Side effect**	**Pharmacological mechanism**	**Possible solutions**
NSAIDs	Bronchospasm	Inhibition of the production of prostaglandins, favouring the production of leukotrienes	Avoid in patients with asthma who are sensitive to NSAIDs
Cytotoxic agents	Myelosuppression	Cytotoxic effects on bone marrow	• Prophylactic antibacterial and antifungal agents • Use of transfusions or colony-stimulating factors to increase white blood cell counts

ACE, angiotensin-converting enzyme; COPD, chronic obstructive pulmonary disease; COX-2, cyclo-oxygenase 2; INR, international normalised ratio; NSAIDs, non-steroidal anti-inflammatory drugs; PPI, proton pump inhibitor; SSRI, selective serotonin reuptake inhibitor.

Important examples where serious toxicity may arise as a consequence of renal impairment are:

- digoxin
- lithium
- NSAIDs
- metformin
- ACE inhibitors
- aminoglycoside antibiotics.

Differences in hepatic metabolism

Alterations in drug metabolism may also lead to increased plasma concentrations. Metabolism may be altered at the extremes of age, such that neonates conjugate drugs at a relatively slow rate, whereas microsomal enzyme activity in the liver by cytochrome P450 isoenzymes decreases variably with age. An example of this is the prolonged half-life of diazepam with age, and hence the increased propensity to side effects, including oversedation. Hepatic metabolism may be impaired in liver disease and this may lead to the enhanced effects of drugs that are usually cleared by the liver.

Pharmacogenetic differences in the expression of cytochrome P450 isoenzymes may also contribute to variations in metabolism. Approximately 10% of the population express a defective P450 isoenzyme, CYP2D6, which slows down the metabolism of a range of drugs including flecainide, metoclopramide and some antidepressants. Accordingly, patients may vary in the way that they handle drugs. In the case of codeine, defects of CYP2D6 can lead to failure of therapy as metabolic conversion is required for it to act. Similarly, the anticancer effects of tamoxifen can be reduced in patients with defective CYP2D6.

Disorders of metabolism

These include a lack of G6PD in erythrocytes and porphyria. G6PD is an enzyme present in red blood cells, which provides reducing power, thereby maintaining glutathione in the reduced form. This prevents oxidative damage to the cells. The absence of G6PD therefore leads to fragile red blood cell membranes and haemolysis, resulting in anaemia. G6PD deficiency is prevalent in the Mediterranean population and patients are sensitive to the effects of oxidative drugs such as antimalarials, sulphonamides, quinolones, nalidixic acid, nitrofurantoin, sulfasalazine

Figure 6.1 Variation of plasma concentration of digoxin over time. In patients the ideal is to maintain the plasma concentration within the therapeutic window. However, in the renally impaired patient, without a dose reduction, the plasma concentration rises to toxic levels.

and aspirin (refer to the *British National Formulary*), leading to oxidative damage with haemolysis and anaemia.

Individuals with porphyria lack one of the enzymes for haemoglobin synthesis and there is an accumulation of porphyrin precursors, leading to gastrointestinal (GI), neurological and behavioural disturbances. Cytochrome P450 inducers including barbiturates, carbamazepine, griseofulvin and hormonal contraceptives (refer to the *British National Formulary*) tend to provoke an attack by inducing amino laevulinic acid synthase, giving rise to porphyrins.

Immunological responses

Drugs are foreign molecules and some may induce an immunological response. These reactions may be delayed and tend not to be dose related, occurring with the smallest doses of drug. They are usually reversible on cessation of the causative agent. Patients at risk of these responses tend to have a predisposition to allergic disorders and the responses may vary from simple skin rashes to life-threatening anaphylaxis (see Chapter 21). Important examples of causative agents are penicillins and streptokinase.

Penicillins couple to proteins, forming immunogens, which may precipitate hypersensitivity reactions. Management includes stopping the drug and treating the patient with antihistamines, adrenaline and/or parenteral steroids according to severity (see Chapter 21). In the case of penicillins, the allergic reaction is a class effect resulting from the presence of the β-lactam ring in the drug molecule and approximately 10% of penicillin-allergic patients are also sensitive to chemically similar cephalosporins. It is therefore appropriate that non-penicillin, non-cephalosporin antibiotics are chosen for patients with a history of penicillin allergy.

In the case of streptokinase, once patients have been treated with this agent for thrombolysis they are likely to develop antibodies against it. This means that on a subsequent exposure the antibodies may either prevent it from acting or lead to an allergic reaction. It is for this reason that patients do not generally receive streptokinase a second time and usually receive an alternative clot-busting agent for a second heart attack.

The increasing use of monoclonal antibodies (e.g. in immunological diseases and anticancer chemotherapy) is also likely to be associated with increased instances of immunological responses. These drugs are likely to be used in specialist settings and the patient should be observed for the period immediately after administration for hypersensitivity reactions, which might involve skin reactions, breathing problems and hypotension. In some cases corticosteroids and antihistamines are given prophylactically.

Withdrawal responses

The withdrawal of certain drugs may lead to predictable symptoms and patients should be counselled appropriately. This type of reaction tends to result from physiological adaptation during the course of treatment, e.g. chronic treatment with β blockers leads to receptor up-regulation, i.e. an increase in the number of β-adrenoceptors occurs in response to the blockade of existing receptors. Sudden withdrawal of β blockade may therefore result in over-stimulation of β-adrenoceptors. In the heart this may predispose to arrhythmias and is associated with increased mortality. Common examples of drugs where abrupt withdrawal may lead to adverse reactions are given below.

Alcohol

Delirium tremens and seizures occur after chronic excessive alcohol intake. Treatment includes short-term chlordiazepoxide or clomethiazole (inpatients only).

Antidepressants

Selective serotonin reuptake inhibitors (SSRIs, particularly paroxetine), tricyclic antidepressants and monoamine oxidase inhibitors (MAOIs) of 8 weeks' use or more should be withdrawn gradually over at least 4 weeks (up to 6 months after long-term maintenance). Monitor for withdrawal symptoms such as nausea, vomiting, anorexia, headache and panic anxiety (see Chapter 25).

Benzodiazepines

Withdrawal from benzodiazepines requires a gradual reduction of dose to prevent symptoms of confusion, toxic psychosis, convulsions or those similar to delirium tremens following alcohol withdrawal. These symptoms may take from a few hours to 3 weeks to develop with longer-acting agents. Milder symptoms include insomnia, loss of appetite, anxiety, weight loss, tremor, sweating, tinnitus and disturbances of perception. Patients are transferred to the equivalent dose of diazepam (*British National Formulary*). The dose is then reduced by increments of approximately one-eighth of the daily dose (or 2–2.5 mg) every 2 weeks, maintaining the new dose for a longer period if withdrawal symptoms occur. The time taken to withdraw completely from long-term benzodiazepine use can be from 4 weeks to a year or occasionally longer. Specialist counselling may benefit some patients, including education about the risks and benefits of withdrawing from these drugs.

It should be noted that antipsychotics aggravate the symptoms of benzodiazepine withdrawal and should not be used (see the *British National Formulary*).

Anticonvulsants

See Chapter 24.

Opioids

'Cold turkey' may be experienced after opioid addiction but is rare when opioids are prescribed for pain relief. Debilitating diarrhoea may occur; this may be treated with loperamide.

Baclofen

There is a risk of serious withdrawal reactions. The dose should be reduced gradually over at least 1–2 weeks, or longer if symptoms develop (*British National Formulary*).

Corticosteroids

Prolonged use of corticosteroids results in the suppression of endogenous production and treatment should therefore be withdrawn gradually.

Gradual withdrawal is recommended for patients whose disease is unlikely to relapse and who have:

- recently received repeated courses
- taken a short course within 1 year of stopping long-term therapy
- other possible causes of adrenal suppression
- received more than 40 mg prednisolone (or equivalent) daily
- repeat doses given in the evening
- received more than 3 weeks' treatment.

Sympathomimetics

Prolonged use of topical decongestant vasoconstrictors causes tolerance and rebound congestion, probably due in part to down-regulation of α-adrenoceptors.

Antipsychotics

Withdraw gradually after long-term therapy and monitor closely for acute withdrawal syndromes or rapid relapse (*British National Formulary*).

Type A adverse drug reactions

In the simplest case, one may predict many common type A ADRs on the basis of the known pharmacology of the drugs. Some common examples are given in Table 6.1.

Gastrointestinal ADRs

ADRs can occur throughout the GI system and, as indicated above, NSAID-induced damage represents the most significant of all ADRs.

Oral problems

The mouth may be the site of ADRs leading to unpleasant side effects, e.g. drugs with significant antimuscarinic activity (e.g. tricyclic antidepressants, older antihistamines) may lead to a dry mouth, which is a minor problem and may be resolved by selecting an alternative (e.g. an SSRI for depression). Alternatively artificial saliva might be recommended. More significant problems include tooth discoloration with tetracycline (which should be avoided in pregnant patients and in children under 12 years) and gingival hyperplasia with phenytoin and calcium-channel blockers.

Oesophageal disorders

These may be induced by the local effects of drugs such as aspirin, tetracycline, doxycycline and bisphosphonates on the oesophagus, leading to irritation, or by drug-induced relaxation of the gastro-oesophageal sphincter producing reflux (e.g. opioids, calcium channel antagonists, nitrates). Symptoms include dysphagia or odynophagia (difficult or painful swallowing, respectively), heartburn, substernal chest pain or the feeling of something lodged in the throat (see Chapter 8).

Bisphosphonates pose a significant risk of oesophagitis and, in the case of alendronic acid, ibandronic acid and risedronate sodium, patients should be counselled to take the tablets with a full tumbler of water in the sitting or standing position and not to lie down for 30 minutes afterwards. These measures are to prevent the tablet becoming lodged in the oesophagus. When a patient is affected then cessation of the particular drug may be appropriate or, in the case of ulceration and/or reflux, a proton pump inhibitor (PPI) might be prescribed.

NSAID gastrotoxicity

NSAID-induced gastrotoxicity represents the most important ADR and is discussed in Chapter 8.

Antiplatelet drugs and gastrotoxicity

The adenosine diphosphate (ADP) receptor antagonist clopidogrel is used as an alternative antiplatelet agent to low-dose aspirin for patients with aspirin sensitivity. Clopidogrel has been shown to exhibit comparable efficacy and fewer adverse GI effects when compared with low-dose aspirin but may cause GI bleeding in patients at risk and should not be used for patients at risk of GI bleeding (see Chapter 15; Harker *et al.* 1999).

Diarrhoea

Drug-induced diarrhoea is discussed in Chapter 10.

Nausea and vomiting

Drug-induced nausea and vomiting are discussed in Chapter 9.

Constipation

Drug-induced constipation is discussed in Chapter 10.

Malabsorption

As the major role of the GI tract is the digestion and absorption of food, alterations in absorption can arise from adverse drug effects, e.g. the pancreatic lipase inhibitor, orlistat, reduces the absorption of fat and consequently the absorption of fat-soluble vitamins. In some cases it may be appropriate to give vitamin supplements (in particular vitamin D), which should be given at least 2 hours after orlistat. Another example are the bile-binding agents such as colestyramine which also reduce the absorption of fat-soluble vitamins, and supplementation with vitamins A, D, E and K might be appropriate.

Hepatic ADRs

Liver function may be altered by drugs to varying degrees, ranging from mild, reversible and asymptomatic changes identified by routine liver function tests (LFTs) to severe damage, leading to hepatic failure. Drug types and classes associated with altered liver function through to liver failure include:

- antiepileptic drugs
- halothane
- paracetamol
- methotrexate
- amiodarone
- flucloxacillin
- clavulanic acid in co-amoxiclav.

Risk factors for developing drug-induced hepatic dysfunction:

- pre-existing liver disease
- female sex
- age
- genetic variations in the expression of cytochrome P450 isoenzymes
- concurrent treatment with enzyme inducers (see Drug interactions below)
- polypharmacy
- concurrent disease: diabetes mellitus predisposes patients to methotrexate-induced damage
- nutritional status: fasting patients lack glutathione required in the non-toxic pathway of paracetamol metabolism
- alcohol consumption.

Clinical features

The presentation of liver impairment may vary but key features that should raise the suspicion of liver dysfunction include anorexia, nausea, vomiting, jaundice, itching, pale stools and dark urine. Patients who are prescribed drugs that are known to cause liver dysfunction should be counselled to report these symptoms if they occur. Diagnosis may be based on a drug history, clinical features, an LFT and a biopsy.

Paracetamol-induced hepatotoxicity and patient counselling

Paracetamol is the most common cause of drug-induced hepatotoxicity. This is partly due to a lack of awareness of the potential toxicity of paracetamol or its presence in different medicines taken together, leading to accidental ingestion of excessive doses.

Monitoring

The monitoring of liver function is discussed in Chapter 2. It should be noted that elevated LFTs are not always followed by hepatic injury. Generally an increase of two to three times any baseline value would indicate possible drug-induced hepatotoxicity and the need to stop the drug.

Cardiovascular ADRs

Drug-induced cardiovascular disorders are common and often predictable Type A reactions, particularly in patients with pre-existing heart disease. Additional risk factors include undisclosed self-medication with OTC drugs, electrolyte disturbances and impaired renal function.

Drugs used to manage cardiovascular diseases may have predictable cardiovascular consequences, e.g. volume depletion with diuretics or inhibition of autonomic homeostatic mechanisms (e.g. α blockers) are very commonly associated with orthostatic or postural hypotension. This is especially prominent in elderly patients and associated with a high risk of falls. Obviously judicious prescribing might reduce this risk by choosing safer alternative agents and counselling patients to take care when changing posture. In the case of ACE inhibitors and α blockers they also pose a risk of first-dose hypotension (especially if the patient is already taking a diuretic) when the initiation of treatment may lead to a precipitous drop in blood pressure. When these drugs are used the patient should be counselled initially to take the drug when retiring to bed to reduce the problems posed by first-dose hypotension.

Drugs may themselves exacerbate or increase cardiovascular risk. Long-term NSAID usage can be associated with increased risk of coronary disease (Kearney *et al.* 2006), whereas the fluid-retaining properties of NSAIDs may exacerbate chronic heart failure or lead to hypertension. In particular, high-dose regimens of diclofenac and ibuprofen were found to pose a significant risk, with naproxen appearing safer.

The antidiabetic rosiglitazone was withdrawn from therapy in 2010 as it was associated with an increased cardiovascular risk (Nissen and Wolski 2007). Obviously assessing a patient's overall cardiovascular risk is important when deciding on a treatment and identifying drug-induced cardiovascular effects as appropriate.

Reduction in heart rate or slowing of atrioventricular conduction is the aim of using β blockers, rate-limiting calcium-channel blockers or digoxin. However, at high doses or if the patient has conduction problems, this may lead to bradycardia with a reduction in cardiac output. Hence, patients taking digoxin are counselled to ensure that their heart rate does not drop below 60 beats/minute and all negative chronotropic drugs should be used with caution in patients with conduction problems.

The prolongation of the Q–T interval, as revealed by electrocardiogram (ECG), and subsequent risk of life-threatening torsade de pointes arrhythmias, have led to the withdrawal of drugs such as cisapride, terfenadine, thioridazine and astemizole. The CSM/CHM has advised against the co-prescribing of two or more drugs known to prolong the Q–T interval. Drugs associated with Q–T interval prolongation include:

- amiodarone
- sotalol
- disopyramide
- macrolide antibacterial agents
- azole antifungal agents
- tricyclic antidepressants (amitriptyline and imipramine)
- antipsychotic agents (including chlorpromazine, haloperidol).

Risk factors for developing this ADR include:

- female sex
- family history of coronary heart disease
- smoking
- high stress levels

- substance misuse, particularly alcohol or cocaine
- renal or hepatic impairment or slow metabolisers
- metabolic-type drug interactions (due to increased drug levels)
- electrolyte disturbance such as hypokalaemia or hypomagnesaemia, e.g. with laxatives or diuretics
- high doses, particularly of antipsychotics
- polypharmacy and particularly concurrent diuretic treatment
- bradycardia
- cardiovascular disease: hypertension, congestive heart failure
- a history of Q–T interval prolongation.

For further information and a list of drugs that prolong the Q–T interval, see Haddad and Anderson (2002).

Patient counselling

Patients prescribed drugs with the potential to prolong the Q–T interval should be advised to report urgently symptoms of arrhythmia such as dizziness, light-headedness, irregular pulse, palpitations and fainting. Drugs should be stopped immediately and the ECG monitored.

Renal ADRs

The kidneys are responsible for the elimination of many drugs and are common targets for drug-induced toxicity, particularly in elderly patients with age-related renal impairment. Drugs implicated commonly include ACE inhibitors, diuretics and NSAIDs, commonly prescribed for the ageing patient with cardiovascular disease and chronic inflammatory conditions such as rheumatoid arthritis. Common mechanisms for drug-induced renal impairment include:

- reduced renal perfusion, e.g. volume depletion during diuretic therapy
- altered glomerular filtration due to altered tone of renal arterioles in the presence of ACE inhibitors or NSAIDs, which inhibit the effects of angiotensin II or prostaglandins, respectively
- damage to renal tubules due to inflammatory reactions triggered by many drugs, including NSAIDs.

Additional risk factors for renal ADRs include dehydration, cirrhosis or heart failure (due to sodium retention), diabetes, polypharmacy (particularly of nephrotoxic drugs), high doses of the causative agent, hypotension, sepsis and shock.

Clinical features

See Chapter 19.

Patient counselling

- Patients with risk factors for renal disorders as outlined above should report nausea, vomiting and muscle cramps. Urinalysis should be undertaken to check for the presence of protein.
- Patients taking diuretics and/or laxatives are at risk of prerenal failure due to reduced renal perfusion and should therefore report fatigue, postural hypotension and muscle cramps. This is particularly important in elderly patients and those taking additional nephrotoxic drugs. Patients should be referred to their general practitioner (GP) and/or a dose of diuretic omitted when suffering from conditions that may result in dehydration, e.g. excess sweating, diarrhoea and/or vomiting.

Haematological ADRs (Table 6.2)

Drugs such as cytotoxic agents cause predictable suppression of bone marrow and could therefore be considered Type A reactions. Many drugs may, however, unpredictably affect the bone marrow and blood cell production. With the exception of cytotoxics, drug-induced blood dyscrasias are rare but potentially fatal, and therefore health professionals should be aware of drugs known to cause these effects. Drugs can cause aplastic anaemia in which typically all cells lines are affected; they can cause neutropenia (agranulocytosis) with white cells affected and thrombocytopenia in which there is a reduction in platelets. Alerting symptoms include sore throat, mouth ulcers, bruising or bleeding, rash, malaise and fever, or non-specific illness.

Other drug-induced haematological problems include haemolytic anaemia (as discussed above in patients with G6PD deficiency) and megaloblastic anaemia through impaired metabolism of either vitamin B_{12} or folic acid. In this latter case methotrexate's

Table 6.2 A summary of adverse drug reactions involving the haematological system

Haematological disorder	Important examples of causative drugs	Comments
Aplastic anaemia (total or partial failure of the bone marrow)	**Antidiabetic** (tolbutamide) **Antiepileptics** (carbamazepine, phenytoin, lamotrigine) **Anti-inflammatory** (diclofenac, gold, indometacin, penicillamine, piroxicam, sulindac, sulfasalazine) **Antimicrobials** (chloramphenicol, co-trimoxazole, sulphonamides) **Antipsychotics** (chlorpromazine) **Antithyroid agents** (carbimazole, propylthiouracil)	• Reduced red cell (anaemia), white cell (leukopenia) and platelet (thrombocytopenia) counts • Often irreversible despite drug withdrawal
Neutropenia (profound reduction of granulocytes with neutrophil count $<0.5 \times 10^9$/L)	**Antibiotics** (e.g. co-trimoxazole) **Antidepressants** (e.g. imipramine, mianserin) **Antiepileptics** (e.g. carbamazepine, phenytoin) **Anti-inflammatory** (e.g. gold, penicillamine, lefunomide, sulfasalazine, NSAIDs) **Antipsychotics** (e.g. chlorpromazine, clozapine) **Antithyroid drugs** (carbimazole, propylthiouracil)	• Recovery usually 2–3 weeks after drug is withdrawn • Repeat exposure to causative drug not recommended due to sensitisation
Thrombocytopenia (reduced platelets to $<150 \times 10^9$/L)	**Antimicrobials** (e.g. chloramphenicol, co-trimoxazole) **Antiepileptics** (e.g. sodium valproate) **Anti-inflammatory** (e.g. gold, NSAIDs, penicillamine) **Diuretics** (thiazides, furosemide) **Others** (tolbutamide, digitoxin, methyldopa, heparin [less likely with low-molecular-weight heparin], quinidine)	• May present as easy bleeding, bruising or purpura • Prolonged bleeding time but INR remains normal • Usually occurs 7–10 days after drug started • Avoid future exposure to the causative agent • Aspirin and NSAIDs reduce the effects of remaining platelets and therefore should be avoided during thrombocytopenia
Pure red cell aplasia (total or partial failure of red cell production)	Azathioprine, phenytoin, isoniazid, penicillamine, chloramphenicol erythropoietin	Anaemia with a marked reduction in reticulocytes (immature red cells)

NSAIDs, non-steroidal anti-inflammatory drugs; INR, international normalised ratio.

pharmacological action is to interfere with DNA synthesis by acting as a folate antagonist and so megaloblastic anaemia is a dose-dependent ADR. To avoid this, patients may receive folate supplements.

Respiratory ADRs

The most significant respiratory ADR is bronchospasm with β blockers and is discussed in detail in Chapter 22. Other examples include anaphylaxis with bronchospasm, which may be life threatening (see Chapter 21), and ACE inhibitor-induced cough (see Chapter 12). Long-term lung damage may also occur and examples of this include amiodarone leading to pulmonary fibrosis and pneumonitis, and methotrexate also causing pneumonitis. In both cases patients should report any change in respiratory function.

Psychiatric ADRs

These are relatively common and consist mainly of type A reactions predictable from pharmacological activity. Psychiatric and cognitive problems occur with a range of drugs and can be exacerbated by alcohol abuse, liver disease or a history of depression. A number of drugs can induce depression and these include isotretinoin, varenicline (for smoking cessation) and the antimalarial mefloquine, which is contraindicated in neuropsychiatric disorders, including depression, or convulsions. SSRIs have been implicated in inducing suicidal thoughts (Fergusson *et al.* 2005), especially in children, and it is for this reason that they are no longer recommended for use in patients under 18 years of age. Many centrally acting drugs cause sedation and this is particularly true of tricyclic antidepressants, benzodiazepines, barbiturates, opioids, antipsychotic agents and sedating antihistamines. Although this can be an advantage when sedation is required, e.g. depression with insomnia, it can be a particularly debilitating side effect and may lead to a lack of patient compliance. When prescribing, this might be avoided by choosing a safe alternative, e.g. an SSRI for depression. When sedating drugs are used it may help to counsel the patient to take the drug when retiring to bed to reduce the side effect, and in all cases the patient should be counselled about the sedating effects.

Neurological ADRs

Neurological disorders encompass disorders of the nervous system, including the brain, spinal cord and all peripheral nerves. Common examples include the following.

Drug-induced movement disorders

Drugs with antidopaminergic actions (such as antipsychotics and metoclopramide) may lead to a drug-induced form of Parkinson's disease (see Chapter 29). The general approach to the management of this ADR is to withdraw the offending drug and use a safer alternative.

Decreased seizure threshold

Some drugs may reduce the threshold for seizure and increase the risk of convulsions. These drugs include antidepressants, bupropion, mefloquine, chloroquine, sedating antihistamines, tramadol, theophylline and quinolone antibiotics. The risk of convulsions is greatest in patients with a history of epilepsy, brain tumours or trauma, and the drug should be used with caution.

Endocrine ADRs

ADRs may also affect a variety of endocrine control systems such as the thyroid and adrenal glands.

Glucose control

See Chapter 37.

Thyroid dysfunction

See Chapter 38.

Adrenal function

Cushing's syndrome

Cushing's syndrome is caused by prolonged treatment with corticosteroids. Clinical signs include 'moon face', weight gain, excess growth of facial and body hair, raised blood pressure, raised blood glucose levels, osteoporosis, psychiatric symptoms, including depressed mood, and skin thinning.

Adrenal insufficiency

Abrupt withdrawal of corticosteroids following prolonged treatment may lead to headache, dizziness, joint pain, weakness and emotional changes. Abrupt withdrawal from long-term treatment may be more severe and potentially fatal.

Drugs that themselves can precipitate adrenal insufficiency include the antifungal agent ketoconazole and rifampicin.

Hyperprolactinaemia

Prolactin is synthesised and stored in the anterior pituitary gland, being released following childbirth, stimulating milk production and progesterone production by the corpus luteum in the ovary. Drug-induced hyperprolactinaemia may occur in patients taking drugs that increase serotonin (5-hydroxytryptamine or 5HT) or reduce dopamine effects (e.g. phenothiazines), leading to galactorrhoea (abnormal milk production), amenorrhoea, impotence or infertility. The condition is usually reversible on cessation of treatment.

Syndrome of inappropriate secretion of antidiuretic hormone (SIADH)

Some drugs can cause an inappropriate secretion of the antidiuretic hormone (ADH or vasopressin) from the pituitary gland, leading to increased reabsorption of water in the kidneys and an increase in extracellular volume with dilute plasma. Symptoms include confusion, weakness, lethargy, weight gain, headache, nausea and vomiting, and ultimately convulsions, coma and death. Monitoring of baseline serum sodium levels is prudent in patients prescribed drugs known to cause SIADH, particularly antipsychotics, carbamazepine and antidepressants (particularly SSRIs), especially if co-prescribed with other drugs that may cause hyponatraemia (see Chapter 2).

Dermatological ADRs (Table 6.3)

The skin is a major site of ADRs, from trivial rashes right through to life-threatening reactions. Any drug, chemical, herb or pharmaceutical excipient has the potential to cause a dermatological reaction. The mechanisms involved are often unknown but tend to result from an allergic or toxic reaction or exacerbation of a pre-existing inflammatory condition.

Allergic reactions such as urticaria may persist for a long time after a drug is stopped or may occasionally fail to develop for up to a week after a drug is withdrawn. The drugs most commonly implicated in ADRs include penicillins, NSAIDs, phenytoin, gold, chlorpromazine and cytotoxic agents.

Identification of the causative agent of a dermatological reaction can be difficult, as rechallenge is not appropriate, with the possible exception of fixed drug eruptions. When making a diagnosis, it is important to consider the information included in summaries of product characteristics (SPCs), previous case reports, the pattern of eruption, together with consideration of a temporal relationship between drug administration and ADR development. A temporal relationship may be apparent in some cases but in others a reaction may take anything from hours to years to develop. Any serious skin reaction should be reported to the CHM/MHRA on a Yellow Card, particularly angioedema, bullous eruption, epidermal necrolysis and generalised exfoliation. In addition, any dermatological reactions suspected to result from new drugs should be reported.

Some important dermatological skin reactions are summarised in Table 6.3.

Table 6.3 A summary of adverse drug reactions involving the skin

Dermatological disorder	Important examples of causative drugs	Comments
Urticaria	Penicillins, NSAIDs, ACE inhibitors	Itchy, weal-and-flare rash. Should respond to oral antihistamines
Erythematous eruptions	Penicillins, NSAIDs	Reddening, may resemble measles as a maculopapular rash
Stevens–Johnson syndrome	Co-trimoxazole, phenytoin, lamotrigine, carbamazepine	May be preceded by a flu-like illness. Large fluid-filled mucosal blisters. May develop into toxic epidermal necrolysis In the case of carbamazepine there is a genetic association with an increased risk of Stevens–Johnson syndrome and this is associated with the HLA-B*1502 allele. Patients of Thai or Han Chinese origin should be screened for this
Toxic epidermal necrolysis	Co-trimoxazole, carbamazepine, phenytoin	Rare but may be fatal with blistering and skin peeling off
Psoriasis	β blockers, chloroquine, lithium	These drugs may exacerbate the condition
Photosensitivity	Thiazides, isotretinoin, amiodarone	Patients should avoid direct sunlight or wear sunblock

ACE, angiotensin-converting enzyme; NSAID, non-steroidal anti-inflammatory drug.

Patient counselling

- Educate patients to avoid direct sunlight and sunbeds, wear protective clothing and use high-protection factor sunscreen during and for a few months after receiving photosensitising drugs.
- Patients should be aware of previous allergic reactions to drugs and encouraged to report them to health professionals. The distinction between traditional side effects and allergy should be made to avoid confusion.

Musculoskeletal ADRs

Drugs may adversely affect muscles, bone and connective tissues in a number of ways, from fluid retention in muscle producing mild aches and pains, to debilitating osteoporosis or life-threatening rhabdomyolysis. It is important to be aware of drugs causing musculoskeletal pathology because early recognition and cessation of the drug can prevent unnecessary suffering and uncertainty, while improving the outcome for patients.

Rhabdomyolysis

This is the breakdown of skeletal muscle leading to the release of myoglobin, which has the potential to block renal tubules and result in renal failure. Rhabdomyolysis may follow myopathy and so it is important that patients reporting muscle pain associated with drug therapy are investigated. Important examples of drugs causing myopathy include fibrates and statins. The co-prescribing of these drugs increases the risk of myopathy.

Patient counselling

- Patients taking statins and/or fibrates should report muscle weakness, pain or tenderness.
- To prevent drug-induced osteoporosis, patients prescribed long-term steroid courses should be advised to stop smoking, limit alcohol consumption, take regular weight-bearing exercise, and ensure an adequate calcium and vitamin D intake.
- Patients should stop taking quinolone antibiotics at the first sign of tendon damage such as pain or inflammation. The affected limb should be rested until tendon symptoms have resolved.

- Young patients prescribed minocycline for more than 6 months should report symptoms such as arthralgia, fever, rash and pleuritic pain, which may indicate systemic lupus erythematosus (SLE).

Monitoring for ADRs

- ECG monitoring should be considered for patients taking tricyclic antidepressants and other drugs that prolong the Q–T interval, and particularly in the presence of additional risk factors such as coronary heart disease. Consider also regular monitoring of potassium levels and the avoidance, if possible, of drugs known to cause hypokalaemia, such as high-dose β_2-adrenoceptor agonists or diuretics (see Chapter 2).
- Patients prescribed treatment long term should be monitored regularly for adverse effects, e.g. patients taking minocycline for longer than 6 months should be monitored for hepatotoxicity, pigmentation and SLE.
- Consider drugs for which regular blood tests are recommended. Common tests include LFTs, full blood counts, renal function or thyroid function tests (see Chapter 2). Monitoring of renal and hepatic function is particularly important for elderly patients taking prescribed drugs.

Reporting of suspected ADRs

Doctors, dentists, coroners, pharmacists, nurses and patients may submit Yellow Cards to the CHM/MHRA for all suspected ADRs produced by new (black triangle) drugs and serious ADRs for all other drugs.

The lessons from rofecoxib

Rofecoxib is a selective cyclo-oxygenase-2 (COX-2) inhibitor that was introduced in the late 1990s to selectively inhibit this 'pathological' isoform of the enzyme associated with inflammation, and leave the 'physiological' isoform responsible for gastroprotection unaffected, so reducing the incidence of peptic ulceration. Indeed it was hailed as a 'wonder drug'. However, in 2000 the VIGOR trial indicated that rofecoxib was associated with increased cardiovascular events compared with the naproxen control (Bombardier *et al.* 2000). One interpretation at the time was that naproxen was, in comparison, actually protective and that rofecoxib was safe. This resulted in further studies which indicated that rofecoxib increased cardiovascular risk by 1.5- to

3.6-fold and that between 1999 and 2004 this may have led to 88 000–140 000 excess cases of severe coronary artery disease in the USA (Graham *et al.* 2005). Consequently rofecoxib was immediately withdrawn from the market. Although this adverse safety profile appeared confined to rofecoxib, patients should be assessed for cardiovascular risk when using COX-2 inhibitors such as celecoxib. Further work has also indicated a small but significant increase in cardiovascular risk for NSAIDs when used long term and at high doses (low-dose and occasional use being regarded as safe) (Kearney *et al.* 2006). The risk is greatest for diclofenac with naproxen being regarded as safe.

The clear lesson learnt from the rofecoxib story is to exercise caution in all areas of drug safety, especially with new drugs, even if their introduction to the market appears to be a landmark in therapeutics. The second lesson is that careful analysis can reveal safety issues with well-established drugs, hence the need to use NSAIDs with appropriate caution.

Practice points

- Health professionals should always consider the adverse effects of drugs, including OTC and herbal supplements when making a diagnosis. Early identification of ADRs may improve the outcome for the patient and prevent unnecessary treatment and intervention.
- Always check the medication history when presented with a rash. Consider drugs stopped recently.
- Take care to identify drug allergies because reintroduction may be more severe. Drug allergies should be recorded prominently on all patient medication records.
- Prescribe a drug only when there is a good indication.
- NSAID-induced gastric damage is a major ADR. To reduce the risk:

    - only one NSAID should be prescribed at any one time
    - a less toxic agent such as ibuprofen should be used first line
    - the lowest effective dose is recommended
    - the maximum daily dose should not be exceeded
    - patients at risk should be prescribed prophylaxis (see Chapter 8)
    - long term, repeat prescriptions should be reviewed
    - patients should be counselled to report warning symptoms (see above).

- Ideally, NSAIDs should be avoided in patients with coronary heart disease and particularly congestive heart failure and hypertension, due to an increase in fluid retention and potential for increased cardiovascular risk. If essential, the lowest effective dose should be prescribed and drugs with a long elimination half-life avoided.
- The greatest bone loss induced by corticosteroid therapy occurs during the first 6–12 months. Early preventive steps are therefore important. Patients taking prednisolone 7.5 mg or more daily for 3 months or more, particularly if aged over 65 years, should be assessed for prophylaxis with hormone replacement therapy, bisphosphonate or calcitriol as appropriate (see Chapter 31).
- Always use the lowest effective dose of all drugs.
- Withdraw drugs associated with withdrawal symptoms gradually.
- Increased monitoring and education of patients to improve the recognition and reporting of suspected ADRs are important issues for preventing ADRs (Avery *et al.* 2002).

Drug interactions

Drug interactions may simply be thought of as the actions of one drug being enhanced or inhibited by the presence or actions of another drug or exogenous substance. These may be adverse or beneficial. In addition to recognising the potential for prescribed medicines to interact, one must always bear in mind the potential for OTC medicines, foods and the constituents of herbal remedies to interact with them.

Although the number of established interactions is extremely large, their importance varies from trivial to potentially life threatening. On the face of it, it is difficult to predict straightforwardly the importance of an interaction but this comes with clinical experience. How does one deal with interactions? Clearly there are a small number of life-threatening combinations that should be avoided. Other interactions require vigilance and careful monitoring, e.g. measuring the international normalised ratio (INR) with warfarin when co-prescribed with an interacting drug and responding with appropriate dosage alterations. In other cases, an interaction may be extremely rare but established in the literature, and in such cases vigilance is important because being over-cautious might result in a patient not receiving a drug when the likelihood of an interaction is very small. As with all drug usage, it is the balance between the beneficial and the adverse effects.

In practice, drug interactions are continually being identified by automated systems and databases and it is often difficult to differentiate between clinically significant and trivial interactions. The *British National Formulary* is also a valuable resource for interactions but does not necessarily indicate the likelihood of an interaction or how to deal with it. The reader is referred to *Stockley's Drug Interactions* (Baxter 2013) for evidence-based information presented in a user-friendly reference with a concise summary of reported drug interactions. In the following chapters an attempt is made to highlight common, serious and clinically significant drug interactions relevant to each section.

Mechanisms of drug interactions

When considering drug interactions the following, in particular, may alert the practitioner to potential problems, which may predispose towards an interaction:

- drugs with a narrow therapeutic window: anticoagulants, anticonvulsants, digoxin, lithium, theophylline and cytotoxic agents
- metabolic enzyme inducers and inhibitors

- drugs with similar pharmacological effects
- extremes of age.

As with ADRs, the mechanisms of interactions are often pharmacological or pharmacokinetic. In one sense the pharmacological interactions are the easiest ones to predict and respond to, e.g. one would expect the actions of a β_2-adrenoceptor agonist for asthma to be opposed by the concurrent use of a β blocker. This is one reason why β blockers are avoided in asthma. Other examples of pharmacological interactions are given in Table 6.4.

Pharmacokinetic interactions

These follow the established pattern of ADME.

Absorption

Absorption reactions may result in a change in either the rate of drug absorption or the total amount of drug absorbed. The following are some key mechanisms.

Acid suppression

Drug absorption occurs best with the uncharged form, which is determined by the individual pK_a for a drug. Accordingly, changes in pH (e.g. rises in the presence of antacids and acid suppressors) may influence the absorption of other drugs. The importance of other interactions resulting from changes in gastric pH is uncertain due to the involvement of additional mechanisms affecting absorption. It is therefore advisable to separate in time the administration of drugs such as antacids, H_2-receptor antagonists and PPIs from other drugs (see Chapter 8).

Binding of drugs

The chemical binding of co-prescribed drugs or drugs with metals in the diet may prevent the drug from being absorbed. A classic example of this is the chelation of tetracyclines with metallic cations, e.g. calcium in dairy products or iron in iron replacement therapy. The simple solution to preventing an interaction is to separate the doses of tetracycline from iron administration or dairy products consumption by 2–3 hours. Another example is colestyramine, which binds to and reduces the absorption of digoxin (see Chapters 11 and 16) and once again concurrent drugs should be taken 1 hour before or 4–6 hours after colestyramine.

Table 6.4 Examples of pharmacodynamic interactions

Interacting drugs	Consequences	Explanation
β-adrenoceptor agonists and β blockers	Antagonism	These agents will oppose each other
Adrenaline (epinephrine) and β blockers	Antagonism	• Adrenaline used in anaphylaxis treatment will be opposed by β blockers • Risk of hypertensive crisis (especially with non-selective β blockers) as the vasoconstrictor activity of adrenaline via α-adrenoceptors will no longer be opposed by $β_2$-adrenoceptor-mediated vasodilatation
β blockers and verapamil	Addition of actions	The combined negative inotropic and chronotropic effects may lead to asystole
Nitrates and sildenafil, tadalafil or vardenafil	Potentiation, leading to severe hypotension	Nitrates act via cGMP, the metabolism of which is prevented by the phosphodiesterase inhibitors. These drugs should be avoided in combination
Antihypertensives	Potentiation, leading to a severe hypotension or used clinically for more effective blood pressure control	Summation of actions (Chapter 12)
Antihypertensives and oral sympathomimetic decongestants	Opposing actions	Avoid sympathomimetics in hypertension, particularly if poorly controlled
SSRIs and $5HT_1$-receptor agonists	Serotonin syndrome (Chapter 25)	SSRIs will prevent the breakdown of endogenous 5HT, leading to over-stimulation of serotonergic system
Betahistine and antihistamines	Antagonism	Betahistine is a histaminergic agent with actions opposed by antihistamines
Warfarin and vitamin K	Antagonism	Warfarin is a vitamin K antagonist
Hypoglycaemic drugs and corticosteroids	Antagonism	Corticosteroids have a diabetogenic effect
Alcohol and sedative agents (including sedative antihistamines)	Potentiation	Potentiation
Potassium-sparing diuretics, ACE inhibitors and potassium	Potentiation, leading to hyperkalaemia	All cause potassium retention
Levodopa activity and some antipsychotic and antiemetic drugs	Antagonism	Some antipsychotic drugs may induce Parkinsonism
Drugs that cause Q–T interval prolongation (e.g. amiodarone, sotalol), macrolide antibacterial agents, azole antifungal agents, tricyclic antidepressants (amitriptyline and imipramine), antipsychotic agents (including chlorpromazine, haloperidol)	Potentiation	Risk of torsade de pointes, arrhythmia and potentially fatal ventricular fibrillation
Drugs with antimuscarinic side effects (e.g. tricyclic antidepressants; certain older antihistamines, e.g. promethazine, see above)	Enhanced antimuscarinic side effects	Side effects include blurred vision, urinary retention, dry mouth and possibly cardiac effects

5HT, 5-hydroxytryptamine or serotonin; ACE, angiotensin-converting enzyme; cGMP, guanosine cyclic 3′:5′-monophosphate; SSRI, selective serotonin reuptake inhibitor.

Altered gastric motility

Gastric emptying determines the rate of movement of drugs into the small intestines, the site at which many drugs are absorbed. Accordingly changes in gastric emptying may influence the rate of drug absorption, e.g. metoclopramide accelerates gastric emptying and is used to enhance the rate of onset of action of paracetamol in some compound antimigraine preparations.

Altered bacterial flora

Broad-spectrum antibiotics often alter the balance of gut bacteria and this may also lead to indirect drug interactions, e.g. the use of erythromycin may inhibit the production of vitamin K by gut bacteria and, if the patient is taking the vitamin K antagonist warfarin, this can enhance the actions of warfarin leading to toxicity.

Distribution

Protein-binding interactions

This type of interaction typically involves two drugs competing for plasma protein or tissue binding. The resulting interaction may lead to displacement from binding sites and increased plasma concentrations. However, the rise in plasma concentration is often offset by enhanced elimination. Accordingly, the clinical significance of this type of interaction tends to be limited. An example of this is the interaction occurring between valproate and phenytoin, where phenytoin may be displaced from plasma protein binding by the former.

Metabolism

Although drug metabolism occurs at a range of sites, hepatic metabolism, and particularly that involving cytochrome P450-dependent mechanisms, represents the most common site of interaction. Alterations in drug metabolism can occur via the induction or inhibition of cytochrome P450-dependent enzymes. As this family comprises a range of isoenzymes, there is added complexity because some forms will be affected by specific inhibitors or inducers and others will not. Accordingly it is difficult to predict which drugs will interact in this way. Having said that, as indicated below, certain drugs are established as either enzyme inhibitors or inducers and should ring alarm bells for potential interactions.

Enzyme inhibition

Some drugs inhibit cytochrome P450 enzymes, resulting in reduced metabolism of other drugs. These are dose dependent and interactions generally develop relatively rapidly with an increase in plasma concentrations (Figure 6.2) and pharmacological effects of the affected drug. Important examples of drugs that may inhibit the various isoenzymes include:

- cimetidine
- ciprofloxacin
- erythromycin
- clarithromycin
- metronidazole
- fluoxetine
- ketoconazole
- fluconazole
- itraconazole
- grapefruit juice
- verapamil
- omeprazole.

Enzyme induction

This forms an extremely common mechanism for drug interactions and leads to increased metabolism of the affected drug, reducing plasma concentrations (Figure 6.2) and therapeutic effects. The result may be failure of treatment and an important example of this occurs with oral contraceptives when used with inducing agents such as rifampicin or carbamazepine. An increased dose may be required due to the increased metabolism of a co-prescribed drug.

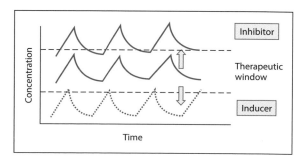

Figure 6.2 Plasma concentration–time for a theoretical drug with a narrow therapeutic window. Enzyme inhibitors may increase the plasma concentrations leading to toxic levels and inducers may reduce concentrations to subtherapeutic levels.

In addition, autoinduction occurs, whereby a drug enhances its own metabolism, so that the doses need to be built up. Important examples of this include barbiturates and carbamazepine. Enzyme induction involves an increase in the amount of microsomal enzymes and cytochrome P450 levels in liver cells. Such interactions take from days to 2–3 weeks to develop and also to reverse when a drug is stopped. Good monitoring is essential, particularly as any change in dose may need to be corrected on cessation of the enzyme inducer to prevent overdose.

Agents associated with induction include:

- barbiturates
- rifampicin
- omeprazole
- phenytoin
- ethanol
- carbamazepine
- St John's wort
- tobacco and cannabis smoke (polycyclic hydrocarbons).

Metabolic conversion

Some drug interactions also occur at the level of drug activation from a prodrug to the active metabolite. A key example of this is the interaction between the antiplatelet drug clopidogrel and omeprazole. Clopidogrel requires conversion to its active metabolite via cytochrome P450-dependent monooxygenases and this conversion is thought to be prevented by the omeprazole and esomeprazole. This is a clinically important interaction and could potentially lead to failure of therapy, with thrombus formation, and so the guidance is to avoid co-prescription and, when a proton pump is required, to use pantoprazole or an H_2 receptor antagonist such as ranitidine (but not cimetidine), which are thought not to interact with clopidogrel.

Renal excretion

The weak acid and weak base transporters in the proximal convoluted tubules may be the site of drug interactions, where there is competition for excretion. One very important example of this occurs between methothrexate and certain NSAIDs, and this may result in methotrexate toxicity as its excretion is reduced. Hence, patients taking methotrexate should not take NSAIDs, even as OTC medicines, without the advice of their doctor.

Excretion of drugs via the weak acid and weak base transporters is also pH dependent, such that alkaline urine enhances the excretion of weak acids and vice versa. This is generally of minor significance but can lead to differences in excretion rate between individuals and was previously employed to enhance drug elimination in overdose when alkaline diuresis was used to enhance the elimination of salicylates.

Conclusions

The management of ADRs and drug interactions remains central to the prevention of drug-related problems. Key issues include the implementation of updated computer warning systems to support health professionals in interpreting the ever-increasing number of potential drug interactions, together with the avoidance of polypharmacy, particularly in elderly patients.

Summary of some key interactions

As indicated above there are numerous drug interactions of varying importance and some key drug interactions include:

- warfarin and NSAIDs: leading to enhanced bleeding
- warfarin and antibiotics (especially erythromycin and ciprofloxacin): leading to enhanced bleeding
- NSAIDs and methotrexate: leading to methotrexate toxicity
- ACE inhibitors and potassium/potassium-sparing diuretics: risk of hyperkalaemia
- verapamil and β blockers: risk of asystole
- digoxin and amiodarone: risk of digoxin toxicity
- digoxin and verapamil: risk of digoxin toxicity
- oral contraceptives and certain inducing agents (e.g. rifampicin, carbamazaepine and phenytoin): risk of failure of contraception
- statins and macrolides: risk of toxicity and myopathy, should be avoided.

Practice points

- The key point is clearly vigilance to any changes in a patient's condition that may point to an ADR or interaction.
- Become familiar with clinically significant interactions.
- Warfarin, lithium, theophylline and digoxin therapy should always alert practitioners to be vigilant for ADRs or interactions.
- The change to a patient's therapy that involves a drug known to influence metabolism should prompt a review of all concurrent drugs, whether prescribed, OTC or herbal remedies.
- Consider the pharmacology of drugs when prescribing to allow for the prediction of pharmacodynamic reactions. Avoid using drugs with similar pharmacology.
- It is good practice to be familiar with common interactions as current computer systems have been found to be lacking in the management of drug interactions.
- Patients should always be questioned about their use of OTC and herbal medicines.

CASE STUDIES

Case 1

A man returning from 6 months in India reports a scaly rash on his knees and elbows.

What is the most likely cause of this rash?

- Possibly drug-induced psoriasis if the patient took chloroquine for malaria prophylaxis.

Case 2

A man prescribed a prolonged course (more than 14 days) of co-amoxiclav for a persistent chest infection reports vomiting, general malaise and pruritus.

What is the likely cause of his symptoms?

- Clavulanic acid-induced cholestatic hepatitis should be suspected.

Case 3

A woman requests that her GP give her a prescription for antibiotics to treat cystitis. On further questioning the symptoms include polyuria, loin pain and bloodstained urine. There is no pain on urination and no clouding or offensive smell. The only medication that the woman takes are painkillers that she buys from the supermarket for headaches.

- These symptoms may point to analgesic nephropathy because cystitis normally presents with a burning pain on urination and/or clouding and an offensive smell. Cystitis is more common, but, in view of the symptoms, together with the chronic use of painkillers, further investigation is required. Antibiotics may not be appropriate.

(continued)

(continued)

Case 4

A middle-aged man requests aspirin tablets to treat pain.

What further questions should be asked?

- Has he taken it before?
- This real but hard-to-believe case turned out to be a request for analgesia to treat stomach pain. On further questioning about the nature of the pain, the patient reported a past history of peptic ulcer disease, which he thought had returned.

Case 5

A 65-year-old woman presents with a chesty cough of 2–3 weeks' duration. She takes ibuprofen and methotrexate.

- This case includes a possible interaction between ibuprofen and methotrexate, leading to reduced clearance of methotrexate with an increased risk of methotrexate toxicity. The combination of methotrexate and ibuprofen is, however, often used without problems but patients should be closely monitored. Signs of infection may indicate a methotrexate-induced blood dyscrasia. In this example, a full blood count is required. The cough may also suggest pulmonary toxicity with methotrexate.

Case 6

A 41-year-old woman has been taking imipramine since the birth of her baby, now 2 years old. She has been troubled with a persistent sore throat and has white spots on the back of her tongue and is feeling tired and run-down.

- On checking the SPC for imipramine, you are alerted to the possibility of agranulocytosis and order a full blood count to be carried out. This is a sensible precaution.

Case 7

A 44-year-old woman prescribed nifedipine for Raynaud's phenomenon reports palpitations. She has been drinking grapefruit juice recently.

- This case illustrates a possible interaction between nifedipine and grapefruit juice. The mechanism is thought to involve inhibition of cytochrome P450 isoenzymes by components of grapefruit juice and therefore increased levels of nifedipine.

Case 8

A man has been taking timolol tablets long term for the treatment of hypertension. A colleague prescribed an adrenaline injection for emergency treatment of peanut allergy over the last few years. The patient has administered a single dose in the last year without apparent problems.

- In this case, the blockade of β-adrenoceptors will render the adrenaline less effective but could lead to unopposed α-adrenoceptor vasoconstriction. A number of antihypertensives are available, and the timolol should be gradually withdrawn.

Case 9

A 22-year-old woman requests some medicine for a dry cough. The counter assistant asks the pharmacist if it is appropriate to sell a product containing dextromethorphan to this woman. Her records indicate that she is taking paroxetine.

- This is a rare but potentially serious drug interaction, due to the risk of the patient developing a serotonin-like syndrome (see Chapter 25). Symptoms include tremor, confusion, tachycardia, hypertension and abnormal movements. It would therefore not be appropriate to recommend this product with paroxetine.

References

Avery AJ, Sheikh A, Hurwitz B *et al.* (2002). Safer medicines management in primary care. *Br J Gen Pract* 52: suppl S17–S22. pmid: 12389765.

Baxter K, ed. (2013). *Stockley's Drug Interactions,* 10th edn. London: Pharmaceutical Press.

Bombardier C, Laine C, Reicin A *et al.* (2000). Comparison of upper gastrointestinal toxicity of rofecoxib and naproxen in patients with rheumatoid arthritis. VIGOR Study Group. *N Engl J Med* 343: 1520–1528. pmid: 11087881.

British National Formulary, latest edition. London: British Medical Association and Royal Pharmaceutical Society of Great Britain.

Fergusson D, Doucette S, Glass KC *et al.* (2005). Association between suicide attempts and selective serotonin reuptake inhibitors: systematic review of randomised controlled trials. *BMJ* 330: 396–399. pmid: 15718539.

Graham DJ, Campen D, Hui R *et al.* (2005). Risk of acute myocardial infarction and sudden cardiac death in patients treated with cyclo-oxygenase 2 selective and non-selective non-steroidal anti-inflammatory drugs: nested case-control study. *Lancet* 365: 475–481. pmid: 15705456.

Haddad PM, Anderson IM (2002). Antipsychotic-related QTc prolongation, torsade de pointes and sudden death. *Drugs* 62: 1649–1671. pmid: 12109926.

Harker LA, Boissel JP, Pilgrim AJ *et al.* (1999). Comparative safety and tolerability of clopidogrel and aspirin. Results from CAPRIE. *Drug Safety* 21: 325–335.

Kearney PM, Baigent C, Godwin J *et al.* (2006). Do selective cyclo-oxygenase-2 inhibitors and traditional non-steroidal anti-inflammatory drugs increase the risk of atherothrombosis? Meta-analysis of randomised trials. *BMJ* 332: 1302–1308. pmid: 16740558.

Lee A, ed. (2006). *Adverse Drug Reactions,* 2nd edn. London: Pharmaceutical Press.

Nissen SE, Wolski K (2007). Effect of rosiglitazone on the risk of myocardial infarction and death from cardiovascular causes. *N Engl J Med* 356: 2457–2471. pmid: 17517853.

Piromhamed M, James S, Meakin S *et al.* (2004). Adverse drug reactions as cause of admission to hospital: prospective analysis of 18 820 patients. *BMJ* 329: 15–19. pmid: 15231615.

Further reading

Bhatia P, O'Reilly JF, Li-Kam-Wa E (2001). Adverse reactions and the respiratory system. *Primary Care Respir J* 10: 39–43.

Dean T (2000). Withdrawing drugs not the solution. *Prescriber* 11: 11.

Merlo J, Liedholm H, Lindblad U *et al.* (2001). Prescriptions with potential drug interactions dispensed at Swedish pharmacies in January 1999: cross sectional study. *BMJ* 323: 427–428. pmid: 11520839.

Sipilä J, Klaukka T, Martikainen J *et al.* (1995). Occurrence of potentially harmful drug combinations among Finnish primary care patients. *Int Pharm J* 9: 104–107.

Stockley IH (2000). Interaction warnings. *Prescriber* 11: 120.

7

Clinical pharmacokinetics

Pharmacokinetics is the study of how the body handles a drug from absorption, distribution and metabolism to excretion (ADME). The interaction of these processes determines both the plasma concentration and how long a drug persists in the blood. Clinical pharmacokinetics is the application of this area of pharmacology and is used to construct dosage regimens and, in the context of therapeutics, it takes account of the variations between individual patients.

Basic pharmacokinetic principles

Absorption and bioavailability

Drugs are administered by various routes, including orally, intravenously, intramuscularly, subcutaneously, by inhalation and rectally. Clearly, the oral route is the most convenient and preferred by patients but it can be less predictable compared with the intravenous route, because absorption can be affected by the presence of food in the stomach, acidic pH, gastric emptying and 'first-pass' metabolism. This last complication is due to absorbed drugs passing straight to the liver where they may be extensively metabolised and their entrance to the systemic circulation is limited. Common examples of drugs undergoing first-pass metabolism include morphine, propranolol and glyceryl trinitrate (GTN); indeed GTN is given as a sublingual spray to overcome this problem. Interestingly, in the case of statins, first-pass metabolism is an advantage

because it limits the actions of statins to the liver (see Chapter 13).

The above processes limit the amount of drug administered reaching the systemic circulation. To account for this, the bioavailability of the drug is considered. This is the fraction of drug administered that reaches the systemic circulation, i.e. the fraction absorbed. Bioavailability (F) is calculated from the ratio of the area under the curve (AUC) of the oral dose to the AUC of an intravenous dose:

$$F = \frac{\text{AUC oral}}{\text{AUC i.v.}}$$

For example, the F for digoxin tablets is 0.70 (i.e. 70% is absorbed) and so if 250 micrograms are given

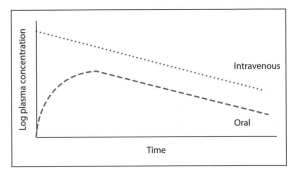

Figure 7.1 A comparison of the log plasma concentration–time plot for a drug via the intravenous and the oral routes. The oral route shows a rising phase as the drug is absorbed. As the drug has a bioavailability <1, the area under the curve (AUC) under the oral plot is proportionally less than under the intravenous plot.

orally then 70% of the dose ($0.70 \times 250 = 175$ micrograms) enters the circulation. This can then be applied to determine the amount of a drug required. So:

$$\text{Dose given} = \frac{\text{Amount needed}}{F}$$

Salt factor

In addition to bioavailability, some medicines are made up of active drug and inert salts. The best example is aminophylline, which is the salt of theophylline, so 80% of the amount of aminophylline is theophylline. This fraction is termed the 'salt factor' or S. So:

$$\text{Amount} = S \times \text{Dose}$$

Amount of drug administered

To take account of F and S the following is applied:

$$\text{Amount} = \text{Dose} \times F \times S$$

Volume of distribution

The volume of distribution (V_d) of a drug is the apparent volume in which a drug is dissolved in the body to give the plasma concentration measured:

$$V_d = \frac{\text{Amount in body}}{\text{Concentration}} = \frac{\text{Dose}}{\begin{array}{c}\text{Concentration}\\\text{at } t = 0\end{array}}$$

where t is time.

The volume of distribution and (therefore) plasma concentration are determined by where the drug goes in the bodily fluids. A widely distributed drug (e.g. one that moves into fat or other tissues) or one that has extensive protein binding has a high V_d and one that is largely retained in the plasma or has low binding has a low value. A commonly encountered drug with a high V_d is digoxin and this reflects wide tissue distribution. In the case of digoxin, a population average V_d is 7.3 L/kg body mass, so for a 70-kg person this would equate to a V_d of 511 L. This value clearly greatly exceeds body volume and is due to the plasma concentration being lower as a result of wide sequestration in the tissues. The V_d is not merely of scientific interest because it is applied clinically in determining loading doses (see later).

Elimination

Elimination is the removal of the active drug from the body and is largely made up of hepatic metabolism and renal excretion. Generally speaking, it is the sum of these two components, the contributions of which vary greatly. Indeed, knowledge of the routes of elimination is essential for drug choice in renal and hepatic impairment, e.g. digoxin is cleared predominantly (about two-thirds) by the renal route and so doses of digoxin are determined in relation to renal function. The dihydropyridine drug amlodipine is cleared via the hepatic route and is therefore a suitable antihypertensive for patients with renal disease because its elimination is not impaired.

Clearance

Clearance (CL) is a measure of the rate of elimination and is largely made up of renal and hepatic clearance. It is defined as the volume of plasma cleared of a drug in unit time and usually expressed in litres per hour or day. The clearance of drug determines the amount of drug required in a maintenance regimen (see later).

Kinetics of elimination

Most drugs illustrate first-order kinetics and the plasma concentration undergoes an exponential decay (analogous to radioactive decay), so there is a logarithmic relationship between plasma concentration and time (Figure 7.2).

Owing to first-order kinetics, the rate of elimination is proportional to the concentration of drug:

$$C_t = C_0 e^{-kt}$$

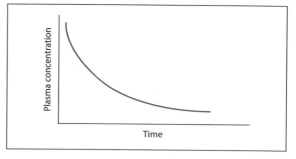

Figure 7.2 The plasma concentration–time plot for a drug illustrating exponential decay owing to first-order kinetics.

where C_t is the concentration at time t, C_0 the concentration at $t = 0$ and k the rate constant (per minute or hour).

This equation is applied to predict plasma concentrations when the concentration at time 0 is known; it may also be used to estimate the time to reach a safe concentration from a toxic level, e.g. if the plasma concentration of a drug such as digoxin is too high, it enables the time for withholding doses to be calculated to reach safe levels.

Rate constant

First-order kinetics involves a rate constant (k) and this is simply the fraction of drug eliminated per unit time: when k is 0.1/day, 10% is eliminated per day. This can be applied mathematically as the clearance per unit time is the fraction of V_d that is cleared per unit time. So:

$$k = \frac{CL}{V_d}$$

or

$$CL = k \times V_d$$

Half-life

This is simply the time for the plasma concentration to decrease by 50%. Therefore at the half-life ($t_{1/2}$):

$$C_t = 0.5\, C_0$$

So:

$$0.5\, C_0 = C_0 e^{-kt}$$
$$\ln 0.5 = -kt$$
$$-0.693 = -kt$$
$$\text{So } t_{1/2} = \frac{0.693}{k}$$

Regimens

Pharmacokinetics is applied in the construction of dosing regimens, the purpose of which is to maintain the plasma concentration within the therapeutic window, which is the desired range between toxicity and sub-therapeutic levels. The aim is also to limit the differences between peaks and troughs (Figure 7.3).

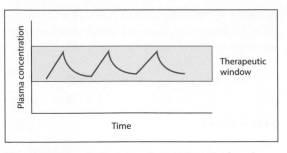

Figure 7.3 The plasma-concentration–time plot for a drug regimen to illustrate the usual approach of maintaining the peaks and troughs within the therapeutic window, to maintain clinical effectiveness and prevent toxicity.

To achieve a steady state within the therapeutic window, regimens are generally based on:

- once daily
- twice daily
- three times daily, often based around 'breakfast, lunch and dinner'
- four times daily.

A once-daily interval is favoured as the most convenient and is likely to achieve the best compliance. However, the above applies to a stable regimen, and at the start of therapy it will take time to achieve steady-state concentration (C_{ss}). A general rule is that it takes five half-lives to reach steady state (Figure 7.4).

The explanation to this rule of thumb is provided in Table 7.1, in which the amount present after each half-life is added cumulatively until the amount approaches 100%.

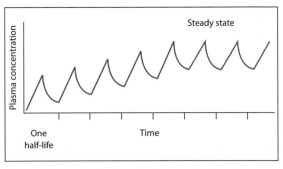

Figure 7.4 The plasma-concentration–time plot for a drug at the start of an oral regimen, when it takes approximately five half-lives to reach steady-state concentration.

Table 7.1 Demonstration that steady state is reached after approximately five half-lives		
Dose	**Amount present in the body after one $t_{1/2}$ from dose (%)**	**Percentage of C_{ss}**
First	50	50
Second	50 + 25	75
Third	50 + 37.5	87.5
Fourth	50 + 43.8	93.8
Fifth	50 + 46.9	96.9

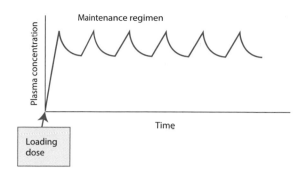

Figure 7.5 The plasma-concentration–time plot for a drug following a loading dose to raise the plasma concentration to therapeutic levels, before the maintenance regimen.

Loading doses

This rule is clinically significant because drugs with a short half-life will soon reach C_{ss}. However, for drugs with long half-lives the time to attain C_{ss} will be prolonged, e.g. digoxin has a half-life of 40 hours and will therefore take 200 hours or over 8 days to reach C_{ss}. Digoxin is widely used to control ventricular rate in atrial fibrillation and the therapeutic effect is required urgently. Therefore, to overcome the delay, drugs with long half-lives or drugs that require immediate action (e.g. lidocaine in ventricular ectopic beats) are often given as a loading dose to take the plasma concentrations quickly up to a desired level (Figure 7.5).

To calculate a loading dose, the amount required is determined by the desired (safe) plasma concentration multiplied by the volume of distribution:

$$\text{Amount required} = \text{target concentration} \times V_d.$$

The dose required must then take account of F and S as follows:

$$\text{Loading dose} = \frac{\text{Amount required}}{F \times S}$$

Maintenance doses

Many therapies involve a maintenance dose to maintain the C_{ss} within the therapeutic window. The maintenance dose equals the amount of drug eliminated per dosage interval and maintains the steady state. Therefore the rate of input equals the rate of output.

To consider maintenance dosing, the pharmacokinetics are analogous to a continuous infusion, which involves an increase in plasma concentration followed by a plateau at the steady state where input equals output (Figure 7.6).

So the maintenance dose equals the amount removed. Therefore, we have the relationship:

$$\text{Infusion rate} = \text{CL} \times C_{ss}$$

This can then be applied to the oral dosing and the 'infusion' rate equates to the dose per dosage interval (tau or τ). Therefore for an oral regimen there is the important equation:

$$\text{Dose} = \frac{[\text{CL} \times C_{ss} \times \tau]}{F}$$

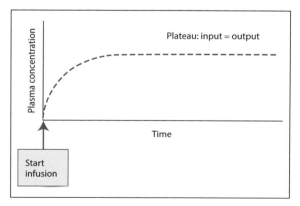

Figure 7.6 The plasma-concentration–time plot for a drug administered by intravenous infusion. At plateau the rate of input equals the rate of output and the steady-state plasma concentration is achieved.

For drugs that display first-order kinetics, the relationship between dose and plasma concentration is clearly linear, so doubling the dose will double the concentration, whereas halving the dose will halve the concentration.

Peak and trough concentrations

The steady-state plasma concentration is the time-averaged concentration, i.e. the mean plasma concentration. For drugs with a wide therapeutic window C_{ss} is appropriate but, for drugs with a narrow therapeutic window, it is important to consider the maximum (C_{max}) or peak and minimum (C_{min}) or trough concentrations (Figure 7.7). In many instances C_{max} and C_{min} should be maintained within the therapeutic window, usually by altering the dose or the dosage interval.

The following equations are used to determine peak and trough plasma concentrations (Winter 2004):

$$\text{Peak } C_{ss} = \frac{F \times \text{Dose}}{V_d(1 - e^{-kt})}$$

$$\text{Trough } C_{ss} = \frac{F \times \text{Dose}}{V_d(1 - e^{-kt})} \times e^{-kt}$$

Dosage interval (tau)

As indicated above, the dosage interval determines the peaks and troughs. For drugs with a long half-life the dosage interval is 24 hours and the dose required equals the amount eliminated in 24 hours. However, for drugs with a relatively short half-life and a narrow therapeutic window, the dosage interval may be determined from the half-life in relation to the magnitude of the therapeutic window, e.g. for theophylline, the C_{max} is 20 mg/L and the C_{min} is 10 mg/L, so the width of the therapeutic window is 10 mg/L and it would take one half-life for the plasma concentration to drop from C_{max} to C_{min}. Therefore, the dosage interval chosen is less than one half-life and this will ensure that the plasma concentration remains within the safe area (Figure 7.8).

An exception to this approach is the aminoglycosides, such as gentamicin, where, although the peak plasma concentration is within the therapeutic window, the trough concentration is chosen to be subtherapeutic to avoid toxicity, e.g. the trough concentration for gentamicin is <2 mg/L and the peak

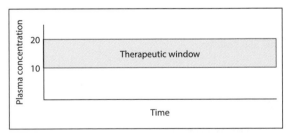

Figure 7.8 A plasma-concentration–time plot to illustrate the therapeutic window in relation to dosage intervals. In the case of theophylline, the maximum concentration is 20 mg/L and the minimum 10 mg/L. The time to drop from 20 mg/L to 10 mg/L is logically one half-life. Therefore, to maintain a plasma concentration within the therapeutic window, the dosage interval should be less than one half-life.

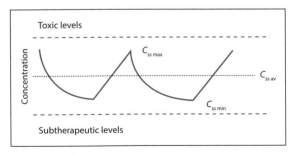

Figure 7.7 Time-averaged steady-state concentration in relation to peak and trough concentrations.

is in the range 5–10 mg/L. Once again the dosage interval is determined by the half-life, e.g. if the peak plasma concentration after an intravenous dose were 8 mg/L then the time to decrease to 2 mg/L would be two half-lives, so the dosage interval would be chosen to be over two half-lives (Figure 7.9).

Real life clinical pharmacokinetics

In spite of the precise science surrounding pharmacokinetic models, patients do not always conform to mathematical equations and this is a result of individual variations that may alter pharmacokinetics, including:

- renal function
- hepatic function
- drug metabolism (including genetics)
- disease
- drug interactions.

Population variables

To take account of individual variation, in terms of renal function and weight there are empirical population-based equations that enable one to calculate a reasonable estimate of volume of distribution and clearance for a drug. The population-based equations are specific to a drug and are useful for recommending a regimen for a patient, the V_d (Example 2) helping to determine the loading dose and CL (Example 3) the maintenance dose.

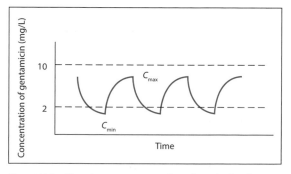

Figure 7.9 The plasma-concentration–time plot for the aminoglycoside gentamicin, where the peak (C_{max}) is usually between 5 and 10 mg/L for clinical effects, but the trough (C_{min}) is subtherapeutic to prevent adverse effects. If the peak is 8 mg/L, a dosage interval of two times the half-life will mean that the trough is 2 mg/L or less.

Applications of population-based equations

Population-based equations are used to predict pharmacokinetics and may be used to recommend dosages, e.g. given the patient below (Example 2), we now know that his V_d is 415 L. Therefore to determine his loading dose, we can carry out the following:

$$\text{Loading dose} = \frac{C_{ss} \times 415}{F}$$

$$\text{So loading dose} = \frac{1.5 \times 415}{0.7}$$

Loading dose = 889 micrograms and using available tablets one might recommend the loading dose as 7 × 125 microgram tablets and a 62.5 microgram tablet = 937.5 micrograms.

EXAMPLE 2

The V_d for digoxin is given by the equation (Winter 2004):

$$V_d\,(\text{L}) = (3.8)\,(\text{weight in kg}) + (3.1)\,(\,CL_{cr}\text{ in mL/minute}\,)$$

As digoxin is largely eliminated by the renal route, an estimate of renal function, i.e. creatinine clearance (CL_{cr}) is used to estimate CL. This is obtained from the Cockcroft–Gault equation:

$$CL_{cr} = \frac{[1.23\,(140 - \text{Age})\times \text{weight}]}{[\text{Serum creatinine}]}$$

In females, 1.04 replaces 1.23.

So for a 70-year-old man, who weighs 70 kg and has a plasma creatinine = $125\,\mu\text{mol}/\text{L}$, his V_d for digoxin is given by:

$$V_d\,(\text{L}) = (3.8)\,(\text{weight in kg}) + (3.1)\,(\,CL_{cr}\text{ in mL/minutes}\,)$$

(Note that, although the CL_{cr} is given in mL/minute, the calculated V_d is in litres).

(continued)

(continued)

$$V_d (L) = (3.8 \times 70) + 3.1(CL_{cr})$$

$$CL_{cr} = \frac{[1.23(140 - 70) \times 70]}{125}$$
$$= 48.2 \text{ mL/min}$$

Therefore $V_d = 266 + 3.1(48.2) = 415$ L

EXAMPLE 3

For digoxin the clearance (CL) is given by the equation (Winter 2004):

$$CL (\text{mL/minute}) = (0.8 \text{ mL/kg per minute})$$
$$(\text{weight in kg}) + CL_{cr}(\text{mL/minute})$$

So for a 70-year-old man, who weighs 70 kg and has a plasma creatinine 125 µmol/L his CL for digoxin is given by:

$$CL_{dig} = (0.8) \times (70) + CL_{cr}$$

$$CL_{dig} = 56 + \frac{[1.23(140 - 70) \times 70]}{125}$$

$$CL_{dig} = 104.2 \text{ mL/minute} = 6.25 \text{ L/hour}$$

Population-based equations may also take account of disease states and drug interactions, e.g. in chronic heart failure the clearance for digoxin is reduced and the population-derived equation is:

$$CL (\text{L/hour}) = (0.33 \times \text{weight in kg}) +$$
$$0.9\,CL_{cr} (\text{mL/minute})$$

In hyperthyroidism the CL for digoxin is increased 1.3 fold, and in hypothyroidism it is reduced 0.7 fold (Winter 2004).

EXAMPLE 4

The patient in Examples 2 and 3 was receiving 312.5 micrograms digoxin/day and his plasma digoxin concentration was found to be 2.5 micrograms/L. In practice the digoxin

would be stopped until therapeutic levels (<2 micrograms/L) returned but the data allow for a dosage alteration. Given:

$$\text{Dose rate} = C_{ss} \times CL$$

$$\text{Then } 312.5 \times F = C_{ss} \times CL \text{ (per day)}$$

$$312.5 \times 0.7 = 2.5 \times CL$$

$$\text{Therefore } CL = \frac{218.8}{2.5} = 87.5 \text{ L/day}$$

Therefore the new daily dose to attain a C_{ss} of 1.5 should be:

$$\text{Daily dose} \times F = C_{ss} \times CL$$

$$\text{Daily dose} = \frac{[1.5 \times 87.5]}{0.7}$$
$$= 187.5 \text{ micrograms/day}$$

and so he could be given a new regimen of 125 micrograms plus 62.5 micrograms tablets, which equals 187.5 micrograms/day.

Similarly, using the CL one can calculate the maintenance dose given:

$$\text{Dose rate} = C_{ss} \times CL$$

From Example 3, dose rate = 1.5 × 6.25 (L/hour) = 9.375 micrograms/hour. As digoxin is given daily the patient requires 24 × 9.375 micrograms/day = 225 micrograms/day. To take account of F the oral dose must be 225/0.7 = 321 micrograms, and to account for available tablets he should receive 250 mg and 62.5 micrograms tablets, as a dose of 312.5 micrograms/day.

Revising a regimen

Once a patient has been prescribed a regimen based on population data, he or she may actually handle the drug in a different manner and this will result in a different plasma concentration from predicted. The difference is due to the clearance being at a different rate. If clearance is greater than predicted then C_{ss} will be lower, and if it is less than predicted then the C_{ss} will be higher. An actual measurement of the C_{ss}

for this patient can be used to determine the revised dosage. If the C_{ss} is measured then, as we know the dose rate (Example 4, above), we can calculate the patient's actual clearance. This actual (as opposed to population-based) value enables the new maintenance dose to be determined.

Zero-order kinetics

Most drugs show first-order kinetics with the rate of elimination being proportional to the concentration of the drug. However, for some drugs, notably the antiepileptic drug phenytoin and ethanol, the enzymes responsible for their elimination become saturated, so the rate of elimination is no longer proportional to the drug's concentration. This means that these drugs exhibit zero-order kinetics with the rate of elimination not being proportional to the drug concentration, so small changes in their dosage lead to disproportionate increases in plasma concentrations. Controlling the dose of phenytoin is therefore difficult to achieve. The pharmacokinetics of phenytoin are described by Michaelis–Menten enzyme kinetics (Figure 7.10), where V_{max} relates to the maximum rate of elimination and K_m is analogous to the affinity of the metabolizing enzymes for phenytoin.

The consequence of the zero-order kinetics is a dose–plasma concentration profile that varies between individuals due to variability in V_{max} (Figure 7.11).

In constructing regimens for phenytoin the loading dose is calculated in the usual way by $(C_{ss} \times V_d)$, because this is independent of metabolism. However,

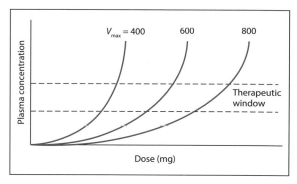

Figure 7.11 Plasma-concentration–time plots for three different patients (with different V_{max} values) demonstrating the variation between individuals. The zero-order kinetics means that increases in dosage cause a disproportionate rise in plasma concentration.

the maintenance dose is calculated from a modified form of the Michaelis–Menten equation:

$$\frac{[S \times F \times \text{Dose}]}{t} = \frac{t[V_{max} \times C_{ss}]}{K_m + C_{ss}}$$

where V_{max} and K_m are obtained from population averages. When adjusting regimens (i.e. once the plasma concentration is known in relation to the dosage), one can calculate the patient's individual V_{max}, assuming that this is more variable and the population K_m is fixed.

Therapeutic drug monitoring (Appendix 2)

The major clinical application of pharmacokinetics is in therapeutic drug monitoring (TDM), which involves taking a blood sample and measuring the concentration of a specific drug. This enables a dosage regimen to be altered in relation to a patient's individual clearance and also detects toxic dosing, subtherapeutic dosing and non-compliance. The sample is taken at a specific time point post-dose (to allow the drug to distribute) or immediately pre-dose. Therapeutic drug monitoring is generally used for drugs with a narrow therapeutic window such as:

- theophylline
- lithium
- phenytoin

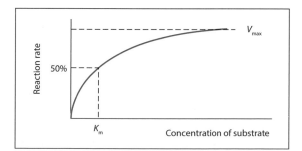

Figure 7.10 The Michaelis–Menten enzyme kinetics plot of reaction rate against concentration of substrate, where V_{max} relates to the maximum rate of elimination and K_m is analogous to the affinity of the metabolizing enzymes.

- gentamicin
- ciclosporin.

In the case of drugs that show first-order kinetics the dose may be adjusted:

$$\text{New dose} = \frac{\text{Target } C_{ss}}{\text{Measured } C_{ss}} \times \text{Current dose}$$

Practice points

- When determining oral doses, one should take account of the salt factor and bioavailability.
- Population-based equations are used to estimate V_d and CL.

- V_d is used to calculate loading doses.
- Clearance is used to calculate maintenance doses.
- A patient's actual data can be used to determine actual parameters.
- Regimens are generally based on 6-, 8-, 12- and 24-hourly dosing.
- The $t_{1/2}$ determines the dose interval.

References

Winter ME, ed. (2004). *Basic Clinical Pharmacokinetics*, 4th edn. Philadelphia: Lippincott, Williams & Wilkins.

Gastrointestinal diseases

Dyspepsia and peptic ulcer disease

Dyspepsia describes upper gastrointestinal symptoms, including heartburn, acidity, nausea, discomfort and wind, and may be referred to as 'indigestion' by the patient.

Disease characteristics

The major problem is one of acidity, in the form of increased acid secretion, reflux of corrosive gastric contents or gastric damage. Clinically, upper gastrointestinal problems encompass simple to serious diseases:

- Gastro-oesophageal reflux disease (GORD) is reflux of the gastric contents into the oesophagus, which leads to erosion (reflux oesophagitis). Contact oesophagitis also occurs and is induced by contact with certain drugs (Chapter 6).
- Gastritis: inflammation of the stomach.
- Peptic ulceration: gastric and duodenal.
- Drug-induced peptic damage (largely non-steroidal anti-inflammatory drugs [NSAIDs] and oral steroids).
- Zollinger–Ellison syndrome: a rare gastrin-secreting tumour of D-cells and G-cells of the pancreas.

A patient presenting with symptoms of dyspepsia ('indigestion'), which may include upper abdominal or epigastric pain, requires differential diagnosis from cardiac problems (see Chapter 1). In the context of primary care, there may be alerting clinical features that may suggest more serious underlying pathology, such as carcinoma, which must be excluded and these include:

- age (patients aged >45 years of age with new or changed symptoms or aged >55 years)
- weight loss
- anaemia
- dysphagia (difficulty in swallowing)
- haematemesis (vomiting blood)
- melaena (tarry stools)
- upper abdominal masses
- persistent symptoms with repeat requests for over-the-counter (OTC) remedies
- onset of new or changed symptoms.

Gastro-oesophageal reflux disease (Figure 8.1)

As the name implies, this is due to the reflux of gastric contents into the oesophagus, causing erosion, which leads to pain, experienced as 'heartburn', although sometimes there may be back or shoulder pain. There may occasionally be wheezing and a cough or an exacerbation of asthma. This condition must be distinguished from oesophageal carcinoma,

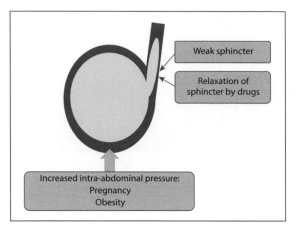

Figure 8.1 Gastro-oesophageal reflux disease and its causes.

although dysphagia is also a leading feature of the latter. GORD may be caused or exacerbated by an increase in abdominal pressure (due to overeating, obesity or pregnancy) or incompetence of the gastro-oesophageal sphincter as a result of a hiatus hernia or drugs (e.g. nitrates, antimuscarinic agents, theophylline, opioids and calcium-channel blockers). Reflux oesophagitis may lead to Barrett's oesophagus, a premalignant condition.

Contact oesophagitis

This is caused by local damage resulting from drugs (see Chapter 6).

Peptic ulceration

Peptic ulceration includes both gastric and duodenal ulceration and is characterised by erosion of the inner lining, which may perforate as a serious complication or erode a major blood vessel, causing haematemesis (vomiting of blood). The leading clinical features of peptic ulceration include:

- epigastric pain, which may be precisely located by the patient by pointing
- hunger pain, which is relieved by eating
- night pain, which is relieved by food, milk or antacids
- waterbrash, which is the appearance of saliva in the mouth
- nausea and, less frequently, vomiting.

It may also present as anaemia (see Chapter 18) due to chronic blood loss or as melaena (tarry stools) due to bleeding.

It is now well established that infection with the Gram-negative bacterium *Helicobacter pylori* is the cause of up to 95% of cases in duodenal ulceration and 70–80% of gastric ulceration. The infection leads to chronic inflammation and gastric damage, leading to ulceration. There is no evidence that emotional stress or eating spicy foods leads to peptic ulceration. Indeed in 2005 the Nobel Prize for medicine was awarded to two Australian doctors (R Marshall and B Warren) who made the controversial proposal in the 1980s that ulceration was associated with this bacterium.

The other leading cause of ulceration is the use of NSAIDs and, to a much lesser extent, oral steroids, generally with concomitant NSAID therapy. The explanation for the ulcerogenic effect of NSAIDs is that prostanoids synthesised in the stomach are cytoprotective by inhibiting acid release and stimulating the production and release of protective mucus and bicarbonate (Figure 8.2 and Table 8.1). These cytoprotective prostanoids are produced by the constitutive cyclo-oxygenase 1 (COX-1), which is inhibited by NSAIDs, so NSAIDs alter the balance in favour of increased acid activity, predisposing towards gastric damage. This important adverse drug reaction led to the development of selective COX-2 inhibitors ('coxibs': celecoxib; etodolac and meloxicam), which inhibit COX-2, associated with inflammation, but leave COX-1 largely unaffected. However, these agents still appear to cause some gastric damage and their early promise was not fully realised.

Goals of treatment

Depending on the conditions, the general goals are symptomatic relief or cure. Symptomatic relief may involve lifestyle changes, avoidance of causative drugs, suppression of acid release or activity, and mucosal protection. Cure may involve suppression of acid release to allow natural healing and, if appropriate, eradication of *H. pylori* infection. This latter goal is also aimed at reducing the possibility of developing gastric carcinomas, because *H. pylori* is regarded as a carcinogen.

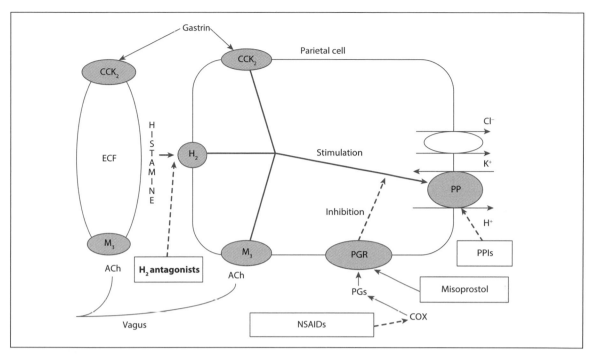

Figure 8.2 Parietal cell and the regulation of acid release. ACh, acetylcholine; CCK, cholecystokinin; ECF, enterochromaffin-like cell; M, muscarinic receptor; H_2, histamine H_2-receptor; PGs, prostanoids; PGR, prostanoid receptor; CCK, cholecystokinin receptor on which gastrin acts; PP, proton pump.

Table 8.1 Regulation of gastric acid production	
Increase acid release	**Reduce acid release**
Histamine via H_2-receptors	Prostaglandins E_2 and I_2 (which are also cytoprotective via mucus and bicarbonate release). Their production is inhibited by NSAIDs
Gastrin via CCK receptors	
Acetylcholine via M_3-receptors and histamine release	

NSAIDs, non-steroidal anti-inflammatory drugs; CCK, cholecystokinin

Pharmacological basis of management

Control of acid secretion

In order to understand the mechanisms of drug action, the control of acid secretion must be considered. Figure 8.2 and Table 8.1 show that the release of protons via the proton pump is regulated physiologically.

Antacids

As the name implies, antacids are anti-acid. A variety of preparations are available that raise pH:

Sodium bicarbonate: $HCO_3^- + H^+ \rightarrow CO_2 + H_2O$

with the 'belching' of CO_2, which makes it less suitable in patients who have flatulence.

Magnesium hydroxide ($Mg(OH)_2$) and aluminium hydroxide ($Al(OH)_3$) are also used:

$$Al(OH)_3 + 3HCl \rightarrow AlCl_3 + 3H_2O$$

$$Mg(OH)_2 + 2HCl \rightarrow MgCl_2 + 2H_2O.$$

To complicate matters, aluminium compounds are constipating and magnesium salts are laxative, and so they are often used in combination to negate these effects. The use of calcium salts (including ingestion of milk) may in fact stimulate gastrin release and so increase acid secretion, leading to an exacerbation of ulceration.

Antacids provide rapid relief of dyspepsia, removing the symptoms, but they do not lead to a cure. Liquid preparations have a faster onset of action.

Alginates

These are mucopolysaccharides and may be combined with antacids (e.g. Gaviscon, Peptac preparations). The alginic acid, when combined with saliva, forms a viscous foam that floats on the gastric contents, forming a raft that protects the oesophagus during reflux.

H_2-receptor antagonists, e.g. famotidine, ranitidine

These are competitive antagonists at the histamine H_2-receptor and inhibit histamine-induced gastric acid secretion (see Figure 8.2). Accordingly, they provide symptomatic relief and in the long term promote ulcer healing, but, if *H. pylori* infection has not been eliminated, then relapse on discontinuation is common. They are most active against basal, as opposed to stimulus-evoked, acid release and are most effective when given at night. Ranitidine and famotidine have fewer interactions than the older agent cimetidine. Low doses are available over-the-counter for short-term relief of dyspepsia (<2 weeks) and higher doses are prescription-only medicines (POMs).

Proton pump inhibitors, e.g. lansoprazole, omeprazole (esomeprazole as its S-isomer), pantoprazole, rabeprazole

These newer drugs are widely used and act via irreversible inhibition of the proton pump (H^+/K^+ ATPase) and hence suppress proton secretion (see Figure 8.2). This leads to a greater than 90% inhibition of acid secretion which is long lasting

(24 hours). The pK_a value of proton pump inhibitors (PPIs) is such that they are converted to active drugs at acid pH, which means that their actions are largely confined to the gastric mucosa, leading to selectivity. However, to achieve this, they must be formulated in gastro-resistant capsules or granules to avoid being degraded as the drug enters the stomach and the pH-dependent formulation means they are released into the duodenum. Following absorption in the duodenum they then act systemically and are activated in the region of the parietal cells. The safety and efficacy of PPIs is so well established that omeprazole and pantoprazole are now available over-the-counter for a maximum of 4 weeks usage. Esomeprazole is the active enantiomer of omeprazole but there is no convincing evidence that it is superior to omeprazole. In 2015 it became available in the UK on a general sales licence.

Prostaglandin analogues, e.g. misoprostol

This is a stable prostaglandin analogue E_1, which inhibits the release of acid (see Figure 8.2) and is also cytoprotective by stimulating the release of mucus and bicarbonate.

Bismuth chelate

These agents are rarely used but bismuth chelate is thought to kill *H. pylori*, coat the ulcer, absorb pepsin, increase prostaglandin production and increase bicarbonate secretion, thereby bringing about ulcer healing.

Prokinetic drugs, e.g. metoclopramide

These agents facilitate the movement of gastric contents from the stomach to the duodenum. Metoclopramide acts locally to increase gastric motility and promote emptying and will provide symptomatic relief of 'bloating'. Prokinetics drugs are now rarely used and the use of metoclopramide is now restricted due to neurological side effects.

Choice of drugs (Figure 8.3)

This is related to the disease and goals of treatment, because occasional heartburn may be effectively relieved by simple antacids or low-dose H_2-receptor antagonists, with the antacids having immediate

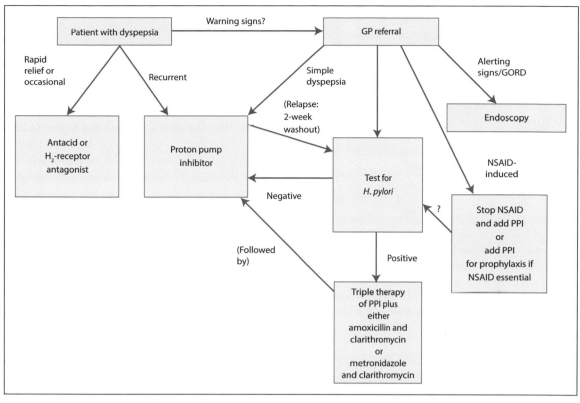

Figure 8.3 Principles of dyspepsia management. The summary indicates the role of OTC medicines and the need for general practitioner (GP) referral with appropriate investigations. The diagram takes account of National Institute for Health and Care Excellence (2014) guidance but full guidance should be consulted for details of patient management. GORD, gastro-oesophageal reflux disease; NSAID, non-steroidal anti-inflammatory drug; PPI, proton pump inhibitor.

effects. In more serious disease, the first issue is to establish the nature of the complaint because the diagnosis will determine the most appropriate treatment. In the meantime symptomatic relief with antacids, alginates, H_2-receptor antagonists or PPIs is appropriate, depending on the severity. Diagnosis may involve the ^{13}C-urea breath test, serological tests for antibodies to *H. pylori* (these may give false-positive results because they indicate past and not necessarily current infection) or stool antigen testing for *H. pylori* infection, and possibly gastroscopy and barium contrast radiology. PPIs should be withheld for 2 weeks prior to the breath test or antigen testing as they may interfere with detection.

The urea breath test involves administering a tablet containing isotope ^{13}C-labelled urea, because *H. pylori* possesses urease activity, which leads to the production of labelled $^{13}CO_2$ in the presence of infection. The $^{13}CO_2$ readily and rapidly passes across the stomach wall and is absorbed into the bloodstream and appears in the breath, where it may be detected by mass spectroscopy, indicating infection (Figure 8.4).

Gastro-oesophageal reflux disease

The initial approach is lifestyle changes such as reducing overeating, weight reduction if appropriate, reducing the intake of fatty foods and chocolate (which may lubricate the gastro-oesophageal sphincter), smoking cessation, reducing alcohol intake and avoiding tight clothes. If lifestyle changes are inadequate, antacids and then antacids plus alginates will provide rapid relief but limited healing. H_2-receptor antagonists may be used to provide relief in mild-to-moderate disease but are much less effective than PPIs. If symptoms persist, then PPIs are the most effective agents; they remove symptoms and allow healing. They may initially be used for 4–8 weeks, after which a lower

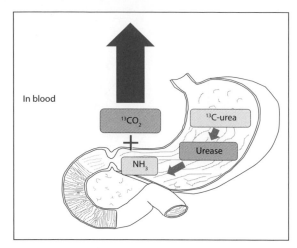

Figure 8.4 The ^{13}C-urea breath test, in which ^{13}C-labelled urea is given as a drink and the presence of urease from *Helicobacter pylori* leads to its metabolism to ^{13}CO$_2$ and ammonia. The ^{13}CO$_2$ is absorbed into the bloodstream and exhaled, such that its presence in the breath is diagnostic of *H. pylori* infection.

maintenance dose should be tried. Prokinetic drugs may also be used, especially when the symptoms include postprandial bloating, nausea and belching.

Non-H. pylori *dyspepsia*

In the absence of proven *H. pylori* infection, the logical approach to dyspepsia, due to gastritis or ulceration, is a stepped approach, stepping up or down as appropriate:

- Step 1: antacid or alginate and antacid.
- Step 2: H$_2$-receptor antagonist.
- Step 3: PPI.

PPIs are the most effective agents and current National Institute for Health and Care Excellence (NICE) guidelines (2014) indicate that PPIs should be used empirically in uninvestigated dyspepsia.

H. pylori *infection*

In patients who are infected with *H. pylori* eradication is the logical course. This may be achieved by a number of different regimens, which involve antibiotics and anti-secretory agents ('triple therapy'), and these are associated with 90% eradication rates. Typically, triple therapy involves a PPI (or sometimes ranitidine or ranitidine bismuth citrate) plus two antibacterial agents from either clarithromycin and amoxicillin or clarithromycin and metronidazole for 1 week. There is significant resistance to metronidazole: patients who have recently received this for other conditions may be harbouring resistant organisms and so this agent should be avoided. In patients who are allergic to penicillin and who have recently received clarithromycin, then tetracycline may be used with metronidazole. Eradication is confirmed by a urea breath test; serology is inappropriate because antibodies to *H. pylori* may persist in the plasma. After eradication, PPIs may be required for 4–8 weeks after triple therapy to promote further healing, especially if the ulcer was associated with bleeding or NSAID usage.

NSAID-induced ulceration

After *H. pylori* infection, NSAID use is the next most common cause of ulceration. Gastric damage due to NSAIDs is highest in older patients and is more often associated with certain NSAIDs, such as aspirin, naproxen and piroxicam, whereas ibuprofen, etodolac and nabumetone appear to cause fewer gastric side effects. It should be recognised that low-dose aspirin (75 mg) for antiplatelet therapy is also associated with a significant incidence of gastric side effects. For patients with NSAID-induced damage it is quite common for them also to have *H. pylori* infection which may predispose towards damage, so should be investigated.

For NSAID-induced damage, the initial approach is to stop the NSAID if this is possible and switch to paracetamol for pain relief if this is required. Healing may be brought about by using either an H$_2$-receptor antagonist, as a cheap first-choice drug, or a PPI.

If the patient must continue with the NSAID or is initially identified as being at a high risk (>65 years, previous ulcer, concomitant oral steroids, concomitant anticoagulants, selective serotonin reuptake inhibitors [SSRIs] or venlafaxine) then prophylaxis is required, for which omeprazole, lansoprazole and misoprostol are currently licensed. According to Yeomans *et al.* (1998), ranitidine is less effective than omeprazole at preventing and healing NSAID-induced ulceration. Misoprostol carries the compliance problem of being required two to four times daily and often causes diarrhoea, but is available in combination with either naproxen or diclofenac. Misoprostol should not be given to women of childbearing age because it may cause uterine contractions and leads to abortions in pregnancy.

Other considerations

Other considerations concerning drug choice are detailed in Table 8.2.

Significant drug interactions

Cimetidine inhibits cytochrome P450 and therefore the metabolism of other drugs, resulting in important drug interactions. Similarly, omeprazole and lansoprazole also inhibit some isoforms of hepatic cytochrome P450. In addition, by altering gastric pH, many drugs used in dyspepsia may alter the absorption of other drugs and their administration should be separated. Examples of some important interactions of drugs used in dyspepsia and the management of peptic ulceration are detailed in Table 8.3.

Over-the-counter considerations

OTC antacids, low doses of H_2-receptor antagonists and low-dose omeprazole (/esomeprazole) or pantoprazole have important roles in the symptomatic relief of dyspepsia but their use is limited (to 2 weeks with H_2-receptor antagonists and to 4 weeks for PPIs), after which time referral should be made if symptoms persist. Antacids and H_2-receptor antagonists are recommended for occasional symptoms and omeprazole is used for recurrent dyspepsia.

Counselling

In patients with dyspepsia general counselling should be directed at lifestyle advice. Altering the diet to

Table 8.2 Considerations of drug choice for dyspepsia in concurrent conditions	
Condition	**Implications for treatment**
Heart failure	Patients should avoid antacids with a high sodium content, especially if they are also receiving diuretics
Prophylaxis of myocardial infarction and stroke with antiplatelet drugs	Low-dose aspirin is associated with gastric bleeding. Clopidogrel is an antiplatelet drug that is used as an alternative to low-dose aspirin. Although it is used when aspirin is contraindicated, there is evidence that, by inhibiting platelet aggregation, it may also cause gastric bleeding and should not necessarily be regarded as a safe alternative to aspirin in this respect. The activity of clopidogrel is reduced by omeprazole and esomeprazole and these combinations should be avoided. Indeed, low-dose aspirin with a PPI for prophylaxis would be preferred
Women of childbearing age	This is a contraindication for misoprostol, a prostaglandin agonist that may cause uterine contractions and subsequent abortion. If misoprostol must be used then effective contraceptive measures should be taken
Pregnancy	This is associated with an increase in GORD due to increases in intra-abdominal pressure. Alginates are the first-line drugs with efficacy and are safe. If alginates fail, then ranitidine or omeprazole are considered as safe
Breastfeeding	Antacids, ranitidine or nizatidine is preferred. The BNF should be consulted: some of the other agents are not recommended by their manufacturers until their safety has been established
Renal impairment	Patients should avoid antacids with a high sodium content
Liver disease	Most agents require dose reductions; the BNF should be consulted. Ranitidine is often used for gastroprotection
Parkinson's disease	Avoid metoclopramide and domperidone due to extrapyramidal effects (although domperidone is recommended for levodopa-induced nausea). Metoclopramide may antagonise levodopa
Depression	SSRIs may impair blood clotting, leading to excess bleeding. Accordingly, they should be used with care in patients with gastric damage or with drugs that also impair clotting

BNF, *British National Formulary*; GORD, gastro-oesophageal reflux disease; PPI, proton pump inhibitor; SSRIs, selective serotonin reuptake inhibitors.

Table 8.3 Examples of some important interactions of drugs used for upper gastrointestinal disease

Interacting drugs	Consequences	Comments
Cimetidine with warfarin, phenytoin, theophylline, carbamazepine tricyclic antidepressants, diltiazem and nifedipine; antiarrhythmics (including amiodarone, flecainide, lidocaine and quinidine) and erythromycin	Cimetidine has been shown to increase the plasma concentration of a number of different drugs, leading to clinically significant interactions	• Monitoring the effects is appropriate and dose reductions may be required for the drug affected • With carbamazepine there are transient increases in the first few days • Generally speaking, these interactions are confined to cimetidine. Other H_2-receptor antagonists do not interact in this way, and so they should be regarded as safe alternatives
Omeprazole or esomeprazole with clopidogrel (Chapter 6)	Reduced antiplatelet effects of clopidogrel with increased risk of thrombus formation	• Avoid these combinations • Clopidogrel with ranitidine or pantoprazole appear safe
Cimetidine or ranitidine with ketoconazole and itraconazole	Reduced absorption of the imidazoles	• Separate dosing by 2–3 hours • Fluconazole appears unaffected
Antacids with ACE inhibitors, chlorpromazine, ciprofloxacin, digoxin, ketoconazole, itraconazole, H_2-receptor antagonists, iron, rifampicin and tetracyclines	Antacids may reduce the absorption of these drugs	Their administration should be separated by 1–3 hours and in the case of ciprofloxacin by 2–6 hours
Sodium-containing antacids with lithium	Sodium may decrease lithium levels	Magnesium or aluminium salts would be appropriate
Omeprazole with benzodiazepines, ciclosporin, digoxin, phenytoin and warfarin	Evidence points to omeprazole having, on occasion, increased the concentration of these drugs	• Omeprazole may inhibit isoforms of cytochrome P450 • Monitoring is appropriate, especially when starting or finishing treatment
Omeprazole with macrolides	• Clarithromycin increases the plasma concentration of omeprazole, which may be beneficial • Erythromycin may reduce the effects of omeprazole	
Lansoprazole with amoxicillin; clarithromycin with metronidazole	Glossitis, stomatitis and black tongue coloration have been reported	Monitoring is appropriate
Metronidazole with alcohol	Disulfiram-like reaction	Alcohol should be avoided with metronidazole

ACE, angiotensin-converting enzyme.

avoid large meals, fatty foods and hot spicy food, and reducing alcohol consumption and smoking cessation should reduce provoking factors. Patients with GORD may (or may not) benefit from raising the head of the bed. Patients taking NSAIDs and other drugs such as doxycycline, tetracycline and bisphosphonates, which may cause contact oesophagitis, should be advised to take their medicine while standing or sitting with a glass of water; NSAIDs may be best taken after food but the effectiveness of this is debatable.

Patients taking NSAIDs should be instructed to tell their GP and pharmacist that they are taking these agents, even if purchased over-the-counter. Of course they should be avoided if possible in patients with dyspepsia or with a risk of peptic ulceration.

Patients should be advised to report alerting symptoms such as:

- unexplained weight loss
- vomiting blood (with a ground-coffee appearance)
- melaena – black tarry stools that contain blood
- dysphagia (difficulty in swallowing).

Antacids

- These will cause immediate relief but normal doses are unlikely to lead to ulcer healing.
- These are most effective when taken 1 hour after food. If they are taken earlier they may be emptied from the stomach.
- Magnesium salts alone may cause diarrhoea.
- Aluminium salts alone may cause constipation.
- Calcium salts will actually stimulate acid release.
- Their administration should be separated in time from a range of other drugs.

Alginates

These should be taken after food and when retiring to bed.

H_2-receptor antagonists

- When used over-the-counter for occasional dyspepsia, H_2-receptor antagonists should not be used for more than 2 weeks without consulting the GP.
- They should be taken regularly for prevention and not just for symptomatic relief.
- For ulceration, they are most effective when taken at night; a daily dose taken at night is effective at ulcer healing.
- Their actions may be suppressed by food, which stimulates acid secretion.
- Cimetidine may inhibit the metabolism of warfarin, phenytoin and theophylline, and it may increase their plasma concentrations.
- Cimetidine may occasionally cause impotence and gynaecomastia in males due to anti-androgenic actions.

Proton pump inhibitors

- PPIs should be taken regularly for prevention and not just for symptomatic relief.

- PPIs should be swallowed whole (as they are prepared as gastro-resistant capsules).
- Relief may take several days for full effects; in the meantime a simple antacid might be used.
- Low-dose omeprazole, pantoprazole and esomeprazole are available over-the-counter for the relief of recurrent dyspepsia.
- If OTC omeprazole is required for more than 4 weeks the patient should be referred to their GP.
- OTC omeprazole should not be used alongside H_2-receptor antagonists.
- They may cause diarrhoea (sometimes secondary to campylobacter infection).

Misoprostol

- Diarrhoea is a common side effect.
- Misoprostol should not be taken by women of childbearing age who may be pregnant or become pregnant.

Bismuth chelate

- This may blacken stools and tongue.
- Bismuth chelate should be taken on an empty stomach, avoiding milk and antacids because they prevent the drug coating the ulcer.

Triple therapy for H. pylori eradication

- Eradication of the bacteria causing an ulcer is the most effective treatment to prevent a relapse.
- The course should be completed for eradication.
- The course is associated with a high incidence of side effects, including diarrhoea.
- Is the patient allergic to any antibiotics?
- Avoid alcohol with metronidazole, as there is a risk of a disulfiram-type reaction.

Guidance should be given for when to take the drugs, because this may appear complicated in triple therapy.

Self-assessment

For the following questions concerning dyspepsia, choose the most appropriate answer:

1 *A positive* ^{13}*C-urea breath tests indicates which one of the following?*

A Increased production of gastric acid
B Bleeding in the stomach
C NSAID-induced damage
D Inhibition of the proton pump
E Infection with *H. pylori*

2 *Which one of the following is a possible side effect of taking a proton pump inhibitor?*

A Antimuscarinic side effects
B Substantial drug interactions through enzyme induction
C Hypokalaemia
D Risk of food poisoning
E Hyperglycaemia

3 *Which one of the following is an appropriate therapy for* H. pylori *infection?*

A An antacid, a H$_2$-receptor antagonist and a proton pump inhibitor
B A prostaglandin analogue (misoprostol), a H$_2$-receptor antagonist and a proton pump inhibitor
C A penicillin (amoxicillin), a macrolide (clarithromycin) and a proton pump inhibitor
D A penicillin (amoxicillin), a macrolide (clarithromycin) and gentamicin
E A H$_2$-receptor antagonist, a proton pump inhibitor and a penicillin (amoxicillin)

4 *Which one of the following best explains NSAID-induced gastric damage?*

A NSAIDs directly activate the proton pump
B NSAIDs have antimuscarinic properties
C NSAIDs release gastrin

D NSAIDs reduce the production of cytoprotective prostanoids
E NSAIDs are local irritants

5 *The prostanoid analogue, misoprostol, is contraindicated in which group of patients?*

A Patients with asthma
B Patients taking NSAIDs
C Patients with arthritis
D Females of childbearing age
E Females past the menopause

Practice points

- Frequent requests for OTC remedies for dyspepsia should prompt referral.
- Peptic ulceration is largely due to *H. pylori* infection (which should be eradicated).
- NSAID-induced peptic damage is a very important adverse drug reaction. Patients should be asked about their use of OTC NSAIDs, and it should be recognised that low-dose aspirin may cause ulceration.
- Cyclo-oxygenase 2 (COX-2) inhibitors may cause gastric damage and should not be used in active ulceration.
- Drugs that alter gastric pH may alter the absorption of other drugs.
- Omeprazole and esomeprazole are thought to reduce the effectiveness of clopidogrel and should be avoided.
- If PPIs are used, the cheapest agent should be chosen.

CASE STUDIES

Case 1

A 30-year-old man visited his local pharmacy and complained of 'heartburn'. After interviewing the patient, the pharmacist recommended that he should take ranitidine for 2 weeks and that, if his symptoms persisted after this time, he should consult his general practitioner.

What might be the cause of the 'heartburn'?

- Poorly defined symptom.
- 'Heartburn' tends to indicate reflux.

What lifestyle advice might be helpful?

- Avoid known precipitants (e.g. alcohol, chocolate, spicy foods).
- Don't wear belts.
- Eat smaller meals and avoid eating late at night.
- Prop up the head of the bed.

How does ranitidine act?

- Histamine H_2-receptor antagonism and so suppresses acid production.

Why wasn't the patient sent immediately to his GP?

- No alerting symptoms (such as vomiting blood, tarry stools, weight loss, masses, difficulty swallowing).
- Heartburn should resolve with lifestyle advice and ranitidine.
- Refer to GP after 2 weeks, and this may require investigation and/or the use of PPIs.

Case 2

Mrs OA is a 57-year-old woman with a 5-year history of osteoarthritis managed by naproxen. She also receiving simvastatin 40 mg (o.n.) to manage hypercholesterolaemia. However, she has developed sharp, stabbing pains and is feeling generally unwell. On questioning she admitted to melaena, and a subsequent full blood profile is detailed below:

Variable	Result	Normal range
Haemoglobin	8 g/dL	11.5–16 g/dL
Haematocrit	32%	35–47%
Mean corpuscular volume (MCV)	70 fL	76–96 fL
White cell count	7×10^9 cells/L	$4–11 \times 10^9$ cells/L
Platelet count	250×10^9 cells/L	$150–400 \times 10^9$ cells/L
Ferritin	5 micrograms/L	20–300 micrograms/L

In addition a ^{13}C-urea breath test was positive.

Based on the clinical presentation and tests results, what appears to be wrong with the patient?

- Gastrointestinal bleeding secondary to peptic ulceration and, given the use of naproxen, this is probably NSAID-induced ulceration. The patient is also infected with *H. pylori* and this may have promoted the NSAID-induced damage.
- The full blood count also indicates microcytic anaemia (as shown by the reduced mean corpuscular volume) and is associated with iron-deficiency anaemia. This condition is likely due to chronic blood loss as a consequence of the ulcer, leading to depletion of iron stores.

(continued)

(continued)

How should this patient be managed?

- The naproxen should be stopped and replaced with paracetamol 1 g (q.d.s.)
- Triple therapy with:

  - PPI for possibly 1 month afterwards?
  - Clarithromycin should be avoided due to interaction with simvastatin

- $FeSO_4$ 200 mg (t.d.s.) to restore iron balance.

Following the successful treatment of your patient, she asks your advice as to whether Voltarol gel (diclofenac) would help her condition.

What advice should you give?

- Topical NSAIDs can be effective to provide some degree of relief and are generally considered safe in a patient with history of peptic ulceration.

References

British National Formulary, latest edition. London: British Medical Association and Royal Pharmaceutical Society of Great Britain.

Brunton L, Chabneer BA, eds (2011). *Goodman & Gilman's The Pharmacological Basis of Therapeutics,* 12th edn. New York: McGraw-Hill.

National Institute for Health and Care Excellence (2014). *Dyspepsia and gastro-oesophageal reflux disease.*

NICE Clinical Guideline no. 184. London: NICE. Available at: via www.nice.org.uk.

Rang HP, Ritter JM, Flower RJ, Henderson G (2015). *Rang and Dale's Pharmacology,* 8th edn. Elsevier.

Yeomans ND, Tulassay Z, Juhasz L *et al.* (1998). A comparison of omeprazole with ranitidine for ulcers associated with nonsteroidal antiinflammatory drugs. *N Engl J Med* 338: 719–726. pmid: 9494148.

9

Nausea and vomiting

Clinical characteristics

Nausea (the desire to vomit) and vomiting are common occurrences and may reflect simple disease, e.g. after exposure to bacterial toxins, be associated with motion as occurs in travel sickness or reflect more serious underlying pathology. Causes of nausea and vomiting include:

- alcohol (the most common)
- viral and bacterial gastrointestinal infections
- motion sickness
- drugs (such as anticancer drugs, digoxin, erythromycin, levodopa, opioids, selective serotonin reuptake inhibitors [SSRIs], non-steroidal anti-inflammatory drugs [NSAIDs], theophylline, iron salts)
- peptic ulceration
- renal failure with uraemia
- myocardial infarction
- pregnancy
- migraine
- vestibular disorders including Ménière's disease
- head trauma.

Given the range of causative factors, there are several mechanisms of nausea, including local irritation of the stomach involving visceral afferent fibres, the central effects of toxins on the chemoreceptor trigger zone (CTZ), and the conflict between visual and balance information, which is thought to occur in motion sickness. The vomiting pathway is under common, central control, leading to a highly coordinated physiological response, involving respiratory, salivary and gastric control, and resulting in the expulsion of gastric contents. Vomiting is under the control of the vomiting centre, which receives a direct input from visceral afferent nerves and is also regulated by the CTZ. The CTZ is, in turn, sensitive to circulating drugs and toxins, and receives input from the vestibular nuclei, which are linked to the labyrinth of the inner ear. The centres involved in vomiting and their receptors are summarised in Table 9.1.

In the context of gastrointestinal infections, the vomit response may be appropriate for removal of the infective agents, whereas drug-induced nausea may lead to a lack of compliance and failure of treatment. Prolonged vomiting may lead to electrolyte disturbances (including hyponatraemia, hypokalaemia and alkalosis) and dehydration.

Pharmacological basis of management

When vomiting is undesirable, removal of any precipitating factors is the first approach and antiemetic agents may be appropriate. Antiemetic drugs encompass a range of different drug classes, with different sites of action. The site of action determines the circumstances in which an agent is effective.

Table 9.1 Summary of the different stimuli, pathways and receptors in vomiting

Stimuli	Site	Receptors
Toxins, irritation, drugs and mechanical	Visceral afferent nerves in the gastrointestinal tract and pharynx	$5HT_3$ Dopamine D_2
Toxins and drugs	Chemoreceptor trigger zone	$5HT_3$ Dopamine D_2
Motion	Labyrinth and vestibular nuclei	Histamine H_1 Muscarinic
Inputs from visceral afferents, vestibular apparatus, chemoreceptor trigger zone	Vomiting centre	Muscarinic Histamine H_1 $5HT_3$

5HT, 5-hydroxytryptamine (serotonin).

Histamine H_1-receptor antagonists, e.g. cinnarizine, cyclizine, promethazine (a phenothiazine)

These older, sedative antihistamines also have appreciable antimuscarinic activity, which contributes towards their use as antiemetics. This is shown by the fact that the 'old antihistamine', chlorphenamine, which lacks antimuscarinic activity, is not antiemetic. They act on the vestibular nuclei and are effective in motion sickness.

Antimuscarinic agents, e.g. hyoscine (but also including other groups such as antihistamines and prochlorperazine)

Antimuscarinic agents act in both the vomiting centre and the vestibular apparatus, making them highly effective in motion sickness. They will also reduce gastrointestinal motility. However, substantial antimuscarinic side effects limit their usefulness.

Histamine analogues, e.g. betahistine

This is a histamine H_1-receptor partial agonist and H_2-receptor antagonist, which has been suggested to increase blood flow to the inner ear and/or decrease endolymph pressure. It is used in vertigo and Ménière's disease.

Dopamine receptor antagonists, e.g. domperidone, metoclopramide, phenothiazines such as prochlorperazine

These act in the CTZ but some may have unwanted central nervous system (CNS) effects (less so with domperidone), which may include extrapyramidal effects and drug-induced Parkinsonism. The potential for neurological side effects of metoclopramide mean that its use is restricted and limited to the short term. Domperidone is associated with cardiac effects and is used with caution. Metoclopramide may also act at 5-hydroxytryptamine (serotonin) $5HT_3$-receptors when used at high doses. The prokinetic effects of domperidone and metoclopramide may increase gastric emptying, reducing any feelings of fullness and nausea. They are effective against anticancer drug-induced emesis.

5-Hydroxytryptamine receptor antagonists, e.g. ondansetron (also metoclopramide)

These block 5HT, acting at $5HT_3$-receptors in the gut and CNS, and are particularly effective against anticancer drugs, which may cause the release of 5HT in the gastrointestinal tract, and also in postoperative nausea and vomiting.

Steroids, e.g. dexamethasone

The mechanism of antiemetic actions of steroids is unknown.

Neurokinin receptor antagonists, e.g. aprepitant

These are novel agents which block the actions of neuropeptides such as Substance P at the neurokinin NK_1 receptors in the vomiting centre. They are used alongside steroids and $5HT_3$ receptor antagonists in anticancer chemotherapy.

Nabilone

This is a cannabinoid receptor agonist with effects that may be mediated via opioid receptors in the CTZ.

Choice of drugs

The initial approach is to remove, if possible, any stimuli that may provoke nausea and vomiting. In the case of infection or alcohol intoxication vomiting may be considered an appropriate response to eliminate the noxious agents. Not all antiemetics are effective for all conditions, e.g. $5HT_3$- and dopamine receptor antagonists are ineffective in motion sickness. Some logical drug choices are summarised in Table 9.2.

Other considerations

In addition to selecting the most appropriate antiemetic to suit a specific cause other considerations are as follows.

- Asthma and peptic ulceration are relative contraindications to using betahistine, which is a histamine analogue and may worsen these conditions through the stimulation of histamine H_1- and H_2-receptors, respectively.
- Antimuscarinic side effects such as blurred vision, urinary retention and constipation of the antihistamines (and of course the antimuscarinic drugs) may be unacceptable, especially if a patient already has, for example, problems of micturition or constipation. Closed-angle glaucoma is a contraindication to using hyoscine. They should also be avoided if there is a risk of dementia in elderly people.
- Sedation may be a desired or undesired side effect of the antihistamines and hyoscine, which would preclude driving. Of the antihistamines, cinnarizine is the least sedating.
- Extrapyramidal effects may occur with phenothiazines (including prochlorperazine), cinnarizine and metoclopramide. These agents may uncover or worsen existing Parkinson's disease. These effects are far less common with domperidone, which does not extensively penetrate

Table 9.2 Some drug choices in nausea and vomiting

Condition	Drug choice	Comment
Motion sickness	Antimuscarinic agents/antiemetic antihistamines	Hyoscine is the most effective but its use is limited by the antimuscarinic side effects
Vestibular disorders	Prochlorperazine or cinnarizine for acute attacks of vertigo. Betahistine is indicated for prophylaxis of Ménière's disease	Prolonged use of cinnarizine in Ménière's disease may render it less effective
Anticancer drugs	$5HT_3$-receptor antagonists, domperidone, metoclopramide, nabilone and dexamethasone	The effects of $5HT_3$-receptor antagonists are enhanced by high doses of dexamethasone. The benzodiazepine lorazepam is also used; it may induce a degree of amnesia, reducing the anticipatory nausea associated with subsequent treatment
Use of 5HT-related drugs such as triptans and SSRIs	$5HT_3$-receptor antagonists	$5HT_3$-receptor antagonists will oppose the serotonergic effects of triptans and SSRIs that are associated with transient nausea
Migraine	Metoclopramide, domperidone, prochlorperazine and buclizine	The prokinetic effects of metoclopramide may enhance the rate of onset of concomitant analgesics. They should also be taken as early as possible in an attack before gastrointestinal motility is reduced
Radiotherapy	$5HT_3$-receptor antagonists and dopamine receptor antagonists are used	

(continued)

Table 9.2 *(continued)*		
Condition	**Drug choice**	**Comment**
Postoperative nausea and vomiting (due to surgical procedures and the use of opioids)	5HT$_3$-receptor antagonists, phenothiazines and cyclizine	
Myocardial infarction	Cyclizine, prochlorperazine or metoclopramide	Cyclizine should be used only if left ventricular function is satisfactory
Cardiac disorders	Domperidone	Domperidone is associated with Q–T interval prolongation and should be avoided in patients with conduction disorders or cardiac disease
Head trauma	Dexamethasone	
Renal failure with uraemia	Dopamine receptor antagonists	
Peptic ulceration	Treat the ulcer (Chapter 8) with proton pump inhibitors or H$_2$-receptor antagonists	
Pregnancy	Antihistamine or a phenothiazine; promethazine is widely used	Vomiting in pregnancy that is potentially life threatening requires rehydration and may need short-term drug treatment under expert supervision
Levodopa-induced nausea in Parkinson's disease	Domperidone	Domperidone does not extensively penetrate the blood–brain barrier and so will not reduce the effectiveness of levodopa in Parkinson's disease

5HT, 5-hydroxytryptamine (serotonin); SSRIs, selective serotonin reuptake inhibitors.

the blood–brain barrier. The phenothiazines will antagonise and reduce the effects of levodopa in patients being treated for Parkinson's disease.

- Young children represent a particular group at risk from vomiting and may require referral at an early stage to prevent dehydration. Projectile vomiting in the first 2 months of life may be caused by pyloric stenosis and requires investigation. Motion sickness is common in children and the following over-the-counter (OTC) availabilities should be noted:

  - promethazine hydrochloride: 2 years and over
  - hyoscine: 4 years and over
  - cinnarizine: 5 years and over.

- Promethazine hydrochloride (Phenergan) is available as a syrup and has the advantage of convenient administration to a toddler but may be misused for sedation in children.
- Timing and duration of antiemetics for motion sickness: in choosing an antihistamine for motion sickness the timings shown in Table 9.3 may be helpful.

- Severe vomiting may preclude effective oral administration and transdermal, intramuscular or rectal administration may be preferred.
- Patients receiving diuretics and who are vomiting are at particular risk of dehydration and should be advised to seek advice at an early stage, which may include withholding the diuretic, the use of oral rehydration therapy and the prescription of appropriate antiemetic drugs.

Important interactions

The interactions with antiemetics are reasonably logical. As indicated above, the dopamine receptor antagonists, except domperidone, may antagonise levodopa in Parkinson's disease. The antihistamines that are antiemetic are all sedating and so will synergise with other CNS depressants. In addition, their antimuscarinic actions (and those of hyoscine) will be enhanced by other drugs with pronounced muscarinic binding (e.g. tricyclic antidepressants). The combination of betahistine with antihistamines is not appropriate as the former is a histamine analogue.

Table 9.3 Dosage timings for drugs used in motion sickness		
Antiemetic	**Time of dose before travel**	**Dosage interval**
Promethazine hydrochloride	Night before travel and also on the morning of travel if required	6–8 hours as required
Hyoscine	30 minutes	6 hours
Cinnarizine	2 hours	8 hours

Information in this table was derived from Goodyer (2001), Blenkinsopp *et al.* (2014) and the *British National Formulary*.

Counselling

If the patient is taking other drugs for unrelated conditions, attention should be paid to ensure that measures are taken to overcome the problems of a missed or vomited dose.

Travel sickness

- Any medication should be taken before the journey (promethazine may be taken the night before).
- Measures that may help to reduce motion sickness include looking at the horizon and not reading.
- Patients taking anti-motion sickness preparations should be informed of their sedating properties and duration of action. This may be important as a patient may take an antiemetic for a sea crossing or a flight and may wish to drive on arrival at the destination.

Hyoscine

- This may cause drowsiness, dry mouth, blurred vision and constipation.
- The effects of patches may persist for up to 24 hours after removal.
- Avoid alcohol while taking hyoscine.
- Patients should wash their hands after handling patches.

Antihistamines

- Some antihistamines are associated with antimuscarinic side effects.
- Patients taking sedating antihistamines or prochlorperazine should be advised that their ability to drive or operate machinery may be impaired. The sedation will be enhanced by alcohol.

Ondansetron

Zofran melts should be placed on the tongue and allowed to disperse before swallowing.

Nabilone

Patients should be warned of the possible adverse effects such as euphoria, hallucinations and difficulties in concentrating.

Herbal remedies

Ginger is advocated in the prevention of nausea and vomiting in a range of conditions including pregnancy, motion sickness and chemotherapy, but not postoperatively. There is evidence to support its use with effects significantly better than placebo (Ernst and Pittler 2000; Vutyavanich *et al.* 2001).

Over-the-counter considerations

OTC antiemetics play a major role in the management of motion sickness. The pharmacist should be mindful of potential misuse, such as using them for sedation.

Practice points

- Antiemetics should be used only when they are essential.
- Antiemetics have different sites of action. Each class is effective only against certain forms of nausea and vomiting.

References

Blenkinsopp A, Paxton P, Blenkinsopp J (2014). *Symptoms in the Pharmacy: a guide to the management of common illnesses*, 7th edn. Oxford: Wiley Blackwell.

British National Formulary, latest edition. London: British Medical Association and Royal Pharmaceutical Society of Great Britain.

Ernst E, Pittler MH (2000). Efficacy of ginger for nausea and vomiting: a systematic review of randomized clinical trials. *Br J Anaesth* 84: 367–371. pmid: 10793599.

Goodyer L (2001). Health problems associated with air and sea transport. *Pharm J*, 267: 464–469.

Vutyavanich T, Kraisarin T, Ruangsri RA (2001). Ginger for nausea and vomiting in pregnancy: randomized, double-masked, placebo-controlled trial. *Obstet Gynecol* 97: 577–582. pmid: 11275030.

Further reading

Veysey M, McNair A (2001). Drug treatment of nausea and vomiting. *Prescriber*, 12: 41–50.

10

Lower gastrointestinal problems

Diarrhoea

Diarrhoea is characterised by the passing of soft or watery stools at an increased frequency (more than three times a day). It is a common and debilitating condition, and in extreme circumstances can be life threatening, with some 5 million deaths annually worldwide due to dehydration. Prolonged diarrhoea, altered bowel habits or the passing of blood should all warrant referral (see Chapter 1). Diarrhoea may be acute, e.g. due to infection, or chronic, e.g. associated with other gastrointestinal pathologies.

Causes

Acute diarrhoea is often the result of bacterial or viral infections. In this regard, rotaviruses cause damage to small-bowel villi and adhesive enterotoxigenic bacteria (such as cholera, *Escherichia coli, Yersinia enterocolitica)* adhere to the brush border, and increase epithelial adenosine cyclic 3':5'-monophosphate (cAMP) levels, leading to Cl^- and Na^+ secretion, which is followed by water secretion from the lower gastrointestinal tract. Other agents such as *Shigella* species release cytotoxins, causing ulceration of the mucosa. Additional pathogens that may cause diarrhoea include amoebae and *Giardia* spp.

Other causes of diarrhoea include the following:

- Broad-spectrum antibiotics may alter the natural gut flora, leading to superinfection. An important example of this is pseudomembranous colitis, which is a rare but serious complication of treatment with broad-spectrum antibiotics, especially clindamycin. It involves the growth of *Clostridium difficile,* which may lead to colitis, with the possibility of toxic megacolon and perforation of the bowel.
- Proton pump inhibitors (PPIs) may suppress acid secretion sufficiently to cause achlorhydria (an absence of hydrochloric acid), which may allow infection, e.g. by *Campylobacter* spp.
- Orlistat, an antiobesity drug, inhibits pancreatic lipases to prevent the breakdown of fat and this may lead to steatorrhoea (fatty diarrhoea), which may be part of its therapeutic action by ensuring that the patient avoids fatty food.
- Misoprostol activates prostanoid receptors in the intestines, increasing cAMP, which may lead to secretory diarrhoea.

Other drug-induced causes include non-steroidal anti-inflammatory drugs (NSAIDs), magnesium salts, withdrawal in opioid dependence, digoxin toxicity, acarbose, metformin and iron salts.

Chronic diarrhoea may be associated with:

- irritable bowel syndrome (IBS): see later
- ulcerative colitis: see later
- Crohn's disease: see later.

Pharmacological basis of management

The first step in the management of acute diarrhoea, where a simple cause such as an adverse drug reaction can be identified, is to remove the cause and the condition may resolve. The patient should continue normal feeding with simple foods such as boiled rice, and infants should continue with breast or formula milk feeds. The first active measure is oral rehydration therapy (ORT).

Oral rehydration therapy

The major adverse effect of diarrhoea is dehydration with electrolyte disturbances (which may increase the risk of adverse drug reactions with drugs such as diuretics, lithium and digoxin), and rehydration is an important goal. This may be achieved by ORT using an approved and specific mixture of electrolytes and glucose. ORT should be considered for all patients. Soft drinks do not substitute for ORT because they do not have the correct composition. The ORT must be made up to the correct osmolality, because a hyperosmotic mixture may promote further water loss from the gastrointestinal tract. The presence of glucose in ORT is to allow sodium to be co-transported with glucose by a specific transporter on the epithelial cells and this will be followed by water, leading to rehydration.

Antibiotics

Many simple gastrointestinal infections, especially in children, are viral and antibiotics are of no value. If a bacterial causative organism is identified by stool cultures then an appropriate antibiotic can be used. In the case of travellers' diarrhoea (associated with foreign travel and ingestion of contaminated food or water), ciprofloxacin is often effective and is sometimes provided to travellers to take at the start of an attack of diarrhoea. In the case of pseudomembranous colitis, metronidazole and vancomycin are indicated. Giardiasis and amoebic dysentery may be treated with metronidazole, *Salmonella* spp. with ciprofloxacin and cholera with tetracycline.

Antimotility agents

Opioids (codeine and loperamide) and antimuscarinic agents

These agents provide symptomatic relief by reducing the motility of the lower gastrointestinal tract, allowing reabsorption of fluid and reducing the passage of watery stools. The relief allows bowel control and prevents diarrhoea from interfering with daily activities. They should be used in addition to ORT. The use of antimotility agents does not alter the time course of the diarrhoea; indeed, diarrhoea may serve to eliminate the causative organisms from the body. Antimotility agents should not be used in children or in adults with severe inflammatory bowel disease where they may cause obstruction, leading to megacolon.

Opioids reduce tone and peristaltic movements of gastrointestinal muscle by presynaptic inhibition of acetylcholine release from the parasympathetic nerves and this is mediated via μ-opioid receptors. Loperamide is an opioid that is widely used and its efficient enterohepatic cycling means that it is largely retained in the gastrointestinal tract, which limits its systemic action. Furthermore, it does not penetrate the blood–brain barrier, and therefore does not have central opioid effects. Codeine and morphine (in kaolin and morphine mixture) are also available but their use is limited by the potential for central opioid effects. Kaolin may also absorb water and interfere with rehydration or increase the risk of obstruction with opioids.

Atropine is present in co-phenotrope and will reduce peristalsis through inhibition of muscarinic receptors on the gastrointestinal muscle. Its use is limited by the obvious widespread antimuscarinic effects.

Probiotics

Antibiotic-associated diarrhoea is due to alterations in gastrointestinal flora, allowing the outgrowth of pathogenic bacteria. A trial in elderly patients has indicated that a course of preventive treatment with probiotic drinks containing lactobacilli reduces the incidence of antibiotic-associated diarrhoea, including *C. difficile* infections (Hickson *et al.* 2007). A similar trial in young children has also indicated that some but not all probiotic preparations reduce the duration of acute diarrhoea (Canani *et al.* 2007).

Counselling

Patients taking diuretics are at increased risk of dehydration and electrolyte disturbances, and may be advised to consult their general practitioner (GP) or omit doses. In patients with diarrhoea it is worth enquiring about drug use and asking about the use of laxatives.

Oral rehydration therapy

- This should be made up with the correct amount of freshly boiled and cooled water.
- The amount required depends on the number of watery stools passed.
- Once reconstituted, ORT may be stored refrigerated for 24 hours.

Antibiotics

- Many cases of diarrhoea are viral, so antibiotics are unlikely to be effective.
- Patients who are taking antibiotics (especially clindamycin) and then develop diarrhoea that is severe or bloody should consult their GP immediately.

Opioids

These are effective at symptomatic relief but will not shorten the course of the diarrhoea.

Constipation

Once again, this is a condition with a range of causes and is defined as altered bowel habits with reduced frequency (e.g. fewer than three motions per week) and the passing of hardened faeces. In the simplest case, constipation may reflect a diet lacking adequate roughage. Other causes may be: psychological; result from painful defecation associated with haemorrhoids or anal fissure, irritable bowel syndrome (IBS); pregnancy; postoperative (secondary to immobility, dehydration or constipating drugs); associated with ageing; caused by serious bowel pathology such as carcinoma of the bowel; secondary fluid restriction in renal failure (see Chapter 19); or induced by drug treatment. Drugs that may cause constipation include:

- opioids – when used as analgesics, antitussives or antidiarrhoeal agents
- tricyclic antidepressants

- antimuscarinic agents, including phenothiazines and older antihistamines
- aluminium salts, as antacids and also when used as phosphate binders in renal failure
- iron
- diuretics
- calcium-channel blockers
- lithium.

The explanation for the constipating effects of opioids is straightforward: the effects result from the presynaptic inhibition of the parasympathetic nerves responsible for gastrointestinal motility, which underlies their use as antidiarrhoeal agents, as discussed above. The constipating action of antimuscarinic agents, including tricyclic antidepressants, is through postsynaptic inhibition of parasympathetic activity, as mentioned above. Diuretics may cause constipation secondary to dehydration and calcium-channel blockers may cause direct relaxation of the gastrointestinal smooth muscle.

In the absence of an obvious cause, constipation, especially in older patients, should warrant referral resulting from the possibility of carcinoma of the bowel.

Management

The best approach to constipation is a balanced diet with non-starch polysaccharides (NSPs) and fluid or adding bulking agents (e.g. methylcellulose, ispaghula husk) to the diet. Exercise might also help. Otherwise laxatives may be indicated.

Osmotic laxatives: lactulose, macrogols, magnesium salts

Lactulose is a disaccharide of galactose and fructose and enters the colon unchanged, where it is converted by bacteria to lactic and acetic acids, which osmotically raise the fluid volume. This increase in fluid volume leads to larger and softer stools.

Macrogols such as polyethylene glycol as polymers absorb and retain fluid in the gastrointestinal tract and so increase the volume of the stools.

Magnesium salts also have an osmotic effect, resulting in a laxative action; this occurs when magnesium is used as an antacid. Magnesium salts release cholecystokinin, which increases gastrointestinal motility.

Stimulant laxatives: dantron, senna extracts

These provide rapid relief of symptoms. Senna extracts enter the colon and are metabolised to anthracene derivatives which stimulate gastrointestinal activity by irritation. Dantron and sodium picosulphate are also irritants that stimulate lower gastrointestinal activity. Dantron is a carcinogen in animal tests and its use is limited to elderly people and terminally ill patients.

Counselling

- Patients should not expect to pass a motion every day – once every 3 days is within the normal range; it is change in bowel habits that is significant.
- A diet rich in NSPs and with plenty of water is likely to prevent constipation.
- Lactulose will take 2 days to have an effect.
- Stimulant laxatives given orally take approximately 8–12 hours for an effect; when given as suppositories their action is more rapid.

Irritable bowel syndrome

This is a common, long-standing bowel disorder (present for at least 3 days per month in the last 3 months) with pain, discomfort (both of which may be relieved by defecation), and episodes of diarrhoea and/or constipation; diagnosis is based on the Rome III criteria (see Spiller *et al.* 2007). The cause of IBS is poorly understood but may have a psychological basis and be associated with depression and stress. It is not thought to be associated with altered gastrointestinal motility but there may be a change in sensitivity of visceral nerves; there is also the concept of a 'brain–gut' interaction. Detailed guidance on IBS and its management has been produced by the British Society of Gastroenterology (Spiller *et al.* 2007) and also the National Institute for Care and Health Excellence (NICE 2015).

Pharmacological management

For constipating symptoms

Currently IBS is managed by adding NSPs (such as ispaghula) to the diet when constipation is a leading feature. In this respect, bran fibre is avoided because its fermentation may exacerbate any distension. Laxatives (e.g. macrogols) are used to overcome constipation but NICE (2015) does not advocate lactulose as a suitable agent.

For bloating and pain

Antispasmodic agents such as antimuscarinic agents and mebeverine are used for the relief of the pain and distension as required. Mebeverine is the most widely used agent and is appropriate for disease with pain and bloating. It causes direct relaxation of gastrointestinal smooth muscle and this is thought to be due to phosphodiesterase inhibition. Dicycloverine is an antimuscarinic agent and inhibits parasympathetic activity, so reducing smooth-muscle tone in the lower gastrointestinal tract. Peppermint oil is also widely used and its effectiveness compared with placebo has been established (Ford *et al.* 2008).

Tricyclic antidepressants, such as amitriptyline, are used at low doses and may be effective through their constipating antimuscarinic effects and analgesic effects. They may potentially improve depression (although as the dose is low this may be unlikely) and alter visceral nerve activity. The British Society of Gastroenterology guidelines point to tricyclic antidepressants as being the most effective drugs in the management of IBS. In addition, selective serotonin reuptake inhibitors (SSRIs) are of proven benefit for improving quality of life in patients with IBS. If pharmacological treatment fails, then NICE (2015) suggest that cognitive-behavioural therapy may be of value.

For diarrhoeal symptoms

Any diarrhoea may be managed by loperamide as required.

Counselling

- Patients should be reminded of the importance of a healthy diet (but limiting fruit to three portions per day) combined with exercise (see Chapter 3).
- Ensure adequate fluid intake.
- Oats may be beneficial in patients with bloating.
- Probiotics may be considered for a trial period.
- Exclusion of agents that exacerbate the condition may help. Avoidance of excessive caffeine and lactose in milk may help.

- Mebeverine should be taken 20 minutes before meals.
- If a tricyclic antidepressant is used, it should be pointed out that it is being used for its benefits in IBS as opposed to antidepressant actions (which require higher doses).

Ispaghula

- Ispaghula husk (Fybogel) should be taken with water and not at bedtime.
- Maintain adequate fluid intake.
- Flatulence and abdominal bloating may be worse on starting the treatment. The dose may be reduced to once daily for a few days if necessary.

Inflammatory bowel disease

This condition encompasses both ulcerative colitis and Crohn's disease, distinct inflammatory conditions that represent a high degree of morbidity and run relapsing–remitting courses. In both cases the causes are unclear and possibilities include genetics, microbial and environmental aetiologies, perhaps with an altered or inappropriate immune response to antigens in the gastrointestinal tract.

Clinical features of ulcerative colitis and Crohn's disease

These may include:

- diarrhoea
- faecal incontinence
- rectal bleeding, bloody diarrhoea
- passing of mucus
- cramping pains
- weight loss
- in Crohn's disease there may also be mouth ulcers and anal skin tags
- in Crohn's disease there may be malabsorption, leading to deficiencies of folate, vitamin B_{12} and iron associated with megaloblastic and iron-deficiency anaemia, respectively; blood loss in ulcerative colitis may also lead to iron-deficiency anaemia (see Chapter 18)

- inflammatory bowel disease (IBD) may also occasionally be associated with arthritis, iritis, uveitis and an increased risk of thromboembolism.

Ulcerative colitis

Ulcerative colitis is characterised by inflammation that involves the rectum and spreads to the colon. In ulcerative colitis the inflammation tends to be superficial, affecting the mucosa.

Crohn's disease

Crohn's disease is an inflammatory condition which may affect any part of the gastrointestinal tract but mostly the ileum and/or colon are involved. The cause(s) of Crohn's disease are unclear but may be related to genetic predisposition, environmental factors and the balance between gut flora and the immune system. The features of Crohn's disease and any associated deficiencies reflect the region of the gastrointestinal tract affected. In Crohn's disease T lymphocytes are activated, leading to transmural inflammation, and the extensive involvement may lead to the formation of fistulae.

Pharmacological basis of management

Drugs used in IBD are intended to suppress or prevent the inflammatory response.

5-Aminosalicylates: balsalazide, mesalazine, olsalazine and sulfasalazine

5-Aminosalicylates yield 5-aminosalicylic acid (5ASA), which is the mainstay of therapy for ulcerative colitis, especially in milder disease. 5ASAs are used in Crohn's disease but they are less effective compared with corticosteroids and so their use is limited. Sulfasalazine (5ASA joined to sulfapyridine), olsalazine (two joined molecules of 5ASA) and balsalazide (a prodrug) are metabolised in the colon by gut flora to 5ASA, whereas mesalazine undergoes pH-sensitive cleavages of its enteric coat to yield 5ASA. The liberated 5ASA is thought to act via the inhibition of leukotriene and prostanoid formation, scavenging free radicals and decreasing neutrophil chemotaxis.

Sulfapyridine, derived from sulfasalazine, is a sulphonamide and is unsuitable for patients who are intolerant of sulphonamide: it leads to side effects that include reversible male infertility. Alternative agents such as mesalazine do not affect fertility. The sulfasalazine-derived sulphonamide is a risk factor for megaloblastic anaemia due to its antifolate properties. The release of 5ASA renders all of these agents unsuitable for patients who cannot tolerate salicylates, e.g. patients with asthma who are sensitive to aspirin. They may also cause interstitial nephritis and should be avoided in renal impairment.

The *British National Formulary* recommends that, for patients taking sulfasalazine, a full blood count and a liver function test should be carried out every month for 3 months at the start of treatment.

Significant interactions of 5-aminosalicylates are summarised in Table 10.1.

Corticosteroids

Corticosteroids are used in order to induce a remission in ulcerative colitis and Crohn's disease, especially in more severe disease. Steroid-induced side effects limit their long-term use for maintenance therapy. Oral prednisolone is widely used and more recently enteric-coated budesonide has been developed: this has poor absorption and extensive first-pass metabolism, both of which will limit its systemic side effects. Oral budesonide is intended for Crohn's disease, affecting ileal and ascending colonic regions. Enemas (prednisolone, budesonide and hydrocortisone) are used in more distal or rectal inflammation, and intravenous hydrocortisone is used in severe disease. The beneficial effects of corticosteroids are via their well-established anti-inflammatory and immunosuppressive actions.

Immunosuppressants: azathioprine, ciclosporin, methotrexate

The role of immunosuppressants in IBD is less clear but they may have a role in refractory disease and for steroid sparing. In this regard both azathioprine and intravenous ciclosporin are used for inducing remissions. If ciclosporin is given there is an increased risk of *Pneumocystis jiroveci* and prophylaxis may be required. Methotrexate is also effective in Crohn's disease for inducing a remission or maintenance but not in ulcerative colitis.

Tumour necrosis factor alpha (TNF-α) antibodies: infliximab and adalimumab

These are monoclonal antibodies that neutralise the proinflammatory cytokine, tumour necrosis factor alpha (TNF-α), which is implicated in the pathology of Crohn's disease, possibly via leukocyte recruitment. The ACCENT I trial (ACCENT I Study Group 2002) indicated that patients who show an initial response to a single dose of infliximab are likely to benefit from repeated doses of this agent, leading to remission and discontinuation of corticosteroids. Infliximab has been identified as a risk factor for developing tuberculosis.

The NICE guidelines (2012) recommended that these monoclonal antibodies can be used in patients

Table 10.1 Some important drug interactions of 5-aminosalicylates		
Drugs	**Consequences**	**Comments**
Mesalazine, olsalazine or sulfasalazine with azathioprine	5ASA may reduce the clearance of azathioprine with enhanced side effects such as bone marrow suppression	Their concurrent use should be monitored and the dose of azathioprine may need to be reduced
Sulfasalazine with antibiotics	Ampicillin and rifampicin have been shown to eradicate gut bacteria and reduce the release of 5ASA from sulfasalazine	The effectiveness of sulfasalazine may be reduced by concurrent antibiotics. Metronidazole does not appear to interact with sulfasalazine
Sulfasalazine with digoxin	The plasma levels of digoxin may be reduced	The levels or effectiveness of digoxin should be monitored

5ASA, 5-aminosalicylic acid.

with severe Crohn's disease that is refractory to immunosuppressants and corticosteroids, where the disease is not fistulating and when surgery is not possible.

Loperamide

This may be of some use in diarrhoea associated with mild IBD but should be used with caution in more severe disease due to the risk of toxic megacolon.

Colestyramine

Colestryramine binds bile salts and may reduce diarrhoea due to malabsorption of bile salts in Crohn's disease.

Fish oils

Fish oils have been advocated in ulcerative colitis and Crohn's disease but there is no evidence to support their effectiveness.

Nutritional therapy

In Crohn's disease it is well established that parental nutrition allows the gastrointestinal tract to recover ('bowel rest') and results in patients entering remission without the need for steroids. Similarly, elemental feeding with simple, predigested foods is also effective in the management of Crohn's disease.

Probiotics

A small-scale trial has reported that non-pathogenic *Escherichia coli* (Nissle 1917) was as effective as mesalazine in maintaining a long-term remission in patients with ulcerative colitis (Rembacken *et al.* 1999). The authors' explanations for the beneficial effects of *Escherichia coli* were that it may have blocked the binding of adhesive bacteria, produced toxins against pathogenic bacteria or altered the local environment. There is no evidence that probiotics are of benefit in Crohn's disease.

Vitamins and minerals

As IBD may be associated with malabsorption of iron, folate and vitamin B_{12}, leading to anaemia, it may be necessary to give appropriate oral or parenteral supplements of these nutrients. Patients taking corticosteroids are at risk of osteoporosis and may benefit from calcium supplementation.

Counselling

- Crohn's and Colitis UK provides patient information and support. It produces a 'Can't Wait' card, which is recognised by many shops and is intended to help patients gain access to a toilet in an emergency.
- Smoking makes Crohn's disease (but not ulcerative colitis) worse.
- IBD may be exacerbated by NSAIDs.
- IBD may be exacerbated by alcohol.
- The effectiveness of dietary modifications is less clear but patients may identify by trial and error which foods exacerbate their condition. Wheat and dairy products may be implicated.
- Patients taking aminosalicylates should report any sore throats, fevers, easy bruising or bleeding due to the risk of blood dyscrasia.
- Aminosalicylates are associated with side effects including rashes, headaches and diarrhoea.
- Sulfasalazine may colour urine orange and discolour soft contact lenses.
- Mesalazine and balsalazide tablets should be swallowed whole.
- Patients should be maintained on the same brand of enteric-coated mesalazine.

Self-assessment

For the following questions concerning lower GI conditions, choose the most appropriate answer:

1 *Which one of the following is most likely to cause constipation?*

    A Proton pump inhibitor (omeprazole)
    B Prokinetic drug (metoclopramide)
    C Opioid receptor agonist (morphine)
    D Acetylcholinesterase inhibitor (neostigmine)
    E An SSRI antidepressant (such as fluoxetine)

2 *Which one of the following is used to manage inflammatory bowel disease?*

    A PPAR γ-agonists
    B A prokinetic drug (metoclopramide)
    C A 5-amino-salicylate (such as mesalazine)
    D An NSAID (such as aspirin)
    E A sulphonamide

Practice points

- Changes in bowel habits, including rectal bleeding, should lead to referral to the GP.
- ORT plays a major role in the treatment of diarrhoea.
- Antidiarrhoeal agents provide symptomatic relief but do not alter the course of the diarrhoea.
- Diarrhoea is an important side effect of antibiotic treatment and, if severe (especially with clindamycin), should lead to prompt referral.
- Constipation is best managed by a healthy diet, adequate fluid intake and exercise.
- Patients receiving chronic opioid treatment should receive a laxative.
- Be vigilant of laxative abuse in eating disorders.
- IBS is poorly defined and is managed according to its leading symptoms.
- Ulcerative colitis and Crohn's disease are distinct relapsing–remitting diseases with high morbidity.
- 5-Aminosalicylates are associated with blood dyscrasias.

CASE STUDY

A 24-year-old woman had developed Crohn's disease and was prescribed:

Budesonide 3 mg (t.d.s.)
Mesalazine 800 mg (t.d.s.)
Folic acid 5 mg (o.d.)
$FeSO_4$ 200 mg (t.d.s.)

What are the typical clinical features of Crohn's disease?

- Diarrhoea
- Faecal incontinence
- Rectal bleeding, bloody diarrhoea
- Passing of mucus
- Cramping pains
- Weight loss
- May have mouth ulcers and anal skin tags
- Malabsorption, leading to deficiencies of folate, vitamin B_{12} and iron associated with megaloblastic and iron-deficiency anaemia, respectively.

What advantage does budesonide have over prednisolone?

- Budesonide has fewer systemic effects as it undergoes extensive first-pass metabolism, which limits its systemic effects.

Why were folic acid and ferrous sulphate included in the prescription?

- To prevent problems associated with malabsorption, leading to deficiencies of folate, and iron associated with megaloblastic and iron-deficiency anaemia, respectively.

  After several months the budesonide failed to control her condition and was stopped.

Devise an appropriate treatment plan for this patient.

- Consider azathioprine or methotrexate or ciclosporin.
- An elemental diet may be helpful.
- Finally infliximab may be considered for unresponsive disease.

References

ACCENT I Study Group (2002). Maintenance infliximab for Crohn's disease: the ACCENT I randomised trial. *Lancet* 359: 1541–9.

British National Formulary, latest edition. London: British Medical Association and Royal Pharmaceutical Society of Great Britain.

Carani RB, Cirillo P, Terrin G et al. (2007). Probiotics for treatment of acute diarrhoea in children: randomised clinical trial of five different preparations. *BMJ* 335: 340–345. pmid: 17690340.

Ford AC, Talley NJ, Spiegal BMR et al. (2008). Effect of fibre, antispasmodics, and peppermint oil in the treatment of irritable bowel syndrome: systematic review and meta-analysis. *BMJ* 337: 2313–2324.

Hickson M, D'Souza AL, Muthu N et al. (2007). Use of probiotic *Lactobacillus* preparation to prevent diarrhoea associated with antibiotics: randomised double blind placebo controlled trial. *BMJ*, 335: 80–84. pmid: 17604300.

National Institute for Health and Care Excellence (2002). *Guidance on the use of infliximab for Crohn's disease.* Technology appraisal no. 40. London: NICE. Available at: via www.nice.org.uk

National Institute for Health and Care Excellence (2012). *Crohn's disease: management in adults, children and young people.* Clinical Guideline no 152. London: NICE. www.nice.org.uk

National Institute for Health and Care Excellence (2015). *Irritable bowel syndrome in adults: diagnosis and management of irritable bowel syndrome in primary care.* Clinical Guideline no 61. London: NICE. www.nice.org.uk

Rembacken BJ, Snelling AM, Hawkey PM et al. (1999). Non-pathogenic *Escherichia coli* versus mesalazine for the treatment of ulcerative colitis: a randomised trial. *Lancet* 354: 635–639. pmid: 10466665.

Spiller R, Aziz Q, Creed F et al. (2007). Guidelines for the management of irritable bowel syndrome: mechanisms and practical management. *Gut* 56: 1770–1798. pmid: 17488783.

Online resources

www.crohnsandcolitis.org.uk
The website of Crohn's and Colitis UK, which provides patient information and support (accessed July 2015).

11

The liver patient

Hepatic impairment may result from infection (e.g. hepatitis), may be drug-induced (see Chapter 6) or associated with chronic alcohol abuse. Liver disease may be acute or chronic and ranges from hepatic impairment through to liver failure. Liver disease may have the following clinical features:

- Jaundice: impaired excretion of bilirubin into the bile by the liver leads to hyperbilirubinaemia, resulting in yellow coloration of the skin and sclera of the eyes.
- Hypoproteinaemia: the ability of the liver to synthesise proteins, including clotting factors, is impaired and leads to a reduction in plasma proteins.
- Decreased clotting: this occurs as a consequence of impaired synthesis of clotting factors, and may lead to easy bruising and bleeding.
- Ascites: this is the accumulation of fluid in the peritoneal cavity and in part is due to oedema secondary to hypoproteinaemia and sodium retention caused by secondary hyperaldosteronism, and also portal hypertension.
- Spider naevi: this is a sign of chronic liver failure and may be an early sign of alcoholic liver disease.

- Pruritus: hyperbilirubinaemia of jaundice leads to itching.
- Nausea.
- Digital clubbing: this may be a non-specific sign in chronic liver failure and its cause is unknown. There may also be white nails due to hypoalbuminaemia.
- Portal hypertension: this is associated with chronic liver failure due to liver fibrosis altering the haemodynamics and may result in bleeding oesophageal varices.
- Gynaecomastia: breast development, possibly due to reduced metabolism of oestrogens.
- Hypoglycaemia: reduced glucose output from the liver's glycogen stores.
- Encephalopathy: this is associated with both acute and chronic liver failure, leading to neuropsychiatric symptoms including changes in personality, disorientation, confusion and drowsiness. The causes of encephalopathy are not fully established but nitrogenous products and false neurotransmitters are believed to contribute. The gut flora are believed to produce many nitrogenous products, including ammonia, which are normally cleared by the liver. In liver failure these toxins are not adequately cleared and may exert neurological effects.

The effects of hepatic impairment

As the liver represents a major site of drug metabolism and elimination, hepatic impairment has significant implications for drugs that are extensively cleared by the liver. On the basis of liver function tests (see Chapter 2) it is difficult to predict systematically how a patient will handle various drugs. Most drug monographs in the *British National Formulary* deal with prescribing issues associated with hepatic impairment and detail which drugs are affected and how to alter or choose drug treatment. Measures include avoiding certain drugs, selecting alternative drugs that are not extensively eliminated by the liver and reducing doses.

In addition to the role of the liver in drug elimination, its other metabolic activities will be disrupted. In particular, the liver synthesises a number of clotting factors and so their synthesis will be reduced, leading to an increased bleeding tendency. This will have important implications for the use of the oral anticoagulant warfarin, which is also metabolised by the liver. In patients with hepatic impairment receiving warfarin their international normalised ratio or INR (which may be elevated before treatment) should be closely monitored and the dose altered accordingly. Hypoproteinaemia will also reduce the plasma protein binding of certain drugs, increasing their free plasma concentration.

Pharmacological management of liver failure

Ascites

In addition to paracentesis (draining off the fluid), patients should have a sodium-restricted diet to limit sodium retention and fluid accumulation. Given the role of aldosterone in secondary hyperaldosteronism, the aldosterone receptor antagonist and potassium-sparing diuretic spironolactone is also used. However, spironolactone may cause gynaecomastia and in liver patients who already have gynaecomastia an alternative potassium-sparing diuretic such as amiloride should be used. Additional diuresis may be provided by loop diuretics. Fluid-retaining drugs such as corticosteroids and non-steroidal anti-inflammatory drugs (NSAIDs) should be avoided. A complication of ascites is spontaneous bacterial peritonitis, for which antimicrobial agents may be used.

Hepatic encephalopathy

To limit the production of nitrogenous products, protein in the diet may be restricted. To limit the production of these toxins, gut flora are eradicated with antibacterial agents such as neomycin or metronidazole. The osmotic laxative lactulose (see Chapter 10) is also routinely used in high doses and its beneficial effects may be via regular clearing of the bowel of toxins and/or alterations in the environment for the gut flora.

Sensitivity to centrally acting drugs

Patients with liver disease are especially sensitive to centrally acting drugs such as benzodiazepines, antipsychotic agents and opioids. These drugs should be used with great care, as there is a risk of precipitating a coma.

Hyperbilirubinaemia

Increased levels of bilirubin in the plasma give rise to jaundice and associated pruritus. In order to enhance the removal of bilirubin from the body, colestyramine is used as a bile-binding agent (see Chapter 13). Colestyramine binds bile in the intestines and so prevents the reabsorption of excreted bile and leads to enhanced overall excretion. This should limit the jaundice and associated symptoms. However, as discussed in Chapter 13, the binding nature of colestyramine gives rise to a range of interactions with other drugs and those affected should be given at different times.

Pruritus

As commented above, colestyramine reduces bilirubin levels and limits pruritus. Other measures to limit pruritus are the use of menthol in aqueous cream for its local cooling effect and oral antihistamines for patients with mild liver disease. Sedating antihistamines are used with caution especially at night if itching is preventing the patient from sleeping. Non-sedating antihistamines can also be of benefit. The 5-hydroxytryptamine (serotonin) $5HT_3$-receptor antagonist ondansetron has been shown to have a small beneficial effect in managing pruritus associated with jaundice (Muller *et al.* 1998).

Gastric bleeding

An increased bleeding tendency means that gastric bleeding is more common in liver impairment and to this end antisecretory agents such as ranitidine may be prescribed to reduce the production of gastric acid.

Bleeding oesophageal varices

The bleeding from oesophageal varices is a medical emergency. To limit bleeding, vasopressin is infused and causes vasoconstriction. Octreotide, a somatostatin analogue, is also widely used (unlicensed indication) and is thought to cause vasoconstriction. A β blocker may be used in prophylaxis against bleeding varices and this may be secondary to lowering portal pressure.

Impaired clotting

The impaired clotting, secondary to the impaired synthesis of clotting factors, may be managed by parenteral vitamin K. The patient should of course avoid drugs that may inhibit clotting (anticoagulants, antiplatelet drugs) or cause bleeding (NSAIDs).

Hypoglycaemia

Intravenous glucose may be required to correct hypoglycaemia.

Considerations in alcoholic liver disease

In addition to caution with the use of drugs when there is liver impairment, patients with alcohol dependence may receive drugs to control their addiction (such as disulfiram, acamprosate) and seizures associated with withdrawal reactions (benzodiazepines, principally chlordiazepoxide, and alternatively clomethiazole). Alcoholism is also associated with deficiencies of thiamine (vitamin B_1) and this may lead to Wernicke's encephalopathy with drowsiness, disorientation, nystagmus and ataxia. To prevent this, alcoholic patients are given vitamin B complex.

Over-the-counter considerations

Obviously greater caution should be exercised when using drugs in liver impairment and failure. Other considerations are the salt content in over-the-counter (OTC) preparations (e.g. antacids, effervescent preparation) if the patient is on a salt-restricted diet. The increased bleeding tendency also means that patients are at increased risk of gastric bleeding with aspirin and ibuprofen. NSAIDs may also lead to fluid retention. These increased risks mean that low-dose paracetamol is a safer alternative for pain relief.

Counselling

- Colestyramine should be mixed with water or a drink and can be used in cooking.
- Colestyramine can interfere with the absorption of other drugs, so other drugs should be taken at least 1 hour before or 4–6 hours after the colestyramine.

Self-assessment

For the following questions concerning liver disease, choose the most appropriate answer:

1 *Which one of the following changes is consistent with cholestasis?*

   A Increased INR
   B Increased alkaline phosphatase
   C Decreased γ-glutamyl transpeptidase
   D Increased alanine transaminase
   E Decreased bilirubin

2 *Which one of the following changes is consistent with chronic liver damage?*

   A Increased INR
   B Decreased γ-glutamyl transpeptidase

C Decreased bilirubin

D Decreased platelet count

E Normal albumin

3 *Which one of the following may worsen ascites?*

A An NSAID

B A proton inhibitor

C An osmotic laxative (lactulose)

D A β blocker (such as propranolol)

E An aldosterone-receptor antagonist (spironolactone)

Practice points

- Liver function should always be taken into consideration when using drugs.
- Blood clotting is impaired in liver failure with increased bleeding tendencies and the actions of warfarin will be potentiated.
- Jaundice may be managed by colestyramine, ascites with spironolactone, and encephalopathy by neomycin and lactulose.

Case studies

Case 1

A 25-year-old woman experienced a tonic–clonic (grand mal) seizure for the second time and her neurologist decided to start her on antiepileptic therapy. She is currently taking Yasmin (ethinylestradiol/drospirenone).

Several months later she complained of itching and nausea, and was jaundiced. A liver function test revealed the following:

Variable	Value	Normal range
Bilirubin	50 µmol/L	<20 µmol/L
Alkaline phosphatase	100 iu/L	40–120 iu/L
Alanine aminotransferase	420 iu/L	0–35 iu/L
Aspartate aminotransferase	315 iu/L	0–34 iu/L
γ-Glutamyl transpeptidase	45 iu/L	0–70 iu/L
INR	2.5	1–1.2

INR, international normalised ratio.

What diagnosis would you make?

- Possible drug-induced hepatocellular damage as indicated by elevated levels of the aminotransferases which leak out of damaged hepatocytes.

Explain why the INR is altered and its significance.

- INR measures coagulation activity and, as clotting factors are produced by the liver, they indicate synthetic activity of liver, which in this case is impaired.

What action would you recommend and how should therapy be changed?

- The antiepileptic drug should be stopped under the cover of another agent.

(continued)

(continued)

- Caution hepatic impairment (see the *British National Formulary*, e.g. dose reduction if lamotrigine chosen) but another antiepileptic drug should be tried.
- Symptomatic relief from pruritis (e.g. antihistamine) and nausea (e.g. antiemetic).

Case 2

Mr JT, a regular customer, presents you with a prescription for omeprazole 20mg b.d., which his general practitioner has started him on for a suspected duodenal ulcer. Your patient medication record verifies that you are aware he has a history of alcoholic liver disease with liver impairment.

Are you happy to dispense the prescription?

- As omeprazole is hepatically cleared, a dose of not more than 20 mg daily is recommended in liver disease as bioavailability and half-life can be prolonged.

References

British National Formulary, latest edition. London: British Medical Association and Royal Pharmaceutical Society of Great Britain.

Muller C, Pongratz S, Pidlich J *et al.* (1998). Treatment of pruritus in chronic liver disease with the 5-hydroxytryptamine receptor type 3 antagonist ondansetron: a randomized, placebo-controlled, double-blind cross-over trial. *Eur J Gastroenterol Hepatol* 10: 865–870. pmid: 9831410.

Further reading

North-Lewis P, ed. (2008). *Drugs and the Liver.* London: Pharmaceutical Press.

PART **D**

Cardiovascular diseases

12

Hypertension

Disease characteristics

The cause of essential hypertension is not known but may be multifactorial. Indeed, rather than a disease in its own right, we may view hypertension as blood pressure (BP) that is associated with significant cardiovascular risk. The cut-off point between normal blood pressure and hypertension is arbitrary, and is now generally regarded as a sustained diastolic >90 mmHg or systolic >140 mmHg.

Over the years alterations in many cardiovascular control mechanisms (nitric oxide, endothelins, renin–angiotensin system and sympathetic nervous system) have been proposed as causing essential hypertension but there is no convincing evidence to support a 'universal cause'. Essential hypertension appears to be multifactorial with a combination of genetics, diet, exercise and obesity playing a role. In relation to the latter, the Prospective Studies Collaboration (2009) reported a clear relationship between body mass index and blood pressure.

Far less commonly, hypertension (<10%) may be secondary to another condition: renal disease, renovascular disease, Conn's syndrome (primary hyperaldosteronism), polycythaemia, Cushing's syndrome, hyperthyroidism, phaeochromocytoma and pregnancy, and these should be excluded. Drugs which may cause hypertension include:

- oral contraceptives
- sympathomimetics
- corticosteroids
- non-steroidal anti-inflammatory drugs (NSAIDs)
- ketoconazole
- moclobemide
- erythropoietin
- ciclosporin
- venlafaxine.

Clinical features

Hypertension is almost always asymptomatic and often detected by routine measurement. The main complications are due to end-organ damage, principally left ventricular hypertrophy, ischaemic heart disease, renal failure, retinopathy and peripheral vascular disease. Ultimately, hypertension is a major risk factor for stroke (especially), myocardial infarction and the development of chronic heart failure, hence the need to treat this condition effectively.

Goals of treatment

The clear goal is a reduction in blood pressure and, when this involves drug treatment, this should be with as few side effects as possible. The NICE guidelines (2011) specify a target systolic <140 mmHg and a target diastolic <90 mmHg and the HOT (Hypertension Optimal Treatment) Study Group (1998) indicated that there is little benefit from lowering BP further. In patients with diabetes the target of <140/<80 mmHg is recommended and a lower target of <130/<80 mmHg where there is evidence of end-organ damage.

As a consequence of treatment the following are ideal goals:

- reduction in cardiovascular damage
- preservation of renal function
- limitation or reversal of left ventricular hypertrophy
- prevention of coronary artery disease and chronic heart failure
- reduction in mortality due to stroke and myocardial infarctions.

Pharmacological basis of management

Angiotensin-converting enzyme inhibitors

Angiotensin-converting enzyme (ACE) inhibitors such as enalapril, lisinopril, perindopril and ramipril are now recognised as having an important role in hypertension but are no more effective than other agents (CAPP Study Group 1999). By inhibiting ACE, they lead to reductions in angiotensin II, which in turn leads to:

- reductions in arterial and venous vasoconstriction (reduced total peripheral resistance)
- reduced aldosterone production, which leads to reductions in salt and water retention, hence reduced circulating volume (reduced cardiac output).

Clinical use

ACE inhibitors may cause pronounced first-dose hypotension and are best given initially on retiring at night. A low starting dose should be used and titrated up to the maximum effective and tolerated dose.

The renin–angiotensin system is activated in renovascular disease (atheroma of the renal artery) in order to maintain renal perfusion and filtration. Hence, ACE inhibitors may cause deterioration of renal function in pre-existing renal disease and these patients should be identified by measuring plasma creatinine and should not receive an ACE inhibitor. Conversely, ACE inhibitors are renoprotective in diabetes and reduce the progression of diabetic nephropathy. This makes them drugs of choice in concurrent diabetes.

A build-up of bradykinin, usually broken down by ACE, may produce a troublesome dry cough in some patients (10%) treated with ACE inhibitors.

Angiotensin II receptor antagonists, e.g. candesartan, irbesartan, losartan, valsartan

This class of drugs blocks the action of angiotensin II at the angiotensin (AT_1) receptor. Hence these agents have similar consequences to ACE inhibitors but do not give rise to a cough. The Lifestyle Intervention for Endpoint Reduction in Hypertension (LIFE) trial (2002) reported that losartan was more effective than atenolol at reducing mortality in hypertensive patients, largely through a reduction in the incidence of stroke. In patients with diabetes with hypertension, the effects of losartan were even more impressive at reducing overall mortality, cardiovascular mortality and the development of heart failure. In both classes of hypertensive patients, losartan was also more effective than atenolol at reversing left ventricular hypertrophy. Current guidelines recommend that AT_1-receptor antagonists be used when ACE inhibitors are indicated but not tolerated, e.g. due to a cough.

Renin inhibitors, e.g. aliskiren

This is a new class of antihypertensives which act via direct inhibition of renin to interfere with the renin–angiotensin system. They appear equally effective as the ACE inhibitors but do not give rise to a cough.

Calcium-channel blockers, e.g. amlodipine, diltiazem, felodipine, nifedipine, verapamil

There are three main classes of calcium-channel blockers: (1) verapamil; (2) dihydropyridines – nifedipine, nicardipine, amlodipine, lacidipine, nisoldipine; and

(3) diltiazem. Verapamil exerts most of its effects on the heart compared with dihydropyridine effects, which target arteriolar smooth muscle. The activity of diltiazem is between class 1 and 2. Worldwide, calcium-channel blockers are currently the most widely used antihypertensives and they act principally to inhibit voltage-operated calcium channels on vascular smooth muscle, leading to vasodilatation and a reduction in blood pressure.

Diuretics: thiazides-like agents, e.g. chlorthalidone, indapamide, metolazone

Diuretics are third-line drugs in the management of hypertension and cause a reduction in circulating volume, thus reducing preload and afterload, and hence cardiac work. In addition, they may have direct vascular effects leading to vasodilatation, which further reduces preload and/or afterload.

Thiazides act in the distal convoluted tubule to inhibit Na^+/Cl^- reabsorption, leading to diuresis. Loop diuretics, which are occasionally used when thiazides (except metolazone) are likely to be ineffective in renal impairment, act via inhibition of the $Na^+/K^+/Cl^-$ transporter in the thick ascending limb of the loop of Henle.

The effectiveness of thiazide diuretics has been established over many years and was confirmed by the ALLHAT trial (2002), which demonstrated that they were effective at preventing cardiovascular disease and supported their use. However, in the UK, NICE evaluated the effectiveness of thiazides, and especially in relation to their ability to impair glucose control and exacerbate diabetes, their prominence in therapy was reduced. Despite this, guidance in the US still advocates thiazides as first-line agents.

β blockers: acebutolol, atenolol, bisoprolol, metoprolol, nadolol, pindolol, propranolol

β blockers were once viewed as first-line drugs and have been widely used over many years. Their precise antihypertensive effect is unclear but it is thought to involve a reduction in sympathetic drive to the heart, reducing cardiac output, and a reduction in sympathetically evoked renin release from the kidneys.

However, in 2006 guidance from NICE recommended that they should no longer be used as first-line antihypertensives, based on their reduced effectiveness at reducing cardiovascular outcomes compared with other antihypertensives, as established by the ASCOT trial (2005).

α blockers, e.g. doxazosin, prazosin

These should generally be regarded as agents of last choice, being added to therapy that has not achieved target blood pressure. They are competitive receptor antagonists, inhibiting sympathetic activation of α_1-adrenoceptors on vascular smooth muscle, leading to vasodilatation and a drop in blood pressure. As a result of this non-selective action, they lead to widespread side effects, making them poorly tolerated. They may, however, be useful for patients with diabetes or a lipid disorder (when diuretics or β blockers are sometimes avoided) or in older men with prostatic symptoms.

Centrally acting agents, e.g. clonidine, α-methyldopa, moxonidine

These agents are occasionally used, e.g. α-methyldopa in pregnancy or when other treatments have failed. Their action is on central vasomotor centres and they lead to a decrease in sympathetic output, causing a fall in blood pressure. The interference with the sympathetic nervous system leads to widespread side effects. In the case of clonidine and moxonidine (an imidazoline receptor agonist), they should not be withdrawn suddenly, because there is a risk of a hypertensive crisis. For withdrawal, if moxonidine is used together with a β blocker, then the β blocker should be withdrawn slowly, several days before the centrally acting agent.

The beneficial pharmacological targets of cardiovascular drugs are listed in Table 12.1. Consideration of the distribution in the body of the sites of action for these drugs also explains some of the unwanted but predictable type A adverse drug reactions (Table 12.1).

Management of hypertension

Lifestyle measures play an important role both before and alongside drug therapy. Lifestyle modifications

Table 12.1 Examples of principal type A adverse reactions of drugs used in hypertension

Drug	Pharmacological activity	Unwanted clinical effects
Calcium-channel blockers	Vascular smooth muscle: arteriolar relaxation (mainly dihydropyridines)	Headache, facial flushing, peripheral oedema (ankles), postural hypotension, gum hyperplasia
(1) Verapamil	Smooth muscle: GI tract	Constipation
	Sinus or AV nodes: negative inotrope	Bradycardia or heart block
	Myocardium	Reduced cardiac output
(2) Dihydropyridines	Reflex sympathomimetic stimulation	Tachycardia or palpitations
(3) Diltiazem	Sinus or AV nodes: negative inotrope	Bradycardia or heart block
	Smooth muscle: GI tract	Constipation
Thiazide-like	Act on the Na^+/Cl^- transporter of the renal distal convoluted tubule to cause diuresis and reduce circulating volume. May also have vasodilator actions	• Postural hypotension • Adversely alter lipid profile • May induce diabetes
β blockers Hydrophilic (atenolol, acebutolol)	Myocardium: sympathetic drive mediated by $β_1$-adrenoceptors	Bradycardia, cardiac failure, conduction disorders
	Smooth muscle: bronchoconstriction	Bronchoconstriction
	Reduce lacrimation	Dry eyes
	Peripheral vascular smooth muscle: constriction	Raynaud's phenomenon, impotence
	Lipids	Adversely affect lipid profile: increase LDL and decrease HDL
	Liver and pancreas	Decrease glycogenolysis, and decrease secretion of insulin
Lipophilic (propranolol, timolol, metoprolol, labetalol)	As above + CNS effects	Lethargy, depression, nightmares

AV, atrioventricular; CNS, central nervous system; GI, gastrointestinal; HDL, high-density lipoprotein; LDL, low-density lipoprotein.

may involve weight reduction, reducing fat and salt intake, increasing fruit and oily fish in the diet, increasing exercise and stopping smoking. It has been reported that a sustained weight loss of 4.5 kg was associated with an 8–9 mmHg drop in diastolic and systolic blood pressure (Stevens *et al.* 2001) and made a significant contribution to blood pressure reduction. Particular attention should be paid to alcohol consumption, because excessive alcohol intake is closely associated with hypertension. In many patients the initial treatment will involve lifestyle changes to see whether these bring about a reduction in blood pressure. During this process the patient's blood pressure should be measured on several occasions (typically 14 times and ideally ambulatory) to determine whether hypertension is established and to exclude 'white-coat' hypertension.

Choice of drugs

If lifestyle measures do not bring about a satisfactory reduction, NICE guidelines (2011) suggest that drug treatment should be initiated in patients with blood pressure that is consistently >160/100 mmHg or when 140/90 mmHg and cardiovascular disease is present, in patients with elevated cardiovascular risk (>20% over 10 years) or end-organ damage (such as left ventricular hypertrophy or renal damage).

The management of hypertension has been the subject of controversy with clinical trials giving different results regarding drug choice and the existence of conflicting guidelines. In 2011, NICE guidance was revised to produce a consensus on the management of hypertension (Figure 12.1). The original Cambridge AB/CD rules were modified and simplified as 'A/C' guidelines. These guidelines divide patients into groups under and over 55 years of age, with black patients of any age being treated as the latter group. The rationale for this is that younger patients are deemed to have high renin hypertension and respond best to ACE inhibitors (A) whereas older patients or black patients are initially treated with calcium-channel blockers (C). It is then acknowledged that most patients require more than one drug, so drug treatment is stepped up using an agent from the other group, e.g. patients who are younger than 55 years would normally be initiated on an ACE inhibitor and, if this failed to control their blood pressure, they would then be additionally prescribed a calcium-channel blocker (C) (step 2). After this the third step would involve adding a diuretic (D). In cases of resistance (step 4), an additional diuretic, β blocker or α blocker should be added to therapy. In some cases, the aldosterone antagonist spironolactone is effective because the patient may have undiagnosed Conn's syndrome with high aldosterone. β blockers are also reserved for patients who are intolerant to ACE inhibitors and used in pregnancy.

Concurrent illnesses

In addition to the A/C rules, concurrent illnesses also influence drug choice, for example, asthma is a reason to avoid β blockers. Some reasons to favour or avoid certain antihypertensives are summarised in Table 12.2.

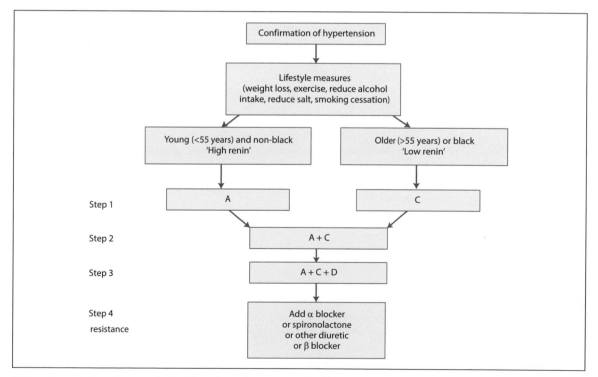

Figure 12.1 National Institute for Health and Care Excellence guidance (NICE 2011) on the management of hypertension using the A/C rules. A, angiotensin-converting enzyme inhibitor; C, calcium-channel blocker; D, diuretic. The stepwise care is shown and, once lifestyle measures have failed to control confirmed hypertension, patients are treated on the basis of age and ethnicity.

Table 12.2 Compelling indications and contraindications for antihypertensives

Condition	Drug indicated	Drugs contraindicated or used with caution
Ischaemic heart disease	β blockers; diltiazem, verapamil, long-acting dihydropyridines	Short-acting formulations of dihydropyridines – associated with increased mortality
Heart failure	ACE inhibitors and AT_1-receptor antagonists; diuretics; β blockers with caution (Chapter 16)	Diltiazem and verapamil – due to negative inotropic effects
Left ventricular hypertrophy (LVH)	The AT_1-receptor antagonist, losartan, has been shown to be particularly effective at reversing LVH (LIFE trial)	
Diabetes mellitus	ACE inhibitors – they are renally and vasoprotective in diabetes (HOPE trial). The AT_1-receptor antagonist, losartan, reduces mortality more than atenolol in diabetic patients with hypertension (LIFE trial). Centrally acting agents and calcium-channel blockers are also suitable	Thiazides and β blockers may cause hyperglycaemia. Thiazides may adversely affect the lipid profile. β blockers may also mask signs of hypoglycaemia (e.g. tachycardia; Chapter 37)
Chronic obstructive pulmonary disease (COPD) and asthma	Centrally acting agents are safe	β blockers are contraindicated in asthma, although in the absence of an alternative, $β_1$-receptor antagonists may be used with extreme caution. In COPD, cardioselective agents are used with caution
History of stroke	Perindopril and indapamide reduce the risk of stroke in both hypertensive and normotensive patients (PROGRESS trial); this may apply to any ACE inhibitor plus a thiazide	
Renal impairment		Thiazides less effective. Dose reduction of hydrophilic β blockers (atenolol, celiprolol, nadolol) may be necessary. Caution with ACE inhibitors. ACE inhibitors and AT_1-receptor antagonists should not be used in renovascular disease
Prostatic hypertrophy	α blocker	Diuretics
Pregnancy	Methyldopa; labetolol, nifedipine (after 20 weeks)	Consider all other agents
Gout	Centrally acting agents safe	Thiazides
Migraine	β blocker; clonidine	
Resistant hypertension	α blocker; minoxidil, hydralazine, sodium nitroprusside	
Depression		Side effect of β blockers, calcium-channel blockers, clonidine and methyldopa
Parkinsonism		Indoramin has extrapyramidal side effects

ACE, angiotensin-converting enzyme; AT_1, angiotensin; HOPE, Heart Outcomes Prevention Evaluation; LIFE, Losartan Intervention for Endpoint Reduction in Hypertension; PROGRESS, Perindopril Protection Against Recurrent Stroke Study.

Hypertension is a major risk factor for cardiovascular disease, so the patient may have other related conditions. Hyperlipidaemia is common in the population at risk of hypertension and should be managed, usually with a statin (see Chapter 13). The NICE guidelines point to using a statin in patients with a 10% or greater 10-year risk of coronary artery disease. In addition, evidence from small-scale studies has also suggested that statins may themselves cause modest reductions in blood pressure and, when used in combination with antihypertensives, may augment the regression of left ventricular hypertrophy, an effect that is independent of lipid lowering (Glorioso *et al.* 1999; Borghi *et al.* 2000; Su *et al.* 2000). In choosing a statin, it is well established that simvastatin can interact with the calcium channel inhibitors amlodipine, verapamil and diltiazem leading to increased plasma concentrations and a risk of statin-induced myopathy. It is for this reason that the maximum dose of simvastatin, when given concurrently with these agents, is 20 mg or atorvastatin may be used in its place.

Diabetes mellitus often coexists with hypertension and, as indicated above, may be a compelling reason to use an ACE inhibitor. Clinical trials certainly suggest that ACE inhibitors are less likely to cause diabetes and they are widely used in patients with diabetes to reduce the chances of renal nephropathy as they are renoprotective. Both thiazides and β blockers may worsen glucose tolerance, so their use in combination is often avoided in diabetes and patients at risk of developing diabetes.

Heart failure is often a consequence of untreated hypertension and, as reviewed in Chapter 16, may well be treated with an ACE inhibitor, diuretic, β blocker or spironolactone, all of which are also indicated for hypertension. In the case of a β blocker, a very low dose would be introduced in heart failure, initially under the supervision of an appropriately experienced clinician.

Drug interactions

Given the diversity of drugs used in the treatment of hypertension there are a range of drug interactions. Some important interactions of antihypertensive drugs are summarised in Table 12.3.

General counselling

As outlined earlier, lifestyle changes (including weight reduction, increased exercise, smoking cessation, a low salt diet and reduction in alcohol consumption) should be advocated. Failure of lifestyle changes alone would then indicate drug treatment. In talking to patients about drug treatment, it should be stressed that the purpose is to lower their blood pressure and this should reduce their risk of having a heart attack,

Table 12.3 Summary of important interactions with drugs used in hypertension

Interacting drugs	Consequences	Comments
β blockers with β agonists	Pharmacological antagonism	Bronchoconstriction may occur due to inhibition of bronchial β_2-adrenoceptors
α Antagonists with calcium-channel blockers or β blockers	Hypotension	Additive effects require close monitoring and counselling
Calcium-channel blockers with β blockers	Some combinations are safe (e.g. felodipine and β blockers). Bradycardia and heart block with verapamil or diltiazem and β blockers (avoid combination or monitor closely); dihydropyridines with β blockers are usually safe but should be monitored	Additive negative inotropic effects. Increased plasma levels of β blockers metabolised by the liver
ACE inhibitors with NSAIDs	Risk of renal impairment	Both associated with renal toxicity
Grapefruit juice with nifedipine (and possibly nicardipine, amlodipine)	Increased effects of calcium-channel blockers	Inhibition of cytochrome P450, therefore reduced metabolism
Alcohol with antihypertensives	• Chronic: increase in BP • Acute: postural hypotension and dizziness	• Evidence of reduced BP when moderate-heavy drinkers take antihypertensives; reduce alcohol intake • Acutely, alcohol causes vasodilatation

ACE, angiotensin-converting enzyme; BP, blood pressure; NSAIDs, non-steroidal anti-inflammatory drugs.

stroke or kidney problems. Although hypertension has no symptoms and the drugs may have side effects, it is important to take the drugs; however, if they find the side effects intolerable, they may find that changing their drug is beneficial.

Diuretics

- Diuretics (or 'water tablets') will cause an increase in urine flow, which may subside after a couple of weeks.
- It is best to take the diuretic in the morning to limit sleep disturbance. A dose may be taken later in the day to avoid the need for urination interfering with social engagements during the day.
- Diuretic use in elderly people is associated with increased incidence of falls.
- Diuretics may cause impotence and this should be discussed with the patient.

ACE inhibitors

- Patients may experience pronounced first-dose hypotension that may be worse if the patient is also taking diuretics; it is best to take the ACE inhibitor on retiring to bed at night. Discuss any cough with their general practitioner (GP). Patients should be encouraged to persist with the ACE inhibitor, because this is an effective treatment.
- Consult a pharmacist before purchasing other medicines or supplements, e.g. avoid the use of potassium salts (salt substitute, effervescent preparations, cystitis treatments) and use NSAIDs with caution.
- If patients experience any lip, facial or tongue swelling (angio-oedema), they should stop taking the ACE inhibitor and seek immediate medical advice.

Calcium-channel blockers

- Calcium-channel blockers may cause flushing, constipation and ankle swelling. Gentle exercise or elevation of the foot may reduce ankle swelling. These side effects should improve after a few weeks. If the side effects become troublesome, patients should discuss this with their general practitioner.
- Avoid grapefruit juice if taking a dihydropyridine.

β blockers

- Male patients may experience impotence.
- Report any additional breathlessness (due to worsening of symptoms or blockade of bronchial β_2-adrenoceptors); cold extremities or peripheral weakness may reflect blockade of vasodilator β_2-adrenoceptors.
- Do not stop taking the tablets suddenly (because this may increase the risk of myocardial infarction). β blockers should be withdrawn gradually over at least a week.

α blockers

- Patients should be alert to first-dose hypotension.
- Patients may also experience urinary incontinence.
- Take care when driving, because of possible drowsiness.

Centrally acting drugs

- Take care when driving, because of possible drowsiness.
- Do not stop taking the tablets suddenly (particularly clonidine).

Monitoring

Home and pharmacy blood pressure measurements

Automated devices are available for home monitoring by the patient. These devices measure blood pressure on different principles from auscultation with a sphygmomanometer. The reliability of automated monitors varies considerably and devices which have been validated by the British Hypertension Society should be used or recommended. Other sources of inaccuracy in home measuring may be poor technique such as cuff placing and inadequate resting before measurement.

'White-coat' hypertension is a well-recognised clinical phenomenon whereby the patient's blood pressure is significantly higher when recorded by a doctor, and is thought to be induced by anxiety. In a proportion of cases, 'white-coat' hypertension is so pronounced that patients who are normotensive under normal conditions may be classed and treated as hypertensive on the basis of measurements made by a doctor. However, 'white-coat' hypertension may be eliminated by nurses or patients themselves measuring blood pressure. In self-measurement, NICE guidance sets a lower level for diagnosis of 135/85 mmHg.

Prior to treatment

The following may be assessed:

- An electrocardiogram (ECG) to test for left ventricular hypertrophy, because up to a third of people with hypertension have left ventricular hypertrophy. There may also be the need for an echocardiogram.
- Electrolytes, especially potassium, because a reduced level may reflect hyperaldosteronism. This is particularly important when initiating diuretics and ACE inhibitors.
- Plasma lipids and glucose: these may be adversely affected by β blockers and diuretics.
- Renal function; plasma creatinine: this will influence drug choice because thiazides, except metolazone, are ineffective in moderate renal failure and ACE inhibitors may make renal impairment worse. Dose reduction with close monitoring is required if estimated glomerular filtration rate (eGFR) is significantly reduced.
- Urinalysis, because protein and/or blood might indicate renal damage.
- Full blood count.
- Liver function test, with mean corpuscular volume to assess for excess alcohol consumption.
- Thyroid function test.

During treatment

- Measurement of blood pressure.
- Monitor renal function and proteinuria (annually).
- Monitor electrolytes, especially potassium, with diuretics and ACE inhibitors.

Over-the-counter considerations

Most patients should be considered for low-dose aspirin therapy because this has been shown to reduce the incidence of myocardial infarction in hypertensive patients. Although NSAIDs should not generally be used with ACE inhibitors or thiazides, low-dose aspirin (75 mg) appears to be safe. Indeed, the HOT trial indicated that low-dose aspirin reduced cardiovascular

events but not stroke. The British Hypertension Society recommends that low-dose aspirin be used in primary prevention in people with hypertension who are aged over 50 years and have controlled BP (<150/90 mmHg), and those with end-organ damage, diabetes or a 15% or greater risk of coronary artery disease over 10 years. Even low-dose aspirin is associated with gastric damage and bleeding, to which the patient should be alerted. Ibuprofen may oppose the beneficial effects of aspirin (see Chapter 15).

There is some evidence that fish oil supplementation may cause a modest reduction in blood pressure, although this has not been universally reported. None the less, fish oil supplementation appears a sensible approach to reducing overall cardiovascular risk and is advocated by the American Heart Association (Kris-Etherton et al. 2002).

Some considerations of over-the-counter (OTC) medicines and their use in hypertension are detailed in Table 12.4.

Alternative remedies

Consideration should be given to herbal preparations and supplements with sympathomimetic activity (see Chapter 4). Diuretic effects of herbal preparations may also increase side effects in combination with antihypertensives.

There has been recent interest in non-pharmacological treatment using devices that aim to lower BP by guiding patients to control their breathing to a rate of 10 breaths/minute for a short period each day. However, the effectiveness of these devices requires confirmation in large trials, although small studies have reported modest BP responses. There is also evidence for a lack of efficacy in patients with diabetes and hypertension (Logtenberg et al. 2007). It could be that these devices may be of benefit in cases of selected patients with mild hypertension or as an adjunct to drug treatment.

Future developments

There has been much recent interest in catheter-based renal denervation. The Symplicity HTN-2 trial in 2010 demonstrated the effectiveness of renal denervation in controlling blood pressure in the management of patients with resistant hypertension.

Table 12.4 Summary of the use of over-the-counter (OTC) medicines in hypertension

OTC medicine	Effects	Comments
Low-dose aspirin	Reduces risk of myocardial infarction and stroke	Need to select high-risk patients due to the risk of gastric damage associated with even low doses. Proton pump inhibitor may be used for prophylaxis
Aspirin or ibuprofen	May reduce effects of captopril	Caution: BP should be monitored
	Aspirin (300 mg) may reduce the effects of enalapril	Paracetamol is a safe alternative analgesic
Antacids	Interaction with ACE inhibitors to reduce their absorption	Separate doses
Cimetidine	May increase plasma concentrations of diltiazem and nifedipine	Ranitidine may be used as an alternative
Systemic sympathomimetic decongestants	Weak pressor effects	Use topical agents (if not swallowed), steam or saline drops

ACE, angiotensin-converting enzyme; BP, blood pressure.

Practice points

- The BHS and NICE have produced joint guidelines. The guidelines recommend the A/C algorithm. β blockers and diuretics are no longer recommended as first-line antihypertensives.
- Most patients do not have their blood pressure adequately controlled by the first drug used.
- Patients should be warned about first-dose hypotension with ACE inhibitors and α blockers (extra caution in combination with diuretics) due to the risk of falls.
- Monitor patients for hypertension secondary to drug treatment, e.g. NSAIDs, oral contraceptives, sympathomimetics, corticosteroids, ketoconazole, moclobemide, venlafaxine and ciclosporin.
- In treatment failure consider OTC drugs, alcohol consumption and compliance.
- The aim of antihypertensive treatment is to reduce cardiovascular risk, reduce/limit end-organ damage, especially kidneys, left ventricular hypertrophy, and reduce the risk of heart failure.
- Aim for blood pressure control without unacceptable side effects, because hypertension is generally asymptomatic.
- Always enquire about side effects, particularly impotence.

Self-assessment

For the following questions concerned with hypertension and its management, choose the most appropriate answer:

1 *Hypertension may be exacerbated by which one of the following?*

  A Non-steroidal anti-inflammatory drugs (such as aspirin)
  B Aldosterone-receptor antagonists (such as spironolactone)
  C Nitrates (such as glyceryl trinitrate)
  D α blockers (such as prazosin)
  E Loop diuretics (such as furosemide)

2 *Untreated hypertension is a risk factor for?*

  A Epilepsy
  B Hypoglycaemia
  C Stomach ulcers
  D Stroke
  E Hypokalaemia

3 *Which one of the following is a first-line antihypertensive?*

  A An ACE inhibitor (such a ramipril)
  B A β-adrenoceptor antagonist (such atenolol)
  C A thiazide diuretic (such as bendroflumethiazide)

D An α-adrenoceptor antagonist (such a prazosin)

E A loop diuretic (such as furosemide)

4 *Which one of the following is a contraindication to using a thiazide-like diuretic (such as indapamide)?*

A Asthma

B Hypoglycaemia

C Chronic heart failure

D Age >55 years

E Gout

5 *Which one of the following is a serious drug interaction?*

A A rate-limiting calcium-channel antagonist plus β-adrenoceptor antagonist

B An ACE inhibitor plus AT_1 receptor antagonist

C An ACE inhibitor plus thiazide diuretic

D An ACE inhibitor plus β-adrenoceptor antagonist

E A β-adrenoceptor antagonist plus AT_1 receptor antagonist

CASE STUDY

Case 1

Mr HT (aged 58) visited his general practitioner for a routine medical check and his blood pressure was measured as 172/100 mmHg in the sitting position. Further questioning and examination revealed:

Weight: 100kg
Height: 1.70m
Marital status: single
FH: father died aged 56 years old ('heart trouble'), mother died 75 years old (colon cancer), 1 sister (alive and well) and 1 brother (type 2 diabetes).
PMH: occasional asthma
Drug history: salbutamol 200 micrograms p.r.n.
Social history: ex-smoker (20 pack years) and admits to 35 units of alcohol a week.

What advice should you give this patient?

● It is important to get the patient to 'own' the problem and to reduce his risks, rather than simply leave it as a problem to be solved with tablets. Reducing alcohol intake (a risk factor for essential hypertension), reduce body mass index (aim for 10% reduction which is achievable), and increase exercise. Consider a healthy diet.

One month later he visits the GP and his blood pressure, based on ambulatory measurements made since his last visit, is now 170/102mmHg and the results of his blood test from the last visit are detailed:
Biochemistry and haematology:

Variable	Value	Reference range
Haemoglobin	15 g/dL	13–18 g/dL
White blood cells	6×10^9/L	4–11×10^9/L
Platelets	200×10^9/L	150–400×10^9/L
Sodium	140 mmol/L	135–145 mmol/L

(continued)

(continued)

Variable	Value	Reference range
Potassium	4.0 mmol/L	3.5–5 mmol/L
Urea	5 mmol/L	2.5–6.7 mmol/L
Glucose (random)	6.2 mmol/L	<11.1 mmol/L
Plasma creatinine	100 μmol/L	<150 μmol/L
Total cholesterol	7.5 mmol/L	<5.2 mmol/L
HDL	1.0 mmol/L	>0.9 mmol/L
Triglycerides	2.0 mmol/L	0.6–1.7 mmol/L
Liver function		
Albumin	40 g/L	36–47 g/L
Bilirubin	10 μmol/L	3–17 μmol/L
Alanine aminotransferase	30 iu/L	3–35 iu/L
Aspartate transaminase	30 iu/L	3–35 iu/L
Alkaline phosphatase	100 iu/L	40–125 iu/L
γ-Glutamyl transpeptidase (GGT)	200 iu/L	<70 iu/L

The GP also performed a 12-lead ECG and no abnormalities were detected.

Why were the above tests carried out?

- To check for diabetes which often coincides with hypertension.
- To exclude electrolyte disturbances (e.g. as in Conn's syndrome, hyperaldosteronism leading to hypertension).
- To check renal function prior to drug treatment.
- To check lipid profile and cardiovascular risk.
- To check liver function: in this case the increase in γ-glutamyl transpeptidase is consistent with high alcohol consumption.
- ECG – to check for left ventricular hypertrophy.

Comment on the findings?

- There is no evidence of diabetes and renal function is fine. However, the patient has hypercholesterolaemia and the increase in γ-glutamyl transpeptidase is consistent with high alcohol consumption.

What further lifestyle advice would you give in light of the results of the tests?

- The γ-glutamyl transpeptidase levels point to excessive alcohol consumption which can lead to increased blood pressure and so there is a need to emphasise reduced alcohol consumption.

He leaves the GP and presents you, the community pharmacist, with the following prescription:

R$_x$
Amlodipine 5 mg (o.d.)

How should you counsel the patient?

- The medicine is to help control his blood pressure.
- Calcium-channel inhibitors may cause oedema as they cause arteriolar vasodilatation, which promotes movement of fluid into the tissues. The patient may notice swollen ankles.
- Also associated with headache and palpitations (caused by reflex tachycardia).

Comment on this choice of agent.

- According to NICE 2011, a calcium-channel blocker should be used as first-line treatment in patients >55 years. Patients <55 years should be started on an ACE inhibitor.

Two months later he visits his GP and his blood pressure is now 160/95mmHg and his new prescription is:

R$_x$
Amlodipine 10 mg (o.d.)
Ramipril 1.25 mg (o.d.)
Simvastatin 20 mg (o.n.)

Why have these changes been made?

- The amlodipine has been increased to maximum daily dose and in light of the target blood pressure not being achieved, the ACE inhibitor ramipril is being added as Step 2 of NICE guidance. Simvastatin has been added in light of his high cholesterol and significant cardiovascular risk. The dose of 20 mg was chosen due to its interaction with amlodipine.

References

ALLHAT Trialists (2002). Major outcomes in high-risk hypertensive patients randomized to angiotensin converting enzyme inhibitor or calcium channel blocker vs diuretic. *JAMA* 288: 2981–2997.

ASCOT Investigators (2005). Prevention of cardiovascular events with an antihypertensive regimen of amlodipine adding perindopril as required versus atenolol adding bendroflumethiazide as required, in the Anglo-Scandinavian Cardiac Outcomes Trial-Blood Pressure Lowering Arm (ASCOT-BPLA): a multicentre randomised controlled trial. *Lancet* 366: 895–906.

British National Formulary, latest edition. London: British Medical Association and Royal Pharmaceutical Society of Great Britain.

CAPP Study Group (1999). Effect of angiotensin-converting-enzyme inhibition compared with conventional therapy on cardiovascular morbidity and mortality in hypertension: the Captopril Prevention Project (CAPPP) randomised trial. *Lancet* 353: 611–616.

HOT Study Group (1998). Effects of intensive blood-pressure lowering and low-dose aspirin in patients with hypertension: principal results of the Hypertension Optimal Treatment (HOT) randomised trial. *Lancet* 351: 1755–1762.

Kris-Etherton PM, Harris WS, Appel LJ (2002). Fish consumption, fish oil, omega-3 fatty acids and cardiovascular disease. *Circulation* 106: 2747–2757. pmid: 12438303.

LIFE (Losartan Intervention for Endpoint Reduction in Hypertension) Study Investigators (2002). Cardiovascular morbidity and mortality in the Losartan Intervention for Endpoint reduction in hypertension study (LIFE): a randomised trial against atenolol. *Lancet* 359: 995–1003.

Logtenberg SJ, Kleefstra N, Houweling ST *et al.* (2007). Effect of device-guided breathing exercises on blood pressure in hypertensive patients with type 2 diabetes mellitus: a randomized controlled trial. *J Hypertens* 25: 241–246. pmid: 17143197.

National Institute for Health and Care Excellence (2006). *Statins for the prevention of cardiovascular disease.* Technology Appraisal 94. London: NICE.

National Institute for Health and Care Excellence (2011). *Hypertension: management of hypertension in adults in primary care.* Clinical Guideline 127. London: NICE.

Prospective Studies Collaboration (2009). Body-mass index and cause-specific mortality in 900 000 adults: collaborative analyses of 57 prospective studies. *Lancet* 373: 1083–1096.

Stevens VJ, Obarzanek E, Cook NR *et al.* (2001). Long- term weight loss and changes in blood pressure: results of the trials of hypertension prevention, phase II. *Ann Intern Med* 134: 1–11. pmid: 11187414.

Symplicity HTN-2 Investigators (2010). Renal sympathetic denervation in patients with treatment-resistant hypertension (The Symplicity HTN-2 Trial): a randomised controlled trial. *Lancet* 376: 1903–1909.

Further reading

Brown MJ (2001). Matching the right drug to the right patient in essential hypertension. *Heart* 86: 113–120. pmid: 11410577.

HOPE (Heart Outcomes Prevention Evaluation) Study Investigators (2000). Effects of an angiotensin-converting-enzyme inhibitor, ramipril, on cardiovascular events in high-risk patients. *N Engl J Med* 342: 145–153.

LIFE Study Investigators (2002). Cardiovascular morbidity and mortality in patients with diabetes in the Losartan Intervention for Endpoint reduction in hypertension study (LIFE): a randomised trial against atenolol. *Lancet* 359: 1004–1010.

PROGRESS Collaborative Group (2001). Randomised trial of a perindopril-based blood pressure-lowering regimen among 6105 individuals with previous stroke or transient ischaemic attack. *Lancet* 358: 1033–1041.

Online resources

www.bhf.org.uk
The website of the British Heart Foundation, providing patient information (accessed July 2015).

13

Lipids and cardiovascular risk

Cardiovascular risk is multifactorial, and derangements of cholesterol levels and the balance between 'good' and 'bad' cholesterol are well established as risk factors. Previously the focus was on treating high levels of cholesterol, but it is now acknowledged that cholesterol-lowering drugs such as the statins are invaluable in reducing cardiovascular risk, even in patients with 'normal' cholesterol levels (Heart Protection Study Collaborative Group, 2002a).

Disease characteristics

Hyperlipidaemia represents hypercholesterolaemia and/or hypertriglyceridaemia and is a major risk factor for atherosclerotic plaque formation on the inner surface of arteries, leading to ischaemic heart disease (IHD), cerebrovascular and peripheral vascular diseases. The cause may be genetic (primary or familial hypercholesterolaemia) or secondary to disease such as liver disease, renal failure, hypothyroidism or poorly controlled diabetes mellitus, or may be induced by drugs including:

- β blockers
- corticosteroids
- thiazide diuretics
- anabolic steroids
- retinoids
- oral contraceptives containing levonorgestrel.

A number of modifiable risk factors may contribute towards or exacerbate this condition:

- hypertension
- smoking
- obesity
- high-fat diet
- excess alcohol consumption
- hyperglycaemia
- reduced physical activity
- infection – this has been proposed as a risk factor associated with a chronic inflammatory response.

These factors should be considered in relation to the lipid profile.

Hypercholesterolaemia

Increased plasma cholesterol or hypercholesterolaemia is a major risk factor for atherosclerosis and is present when cholesterol exceeds the desirable level of 5 mmol/L. However, it is increasingly recognised that it is not necessarily the absolute level of cholesterol which is important but the level in relation to other risk factors (composition of total cholesterol, blood pressure, gender, smoking status, diabetes) and how these give rise to the overall cardiovascular risk. Indeed, decisions to use antihyperlipidaemic agents are now based on the patient's cardiovascular risk rather than absolute levels of total cholesterol.

The transport of lipids and cholesterol through the blood is carried out by one of four main classes of lipoprotein: high-density lipoprotein (HDL), low-density lipoprotein (LDL), very-low-density lipoprotein (VLDL) and chylomicrons. These lipoproteins, each with a different role, comprise a central core of hydrophobic lipid, encased in phospholipid, cholesterol and apolipoproteins. Classification is determined by differences in density, size and proportion of core lipid.

Lipoproteins

In the context of atherogenesis, it is the balance between LDL and HDL that plays a major role:

- LDL ('bad cholesterol') is cholesterol rich and taken up by the liver and tissues, and this involves the LDL receptor. LDL provides cholesterol for cell membranes, steroid synthesis and the production of bile acids. Its uptake into arterial walls is associated with atherogenesis.
- HDL ('good cholesterol') takes up cholesterol from cellular breakdown and prevents its deposition.

Atherogenesis (Figure 13.1)

Especially important in atherosclerosis is a high LDL component or low levels of HDL. Indeed, the ratio LDL:HDL is of clinical importance (ideally <3). Blood vessels express LDL receptors for cellular uptake. However, when injury occurs or in the presence of risk factors (such as smoking), the activated monocytes and macrophages generate reactive oxygen species, which oxidise the LDL, and this damages the LDL receptor so that modified LDL is taken up by macrophages. In turn, these macrophages form foam cells which collect beneath the endothelium, leading to fatty streaks. In the special case of familial hypercholesterolaemia, the LDL receptor is defective and thus LDL is cleared less rapidly and therefore accumulates in the plasma. In contrast to the above role of LDL in atherogenesis, HDL binds cholesterol and removes it from local sites, taking it to the liver. Hence HDL is viewed as 'good cholesterol' and protects against atherogenesis. Accordingly, low levels of HDL will offer less protection and are viewed as an important cardiovascular risk.

The process of atherogenesis is regarded as an inflammatory response to injury and the release of inflammatory mediators leads to altered smooth muscle activity and growth. Over time the changes in the blood vessel lead to the formation of atherosclerotic plaques that are lipid rich and become calcified. This long-term process leads to stenosis or the narrowing of large arteries (e.g. the coronary arteries), whereas rupture of a plaque leads to platelet adhesion and aggregation, which may cause thromboembolic occlusion.

Hypertriglyceridaemia

This is elevated plasma triglyceride levels, which may or may not coexist with hypercholesterolaemia. Elevated levels of triglycerides are often associated with other conditions such as obesity, diabetes mellitus, high doses of thiazides (transiently) and high alcohol intake. Its association with atherosclerosis is less strong compared with that for hypercholesterolaemia, but at very high levels it is associated with pancreatitis.

Clinical features

The patient may have few obvious symptoms and hyperlipidaemia may become apparent only after determination of plasma lipid levels. In severe hyperlipidaemia there may be physical signs such as xanthomas, which are yellowish lipid deposits, especially on the eyelids, cornea and tendons. Coronary artery disease presenting as angina or myocardial infarction (MI) is a secondary manifestation of hyperlipidaemia.

Hyperlipidaemia may be associated with diabetes mellitus, renal failure and hypothyroidism, so blood glucose levels and renal and thyroid functions should be determined to exclude possible contributions from these conditions.

Goals of treatment

The primary objective of treating hyperlipidaemia is to bring about reductions of plasma cholesterol (improving the HDL:LDL ratio) and/or reducing triglyceride levels. This should lead to a reduction in

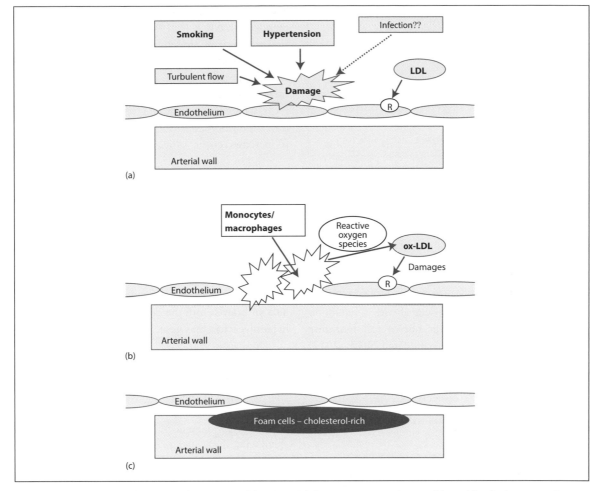

Figure 13.1 Sequence of events in atherogenesis. (a) Various risk factors may cause damage (b) resulting in the generation of reactive oxygen species, which may oxidise the low-density lipoprotein (ox-LDL), damaging the LDL receptor (R), and these changes may lead to (c) foam cells accumulating between the endothelium and arterial wall. ROS, reactive oxygen species.

risk of MI and stroke. The ideal goal would be regression of atherosclerotic lesions. If diet and lifestyle modification fail, the following pharmacological interventions may be considered in addition.

Pharmacological basis of management

HMG-CoA reductase inhibitors or 'statins', e.g. atorvastatin, fluvastatin, pravastatin, rosuvastatin, simvastatin

The statins inhibit the hepatic enzyme, hydroxymethylglutaryl coenzyme A reductase (HMG-CoA reductase), which catalyses the first committed step of cholesterol synthesis in the liver (Figure 13.2). Statins are hepatoselective with extensive first-pass metabolism, which is advantageous because the liver is the main site of cholesterol synthesis, with extrahepatic sites synthesising essential cholesterol.

Fibrates, e.g. bezafibrate, ciprofibrate, fenofibrate, gemofibrozil

Fibrates are activators of peroxisome proliferator-activated receptor α (PPAR-α) and lead to alterations in lipoprotein metabolism. This results in the stimulation of peripheral lipoprotein lipases, which promotes

Figure 13.2 Cholesterol synthesis in the liver. HMG-CoA, hydroxymethylglutaryl coenzyme A.

the breakdown of VLDL (with small reductions in LDL and increases in HDL) and also leads to reductions in triglycerides. The increased biliary excretion of cholesterol predisposes the patient to gallstones and fibrates are therefore contraindicated in gallbladder disease. Their use is associated with a reduction in cardiovascular events but not overall mortality (VA-HIT Trial Study Group 1999) and NICE (2014) does not recommend their routine use in primary or secondary prevention.

Cholesterol absorption inhibitors: ezetimibe

These agents, which may be used alone or in addition to a statin, inhibit the absorption of exogenous and biliary cholesterol in the gastrointestinal tract, bringing about a reduction in total cholesterol and LDL. They may be ideal as an addition to statin therapy, instead of increasing the dose of statin that may be associated with side effects.

Bile acid-binding resins, e.g. colestyramine

These agents bind bile salts in the intestines, preventing both their reabsorption and their cycling. This interruption in bile cycling leads to incorporation of endogenous cholesterol to form bile salts and there is an increase in the number of LDL receptors, which favours the cellular uptake of cholesterol.

Colestyramine is generally used in addition to other agents and can cause a modest fall in plasma cholesterol, which may lead to a reduction in coronary

artery disease. Bile binding agents are not recommended by NICE (2014) for primary or secondary prevention. The binding nature of these agents will reduce the absorption of fat-soluble vitamins (A, D, E and especially K) and other drugs (including warfarin, digoxin, thiazides, levothyroxine and paracetamol), which should not be given at the same time of day. Changes in the absorption of vitamin K may lead to increased effects of warfarin.

Nicotinic acid (niacin)

Vitamin B_3 or its derivatives inhibit hepatic triglyceride production and VLDL secretion. This results in a reduction in LDL and increase in HDL. Nicotinic acid is rarely used due to troublesome adverse effects such as headache and flushing (caused by prostaglandin production, which may be reduced by taking aspirin half an hour before the dose), palpitations, pruritus, hyperglycaemia and gout.

Fish oils

Fish oils rich in omega-3 fatty acids (eicosapentaenoic acid and docosahexaenoic acid) are used for hypertriglyceridaemia, although they do increase levels of LDL. Fish oils are not recommended by NICE (2014) for primary or secondary prevention.

The low incidence of coronary artery disease in Eskimos is attributed to their high dietary intake of omega-3 fatty acids in oily fish. A fish-rich diet following an MI has been demonstrated to reduce mortality and reinfarction significantly. The consumption of at least two portions of oily fish per week or supplementation with fish oils is recommended by the American Heart Association (Kris-Etherton *et al.* 2002). Fish oils should be used with caution in diabetes, haemorrhagic disorders, anticoagulant treatment and aspirin-sensitive asthma.

Antioxidants

The process of atherogenesis involves the production of reactive oxygen species and it was previously thought that antioxidants such as vitamin E might be protective. However, in patients with a high risk of death from cardiovascular disease (diabetes mellitus, ischaemic heart disease, hypertension or arterial disease), the Heart Protection Study Collaborative Group (2002b) found that supplementation with antioxidants, β-carotene, vitamin C or vitamin E did not reduce mortality.

Sitostanol

This is a functional food that is added to certain brands of margarine and prevents the absorption of cholesterol. Additions of sitostanol to the diet reduce LDL by 10–15% and may be helpful as an addition to dietary restrictions or statin therapy.

Choice of drugs

The number of patients who may potentially benefit from treatment with a lipid-lowering drug is enormous. In 2014 the National Institute for Health and Care Excellence (NICE 2014) substantially reduced the threshold for statin therapy, which they recommend should be initiated in patients with cardiovascular disease and for primary prevention in patients with a 10% or greater risk of cardiovascular disease over the next 10 years, as assessed by the patient's risk obtained from QRISK2 (www.qrisk.org). Based on these recommendations then the proportion of the population who could be taking a statin is substantial.

Hypercholesterolaemia and reduction of cardiovascular risk

In hypercholesterolaemia, once dietary changes have been tried, and in patients who have cardiovascular disease or who are at a high risk, statins are the drugs of choice. Statins are of benefit in types IIa and IIb hyperlipoproteinaemia (elevated LDL and LDL/VLDL, respectively). They cause a reduction in plasma cholesterol, whereas the reduction in hepatic cholesterol synthesis leads to an upregulation of hepatic LDL receptors, promoting LDL uptake. However, with the exception of atorvastatin, they are less effective in homozygous familial hypercholesterolaemia, a very rare condition where the LDL receptor is lacking.

The 4S trial (Scandinavian Simvastatin Survival Study Group 1994) reported that simvastatin, in patients who had previously had an MI or had angina, caused a 35% reduction in LDL (increased HDL), and over 5 years this was associated with a 30% reduction in mortality. The WOSCOPS trial (Shepherd *et al.* 1995) also confirmed the effectiveness of pravastatin in primary prevention, with a 20% reduction in cholesterol and a 28% reduction in mortality from coronary artery disease in patients with hypercholesterolaemia. Statins also reduce the progression of carotid artery disease and so reduce the risk of stroke.

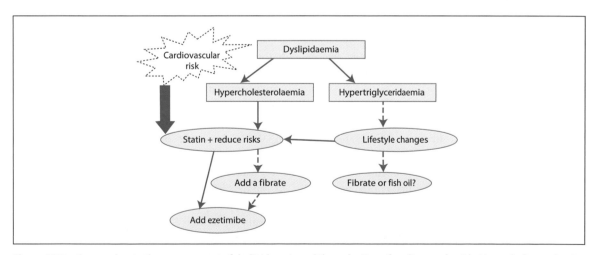

Figure 13.3 Approaches to the management of dyslipidaemia and the reduction of cardiovascular risk. Hypercholesterolemia and high cardiovascular risks (or disease) are reasons to use a statin, with fibrates and ezetimibe being added as appropriate. In the case of hypertriglyceridaemia, lifestyle changes can play a significant role. If drug therapy is required then statins are often used first line whereas fibrates have the greatest effect on triglyceride levels.

The Heart Protection Study Collaborative Group (2002a) has reported substantial benefits of simvastatin in high-risk patients, with marked reductions in events and mortality, and the protection was related to the level of risk rather than plasma lipid level. The PROSPER study (Shepherd *et al.* 2002) has also demonstrated that pravastatin is effective at reducing mortality from coronary artery disease in elderly patients (70–84 years) with a history of, or risk factors for, cardiovascular disease.

The beneficial effects of statins may be due to regression of atherosclerosis, because there is some evidence that not only do they slow down atherosclerosis but they may also cause regression with lipid depletion, leading to stabilisation of lesions. The large-scale ASTEROID (2006) trial has established that high doses of rosuvastatin actually cause regression of coronary atherosclerosis. This is a major goal in the management of cardiovascular disease and it remains to be established whether this is unique to rosuvastatin or due to high intensity therapy.

Although the prototypical statin, simvastatin, has been extensively used over many years, NICE (2014) have recommended that atorvastatin is the agent of choice. The recommendations are that low-intensity therapy (atorvastatin at 20 mg per day) is used in primary prevention and high-intensity therapy (atorvastatin at 80 mg per day) is used in secondary prevention.

In severe hypercholesterolaemia it may be necessary to add the cholesterol absorption inhibitor, ezetimibe.

Hypertriglyceridaemia

As a first step, care should be taken in patients with hypertriglyceridaemia to exclude and modify causes such as excess alcohol intake, obesity and diet. Treatment of hypertriglyceridaemia is less compelling but statins may cause a modest reduction in plasma triglycerides and be considered first-choice agents in moderate hypertriglyceridaemia or combined hyperlipidaemia. Fish oils are also effective in hypertriglyceridaemia. Anion-exchange resins may aggravate hypertriglyceridaemia.

Homocysteinaemia

This condition is also associated with atherosclerosis and is a genetic impairment of vitamins B_6 and B_{12} and folic acid metabolism, which leads to an increase in plasma levels of homocysteine. This induces oxidative stress, which predisposes towards atherosclerosis and thrombogenesis. Folic acid is thought to reduce plasma homocysteine levels and reduce the progression of atherosclerosis.

Concurrent illnesses

Clinically significant hyperlipidaemia that necessitates treatment is likely to occur in the older patient population where a range of other illnesses may coexist. Of specific importance to atherosclerosis are diabetes mellitus and hypertension, both of which should be treated in concert with lipid lowering. Some considerations of drug prescribing in concurrent conditions are summarised in Table 13.1.

Drug interactions

When considering drug choice within the lipid-lowering agents, interactions should be considered (Table 13.2).

In addition to within-group interactions, antihyperlipidaemic drugs show a range of interactions and some important examples are summarised in Table 13.3.

Drug safety

The safety of statins has received much interest and the consensus of expert opinion is that their beneficial effects in reducing cardiovascular risk greatly outweigh their potential for adverse effects. Statins and fibrates are both, to varying degrees, associated with myopathy presenting as muscle pain (myalgia), which may potentially lead to rhabdomyolysis; this is the breakdown of muscle, which may lead to the release of myoglobin and is associated with renal damage. Despite this, the instances of myopathy with elevated creatine kinase are very rare and occur in less than 1 in every 10 000 patients on standard dose statin. The risk is, however, increased with interacting drugs or concomitant fibrates. Statins are also commonly associated with derangements of hepatic transaminases but not liver damage. Therefore, with appropriate counselling and monitoring, statins are regarded as safe medicines.

Table 13.1 Effects of concurrent conditions on drug choice in hyperlipidaemia

Conditions	Effects on drug choice	Comments
Liver disease	A reason to avoid statins and severe disease would be a reason to avoid fibrates	Anion-exchange resins are contraindicated in complete biliary obstruction because they are ineffective
Gallstones	Fibrates can cause gallstones	Avoid in patients who have gallbladder disease
Hypertension	It is well established that thiazides alter lipid profile, by raising cholesterol and triglycerides. Statins may themselves lower blood pressure, when used with antihypertensive drugs	Whether the increase in cholesterol with thiazides is sustained is unclear, but this adverse reaction may have a bearing on the treatment of borderline cases of hyperlipidaemia
Recent heart attack	The PRISM trial (PRISM Investigators 2002) has indicated that patients who are taking a statin before an MI are at increased risk of further cardiac events for the following week if the statin is abruptly withdrawn at the time of the initial event	This effect appeared to be independent of the effects of the statins on plasma lipids and may be due to the loss of other beneficial effects. This suggests that statin therapy should not be withdrawn abruptly in these patients
Renal impairment	May necessitate dose reductions	The risk of rhabdomyolysis is increased in those with renal impairment. Modified-release bezafibrate is not appropriate in renal impairment
Diabetes mellitus	Fibrates improve glucose tolerance with an additive effect in combination with hypoglycaemic agents	A reduction in the dose of hypoglycaemic agent may be necessary, particularly with clofibrate. Nicotinic acid should be used with caution
Gout	Nicotinic acid should be used with caution in gout	
Hypothyroidism	Increased risk of rhabdomyolysis with statins and fibrates	
Pregnancy	Statins, nicotinic acid and fibrates are contraindicated in pregnancy and breastfeeding	With statins, adequate contraception should be used during treatment and for 3 months after stopping
Postmenopausal osteoporosis	Statins may reduce bone turnover (Rejnmark *et al.* 2002)	
Peptic ulcer	Nicotinic acid should be used with caution	

BNF, *British National Formulary;* MI, myocardial infarction; PRISM, Platelet Receptor Inhibition in Ischaemic Syndrome Management.

Table 13.2 Summary of interactions within drugs used in hyperlipidaemia

Interaction	Consequences	Comments
Fibrates and statins	This beneficially results in additional lipid lowering but increases the risk of myopathy	Adverse interaction appears to be rare but the agents should be used with caution or a lower maximum daily dose
Colestyramine with fluvastatin/pravastatin	Increased lipid-lowering effect but reduced bioavailability of the statins	Colestyramine binds these statins and so giving the statins several hours afterwards improves bioavailability

General counselling

In a patient with hyperlipidaemia the counselling should first be directed at lifestyle advice to attempt to reduce plasma cholesterol and other risk factors for atherosclerosis. In relation to hyperlipidaemia it may be worth talking in terms of the blood containing too much of a fatty substance which, over time,

Table 13.3 Summary of interactions with drugs used in hyperlipidaemia

Interacting drugs	Consequences	Comments
Simvastatin and calcium-channel inhibitors	Simvastatin is commonly prescribed along with diltiazem, amlodipine and verapamil. All of these agents can increase the plasma concentration of simvastatin	The maximum daily dose of simvastatin is limited to 20 mg
Warfarin with fibrates or statins	Fibrates and some statins (Chapter 16) may increase the anticoagulant effect of warfarin	INR should be monitored
Warfarin with fish oils	Fish oils may have anticoagulant effects	Additional monitoring of clotting seems appropriate
Simvastatin and macrolides	This can lead to increases in the concentration of simvastatin and the risk of rhabdomyolysis	Avoid this combination. Plasma concentration of other statins may also be increased by macrolides
Simvastatin and grapefruit juice	High consumption of grapefruit juice can increase substantially the plasma concentrations of simvastatin. This is less marked for atorvastatin whereas pravastatin appears unaffected	Patients taking simvastatin should avoid drinking grapefruit juice
Statins or fibrates with ciclosporin	Increased levels of ciclosporin and increased risk of rhabdomyolysis with statins, particularly simvastatin, and fibrates	Simvastatin is contraindicated with ciclosporin and gemfibrozil. Pravastatin does not appear to interact adversely with ciclosporin
Statins with itraconazole	Itraconazole increases the levels of simvastatin with an increased risk of rhabdomyolysis	
Pravastatin with orlistat	Possible increase in levels of pravastatin	

INR, international normalised ratio.

can lead to the patient having a heart attack or stroke. The good news is that, by altering diet, with or without taking drugs, the risk of having a heart attack or stroke is reduced. The patient would be advised to reduce the intake of fatty foods, especially dairy products, and perhaps to consider a Mediterranean diet with plenty of oily fish, fruit and vegetables. Dietary changes alone may cause a modest reduction in plasma cholesterol but this is limited, because only 25–30% of cholesterol is derived from the diet. The importance of smoking cessation should be emphasised. Weight reduction, increased physical activity and reduction of excessive alcohol consumption would all be beneficial.

Patients with suspected familial hypercholesterolaemia should be advised that other members of their family should be screened and counselled.

Specific counselling for lipid-lowering therapy is detailed below.

Statins

- Statins (except atorvastatin which has a prolonged half-life) should be taken at night (this offsets a nocturnal increase in cholesterol synthesis).
- They may cause myopathy (rarely leading to rhabdomyolysis) and so patients should immediately report any unexplained muscle pains, tenderness or weakness to their general practitioner.
- Patients may expect to suffer from headaches, nausea and gastrointestinal pain. These side effects should improve as treatment continues.
- Statins exhibit a number of interactions. Some statins may enhance plasma levels of warfarin (see Chapter 17), and so patients should be advised to inform other healthcare professionals that they are receiving this drug. The international normalised ratio (INR) should

ideally be checked before and 5 days after treatment with an interacting drug.

- Simvastatin may interact with grapefruit juice and patients should be counselled to avoid drinking grapefruit juice.
- It is important to continue with the recommended dietary and lifestyle changes.

Fibrates

- Fibrates may cause myopathy (rarely leading to rhabdomyolysis) and so patients should immediately report any muscle pains to their GP.
- Side effects include rash, urticaria, weight gain, impotence and headache.

Anion-exchange resins

- Take other drugs or supplements 1 hour before or 4–6 hours after colestyramine.
- The powder may be used in sauces or added to fruit juice.
- The dose should be increased gradually and then taken regularly.
- Constipation is a common side effect. Nausea and vomiting, diarrhoea, flatulence and abdominal discomfort may occur but should improve after the first few months of treatment.

Fish oils

- These are best taken with food.
- They may cause occasional nausea and belching.
- Fish oils contain vitamins A and D. Avoid additional supplements containing these vitamins which are stored by the body.

Ispaghula

See Chapter 10.

Monitoring

Liver function

Liver function tests (LFTs) should be carried out before treatment with statins and within 3 months of initiating treatment. Liver function should then be monitored on a fairly regular (6-monthly to yearly) basis. A sustained rise in transaminase levels of three times the upper limit of the reference range would necessitate discontinuation of treatment.

Monitoring advice for patients prescribed fenofibrate indicates that LFTs should be repeated every 3 months for the first year. LFTs are also recommended before initiating long-term treatment with gemfibrozil.

Creatine kinase

A patient reporting muscle pains should have creatine kinase levels measured. A 10-fold elevation would be consistent with myopathy and treatment would be discontinued.

Over-the-counter considerations

Low-dose (10 mg) simvastatin (and other statins may soon follow) has been made available as an over-the-counter (OTC) medicine for patients who are at moderate risk of cardiovascular disease and these have been identified as:

- all men >55 years of age
- men aged 45–55 year of age and women >55 with one of the following:
- patients with a family history of ischaemic heart disease
- smokers
- overweight patients
- south Asians from the Indian subcontinent.

However, this presents a number of issues and the pharmacist should be vigilant for patients who may be presenting with evidence of IHD (such as angina) and should be referred to their doctor. Similarly, patients require full counselling with respect to reporting muscle pains, should be vigilant for signs of heptatoxicity (jaundice, itching, dark urine), and should be aware of significant interactions (which include those with HIV protease inhibitors, ciclosporin, azoles, fibrates, anticoagulants and macrolides). It would also be good practice to suggest that patients document their use of statins with their GP.

Although the wider availability of statins is a significant step in healthcare it does raise some issues. Its OTC use does not, surprisingly, require a cholesterol test or liver function monitoring. Furthermore, the use of simvastatin at 10 mg has not been established by trials as providing protection, e.g. the Heart

Protection Study (2002a) established the efficacy at 40 mg. There is also the issue that patients may buy simvastatin to offset an otherwise unhealthy lifestyle or bingeing and so its use should be alongside appropriate lifestyle advice.

In a patient with IHD or at a high risk from it, it would be sensible to consider low-dose aspirin as an antiplatelet drug and/or referral for a cholesterol test. Some pharmacists offer 'healthy heart checks', including blood pressure and cholesterol measurement, medical history taking and body mass index calculations to estimate the patient's risk of heart disease while providing lifestyle advice before coronary artery disease becomes symptomatic. High-risk patients should be advised to wear support hosiery during long flights to reduce the risk of thromboembolism (see Chapter 17). These can be purchased over-the-counter.

Requests for supplements should be considered in relation to prescribed treatment, e.g. patients taking warfarin should be advised to have their INR checked if they wish to take fish oils. Ideally, general diet and lifestyle advice should be given to all patients requesting food supplements (see Chapters 3 and 4).

Self-assessment

For the following questions concerning lipid-lowering drugs, choose the most appropriate answer:

1 *Statins act via inhibition of which one of the following?*

A HMG-CoA reductase
B Acetylcholine esterase
C Angiotensin-converting enzyme (ACE)
D Renin–angiotensin–aldosterone system
E HMRC

2 *Which one of the following statins can be taken at any time of the day?*

A Atorvastatin
B Fluvastatin
C Pravastatin
D Rosuvastatin
E Simvastatin

3 *Which one of the following can increase the plasma concentration of simvastatin and should be avoided?*

A Alcohol
B Cranberry juice
C Grapefruit juice
D Olive oil
E Raspberries

Practice points

- Monitoring of cholesterol should be carried out in those at increased risk of heart disease.
- Lifestyle and dietary measures should be tried first and continued alongside pharmacological intervention if ineffective alone. The maintenance of dietary measures may need emphasising to the patient.
- Statins have been shown to be effective in both primary and secondary prevention.
- Statins reduce cardiovascular risk irrespective of their cholesterol levels.
- NICE currently advocate atorvastatin at low intensity for primary prevention and high intensity for secondary prevention.
- The use of OTC statins requires full counselling and should be documented with the patient's general practitioner.
- Fibrates are effective in mixed hyperlipidaemia and hypertriglyceridaemia.
- Statins should be taken at night (except atorvastatin) and LFTs performed.
- Low-dose aspirin should be considered for all patients at risk of IHD.
- Health professionals should be alert to reports of muscle pain, tenderness or weakness by patients taking lipid-lowering drugs.
- Serious adverse effects with statins are very rare and patients should be reassured of their benefits.

CASE STUDY

A 58-year-old woman presents you with a prescription for simvastatin (40 mg daily every night). She is also taking atenolol (50 mg daily) having suffered a heart attack last year:

Are you happy to dispense the simvastatin? Justify your decision.

- Yes – there is no interaction with atenolol.

How would you counsel this patient?

- Take the simvastatin at night.
- Report any muscle pain or weakness immediately: rhabdomyolysis is a rare but important side effect.
- She may also initially expect headache, nausea and gastrointestinal pain.
- Discuss cardiovascular risks – give up smoking if appropriate; low-fat diet; moderate exercise; weight reduction if appropriate?
- Was she taking low-dose aspirin? If not, might this be appropriate?
- It is important that she continues to take the statin long term.

Why is the simvastatin to be taken at night?

- Simvastatin is taken at night, when cholesterol synthesis is greatest.

The patient would like to know what this new prescription is for; explain in lay terms why she has this new addition.

- The new medicine is to lower the amount of a fatty substance in her blood called cholesterol which is known to cause heart trouble. Lowering the cholesterol should reduce her chances of another heart attack.

A year later, while being maintained on simvastatin (40 mg daily every night), she presents with a prescription for erythromycin (250 mg four times daily) for sinusitis (she is allergic to penicillin).

How would you respond?

- Simvastatin should not be prescribed with erythromycin owing to the risk of increased plasma concentrations of simvastatin and of myopathy. The prescriber should be contacted and it might be suggested that a non-penicillin/non-cephalosporin antibacterial such as doxycycline be used as an alternative.

References

ASTEROID Trial Group (2006). Effect of very high-intensity statin therapy on regression of coronary atherosclerosis. *JAMA* 295: 1556–1565.

BIP Study Group (2000). Secondary prevention by raising HDL cholesterol and reducing triglycerides in patients with coronary artery disease: the bezafibrate infarction prevention (BIP) study. *Circulation* 102: 21–27.

British National Formulary, latest edition. London: British Medical Association and Royal Pharmaceutical Society of Great Britain.

Heart Protection Study Collaborative Group (2002a). MRC/BHF Heart Protection Study of cholesterol lowering with simvastatin in 20 536 high-risk individuals: randomised placebo-controlled trial. *Lancet* 360: 7–22.

Heart Protection Study Collaborative Group (2002b). MRC/BHF Heart Protection Study of antioxidant vitamin supplementation in 20 536 high-risk individuals: randomised placebo-controlled trial. *Lancet* 360: 23–33.

Kris-Etherton PM, Harris WS, Appel LJ (2002). Fish consumption, fish oil, omega-3 fatty acids and cardiovascular disease. *Circulation* 106: 2747–57. pmid: 12438303.

National Institute for Health and Care Excellence (2014). *Lipid Modification*. Clinical Guideline 181. London: NICE. Available at: www.nice. org.uk.

PRISM Investigators (2002). Withdrawal of statins increases event rates in patients with acute coronary syndromes. *Circulation* 105: 1446–1452.

Scandinavian Simvastatin Survival Study Group (1994). Randomised trial of cholesterol lowering in 4444 patients with coronary heart disease: the Scandinavian Simvastatin Survival Study (4S). *Lancet* 344: 1383–1389.

Shepherd J, Cobbe SM, Ford I *et al.* (1995). Prevention of coronary-heart disease with pravastatin in men with hypercholesterolaemia. *N Engl J Med* 333: 1301–1307. pmid: 7566020.

Shepherd J, Blauw GJ, Murphy MB *et al.* (2002). Pravastatin in elderly individuals at risk of vascular disease (PROSPER): a randomised controlled trial. *Lancet* 360: 1623–1630. pmid: 12457784.

VA-HIT Trial Study Group (1999). Gemfibrozil for the secondary prevention of coronary heart disease in men with low levels of high-density lipoprotein cholesterol. *N Engl J Med* 341: 410–418.

Online resources

www.bhf.org.uk
The website of the British Heart Foundation, providing patient information (accessed July 2015).

www.qrisk.org
QRISK2 website which enables cardiovascular risk to be determined (accessed October 2015).

14

Obesity

Disease characteristics

Worldwide obesity is reaching epidemic proportions and is largely related to an unhealthy lifestyle. With the exception of genetic causes (which are uncommon), obesity simply results from the intake of calories in excess of those required to meet energy demands. Indeed, the excess intake of small amounts of energy (e.g. 100 calories/day) over several years will lead to obesity. However, this apparently simple relationship is not easily modified, making obesity a particularly challenging condition. The complex picture of obesity includes genetics, lack of education, derangements of appetite, immobility, emotional problems, co-morbidity, e.g. hypothyroidism, and drug therapy. Drugs that are associated with weight gain include:

- antipsychotics
- corticosteroids
- hormone replacement therapy
- lithium
- oral contraceptives
- pizotifen
- sodium valproate
- sulphonylureas
- insulin
- glitazones
- tricyclic antidepressants.

In the UK more than half of women and approximately two-thirds of men are overweight or obese and the increased incidence of obesity in children is also of special concern. The main health consequences are hypertension and other cardiovascular disease, type 2 diabetes, gallstones and osteoarthritis. Indeed, alongside hypertension and hypertriglyceridaemia, obesity forms the so-called metabolic syndrome. Obesity has also been shown to increase the risk of various cancers (e.g. Reeves *et al.* 2007) and the World Health Organization has highlighted that, after smoking, obesity is the second most important modifiable risk factor for cancer-related mortality.

The health risks associated with obesity are in part related to the endocrine activity of adipose tissue, leading to the secretion of a wide range of physiological and pathological mediators. Elevated glucose levels and adipose-derived mediators lead to reduced insulin sensitivity associated with prediabetes and this ultimately leads to type 2 diabetes. The Prospective Studies Collaboration (2009) drew a clear relationship between body mass index (BMI), blood pressure and mortality.

Clinical features

In 2014 the National institute for Health and Care Excellence (NICE) produced detailed guidance for the management of obesity in adults and children according to BMI (in kg/m²), and co-morbidities. It is important to note that BMI should not be considered alone due to limitations of only considering weight and height, i.e. the BMI does not take into account body composition and does not assess the body's adiposity. Therefore people with significant muscle mass, such as rugby players, have high BMIs without the associated health risks. It is also important to note that obesity should be thought of as a clinical condition rather than associated with appearance. Classification using BMI and waist measurement is shown in Table 14.1. In addition, the distribution of fat is an issue, with central (abdominal) fat posing a risk factor for cardiovascular disease and diabetes and a more pelvic distribution or 'pear-shape' being seen as relatively protective.

Goals of treatment

Successful treatment will produce gradual weight reduction resulting in improved health and self-esteem. Weekly weight loss should not usually exceed 0.5–1 kg with the aim for an overall weight reduction of 5–10%. The central goal is a reduction in the risk of obesity-related conditions, especially cardiovascular disease and diabetes, and their associated mortality.

Management

General advice on healthy weight, diet and lifestyle

Treatment ranges from support and advice on increasing physical activity and reducing calorie intake to drug treatment and surgery. Clearly any diet regimen

needs to involve reducing calorific intake to below the daily expenditure (typically a deficit of 600 calories/day) and ensuring that it is balanced and benefits from low glycaemic foods and five portions of fruit and vegetables, and is low in fat and alcohol.

There is no convincing evidence that supports the efficacy of fashionable diets over simple calorie restriction, and the main dietary approach should be a calorie-reduced, balanced diet. Fashionable diets may also be associated with nutritional deficits. Examples include liquid-only or 'soup' diets and high-protein, high-fat diets such as the Atkins diet (Mason 2002b).

Additional treatment options include behavioural intervention such as cognitive–behavioural therapy (CBT) and, as a last resort, surgery. The limited availability of CBT means that it is not currently an option for all patients. CBT addresses both cognitive and behavioural aspects of overeating and is therefore important for producing long-term change. Patients need structured guidance to identify and change what may be life-long thinking patterns, attitudes and behaviour such as comfort or binge eating.

Patients who are overweight but have a relatively low waist circumference may benefit from general lifestyle advice as outlined in Chapter 3, together with verbal and written information about reaching a healthy weight and the benefits of this, in terms of reducing cardiovascular risk and the risk of developing diabetes.

Physical activity

All adults are encouraged to take regular exercise because this reduces the risk of type 2 diabetes and cardiovascular disease regardless of weight loss. Recommendations include the following:

- At least 30 minutes of moderate activity on at least 5 days a week in sessions not less than 10 minutes each.
- To prevent obesity 45–60 minutes of exercise per day may be required.
- To sustain target weight 60–90 minutes of exercise per day may be required.
- Ideally activities should form part of daily life, e.g. walking or cycling to work, leaving the bus at an earlier stop, climbing stairs, walking, vigorous housework or gardening.

Table 14.1 Classification of weight using body mass index	
Classification	**BMI (kg/m²)**
Healthy weight	18.5–24.9
Overweight	25–29.9
Obesity I	30–34.9
Obesity II	35–39.9
Obesity III	≥40

BMI, body mass index.

- Reducing periods of inactivity such as watching television and playing computer games.
- Consider the patient's fitness level, current lifestyle and ability, aiming for gradual and manageable change.

Pharmacological management

Treatment for obesity has proven a challenge over the years with a number of drugs being withdrawn due to safety concerns. The only drug in current use is orlistat.

Orlistat

Orlistat irreversibly inhibits pancreatic lipases, thereby reducing fat absorption. A proportion of dietary fat is therefore excreted in faeces. Indeed, the malabsorption of fat leads to steatorrhoea, which is the passing of oily stools and sometimes the loss of bowel control. These adverse effects actually contribute to the actions of orlistat because the patient would tend to avoid food with a high fat content. The malabsorption of fat also leads to reduced absorption of fat-soluble vitamins such as vitamin D, with possible consequences for calcium balance and bone mineralisation.

Drug choice

The NICE (2014) guidelines indicate that drug treatment should be initiated after a period of lifestyle and dietary change, for patients who have not reached their target weight. It should be stressed that lifestyle and dietary changes should be continued alongside drug treatment. Orlistat is recommended for patients with a BMI ≥28.0 kg/m^2 with co-morbidities or BMI ≥30 kg/m^2.

In addition to drug treatment, surgical interventions (bariatric surgery), which may involve stapling, banding or bypassing of the stomach to reduce volume and so restrict intake are used. These procedures appear to be effective in weight loss and also in the prevention of the onset of type 2 diabetes. At the moment surgery is advocated for patients with a BMI >40 kg/m^2 or, in the presence of diabetes or hypertension, a BMI >35 kg/m^2.

Drug interactions (Table 14.2)

Drug interactions involving orlistat occur due to reduced absorption, as might be expected.

Over-the-counter considerations

Orlistat is available as an over-the-counter medicine and pharmacists should be vigilant to its use as a substitute to healthy eating or lifestyle. Pharmacists should also be alert for the misuse of laxatives and herbal preparations, and patients referred to their general practitioner (GP) or local slimming club as appropriate.

Table 14.2 Examples of drug interactions involving orlistat		
Interacting drugs	**Consequences**	**Comments**
Orlistat with:		
Acarbose	Unknown	Manufacturers recommend avoidance of concurrent use
Other antidiabetics, e.g. glipizide, metformin, insulin	Glycaemic control may improve	Blood glucose levels should be monitored and doses of antidiabetic drugs reduced as appropriate
Ciclosporin	Absorption reduced significantly, possibly >50%	Closer monitoring is required and the dose of ciclosporin adjusted as appropriate
Warfarin	Possible increased INR	INR should be monitored closely for the first 4 weeks
Vitamins	Reduced absorption	Multivitamins should be taken at least 2 hours after orlistat or at bedtime

INR, international normalised ratio.

General counselling

The health benefits of losing weight should be emphasised. These include increased mobility and therefore improvement in arthritis, a greater feeling of wellbeing and reduced risk of diseases such as coronary heart disease, type 2 diabetes and some cancers. Advice should be practical and easily incorporated into people's lives, e.g. simple changes can include walking to school or the shops, taking the stairs rather than the lift. Recommended changes should be tailored to individual patients and include the following.

Weight

Ideal weight and waist measurement should be calculated and a realistic target of weight loss given. Weight loss should be no more than 0.5–1 kg/week.

Diet

Modifications to the diet need to be manageable. The recommendations for a healthy, balanced diet are given in Chapter 3.

Exercise

Exercise that is appropriate to the patient's current level of fitness and health should be recommended and preferably something that the person enjoys. The advice of the patient's GP should be sought in the presence of concurrent morbidity such as heart disease, diabetes and arthritis. Patients, including children, should be advised to reduce the time spent watching the television and playing computer games.

Children

The NICE (2014) guidelines recommend that clinical judgement be used do decide when it is necessary to measure the weight and height of children and that BMI charts are referred to. Routine waist measurement is not recommended. Physical activity should include at least 60 minutes of moderate exercise daily or several shorter sessions of at least 10 minutes each. It is useful for pharmacists to liaise with health visitors about local guidelines for dealing with excessive weight gain in children. The NICE guidance does not advocate the use of drug treatments unless there are compelling reasons such as co-morbidities.

Action points

- Setting healthy target weight, with the aim of losing approximately 5–10% of initial weight
- A maximum weight loss of 0.5–1 kg/week.
- Emphasis on long-term lifestyle changes.
- Using a variety of approaches to improve *both* diet and exercise.
- Recommending a healthy balanced diet.
- The provision of safe and realistic advice on increasing activity.
- Addressing techniques for changing behaviour such as encouraging patients to keep a diary and developing strategies to deal with regression to old habits.
- Patients should be given access to continued support.

Specific counselling points

Orlistat

- Should be taken in addition to long-term dietary and lifestyle changes.
- Take immediately before, during or up to one hour after each main meal (max. 360 mg/day).
- Dose should not be taken if a meal is missed or does not contain fat.
- Multivitamins should be taken at least 2 hours after orlistat or at bedtime.
- May cause liquid or oily stools and reducing fat intake should lessen these side effects.
- It should be used regularly, rather than avoided after fatty meals. Some patients might omit a dose after a fatty meal to avoid the unpleasant side effects of fatty stools and this undermines the purpose of the drug treatment (Ali 2002c).
- Other common side effects include respiratory tract infection, headache, gum problems and irregular periods.

Self-assessment

For the following questions concerning the management of obesity, choose the most appropriate answer:

1 *Orlistat acts via which mechanism?*

    A Inhibition of HMG Co-A reductase
    B Stimulation of lipolysis

C Inhibition of the cholesterol transporter

D Inhibition of amylases

E Inhibition of pancreatic lipases

2 *Orlistat is associated with which common side effect?*

A Steatorrhoea

B Steatosis

C Hypokalaemia

D Hyperkalaemia

E Hypertension

Practice points

- Be alert for weight gain as an adverse drug reaction and counsel patients as appropriate. The balance of risks versus benefits of treatment should be considered carefully.
- Signposting to local slimming clubs may help patients find the support that they need to lose weight. Check that these clubs meet best-practice standards set out by NICE.
- Consider setting up an obesity clinic, which could possibly target certain groups more likely to gain excess weight such as ante- and postnatal women, people attempting to stop smoking or menopausal women.
- Obesity should be thought of as a clinical condition rather than associated with appearance.
- Emphasise that exercise produces health benefits even in the absence of weight loss. This may prevent patients from giving up exercise if they are not losing weight.
- Display leaflets and posters supporting health campaigns. These are available from organisations such as the Food Standards Agency and the British Heart Foundation.

CASE STUDY

A 60-year old woman who is visibly obese is having concerns about her health since turning 60. Her general practitioner advised her to lose weight and increase physical activity but she has not reached her target weight and is finding it difficult to exercise because of painful knees. She refuses to be weighed or to allow measurement of her waist circumference. She has a family history of cardiovascular disease, has worked in a smoky environment for many years and had an early menopause. She is currently taking:

amlodipine 10 mg (once daily)
indapamide 2.5 mg (every morning)
atorvastatin 20 mg (once daily)
glucosamine with chondroitin for painful knees.

What risk factors does this patient have?

- Diabetes due to obesity and use of a thiazide-like diuretic.
- Osteoporosis due to early menopause.
- Cardiovascular disease owing to obesity, hyperlipidaemia, passive smoking, family history and early menopause.

What changes to treatment might her GP consider?

- ACE inhibitor: this would be appropriate, especially in view of her risk of diabetes.
- Orlistat: to support weight loss if BMI is sufficiently elevated.

(continued)

(continued)

- Vitamin D supplement if orlistat is prescribed.
- Glucosamine with chondroitin should not be recommended as there is no evidence to support their effectiveness.

Her treatment is changed to:

enalapril 5 mg (once daily)
amlodipine 10 mg (daily)
atorvastatin 20 mg (once daily)
orlistat 120 mg (three times daily).

How would you counsel the patient regarding her new prescription for orlistat?

- Drug-specific counselling for orlistat should focus on its role alongside a healthy, balanced diet and the avoidance of fat. Indeed, consumption of fat will lead to oily stools. The tablets should be taken during or just after a meal. Provide advice on exercise that the patient could try such as swimming, and reinforce healthy eating information. It may help to motivate the patient to lose weight knowing that weight loss may help her painful knees. The patient is likely to be particularly receptive to advice given her health concerns since turning 60. Local slimming clubs could also be recommended.

References

Mason P (2002a). Slimming. (1) OTC weight control products. *Pharm J* 269: 103–105.

Mason P (2002b). Slimming. (2) Popular slimming diets. *Pharm J* 269: 135–137.

National Institute for Health and Care Excellence (2014). *Obesity: identification, assessment and management of overweight and obesity in children, young people and adults*. Clinical Guideline 189. London: NICE.

Prospective Studies Collaboration (2009). Body-mass index and cause-specific mortality in 900 000 adults: collaborative analyses of 57 prospective studies. *Lancet* 373: 1083–1096.

Reeves GK, Pirie K, Beral V *et al.* (2007). Cancer incidence and mortality in relation to body mass index in the Million Women Study: cohort study. *BMJ* 335: 1134–1138. pmid: 17986716.

Rucker D, Padwal R, Li SK *et al.* (2007). Long term pharmacotherapy for obesity and overweight: updated meta-analysis. *BMJ* 335: 1194–1199. pmid: 18006966.

15

Ischaemic heart disease

Disease characteristics

Ischaemic heart disease (IHD), which is also referred to as coronary artery disease (CAD) or coronary heart disease (CHD), is the biggest killer in the Western world and so represents a crucial area for both prevention and treatment. IHD may manifest as either angina or myocardial infarction (MI) and is an important cause of chronic heart failure (see Chapter 16). In both cases, IHD is generally associated with atherosclerosis within the coronary artery, leading to impaired blood flow or thromboembolic occlusion. In angina the reductions in coronary blood flow mean that perfusion does not match demand, leading to ischaemia, which provokes the symptoms. In MI, there is often thromboembolic occlusion of the coronary artery, which may lead to acute left ventricular failure and/or arrhythmias; these are the leading cause of early mortality.

Risk factors for IHD include the following (*modifiable factors):

- male gender
- family history
- smoking*
- diabetes mellitus*

- hypercholesterolaemia*
- hypertension*
- sedentary lifestyle*
- obesity.*

Angina pectoris

Angina may be divided into two groups: stable and unstable. Stable angina reflects atherosclerotic disease, which limits the heart's ability to respond to increased demand and is characterised by symptoms that appear on exertion but are relieved by rest. By contrast, unstable angina is generally due to plaque rupture and the formation of a non-occlusive thromboembolism, or, less commonly, vasospasm (Prinzmetal's angina), both of which give rise to symptoms at rest.

The characteristic feature of angina is a crushing chest pain, which may radiate to the arm and jaw. Of course, chest pain may reflect a number of other causes (see Chapter 1):

- myocardial infarction
- dyspepsia
- musculoskeletal pain
- pulmonary embolism.

A diagnosis may be made on the basis of history and, in the case of stable angina, its provocation by exercise or eating a meal. The pain should be relieved by glyceryl trinitrate (GTN) and in stable angina is relieved by rest. An electrocardiogram (ECG) during an attack would confirm a diagnosis by showing ST-segment depression. Angina may also be secondary to increased cardiac work in anaemia (see Chapter 18) and hyperthyroidism (see Chapter 38), which should be excluded.

Goals of treatment of angina

Angina is a manifestation of IHD and the principal goal of treatment is the reduction of cardiovascular risk. In relation to the management of angina the specific goals are to:

- reduce symptoms
- improve exercise capacity
- reduce the risk of a heart attack
- stabilise or bring about regression of atherosclerotic lesions.

Management of angina

In the first instance, attention should be paid to reducing cardiovascular risk by smoking cessation, weight loss and dietary changes (see Chapters 3, 12 and 13). Treatment options include percutaneous transluminal coronary angioplasty to open the occlusion and the placing of a stent. Stents, which are essentially 'cages' are inserted at the diseased area to hold the vessel open and prevent restenosis. In some cases the stents are impregnated with cytotoxic drugs ('drug-eluting stents') to suppress the growth of blood vessels locally. Alternatively, coronary artery bypass grafting (CABG) is a surgical option in which the diseased artery is bypassed by a saphenous vein or internal mammary artery. CABG has been proved to offer longer-term relief of symptoms but is associated with a degree of operative mortality.

Pharmacological basis of the management of angina

Drug treatment is aimed at reducing cardiac work or improving coronary blood flow. The first group of agents to consider is the nitrates.

Nitrates: GTN, isosorbide mononitrate

Nitrates cause vasodilatation via the release of nitric oxide (NO), which gives rise to an increase in guanosine cyclic 3':5'-monophosphate (cGMP). In the context of angina, their beneficial effect is largely via venodilatation, leading to a decrease in preload and a reduction in cardiac work, although they may also cause coronary vasodilatation to improve coronary flow.

GTN is widely used for rapid symptomatic relief of an attack or may be given before exercise, which may provoke an attack. GTN may be given by a spray under the tongue or as a sublingual tablet. Isosorbide mononitrate tablets may be given orally with the aim of giving longer-term nitrate treatment.

β blockers

These are dealt with in detail in Chapter 12. In the context of angina they should be considered as first-choice drugs for prevention, with their negative inotropic and chronotropic effects reducing cardiac work and preventing symptoms. As coronary flow occurs only during diastole, then by slowing the heart the diastolic period will be increased, as will the time for coronary blood flow. They also have antiarrhythmic effects and reduce the risk of MI.

Calcium-channel blockers, e.g. amlodipine, diltiazem, felodipine, nifedipine, verapamil

Once again, these are dealt with in detail in Chapter 12. The calcium-channel blockers give rise to vasodilatation and improve coronary blood flow, so preventing symptoms. In addition, verapamil, and to a lesser extent diltiazem, also have myocardial-depressant and bradycardic actions, so reducing cardiac work. Verapamil also exerts class IV antiarrhythmic activity.

Angiotensin-converting enzyme inhibitors

Angiotensin-converting enzyme (ACE) inhibitors are dealt with in detail in Chapters 12 and 16. In addition, the Heart Outcome Prevention Evaluation (HOPE) trial (Yusuf et al. 2000) indicated that ramipril reduced mortality in patients with IHD and it may therefore be worth considering the addition of ramipril (or presumably any ACE inhibitor) to treatment of a patient with IHD.

Potassium channel activators: nicorandil

Nicorandil is a combined NO donor and activator of adenosine triphosphate (ATP)-sensitive K⁺ channels. The release of NO leads to an elevation in cGMP levels and the independent activation of ATP-sensitive K⁺ channels leads to vascular smooth-muscle hyperpolarisation with coronary artery vasodilatation and improved coronary flow. The vasodilator actions of nicorandil contribute towards its side effects of flushing and reflex tachycardia.

Ivabradine

This agent inhibits pacemaker sodium and potassium (i-funny (I_f) or 'funny current') currents in the sinoatrial node of the heart. This leads to bradycardia and reduces the work of the heart, which is of benefit in angina. Although its place in therapy has yet to be established, the INITIATIVE trial (2005) indicated that it was equally effective as atenolol but without the side effects associated with β blockers.

Ranolazine

Ranolazine reduces the work of the heart by reducing the late sodium current in the cardiac action potential; the consequence of this is the reduction of calcium entry as sodium is exchanged for calcium. The reduction in intracellular calcium reduces wall tension, which ordinarily impairs coronary microcirculation. The reduction in diastolic wall tension improves coronary blood flow, which is of benefit in ischaemic heart disease. Ranolazine does have the potential to cause the adverse effect of Q–T interval prolongation.

Choice of drugs (Figure 15.1)

All patients with angina are at a high risk of having an MI and so all patients should be considered for antiplatelet treatment with low-dose aspirin and/or clopidogrel. Low-dose aspirin is now well established as playing a major role in the primary and secondary prevention of MI. Aspirin inhibits irreversibly both

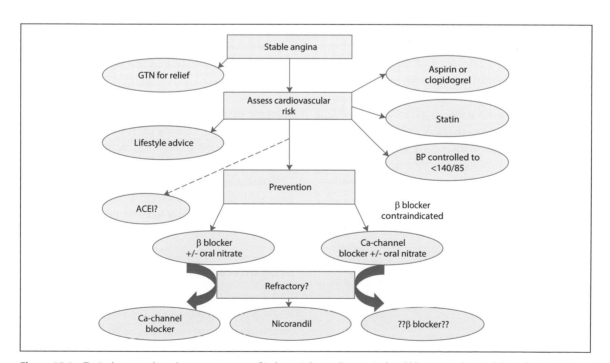

Figure 15.1 Typical approach to the management of ischaemic heart disease. It should be re-emphasised that, if a β blocker is combined with a calcium-channel blocker, this is usually safe with dihydropyridines, **but rate-limiting agents such as verapamil and diltiazem pose a serious risk of asystole and should be avoided**. ACEI, angiotensin-converting enzyme inhibitor; GTN, glyceryl trinitrate.

platelet and endothelial cyclo-oxygenases (COXs). The endothelial cells may regenerate COX but the platelets lack nuclei and cannot, so endothelial production of prostacyclin may be resumed shortly afterwards, although the production of thromboxane is impaired until a new cohort of platelets are produced. This leads to a state that opposes platelet aggregation. Other non-steroidal anti-inflammatory drugs (NSAIDs) may cause reversible inhibition of COX, leading to transient antiplatelet actions, so they are not suitable for primary or secondary prevention. There is some evidence that ibuprofen administered before aspirin may inhibit the actions of aspirin, presumably by protecting COX against aspirin (Catella-Lawson *et al.* 2001).

Clopidogrel is an equally effective alternative antiplatelet drug for patients intolerant of aspirin. Clopidogrel inhibits adenosine diphosphate (ADP)-induced expression of platelet glycoprotein IIb/IIIa, which is involved in aggregation by cross-linking fibrinogen.

Pharmacogenetics and antiplatelet drugs

A significant proportion (around a quarter) of patients are now recognised as being resistant to the protective effects of low-dose aspirin and do not derive benefit from this treatment. This resistance is apparently independent of its action at COX and it appears that patients do not benefit from other antiplatelet drugs. To confound the matter, this cohort of patients is also at a greater risk of cardiovascular events compared with aspirin-sensitive patients (Krasopoulos *et al.* 2008).

A proportion of patients are also unresponsive to clopidogrel. Although the mechanism of this is uncertain, there is a suggestion that some patients may have a deficiency or defect of the paraoxonase-1 (PON1) enzyme which is required for the biotransformation of clopidogrel to its active molecule (Bouman *et al.* 2011). This suggests that pharmacogenetic differences may mean that the drug is less effective or ineffective in some individuals.

Management

Attention should be paid to controlling blood pressure (to obtain a target of 140/85 mmHg; see Chapter 12) and managing hypercholesterolaemia (see Chapter 13).

For symptomatic relief or occasional treatment, a GTN spray or sublingual tablets would be appropriate.

In terms of continuous, the following are the preventive treatments:

- First choice: β blockers should be used for more pronounced stable and unstable angina (but not Prinzmetal's angina). Oral long-acting nitrates may be added.
- Second choice: if a β blocker is ineffective or contraindicated, then verapamil (or diltiazem) would be used or, failing that, a long-acting dihydropyridine. Calcium-channel blockers are particularity effective at reversing vasospasm and are first choice drugs for Prinzmetal's angina.
- In refractory disease: a β blocker may be used with dihydropyridine calcium-channel blockers *but not with verapamil* because there is a severe risk of asystole; diltiazem and β blockers may be used with caution. Nicorandil may also be added to therapy. If two agents fail to control the disease then surgical treatment may be required.

The large-scale IONA clinical trial (Impact Of Nicorandil in Angina) IONA Study Group 2002) has found that in stable angina nicorandil, in addition to standard therapy, reduced the incidence of cardiovascular events. This indicated that nicorandil afforded cardioprotection and it was proposed that by activating cardiac mitochondrial K_{ATP} channels it was able to mimic ischaemic cardiac preconditioning, the natural phenomenon whereby short periods of ischaemia protect the heart. This points to nicorandil as being of particular benefit in IHD.

Some compelling indications and contraindications are indicated in Table 15.1. In addition, patients with unstable angina are likely to be maintained on a low-molecular-weight heparin.

Drug interactions

Within antianginal drugs, the major within-group interaction is between β blockers and verapamil, because in combination they may cause asystole. All of the agents, by acting as vasodilators, may lead to hypotension, with the possibility of a fall in elderly people.

The effectiveness of the clopidogrel is thought to be reduced by omeprazole and esomeprazole, and these combinations should be avoided.

Table 15.1 Other considerations in the choice of antianginal agents

Condition	Drug choice	Comments
Heart failure	β blocker can be used with caution (Chapter 16) Verapamil is contraindicated	
Arrhythmias	May be a reason to use a β blocker or verapamil	Both agents are antiarrhythmic
Chronic obstructive pulmonary disease (COPD) and asthma	Contraindication for β blockers in asthma and caution in COPD	β blockers may lead to bronchospasm
Migraine	β blocker	β blockers are effective in migraine prophylaxis
Diabetes mellitus	May be a reason to avoid β blockers	β blockers may reduce the warning signs of hypoglycaemia
Hyperthyroidism	An indication for a β blocker	For reduction of cardiac effects in hyperthyroidism
Glaucoma	Closed-angle glaucoma is a contraindication for nitrates	
	Chronic simple glaucoma is an indication for a β blocker	In glaucoma, β blocker eye drops are absorbed and should not be used in addition to an oral β blocker

General counselling

Counselling should be directed towards a reduction in cardiovascular risk, with smoking cessation, weight reduction, increased exercise, reduced alcohol intake and dietary changes, to reduce the intake of saturated fats and increase oily fish in the diet or supplementation with fish oils. When explaining the disease to patients, one approach might be to tell them that their heart muscle is not getting enough blood to do the job that it used to do, and that the pains that they experience are similar to muscle cramp.

Nitrates

- GTN sprays or sublingual tablets should be used before an event likely to provoke an attack.
- The patient should be counselled on how to use a GTN spray and supervised in its use.
- GTN sprays or sublingual tablets may cause pronounced hypotension and are best taken while sitting.
- If a patient feels faint after GTN tablets the tablet should be spat out or swallowed; the patient could also bend over and place the head between the knees.

- GTN tablets have a short shelf-life of 8 weeks once opened and should be discarded after this time.
- When taking isosorbide mononitrate or dinitrate, there is a substantial risk of nitrate tolerance. This may be reduced by having a nitrate-free period, usually at night when symptoms are less. Patients may be advised to take their twice-daily nitrate tablets 8 hours apart, at say 8am and 4pm, to give a nitrate-free period. GTN patches should also be removed for several hours each day, perhaps at night.
- If GTN does not relieve an episode of chest pain, medical help should be sought immediately.
- Drugs that cause a dry mouth may reduce the effects of sublingual GTN.

β blockers

See Chapter 12.

Great emphasis should be made to ensure that patients do not stop taking the β blocker suddenly, because this is likely to lead to a worsening of symptoms and may increase their chances of having an MI.

Calcium-channel blockers

See Chapter 12.

Nicorandil

- Nicorandil may affect driving or operating machinery.
- Side effects are related to vasodilatation and may include headache.

Myocardial infarction

MI is often due to the formation of a thrombus at the site of rupture of an atherosclerotic plaque, leading to cardiac ischaemia and damage, with early deaths resulting from arrhythmias and late deaths from damage to the myocardium, which may cause heart failure. The necrotic muscle may rupture, leading to rupture of the ventricles (giving rise to tamponade) or pulmonary oedema if papillary muscles rupture and there is severe mitral regurgitation. Rupture of the septum leads to shunting, which requires surgery.

In full-thickness infarctions, the infarct may undergo thinning and stretch, causing ventricular dilatation and hypertrophy, which may lead to the development of heart failure at a later date.

Symptoms of MI

- Prolonged cardiac pain – chest, throat, arms, epigastrum or back
- Breathlessness
- Collapse
- Anxiety
- Nausea/vomiting.

Signs of MI

- Pallor/sweating/tachycardia (due to sympathetic activation)
- Vomiting/bradycardia (vagal)
- Signs of impaired cardiac function
- Hypotension, oliguria, cold extremities
- Weak pulse
- Lung crepitations
- Some (especially elderly) patients have a 'silent MI' with no signs or symptoms.

Differential diagnosis

- Dyspepsia
- Angina (which is relieved by GTN)
- Musculoskeletal pains
- Panic attacks
- Pulmonary embolism.

Diagnosis

The diagnosis is based on ECG changes (including ST-segment elevation) and increases in cardiac enzymes released by infarcted tissue. These are creatine kinase (CK), troponin T (TrT), aspartate aminotransferase (AST) and lactate dehydrogenase (LDH).

Management

Following the identification of an MI, the 'gold standard' treatment is an emergency angioplasty with stenting. Although the initial management of MI is beyond the scope of this book, a brief summary of additional or alternative measures is given in Table 15.2.

For patients who survive the initial MI the outlook can be good, with on average 80% being alive after 1 year, although the outlook is influenced by the initial presentation and development of heart failure. Therefore, in primary care the central issues are secondary prevention and prevention of long-term complications such as heart failure. All patients should be counselled with respect to lifestyle changes:

- weight reduction
- dietary advice, including increased intake of oily fish
- smoking cessation
- appropriate exercise.

Secondary prevention

In terms of drug treatment for secondary prevention in patients who have already had an MI there are a number of considerations and the following takes account of the National Institute for Health and Care Excellence (NICE) guidelines issued in 2007:

- Antiplatelet therapy with low-dose aspirin (75–150 mg) is established as substantially reducing reinfarction. In patients who are intolerant of aspirin due to asthma, clopidogrel is indicated, and it is equally effective. Low-dose aspirin is associated with gastric damage, and

Table 15.2 Management of a myocardial infarction

Treatment	Comments
Immediate	
Soluble or chewable aspirin (150–300 mg)	This may be given as a first-aid measure as an antiplatelet treatment to reduce further thrombus formation
Oxygen	To reduce hypoxia
Nitrates	To reduce ischaemia, but they have no bearing on mortality
IV morphine or diamorphine with antiemetics (cyclizine (but only if left ventricular function is satisfactory), prochlorperazine or metoclopramide)	• Morphine for relief of dyspnoea; also causes venodilatation to reduce preload and induces a degree of calm • An antiemetic to reduce nausea associated with opioids
Thrombolytic agent (e.g. alteplase, streptokinase, reteplase) as an alternative to angioplasty if this is not available	• Should be given to dissolve the clot as soon as possible (ideally within 90 minutes) and certainly within the first 12 hours, unless contraindicated (including recent surgery, peptic ulceration, current menstruation, pregnancy, recent stroke, history of haemorrhagic stroke) • Streptokinase can be given up to 4 days after an initial dose, but thereafter it should not be given for at least 12 months, if at all • Streptokinase may be ineffective in patients who have recently had a streptococcal sore throat, due to the production of antibodies • Streptokinase may cause an allergic reaction • Certain thrombolytic agents are now licensed for use before admission
Subsequent use of acute treatments	
β blocker	• Intravenous atenolol or metoprolol given early reduces arrhythmias and improves survival • Improves myocardial perfusion and reduces infarct size • Reduces chance of cardiac rupture • If β blockade is contraindicated and in the absence of heart failure, then verapamil might be used
ACE inhibitors	ACE inhibitors are recommended within the first 24 hours if there is evidence of heart failure emerging
Anticoagulants	Heparin given for 7–10 days post-MI after thrombolysis may prevent reinfarction
Nitrates	If systolic blood pressure >100 mmHg they may be given in the first 24 hours to reduce cardiac work
Antiarrhythmics	• Despite arrhythmias complicating post-MI, antiarrhythmics may increase mortality • Antiarrhythmics may be proarrhythmic on the ischaemic myocardium • β blockade is likely to have been initiated • Lidocaine is indicated for ventricular ectopics but is less widely used now
Insulin	Patients with diabetes often receive intensive insulin therapy from admission for 3 months because this reduces mortality

ACE, angiotensin-converting enzyme; MI, myocardial infarction.

prophylaxis with a proton pump inhibitor may be required (see Chapter 8). The addition of aspirin and clopidogrel can result in additive protective effects and they may be used in combination.

• β blockade: all patients should be considered for a β blocker to limit cardiac work and reduce the risk of rupture, to manage stable angina and hypertension and as an antiarrhythmic. β blockers are contraindicated in bradyarrhythmias. Long-term β blockade is well established at reducing reinfarction. If the patient has heart failure, the β blocker may be introduced (after an ACE inhibitor) at a low dose and under expert supervision, and would be contraindicated in severe heart failure.

- ACE inhibitors: all patients with heart failure should receive an ACE inhibitor. NICE guidelines point to an ACE inhibitor also being considered for patients without heart failure after they have been considered for a β blocker.
- Calcium-channel blockers: these should be considered only for patients who are intolerant of β blockers or ACE inhibitors and for the relief of angina and/or hypertension, because there is no evidence that they reduce mortality. Diltiazem or verapamil should be used with caution because of their cardiodepressant actions.
- Statins: these should be considered for all patients. Currently plasma cholesterol should be measured within 24 hours of the MI because it is believed that cholesterol falls for the first 3 months afterwards. Statins are believed to be equally effective to β blockers and antiplatelet drugs in secondary prevention.
- Diuretics: patients with symptomatic heart failure benefit from loop diuretics or thiazides. Patients

in moderate-to-severe failure benefit from the addition of spironolactone.

- Antiarrhythmics: there is no evidence that long-term treatment with these agents confers any benefit in the patient post-MI, but they may be needed in some patients.
- Anticoagulants: these drugs do not appear to have a long-term role in most patients and do not appear to confer any additional benefit to aspirin, except in patients with atrial fibrillation. Fiore *et al.* (2002) have reported that the addition of warfarin to low-dose aspirin does not confer further benefit in the secondary prevention of MI. NICE guidance suggests that moderate intensity warfarin therapy is appropriate for patients who cannot receive antiplatelet drugs.

Additional considerations

There is a high incidence of depression after an MI. In terms of drug treatment this may present a question of drug choice because tricyclic antidepressants have been associated with increased mortality in patients post-MI, especially if class I antiarrhythmics are also used. Currently, selective serotonin reuptake inhibitors (SSRIs, particularly sertraline) are considered more suitable.

A history of IHD may affect other treatments, which are detailed in Table 15.3.

Table 15.3 Examples of conditions that may be affected by a previous myocardial infarction

Condition	Problems	Comments
Migraine	• $5HT_{1D}$-receptor agonists (triptans) are contraindicated in patients with IHD • Ergotamine is contraindicated in IHD	The triptans may cause coronary artery spasm (Chapter 23)
Nicotine addiction	Nicotine replacement products should be avoided immediately post-MI	
Depression	Tricyclic antidepressants are contraindicated after recent MI and used with caution in cardiac disease	SSRIs appear to be more appropriate (Chapter 25)
Hypothyroidism	Levothyroxine	May cause anginal symptoms; monitor and reduce dosage in IHD (Chapter 38)
Impotence	Sildenafil	Risk of severe interactions with nitrates, as sildenafil inhibits phosphodiesterases and prevents the breakdown of cGMP. It is contraindicated after recent MI

5HT, 5-hydroxytryptamine (serotonin); cGMP, guanosine cyclic 3′:5′-monophosphate; IHD, ischaemic heart disease; MI, myocardial infarction; SSRIs, selective serotonin reuptake inhibitors.

Specific counselling

All of the counselling for specific drugs or classes is detailed in other sections:

- β blockers (see Chapters 12 and 16)
- ACE inhibitors (see Chapters 12 and 16)
- statins (see Chapter 13).

The only additional consideration is to advise patients who have received streptokinase to carry a card to alert medical staff who may treat them at a subsequent MI that they have previously received this agent.

Self-assessment

For the following questions concerning the management of ischaemic heart disease, choose the most appropriate answer:

1 *Which one of the following best describes the mechanism of action of β-adrenoceptor antagonists in angina?*

A Coronary vasodilatation
B Venodilatation
C Reduction in heart rate and prolongation of diastole
D Increased force of contraction
E Improved glucose utilisation

2 *Stable angina can be confirmed by which one of the following?*

A Increased levels of B-type natriuretic peptide (BNP)
B Increased levels of cardiac enzymes
C ST-segment depression on an ECG
D ST-segment elevation on an ECG
E The absence of P-waves on an ECG

3 *Nitrates used in angina act via which one of the following?*

A Potassium channels
B cAMP
C cGMP
D BNP
E Calcium channels

4 *Which one of the following does not form a standard secondary prevention regimen post-myocardial infarction?*

A A β-adrenoceptor antagonist
B An ACE inhibitor
C A statin
D An antiplatelet drug
E A nitrate

Practice points
- NICE guidance should be consulted for secondary prevention.
- For secondary prevention after an MI, patients are often prescribed a β blocker, an ACE inhibitor, a statin and an antiplatelet drug.

CASE STUDY

Mr PS (56 years) has recently suffered an MI and is on a cardiac ward. He was initially treated with diamorphine (5 mg i.v.) and cyclizine (50 mg i.v.), and he received an emergency angioplasty. On discharge he is now written up for:

aspirin 75 mg daily
clopidogrel 75 mg daily
atenolol 50 mg daily
atorvastatin 80 mg daily
ramipril 2.5 mg b.d.

(continued)

(continued)

Explain the use of all of the above drugs.

- Diamorphine – pain relief (pain can be severe in MI), and may induce some euphoria
- Cyclizine – H_1-receptor antagonist used as an antiemetic to prevent diamorphine-induced emesis
- Atenolol – an antiarrhythmic: reduces infarct size and cardiac work (risk of cardiac rupture); improves survival
- Atorvastatin – high-intensity therapy for secondary prevention
- Aspirin and clopidogrel are antiplatelet drugs used to reduce the risk of further thrombosis, including thrombus formation on the stent
- Ramipril – all post-MI patients should be discharged on an ACE inhibitor if appropriate.

How would you counsel the patient with regard to treatment with atorvastatin?

- Atorvastatin: the patient should stick to the recommended diet and report muscle pains straight away because they may indicate rhabdomyolysis. Ten per cent of patients have gastrointestinal disturbances. Avoid grapefruit juice.

On presentation of a repeat prescription to his community pharmacist, Mr PS complains of indigestion-type discomfort.

What do you advise?

- Refer to the general practitioner – the discomfort may be due to cardiac symptoms or gastric irritation caused by aspirin. Several years later Mr PS is experiencing chest pains and is prescribed glyceryl trinitrate (GTN) sublingual tablets (500 micrograms as required).

How would you counsel Mr PS?

- Take the GTN when symptoms develop or before provoking event.
- Sit down while taking the GTN.
- Place the tablet under the tongue.
- Spit it out or swallow the tablet if feel faint.
- Keep in the original container and discard after 8 weeks of opening.
- Any headache may be managed with paracetamol. The above treatment is only partially successful and Mr PS is now prescribed verapamil (80 mg three times daily).

Are you happy to dispense the new prescription?

- No – we do not know whether he is still taking atenolol. There is a risk of a serious interaction of β blockers and verapamil, and the cardiac depression could cause asystole.

References

Bouman HJ, Schomig E, van Werkum JW *et al.* (2011). Paraoxonase-1 is a major determinant of clopidogrel efficacy. *Nat Med* 17: 110–117.

Catella-Lawson F, Reilly MP, Kapoor SC *et al.* (2001). Cyclooxygenase inhibitors and the antiplatelet effects of aspirin. *N Engl J Med* 345: 1809–1817. pmid: 11752357.

Fiore LD, Ezekowitz MD, Brophy MT *et al.* (2002). Department of Veterans Affairs Cooperative Studies Program clinical trial comparing combined warfarin and aspirin with aspirin alone in survivors of acute myocardial infarction – primary results of the

CHAMP study. *Circulation* 105: 557–563. pmid: 11827919.

INITIATIVE Investigators (2005). Efficacy of ivabradine, a new selective I_f inhibitor, compared with atenolol in patients with chronic stable angina. *Eur Heart J* 26: 2529–2536.

IONA Study Group (2002). Effect of nicorandil on coronary events in patients with stable angina: the Impact Of Nicorandil in Angina (IONA) randomised trial. *Lancet* 359: 1269–1275.

Krasopoulos G, Brister SJ, Beattie WS *et al.* (2008). Aspirin 'resistance' and risk of cardiovascular morbidity: systematic review and meta-analysis. *BMJ* 33: 195–198.

National Institute for Health and Care Excellence (2007). *MI Secondary Prevention.* Clinical Guideline 48. London: NICE. Available at: www.nice.org.uk.

Yusuf S, Sleight P, Pogue J *et al.* (2000). Effects of an angiotensin converting-enzyme inhibitor, ramipril, on cardiovascular events in high-risk patients. The Heart Outcomes Prevention Evaluation Study Investigators. *N Engl J Med* 342: 145–153. pmid: 10639539.

Further reading

ACE Inhibitor Myocardial Infarction Collaborative Group (1998). Indications for ACE inhibitors in the early treatment of acute myocardial infarction. *Circulation* 97: 2202–2212.

Cohen HW, Gibson G, Alderman MH (2000). Excess risk of myocardial infarction in patients treated with antidepressant medications: association with use of tricyclic agents. *Am J Med* 108: 2–8. pmid: 11059434.

de Bono DP, Hopkins A (1994). The management of acute myocardial infarction: guidelines and audit standards. *J R Coll Phys Lond* 28: 312–317.

ISIS-2 (Second International Study of Infarct Survival) Collaborative Group (1988). Randomised trial of intravenous streptokinase, oral aspirin, both, or neither among 17187 cases of suspected acute myocardial infarction: ISIS-2. *Lancet* ii: 349–360.

McGlynn S, Reid F, McAnaw J *et al.* (2000). Coronary heart disease. *Pharm J* 265: 194–205.

Roose SP (2000). Considerations for the use of anti-depressants in patients with cardiovascular disease. *Am Heart J* 140 (suppl): 584–588.

Saltissi S, Mushahwar S (1995). Myocardial infarction: prophylaxis after infarction. *Prescribers J* 35: 149–158.

Scandinavian Simvastatin Survival Study Group (1994). Randomised trial of cholesterol lowering in 4444 patients with coronary heart disease: the Scandinavian Simvastatin Survival Study (4S). *Lancet* 344: 1383–1389.

Online resources

www.bhf.org.uk
The website of the British Heart Foundation, providing patient information (accessed July 2015).

16

Heart failure

Disease characteristics

In simple terms, heart failure may be viewed as a failure of the heart as a pump to meet circulatory needs and this may be either acute (e.g. following a heart attack or volume loading) or chronic. The underlying cause is failure of the heart muscle, sustained arrhythmias (such as atrial fibrillation) or failure of the heart valves (through infection or ageing-related changes).

The leading causes (70%) of chronic heart failure (CHF) are ischaemic heart disease and hypertension. In the case of hypertension, the increased afterload leads in time to hypertrophy. The cardiac enlargement thus increases the work of the heart and lessens the ejection fraction. Indeed, a compelling reason to treat hypertension is to reduce the likelihood of developing CHF. Heart failure associated with ischaemic heart disease (IHD) results from reduced blood flow, leading to impaired cardiac muscle function, with a reduction in pump performance. Cardiomyopathies due to alcohol abuse, infection and drug treatment (e.g. anthracycline anticancer drugs) may also cause CHF. Other causes of heart failure are pregnancy, anaemia, thyrotoxicosis, excessive infusion of intravenous fluids and fluid-retaining drugs (e.g. non-steroidal anti-inflammatory drugs [NSAIDs], corticosteroids, mineralocorticoids) and these should be excluded.

Both rate-limiting calcium-channel inhibitors (such as verapamil) and standard dose β blockers (such as atenolol) can depress cardiac activity and precipitate or exacerbate cardiac failure.

Underlying pathology

The key change, to which therapy is ideally targeted, is inappropriate neurohormonal adaptation. As a pathophysiological adaptation, in an attempt to compensate for circulatory failure, there is activation of the sympathetic nervous system and the renin–angiotensin–aldosterone system (RAAS), with increased release of antidiuretic hormone (ADH), although there is also a release of atrial natriuretic peptide from the dilated heart. Although these activations may seem logical to restore circulatory function, the increased sympathetic and RAAS activities increase arterial vascular resistance (afterload) and venous return (preload), thus increasing the workload of the heart. The increased sympathetic activity will also attempt to increase the force of cardiac contraction but will predispose towards arrhythmias. The attendant increase in circulating volume, evoked principally by the RAAS, will similarly increase preload and afterload on the heart. Consequent on the increased resistance there is impaired renal function, with additional salt and water retention and further activation of RAAS.

Hence a vicious cycle develops which further impairs the pump activity of the heart. A consequence of these changes is oedema (congestion) at different sites in the body and the term 'congestive heart failure' is also widely used (Figure 16.1).

The neurohormonal activation also leads to myocyte dysfunction, with increased aldosterone activity leading to fibrosis and stiffening of the cardiac muscle, further impairing pump activity.

Classification

Left-sided failure

- This is the most common form of heart failure, and is often secondary to hypertension.
- Left ventricular (systolic) function is impaired, with poor output leading to increased left atrial

and pulmonary venous pressures with pulmonary congestion and oedema.

Right-sided failure

- Right-sided failure is often due to chronic lung disease (cor pulmonale).
- Right ventricular output falls, leading to increased venous pressure, with peripheral oedema.

Biventricular failure

- Both main chambers are affected because left and right ventricular failure often coincide. Diseases such as IHD may have affected both ventricles.
- Often, left ventricular failure leads to pulmonary congestion, which in turn impairs right ventricular function, causing failure on the right side as well.

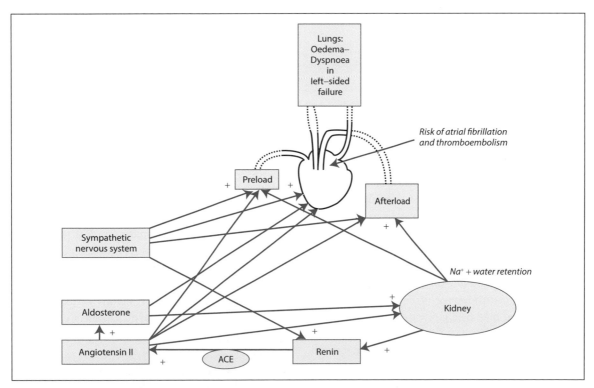

Figure 16.1 Principal pathophysiological changes and interactions in chronic heart failure. Activation of the renin–angiotensin systems leads to increased levels of angiotensin II (via angiotensin-converting enzyme [ACE]) which activates the release of aldosterone, promotes sodium retention, and causes arterial and venous vasoconstriction, and cardiac remodelling. The sympathetic nervous system also stimulates renin release and causes both arterial and venous vasoconstriction. Aldosterone promotes sodium retention and is associated with cardiac fibrosis. Sodium and water retention increase the circulating volume, with increases in preload and afterload.

Clinical features

As one might predict from a failure of the heart to meet circulatory needs, cardiovascular-related features are:

- reduced ejection fraction
- hypotension, leading to tiredness and possibly dizziness
- reduced urine flow
- cold peripheries
- breathlessness
- oedema.

With associated, non-specific symptoms:

- fatigue, listlessness
- poor exercise tolerance (determines grade)
- weight loss or even gain due to oedema.

Clinical staging of heart failure

This is largely stage (New York Heart Association or NYHA) dependent:

- stage I (asymptomatic)
- stage II (slight limitations through breathlessness/ fatigue on normal exertion)
- stage III (marked limitations through breathlessness/fatigue on normal exertion)
- stage IV (breathless at rest).

Left ventricular failure

The key feature is pulmonary oedema, which leads to dyspnoea with a sensation of drowning. There is often marked orthopnoea, because lying down leads to further venous congestion, which is relieved on sitting up or standing. This is particularly pronounced in bed and patients often describe having to go to the window 'to get air'. Using pillows to prop the patient up may relieve orthopnoea in bed and the number of pillows used may be a guide to the severity of this symptom. The pulmonary congestion may also lead to a cough, with sputum, which may or may not be frothy and contain blood.

Right ventricular failure

The leading feature of right ventricular failure is raised venous pressure, which leads to peripheral oedema (typically in the ankles on standing, and which may shift to the sacral regions while lying down). The raised venous pressure will also manifest as raised jugular venous pressure (JVP, which is raised if >4 cm from the clavicular line). The increased venous pressure may also lead to hepatomegaly (enlarged liver), with abdominal discomfort.

Although a diagnosis may be made on clinical features, it should be established by an echocardiogram, in which an ejection fraction of less than 45% is consistent with left ventricular failure. Heart failure may also be suggested by increased plasma levels of B-type natriuretic peptide (BNP), and this is also used as a diagnostic blood test.

Atrial fibrillation

A major and common consequence of cardiac failure is a build-up of back-pressure in the heart, as there is impaired ejection. This often leads to dilatation of the left atrium and the physical distension of the muscle causes disturbances in atrial electrical activity, resulting in atrial fibrillation. This does not greatly impair cardiac function; however, the consequent stasis of blood in the left atria increases the likelihood of thrombi forming. These may dislodge and travel to the cerebral circulation, giving rise to thromboembolic occlusion, resulting in transient ischaemic attacks or stroke.

The key feature of a patient with atrial fibrillation is an irregularly irregular pulse. Atrial fibrillation is readily identified on an electrocardiogram (ECG) as the absence of P waves and irregular QRS complexes.

Goals of treatment

The main goal of treatment is to improve the quality of life by relieving symptoms and, if possible, to reverse or modify the disease processes.

The simplest approach is to treat any underlying causes, such as valvular disease, IHD or atrial fibrillation. In these cases this may involve cardiac surgery.

The principles of medical management using drugs are to:

- decrease cardiac work, which may be achieved by using diuretics or vasodilators
- increase cardiac output, which may be achieved by using positive inotropic agents
- counteract maladaptation: the key goal, which involves blocking and reversing the neurohormonal adaptation; if this is achieved then the outcome should be improved.

Table 16.1 Summary of principal effects of drugs used in heart failure			
Drug	**Pharmacological targets**	**Mechanism**	**Effects**
ACE inhibitors	Renin–angiotensin system (RAS)	Inhibition of ACE	• Decreased arterial and venous vasoconstriction • Decreased blood volume • Decreased compensatory effects of RAS
β blockers	Myocardium	Antagonism of β_1-adrenoceptors	• Reduce sympathetic drive to the heart • Oppose neurohormonal adaptation • Antiarrhythmic actions
Loop diuretics	Kidney: loop of Henle	Inhibition of $Na^+/K^+/2Cl^-$ transporter in loop of Henle	• Na^+ excretion • Decreased blood volume • Decreased plasma K^+
Thiazide diuretics	Kidney: distal convoluted tubule	Inhibition of Na^+/Cl^- reabsorption	• Na^+ excretion • Decreased blood volume • Decreased plasma K^+
Potassium-sparing diuretics (amiloride)	Kidney: aldosterone-responsive segment of distal tubule	Decreased Na^+ permeability due to blockade of Na^+ channels	• Weak diuretic effect (increased Na^+ excretion) with decreased K^+ excretion
Potassium-sparing diuretics (spironolactone, eplenerone)	Kidney: as above	Aldosterone receptor antagonist	• Weak diuretic effect (increased Na^+ excretion) with decreased K^+ excretion • Reverses adverse effects of aldosterone on the heart
Digoxin	Myocardium, AV node	Inhibition of Na^+ pump	• Positive inotropic effects • Induces a degree of AV block
Nitrates	Vascular smooth muscle	Increased cGMP production	• Vasodilatation
α blockers (prazosin or mixed α/β blocker carvedilol)	Sympathetic nervous system	α-adrenoceptor antagonists	• Vasodilatation

ACE, angiotensin-converting enzyme; AV, atrioventricular; cGMP, guanosine cyclic 3′:5′-monophosphate.

If atrial fibrillation is present, additional aims are to control ventricular rate and prevent thrombus formation, reducing the likelihood of a transient ischaemic attack.

Pharmacological basis of management (Table 16.1)

ACE inhibitors, e.g. enalapril, lisinopril, perindopril, ramipril

ACE inhibitors are now recognised as first-line therapy in CHF and may be given to asymptomatic patients. They have been proved to both reduce symptoms and improve prognosis (Cooperative North Scandinavian Enalapril Survival Study [CONSENSUS] trial: Swedeberg, 1987). By inhibiting ACE (Figure 16.2), they lead to reductions in the neurohormonal adaptation due to angiotensin II and aldosterone, with the following consequences:

- reduction in arterial and venous vasoconstriction (reduced after- and preload)
- reduction in salt and water retention, hence reduced circulating volume
- indirect positive inotropic effect
- prevention and reversal of cardiac remodelling due to RAAS.

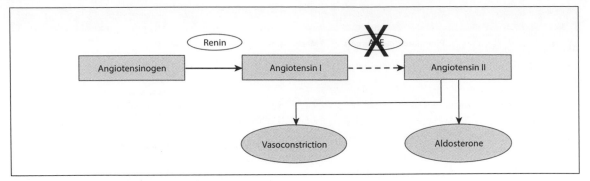

Figure 16.2 Mode of action of ACE inhibitors to interrupt the renin–angiotensin–aldosterone pathway.

Clinical use

By nature of their action, ACE inhibitors may cause severe hypotension (in about 2% of patients) and are best given initially on retiring at night. A low starting dose should be used and titrated up to the maximum tolerated dose. In certain patients at high risk, including those with a systolic blood pressure <90 mmHg, treatment should be initiated in hospital under supervision. There should be close monitoring of creatinine, urea and electrolyte levels before and after each dosage change.

The renin–angiotensin system is activated in renovascular disease in order to maintain renal perfusion and filtration. Hence ACE inhibitors may cause deterioration of renal function in pre-existing renal disease, and these patients should be identified by measurement of plasma creatinine and monitoring of renal function throughout treatment.

Angiotensin II receptor antagonists, e.g. candesartan, irbesartan, losartan, valsartan

This class of drugs blocks the action of angiotensin II at the angiotensin AT_1-receptor, which will also reduce the stimulation of aldosterone release. Hence AT_1-receptor antagonists act in a similar manner to ACE inhibitors but do not give rise to a cough. The ELITE II trial (Pitt *et al.* 2000) reported that losartan was equally effective at reducing mortality in elderly patients with heart failure to captopril, but it was also better tolerated. Similarly, results (Valsartan Heart Failure Trial or Val-HeFt: Cohn and Tognoni 2001) have indicated that valsartan improves the quality of life in patients with heart failure.

β blockers: bisoprolol, carvedilol and metoprolol

β-adrenoceptor antagonists were previously contraindicated in heart failure, because they reduce sympathetic drive to a failing heart or may precipitate failure in compensated failure. However, they play a major role in heart failure to reduce disease progression, symptoms and mortality (CIBIS-II Investigators and Committee 1999; MERIT-HF Study Group 1999). Principally, β blockers:

- reduce sympathetic stimulation, heart rate and oxygen consumption
- reduce sudden death by their antiarrhythmic properties
- oppose the neurohormonal activation which leads to myocyte dysfunction.

In addition, carvedilol causes vasodilatation as it is also an α blocker, and its antioxidant properties may be beneficial.

Clinical usage

Licensed β blockers such as bisoprolol are recognised as first-line agents in heart failure. The key concept is that they are used initially at a very low dose and this is then gradually increased ('start low and go slow') in relation to how well they are tolerated, usually assessed by the patient's blood pressure. However, they should be used with caution in patients with chronic obstructive pulmonary disease (COPD), which is relatively common in the patient population with the highest incidence of heart failure. Their use would also be contraindicated in hypotension and marked bradycardia.

Diuretics: loop diuretics (e.g. furosemide), thiazide and related thiazide-like agents (e.g. bendroflumethiazide, indapamide, metolazone)

Diuretics are the mainstay of drug treatment in heart failure and provide rapid symptomatic relief. Diuretics reduce circulating volume, thus decreasing pre- and afterload, and hence cardiac work. In addition, they may have direct vascular effects leading to venodilatation, which further reduces preload. Diuretics provide relief for the symptoms of congestion but do not affect the progression of the disease.

Thiazides act in the distal convoluted tubule to inhibit Na^+/Cl^- reabsorption. Loop diuretics inhibit the $Na^+/K^+/2Cl^-$ co-transporter in the thick ascending limb of the loop of Henle, inhibiting the establishment of a hyperosmotic interstitium and so reducing the ability of the kidneys to produce concentrated urine, leading to profuse diuresis.

Clinical use

The rational use of diuretics includes situations where there is oedema (peripheral or pulmonary). Thiazides induce modest diuresis and are used in mild failure or in elderly people. Loop diuretics, which are more extensively used, cause very pronounced diuresis and are especially useful in causing rapid relief of pulmonary oedema. Indeed, intravenous furosemide rapidly reduces the dyspnoea associated with pulmonary oedema in acute left ventricular failure. This effect precedes the diuresis and is thought to be due to venodilatation reducing preload on the heart.

Why do thiazides and loop diuretics cause hypokalaemia?

Hypokalaemia is a major side effect of these diuretic agents. By acting on the kidney, largely before the distal tubule, these agents increase the sodium content in the tubular fluid. Under the control of aldosterone, the distal tubule attempts to reabsorb sodium (via amiloride-sensitive sodium channels) but at the cost of excreting potassium. In addition, these agents will also provoke the release of renin and the activation of RAAS, which will further promote the excretion of potassium. By contrast, ACE inhibitors will oppose the aldosterone-sensitive potassium loss and

there is a risk of significant hyperkalaemia if the ACE inhibitor is given in addition to potassium supplements or potassium-sparing diuretics (e.g. amiloride, spironolactone).

Aldosterone receptor antagonists: spironolactone and eplenerone

Aldosterone or mineralocorticoid receptor antagonists are also weak potassium-sparing diuretics used in CHF. They are used at low doses, which do not have pronounced haemodynamic effects but reverse the aldosterone-mediated neurohormonal changes. Even after ACE inhibition, aldosterone levels may still be appreciable, so spironolactone is able to exert substantial beneficial effects. It is thought that they inhibit aldosterone-induced fibrosis, which otherwise stiffens the heart and is associated with arrhythmias. It may also inhibit the adverse effects of aldosterone on autonomic and baroreceptor function. The RALES trial (Pitt *et al.* 1999), in which low-dose spironolactone was added to conventional therapies, indicated that this treatment reduced mortality by 30%.

Digoxin

Digoxin used to be the mainstay of therapy and has been in and out of fashion over many years. Its principal action is as a positive inotrope by inhibiting Na^+/K^+ ATPase (which causes a rise in intracellular sodium, promoting calcium entry, and leading to increased force of contraction). However, digoxin also directly and indirectly (via central vagal activation) impairs atrioventricular conduction. This induction of heart block and bradycardia is beneficial in heart failure with atrial fibrillation because it controls ventricular rate. Indeed, it is now widely believed that digoxin should be reserved for heart failure with atrial fibrillation, or when treatment with an ACE inhibitor and a diuretic is inadequate for patients in sinus rhythm.

Clinical usage

Digoxin improves the patient's symptoms, reduces hospitalisation but does not affect all-cause mortality (DIG trial: Digitalis Investigation Group 1997). Digoxin has a very narrow therapeutic window and is largely renally excreted, which means that renal function should be taken into account, with dose reductions to prevent increased plasma concentrations and toxicity. Digoxin is associated with a range of significant side effects which include:

- anorexia
- nausea
- gastrointestinal disturbances
- visual disturbances
- arrhythmias.

Vasodilators

Nitrates in particular may have a role in CHF because they will cause venodilatation, leading to a reduction in preload. Many patients will also have IHD and so nitrates will be of benefit in these patients. Nitrates may be suitable for people in whom ACE inhibitors are not tolerated, but are contraindicated in hypotension and marked anaemia.

Other vasodilators that may be added on to therapy are α blockers such as prazosin, which will reduce peripheral resistance by opposing sympathetic activity. They are of no proven benefit. The arterial vasorelaxant hydralazine is also used as an add-on drug or for those intolerant of ACE inhibitors.

Other positive inotropes

In addition to digoxin, phosphodiesterase inhibitors (PDEIs) such as milrinone have a limited role. These drugs act to potentiate adenosine cyclic 3':5'-monophosphate (cAMP) in myocytes and so have positive inotropic effects; they are used in end-stage failure on a short-term basis in hospital. It should be noted that their long-term use is associated with increased mortality.

Amines such as dobutamine, which acts as a β agonist, similarly may have a role in the management of acute failure and end-stage failure in the context of specialist hospital care.

Choice of drugs

Both ACE inhibitors and licensed β blockers (initially using a low dose) have central roles and should be used in all cases of left ventricular systolic dysfunction. Although both classes of drug are used 'first line', it is usual to initiate an ACE inhibitor with upwards titration before introducing a β blocker and this is dependent on the patient's blood pressure. If patients are intolerant of ACE inhibitors because of the associated cough, then AT_1-receptor antagonists may be used instead. Combination therapy of an ACE inhibitor and an AT_1-receptor antagonist should be avoided due to the increased risk of adverse events. The purpose of the combination of an ACE inhibitor with a β blocker is to modify the disease. In addition to this combination, diuretics and especially loop diuretics are used for the symptomatic relief of associated oedema.

For patients whose condition is not fully controlled by an ACE inhibitor/β blocker combination, the next step is the introduction of an aldosterone receptor antagonist. If the patient is still refractory to treatment, digoxin is often introduced.

Concurrent disease

Additional considerations when prescribing in CHF:

- Renal impairment may preclude the use of ACE inhibitors and thiazides and lead to a dose reduction with digoxin. In moderate failure higher doses of loop diuretics are required and in anuria their use would be precluded.
- Liver function: close monitoring with ACE inhibitors is important in liver disease. Warfarin and carvedilol should be avoided and a reduced dose of metoprolol may be required. The use of potassium-sparing diuretics may be necessary. This is due to the risk of precipitating coma if hypokalaemia develops during treatment with loop and thiazide diuretics. There is also an increased risk of hypomagnesaemia in alcoholic cirrhosis. Thiazides should be avoided in severe liver disease.
- Atrial fibrillation would be a compelling reason to use digoxin and an indication for an anticoagulant (see Chapter 17). Amiodarone may also be required.
- Asthma would preclude the use of a β blocker because of the risk of bronchospasm. This is

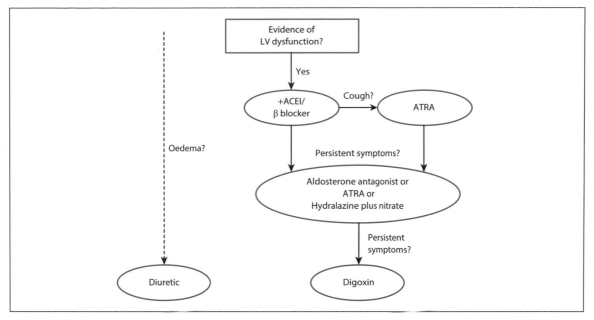

Figure 16.3 Current approaches to the management of chronic heart failure incorporating National Institute for Health and Care Excellence (NICE 2010) guidance. Approaches to managing atrial fibrillation in CHF are also indicated. ACEI, angiotensin-converting enzyme inhibitor; AT, angiotensin; ATRA, angiotensin-receptor antagonists; LV, left ventricular.

less clear cut in the case of COPD, where the beneficial effects of β blockers in heart failure are significant. The current view is that in patients with concurrent COPD the cautious use of cardioselective β blockers is acceptable.

- Diabetes mellitus may be a reason not to use a thiazide (due to risk of hyperglycaemia) but may be a compelling reason to use an ACE inhibitor (see Chapter 37). Blood pressure and plasma glucose concentration should be monitored regularly.

- History of stroke would be an indication for perindopril alone or in combination with indapamide. The PROGRESS Collaborative Group (2001) trial has indicated that perindopril alone or in combination with indapamide reduces the incidence of stroke (both haemorrhagic and thromboembolic) in patients who have previously suffered any type of stroke. It remains to be determined if this is specific to perindopril and indapamide or whether it applies to any ACE inhibitor plus a thiazide. Cerebral haemorrhage would be a contraindication for the use of nitrates.

- Many patients with ischaemic heart disease go on to develop CHF. Many of these patients will be taking a standard dose of a β blocker such as atenolol, which may itself exacerbate the condition and the β blocker should be replaced with a low dose of a licensed agent such as bisoprolol.

- Risk of infection from influenza and pneumonia would be a reason to consider immunisation with influenza and pneumococcal polysaccharide vaccines, respectively.

Additional considerations are: Wolff–Parkinson–White syndrome (contraindication for digoxin); closed-angle glaucoma (contraindication for nitrates); Addison's disease (contraindication for thiazides); and gout (contraindication for thiazides).

CHF may itself influence drug choice in unrelated conditions: important examples are summarised in Table 16.2.

Drug interactions

In the context of drug choice, the interactions between drugs used in CHF should be considered (Table 16.3).

Table 16.2 Examples of how chronic heart failure may influence drug choice in other conditions

Condition	Drugs	Comments
Diabetes	Pioglitazone	May cause oedema and exacerbate CHF and should be avoided
Migraine	$5HT_1$-receptor agonists – triptans and ergotamine	Coronary vasoconstriction in ischaemic heart disease or Prinzmetal's angina. Also contraindicated with nitrates
Glaucoma	Timolol eye drops	Systemic effects of β blockade
Thyroid disease	Levothyroxine	Risk of rapid increase in metabolism and activation of sympathetic nervous system
Bipolar affective disorder	Lithium	Lithium concentrations increased by ACE inhibitors and diuretics
Depression	Tricyclic antidepressants	Prolongation of Q–T interval. Risk of arrhythmias and sudden death
Pain	NSAIDs	Risk of Na^+ and fluid retention, renal failure with ACE inhibitor
	Sodium load from soluble paracetamol	
Indigestion	Antacids	Na^+ content should be considered. Absorption of prescribed drugs may be affected
Infection	Erythromycin, clarithromycin	Prolongation of Q–T interval. Risk of arrhythmias and sudden death. Macrolides interact with amiodarone, warfarin, digoxin and antihyperlipidaemic agents
Menopause	HRT (also oral contraception)	Contraindicated in thromboembolic disorders
Angina, hypertension, Raynaud's phenomenon	Verapamil, diltiazem	May cause or worsen CHF (bradycardia)
COPD	High doses and chronic use of $β_2$-adrenoceptor agonists	Risk of serious hypokalaemia. Regular monitoring required

ACE, angiotensin-converting enzyme; CHF, chronic heart failure; COPD, chronic obstructive pulmonary disease; HRT, hormone replacement therapy; NSAIDs, non-steroidal anti-inflammatory drugs.

Table 16.3 Summary of important interactions within drugs used in chronic heart failure

Interaction	Consequences	Comment
ACE inhibitor with potassium-sparing diuretics or potassium supplements	Hyperkalaemia	ACE inhibitors and potassium-sparing diuretics both oppose aldosterone, leading to potassium retention
Loop diuretics or thiazides with digoxin	Enhanced effects of digoxin	Diuretic-induced hypokalaemia will enhance the actions of digoxin
Digoxin with captopril, telmisartan, amiodarone or spironolactone	Increased plasma concentrations of digoxin	Pharmacokinetic interaction
Digoxin with β blockers	Bradycardia, increased AV block	Addition of actions
Diuretics with vasodilators	Hypotension	Addition of actions

ACE, angiotensin-converting enzyme; AV, atrioventricular.

General counselling

One approach to explaining CHF to a patient is that the heart is simply not able to pump the blood as well as it used to, making exercise more difficult. Patients may notice that they have become increasingly breathless and their ankles swell. In some cases it may be appropriate to avoid mentioning failure, and use of terms such as 'congestion' may be helpful. The purpose of the drug treatment is either to reduce the work of the heart or to make it beat more forcefully. Other points to consider:

- General counselling would follow the lifestyle advice outlined in Chapters 3 and 12.
- If the patient is taking diuretics, it would be worth suggesting cutting out excess salt in the diet, because this would undo the beneficial effects of the diuretic.
- Patients are at risk of developing secondary depression as a consequence of reduced quality of life or with the realisation of the seriousness of their condition. The GP should be alert to this and may wish to consider antidepressant therapy.
- In the presence of orthopnoea, patients would be advised to prop themselves up with pillows in bed at night.
- Patients taking ACE inhibitors, diuretics, α blockers, β blockers and nitrates should be alerted to the problems of hypotension and orthostatic hypotension, and the possibility of having a fall. They should be advised to stand up slowly.
- Patients should be advised to report muscle cramps, pain, nausea or vomiting, which may indicate hypokalaemia. Confusion may point to hyponatraemia.
- Patients should be alert for changes in heart rate and palpitations.

Specific counselling

ACE inhibitors

- Patients may experience pronounced first-dose hypotension; it is best to take the first doses of the ACE inhibitor immediately before retiring to bed at night. First-dose hypotension may be worse if the patient is also taking diuretics and the diuretic may be stopped for a few days before the ACE inhibitor is initiated.
- Discuss any cough with the general practitioner. Patients should be encouraged to persist with the ACE inhibitor, because this is the most effective treatment. The ACE inhibitor could be changed or an angiotensin receptor antagonist used.
- Consult a pharmacist before purchasing other medicines or supplements, e.g. avoid use of potassium salts (salt substitute, effervescent preparations, cystitis treatments), and use caution with NSAIDs.
- ACE inhibitors can very rarely lead to angioedema and patients should be alerted to this and report swollen lips and eyelids.

β blockers

- Beneficial effects may not be immediate and there may be a worsening of symptoms.
- Male patients may experience impotence.
- Report any additional breathlessness (due to worsening of symptoms or blockade of bronchial β_2-adrenoceptors); cold extremities or peripheral weakness may reflect blockade of vasodilator β_2-adrenoceptors.
- Do not suddenly stop taking the tablets.

Diuretics

- Male patients should be informed of possible impotence as a side effect.
- Diuretics (or 'water tablets') will cause an increase in urine flow, usually after 2 hours of taking the dose. This may subside after a couple of weeks. In the case of furosemide, it may be worth pointing out that diuresis may be pronounced.
- It is best to take the diuretic in the morning to limit sleep disturbance. A dose may be taken later in the day to avoid the need for urination interfering with social engagements during the day. If two daily doses are required, they may be taken at 7am and 1pm.
- Omit a dose during periods of diarrhoea and vomiting to prevent dehydration and electrolyte disturbances.
- If appropriate, correction of oedema may be monitored by the patient's weight.

- Sunscreen advice may be appropriate to avoid photosensitivity reactions.

Digoxin

- Patients should be advised to report signs of toxicity, e.g. nausea, vomiting, diarrhoea, disturbances of vision or loss of appetite.
- As digoxin may cause arrhythmias, patients should also report dizziness, an irregular heartbeat or palpitations.
- Ensure the pulse does not fall below 60 beats/minute. If this occurs, the patient should omit the next dose.

Nitrates

Patients may experience a throbbing headache, which should be relieved with paracetamol.

Spironolactone

Male patients may be advised of the small risk of breast enlargement (gynaecomastia), which in itself is harmless.

Hydralazine

Patients should report any weight loss, arthritis or ill health because this may suggest systemic lupus erythematosus.

α blockers

- Patients should be alert to first-dose hypotension.
- Patients may also experience urinary incontinence.

Monitoring

Renal function (creatinine)

- This should be monitored before treatment to determine estimated glomerular filtration (eGFR) rate, because this may be impaired through age or CHF. This is important, because thiazides (except metolazone, which is rarely used) are ineffective in moderate renal failure. Furthermore, digoxin is largely, but not entirely, excreted renally and so in renal impairment there should be a dose reduction, or digitoxin, which is not renally excreted, should be used instead.

- ACE inhibitors are contraindicated in renovascular disease.
- Renal function may deteriorate slightly after initiating an ACE inhibitor or diuretic and this may require dose reduction. eGFR should then be checked after 2 weeks and after each dose change.

Electrolytes

Ideally, potassium levels should be monitored a week after starting diuretic treatment or adjusting treatment and then at least annually once the regimen is stabilised. Sodium may also be affected, presenting as hyponatraemia in which the patient may become confused. Thiazides are also associated with hypomagnesaemia and hypercalcaemia.

Hyperkalaemia

ACE inhibitors, by inhibiting the production of angiotensin II and aldosterone, will tend to cause potassium retention, leading to hyperkalaemia. This may become significant if the ACE inhibitor is taken with a potassium-sparing diuretic or potassium supplements, and their concurrent use is contraindicated or they should be used with great care (e.g. regular monitoring).

Hypokalaemia

Thiazides (especially) and loop diuretics cause hypokalaemia, which is associated with increased fatal arrhythmias. Hypokalaemia is less of a problem if ACE inhibitors are also used because they have the opposite effect (as mentioned above). Hypokalaemia is especially problematic in patients taking digoxin, because hypokalaemia potentiates its pharmacological actions and may lead to toxicity. If hypokalaemia occurs in patients not receiving an ACE inhibitor (unlikely nowadays), the patient may benefit from the addition of a potassium-sparing diuretic or, less commonly, potassium supplements. Digoxin should be withheld until the hypokalaemia is corrected.

Digoxin

Ideally, plasma levels should be measured on a regular basis, although this does not often happen in practice. Plasma concentrations of digoxin should be measured (6–12 hours post-dosing, see Appendix 2) at regular intervals because toxicity is a common occurrence. As commented above, patients or their carers should be told to ensure that their heart rate does not fall below 60 beats/minute, and this will also act as a rough therapeutic monitor.

Over-the-counter considerations (Table 16.4)

The main problems with over-the-counter (OTC) products result from sodium or potassium content, sodium retention or sympathomimetic activity. Due to the complex nature of CHF treatment there is also a great potential for drug interactions. The pharmacist is ideally placed to identify concordance problems, side effects of prescribed medicines or worsening symptoms, and can advise the patient accordingly, e.g. a classic side effect of ACE inhibitors is a persistent cough, which may result in failure of treatment due to poor patient concordance. Patients should be encouraged to continue with the ACE inhibitor despite the cough, because alternative treatments may be less effective.

Alternative medicine

In an attempt to avoid polypharmacy and in the absence of reliable clinical trial data, the concurrent use of herbal drugs and conventional medicines should be discouraged. Many herbal drugs exhibit pharmacological activity and therefore have the potential to produce the undesirable side effects outlined with conventional medicines above, e.g. there is some evidence that herbal medicines may exhibit sympathomimetic activity, diuretic or antiplatelet effects. Food supplements may also interact with conventional medicines (see Chapters 3 and 4).

Self-assessment

For the following questions concerning chronic heart failure, choose the most appropriate answer:

1 *Which one of the following pathophysiological changes occurs in chronic heart failure?*

A Decreased renin levels
B Increased levels of B-type natriuretic peptide (BNP)
C Decreased sympathetic activity
D Increased parasympathetic activity
E Decreased levels of aldosterone

2 *Which one of the following is* not *a clinical feature of left-sided cardiac failure?*

A Breathlessness
B Peripheral oedema
C Orthopnea
D Cardiomegaly
E Reduced exercise tolerance

Table 16.4 Over-the-counter (OTC) medicines to avoid in chronic heart failure	
OTC products	**Comments**
Na⁺: table salt, high-salt foods (bacon, crisps, etc.), soluble preparations, indigestion remedies (Na⁺-free alternatives are available), cystitis treatments	Increased Na⁺ will reduce the effect of treatment or enhance renal impairment with ACE inhibitors
K⁺: salt substitute, cystitis treatments (low-sodium or potassium citrate mixture), some indigestion remedies	Interaction with ACE inhibitors and K⁺-sparing diuretics with a risk of hyperkalaemia
Cough and cold remedies containing decongestants (pseudoephedrine, phenylpropanolamine)	Decongestants may increase blood pressure due to sympathomimetic activity
NSAIDs (aspirin, ibuprofen, ketoprofen) in oral and topical analgesics	In addition to drug interactions, the use of NSAIDs may exacerbate heart failure. Gout may be a side effect of thiazides and ibuprofen would be unsuitable
Laxatives (senna, lactulose)	Chronic use of laxatives may cause electrolyte disturbances
Caffeine (analgesic preparations)	Caffeine may cause myocardial ischaemia

ACE, angiotensin-converting enzyme; NSAIDs, non-steroidal anti-inflammatory drugs.

3 *Which one of the following drugs should be avoided in a patient with chronic heart failure?*

A Rate-limiting calcium-channel inhibitors (such as verapamil)

B Thiazide diuretics (such as bendroflumethiazide)

C Cardiac glycosides (such as digoxin)

D β_2-adrenoceptor agonists (such as salbutamol)

E AT_1 receptor antagonists (such as losartan)

4 *What should be monitored prior to using an angiotensin-converting enzyme (ACE) inhibitor (such as ramipril)?*

A Lung function

B ECG

C eGFR

D Sodium levels

E Haemoglobin levels

5 *Which one of the following is an important adverse effect of taking an ACE inhibitor (such as ramipril)?*

A Hypokalaemia

B Breathlessness

C Peripheral oedema

D Gastric bleeding

E Angioedema

6 *Which one of the following is a contraindication to using an ACE inhibitor (such as ramipril)?*

A Asthma

B Diabetes mellitus

C Atrial fibrillation

D Hyperthyroidism

E Renovascular disease

7 *Which one of the following is a significant adverse effect of loop diuretics (such as furosemide)?*

A Bradycardia

B Hypoglycaemia

C Hypertension

D Stroke

E Hypokalaemia

8 *Which one of the following is a key counselling point when introducing a β blocker for the management of heart failure?*

A Your symptoms may initially worsen

B Take with food

C Take prior to exercise

D Do not drive

E Do not take any aspirin-containing medicines while taking this

9 *Which one of the following concurrent conditions might worsen when a β blocker is used in chronic heart failure?*

A Stable angina

B Ischaemic heart disease

C Chronic obstructive pulmonary disease

D Atrial fibrillation

E Hypertension

10 *In a patient with heart failure which is not controlled by the use of a loop diuretic, an ACE inhibitor and a β blocker combination, which is the next step in therapy?*

A An α blocker (such as prazosin)

B An anticoagulant (such as warfarin)

C An aldosterone-receptor antagonist (such as spironolactone)

D Adrenaline

E A non-selective β blocker (propranolol)

Practice points

- Be observant for symptoms suggestive of heart failure, particularly in high-risk patients such as after a myocardial infarction.
- Treatment should be aimed at relieving symptoms and reducing the risk of death.
- Take steps to prevent readmission to hospital: ensure good symptom control, improve concordance with medicines and diet, reduce alcohol consumption, recognise psychological problems and lack of social support.
- Lower doses of diuretics should be used initially in elderly people due to an increased risk of side effects.
- ACE inhibitors and β blockers improve both symptoms and prognosis and have a major role in the management of CHF as first line agents.

- Regular monitoring is essential, particularly for patients taking digoxin. Potassium-sparing diuretics can cause severe hyperkalaemia in patients taking an ACE inhibitor.
- Angiotensin AT_1-receptor antagonists may have an important role in patients intolerant of ACE inhibitors.
- β blockers are used according to the recommendation 'to start low and go slow'.

- People with CHF are at high risk of developing arrhythmias and of sudden death. Arrhythmias should be investigated and treated as appropriate.
- Be vigilant of the use of OTC medicines and supplements in patients with CHF.
- Patients should be warned about first-dose hypotension with ACE inhibitors and α blockers (extra caution in combination with diuretics).

CASE STUDY

Mr IHD is a 65-year-old man with a history of ischaemic heart disease, which is managed by:

Verapamil 120 mg (t.d.s.)
Glyceryl trinitrate spray 400 micrograms p.r.n.
Aspirin 75 mg (o.d.)
Simvastatin 40 mg (o.n.)
However, he was admitted to hospital with pulmonary oedema secondary to chronic heart failure.

What symptoms are associated with pulmonary oedema?

- Shortness of breath
- Orthopnea
- Cough

What should be prescribed to Mr IHD for the immediate management of pulmonary oedema?

- Add 20–50 mg furosemide i.v.

Following admission to Cardiology, Mr IHD underwent tests which indicated:

Test	Result	Reference range
Full blood count	Normal	
Thyroid status	Normal	
Echocardiogram	Ejection fraction = 38%	>45%
B-type natriuretic peptide (BNP) levels	400 pg/mL	<100 pg/mL
eGFR	70 mL/minute per 1.73m³	>90 mL/minute per 1.73m³
Plasma potassium	4.0 mmol/L	3.5–5 mmol/L

(continued)

(continued)

As Mr IHD is confined to bed in hospital, what is he at risk of and what actions should you take?

- Mr IHD is at risk of deep vein thrombosis and should receive thromboembolic-deterrent (TED) stockings and be treated with a low-molecular-weight heparin (see Chapter 17).

Which drugs should be continued and which drugs should be introduced to therapy?

- Stop verapamil because of its cardiodepressant actions and replace with a dihydropyridine calcium-channel inhibitor (and possibly an oral nitrate?)
- Add ACEI (e.g. ramipril 1.25 o.d.)
- Add furosemide 40 mg (o.m.)
  Simvastatin 40 mg (o.n.) (20 mg if amlodipine prescribed)
  Aspirin or clopidogrel

  One week later, Mr IHD has been stabilised and is ready for discharge into the care of his general practitioner.

Devise a management plan to continue and optimise Mr IHD's treatment for chronic heart failure. Your plan should include regimens, any additional drugs and patient monitoring.

- Upwards titration of ACEI to maximum licensed dose, so long as tolerated. Monitor blood pressure, electrolytes and eGFR.
- As long as his blood pressure is fine, once ACEI established then introduce licensed β blocker (e.g. bisoprolol).
- Bisoprolol: 1.25 mg o.d. with upwards titration – 'start low and go slow'.

  One year later Mr IHD's condition is well controlled. However, his eGFR is now 20 mL/minute per 1.73m^3.

How might this affect his therapy? What actions might you take?

- Reduce the maximum dose of ramipril to 5 mg.

References

CIBIS-II Investigators and Committee (1999). The Cardiac Insufficiency Bisoprolol Study II (CIBIS-II): a randomised trial. *Lancet* 353: 9–13.

Cohn JN, Tognoni G (2001). A randomized trial of the angiotensin receptor blocker valsartan in chronic heart failure. *N Engl J Med* 345: 1667–1675. pmid: 11759645.

Digitalis Investigation Group (1997). The effect of digoxin on mortality and morbidity in patients with heart failure. *N Engl J Med* 336: 525–533.

MERIT-HF Study Group (1999). Effect of metoprolol CR XL in chronic heart failure: Metoprolol CR XL Randomised Intervention Trial in Congestive Heart Failure (MERIT-HF). *Lancet* 353: 2001–2007.

National Institute for Health and Care Excellence (2010). *Chronic Heart Failure: management of chronic heart failure in adults in primary and secondary care.* Clinical guidance 108. London: NICE.

Pitt B, Zannad F, Remme WJ *et al.* (1999). The effect of spironolactone on morbidity and mortality in patients with severe heart failure. *N Engl J Med* 341: 709–717.

Pitt B, Poole-Wilson PA, Segal R *et al.* (2000). Effect of losartan compared with captopril on mortality in patients with symptomatic heart failure: randomised trial – the Losartan Heart Failure Survival Study ELITE II. *Lancet* 355: 1582–1587. pmid: 10821361.

PROGRESS Collaborative Group (2001). Randomised trial of a perindopril-based blood-pressure-lowering regimen among 6105 individuals with previous stroke or transient ischaemic attack. *Lancet* 358: 1033–1041.

Swedeberg K (1987). Effects of enalapril on mortality in severe congestive-heart failure – results of the Cooperative North Scandinavian Enalapril Survival Study (CONSENSUS). *N Engl J Med* 316: 1429–1435. pmid: 2883575.

Further reading

Cleland JGF, Swedberg K, Poole-Wilson PA (1998). Successes and failures of the current treatment of heart failure. *Lancet* 353 (suppl): 19–28.

Cowie MR, Zaphiriou A (2002). Management of chronic heart failure. *BMJ* 325: 422–425. pmid: 12193359.

Perry G, Brown E, Thornton R *et al*. (1997). The effect of digoxin on mortality and morbidity in patients with heart failure. *N Engl J Med* 336: 525–533. pmid: 9036306.

Seed A, McMurry J (2001). Current approaches to treating heart failure. *Prescriber* 12: 75–95.

Online resources

www.bhf.org.uk
The website of the British Heart Foundation, providing patient information (accessed July 2015).

17

Thromboembolic prophylaxis

Thrombosis

Thrombosis is the unwanted formation of blood clots and may be venous or arterial. Venous thrombosis is associated with stasis of blood: the major problem is that the clot may become dislodged and travel to the lungs, leading to a life-threatening pulmonary embolism. By contrast, thrombosis formed at an atherosclerotic site may lead to arterial blockage in the heart (myocardial infarction; see Chapter 15), cerebral vessels or the peripheral circulation, resulting in ischaemia and infarction. In addition, atrial fibrillation is associated with the stasis of blood and the formation of thrombi in the left atria, which may become dislodged and result in embolism of cerebral vessels, leading to a cerebrovascular accident. Other important thrombogenic sites include artificial mechanical heart valves.

Venous thrombosis is largely associated with an inappropriate activation of the clotting cascade; the thrombi formed have a high fibrin but a low platelet content. Once again, arterial thrombosis has different characteristics, with platelet activation playing a central role. This has a bearing on prevention, because venous thrombosis is largely managed by anticoagulants and arterial thrombosis largely by antiplatelet agents (see Chapter 15), although anticoagulants may also have a role in limiting recruitment of the clotting cascade in arterial thrombosis. Thrombosis associated with atrial fibrillation involves activation of both clotting factors and platelets, hence anticoagulants are used.

Risk factors for venous thrombosis include oral contraceptives, hormone replacement therapy, a history of thrombosis, recent surgery, immobility, obesity, pregnancy, malignancy and previous myocardial infarction. Risk factors for arterial thrombosis are detailed in Chapter 15.

Goals of treatment

The goals of treatment are prophylaxis against either arterial or venous thrombosis, and the preventive treatment is targeted at those at risk. Specific targets for treatment with the anticoagulant warfarin are detailed in Table 17.1.

Pharmacological basis of management

Anticoagulants

Injectable anticoagulants: unfractionated heparin and low-molecular-weight heparins (e.g. dalteparin, enoxaparin, tinzaparin)

Heparin is a glycosaminoglycan found naturally in mast cells and the vascular endothelium. Due to the size of this polymer, heparin is poorly absorbed from the gastrointestinal tract and is therefore given by subcutaneous or intravenous injection.

Table 17.1 Target international normalised ratios for various indications for warfarin

Indication	Target INR	Duration of treatment
Pulmonary embolism	2.5	6 months
Proximal deep vein thrombosis	2.5	6 months
Calf vein thrombosis (non-surgical)	2.5	3 months
Postoperative calf vein thrombosis	2.5	6 weeks
Recurrence of deep vein thrombosis or pulmonary embolism in patients not taking warfarin	2.5	Indefinite
Recurrence of deep vein thrombosis or pulmonary embolism in patients already taking warfarin	3.5	Indefinite
Atrial fibrillation	2.5	Long term
Mural thrombosis after an MI	2.5	3 months
Mechanical prosthetic heart valves	2.5–3.5 (depends on valve type)	Lifelong

Information obtained from the oral anticoagulant guidelines of the British Society for Haematology (1998; updated 2005). INR, international normalised ratio; MI, myocardial infarction.

Heparin activates antithrombin III, a natural protein, which inactivates some clotting factors and thrombin by complexing with their serine protease component. Accordingly, the effects of heparin are rapid in onset and are given when anticoagulation is required immediately. Heparin is available as either unfractionated heparin (average molecular mass 15 kDa) or low-molecular-weight heparin (LMWH) (average molecular mass 4.5 kDa). Compared with unfractionated heparins, LMWHs have greater activity against factor Xa and less against thrombin. Unfractionated heparins may also reduce platelet aggregation, which does not occur with LMWHs.

Oral anticoagulants: warfarin

Warfarin is a vitamin K antagonist, which inhibits the enzyme vitamin K epoxide reductase complex required for vitamin K to act as a cofactor in the production of clotting factors. In this regard, vitamin K is essential for the post-translational modification by carboxylation of glutamic acid residues of prothrombin and factors VII, IX and X. Accordingly, warfarin inhibits the hepatic synthesis of these clotting factors and its action is apparent only after several days, once the existing clotting factors have been replaced by these newly synthesised, defective factors. The inhibition persists for 4–5 days after the withdrawal of warfarin.

Oral anticoagulants: thrombin inhibitors (e.g. dabigatran) and factor Xa inhibitors (e.g. apixaban, rivaroxaban)

The difficulty in using warfarin (narrow therapeutic window, the need for monitoring and numerous interactions) has meant that drug discovery has aimed to develop safer oral anticoagulants. Dabigatran has been introduced to therapy and acts via inhibition of thrombin in the coagulation cascade. Apixaban and rivaroxaban are similarly oral anticoagualants which inhibit factor Xa in the coagulation cascade. Experience of these novel drugs is increasing, there are fewer interactions and their actions appear more predictable. As their safety and efficacy are being established they are increasingly replacing warfarin in certain patient groups. Their biggest disadvantage is that, unlike warfarin, they do not a have a selective antagonist to reverse their effects.

Antiplatelet drugs

Aspirin and clopidogrel are dealt with in Chapter 15, in the context of their major role in the primary and secondary prevention of myocardial infarction and cerebrovascular accidents. Dipyridamole is also an antiplatelet drug that is thought to act via phosphodiesterase inhibition and so potentiate cAMP (adenosine cyclic 3′:5′-monophosphate), leading to an inhibition of platelet activation. This mechanism of action will potentiate endogenous prostacyclin and synergise with low-dose aspirin. Antiplatelet drugs are no longer recommended for the prevention of thrombosis in atrial fibrillation.

Clinical use of anticoagulants

Oral anticoagulants have a number of indications to prevent thrombosis, which are listed in Table 17.1. To initiate treatment with warfarin it must be borne in mind that it will take several days for full effects to become apparent, while in the meantime there may be an increased chance of clotting due to lowering of the levels of protein C (a protein generated from a vitamin K-dependent precursor, which destroys certain clotting factors). Therefore, heparin is started at the same time to 'anticoagulate' the patient and this should be continued until the target international normalised ratio (INR) has been achieved and maintained for 2 days.

Use of heparin

Heparin may be used to initiate anticoagulant treatment or is given for a short, defined period for the prevention of postoperative thromboembolism, e.g. after surgery and in particular after orthopaedic surgery. In terms of clinical use, LMWHs have the advantage of once-daily administration by subcutaneous injection.

The anticoagulant effects of unfractionated heparin are monitored daily by the activated partial thromboplastin time (APTT), with a target value of 1.5–2.0, and the dose is altered to maintain this. By contrast, LMWHs do not require monitoring because their effects are predictable (and they do not prolong APTT). In addition, the use of heparin is associated with thrombocytopenia (less so with LMWH) and with sustained use (>5 days) the platelet count should be monitored.

Initiation of warfarin

Before starting warfarin, it is appropriate to monitor liver function and the INR. The INR is the key

anticoagulant screen for warfarin and is the prothrombin time (the normalised time for thromboplastin to cause clotting when added to citrated plasma compared with a standard). The INR is measured during initiation to achieve a target, which depends on the indication (Table 17.1), and should be maintained at this level by altering the dose of warfarin. The INR should be determined daily or on alternate days and then at longer intervals, depending on response (unless a change in clinical condition or administration of other drugs dictates otherwise). Once stabilised, the INR should be monitored at least every 12 weeks.

Warfarin is not indicated for ischaemic stroke without atrial fibrillation. After coronary artery thrombosis, coronary artery bypass grafting or coronary angioplasty, low-dose aspirin (see Chapter 15) and/or heparin should be considered. Heparin is also considered for unstable angina.

When initiating treatment, the patient is typically loaded with warfarin doses of 10 mg, 10 mg and then 5 mg on three consecutive days and the INR should be reviewed on day 4 to determine the maintenance dose. In patients who initially have a higher INR (>1.2), e.g. through age, liver disease or warfarin-potentiating drugs, the loading doses should be reduced.

For patients whose anticoagulant therapy is poorly controlled and who have an elevated INR, a number of procedures may be carried out. These are given in more detail in the *British National Formulary* but, depending on the extent of increase, involve dose reduction or withholding doses, oral or intravenous vitamin K and, in the presence of severe bleeding, the administration of clotting factors or, failing that, fresh frozen plasma. Heparin is reversed with protamine, although it is less effective against LMWHs.

Drug choice

Before initiating warfarin treatment, patients must be identified as able to adhere strictly to the regimen and sufficiently motivated and compliant to ensure that their INR is monitored regularly.

Atrial fibrillation

Oral anticoagulants play a major role in the prevention of thrombosis and associated stroke in atrial fibrillation. In recommending therapy the risk of stroke is associated in relation to the risk of bleed as a consequence of anticoagulation, and this may be carried out by the CHA_2DS_2-VASc score. Traditionally warfarin has been prescribed to patients with a significant risk and now the newer agents such as dabigatran or apixaban may be used. According to NICE (2014) these agents might be considered for older patients and also for patients with co-morbidities such as diabetes, hypertension or heart failure.

In terms of a comparison between warfarin and dabigatran, the RELY trial (2009) established that dabigatran was equally as effective as warfarin when used at 110 mg twice daily and was associated with a lower incidence of major haemorrhage. At the higher dose of 150 mg twice daily it was more effective than warfarin at reducing stroke but with a comparable risk of major haemorrhage.

Anticoagulation following a previous bleed

One of the greatest therapeutic challenges is in managing a patient who has previously had a haemorrhagic stroke while on warfarin for anticoagulation in atrial fibrillation. Once again difficult decisions are required regarding the risk of further bleeds versus the desirability to anticoagulate the patient.

Deep vein thrombosis

Deep vein thrombosis (DVT) is associated with immobility leading to stasis of blood and hypercoagulability: pregnant and postoperative patients are at an increased risk. The major complication is that the thrombus may dislodge and lead to a life-threatening pulmonary embolism. Patients with DVTs should be heparinised and non-pregnant patients should then be initiated on warfarin.

DVTs with the potential to lead to pulmonary embolisms have been a major concern for patients who are immobile in hospital. All inpatients are assessed for their risk of a DVT and supplied with thromboembolic-deterrent (TED) stockings and treated with prophylactic LMWH as appropriate.

'Economy-class syndrome'

This term describes DVT leading to pulmonary embolism associated with prolonged travel; whether it is exacerbated by air travel has yet to be established. It is associated with immobility, and so exercise and wearing compression stockings may be effective. Recommended exercises include short walks, bending and straightening legs, feet and toes, and pressing feet on the ground. Passengers should also avoid excess alcohol and becoming dehydrated. Passengers with a moderate risk for DVT (e.g. pregnancy, heart disease, family history of DVT, hormonal contraception, hormone replacement therapy) may consider low-dose aspirin and support stockings. Recommending low-dose aspirin to all passengers seems unwise, as the risk of gastric bleeding in the general population is greater than the risk of DVT. The Department of Health (2001) advised that patients at high risk due to previous DVT, clotting tendency (thrombophilia), a history of cancer, major surgery in the past 3 months (including hip or knee replacement) or stroke should consult their GP. High-risk patients may be prescribed an LMWH and/or advised to wear compression stockings.

Pregnancy

Warfarin is teratogenic if it is given during the first trimester and particularly after 6 weeks of gestation. During the last few weeks of pregnancy and during delivery warfarin may cross the placenta, leading to a risk of placental or fetal haemorrhage. Vitamin K deficiency of neonates may also be an issue. Warfarin should therefore be avoided during pregnancy and in particular during the first and third trimesters. Heparin does not cross the placenta into the fetus and may be used under expert supervision, although prolonged use is associated with osteoporosis.

Concurrent disease

Warfarin is contraindicated in peptic ulcer disease, severe hypertension and bacterial endocarditis and should not be used in cerebral thrombosis or peripheral arterial occlusion as first-line therapy. It should be used with caution after recent surgery. Warfarin itself is associated with a significant risk of haemorrhagic stroke.

Heparin is also contraindicated in patients with peptic ulcer, severe hypertension in addition to haemophilia and other haemorrhagic disorders, thrombocytopenia, recent cerebral haemorrhage, severe liver disease including oesophageal varices, major trauma or recent surgery.

Hepatic disease

Oral anticoagulants should be avoided in severe liver disease, particularly if the prothrombin time is already prolonged. The dose of heparin should be reduced in severe liver disease.

Renal disease

Oral anticoagulants should be avoided in severe renal impairment. There is an increased risk of bleeding when heparin is given in severe renal impairment.

Monitoring

INR, APTT and platelets

See earlier.

Electrolytes

Heparin inhibits aldosterone secretion and may possibly result in hyperkalaemia. The risk increases with prolonged therapy and in patients with diabetes mellitus, chronic renal failure, acidosis and those taking drugs that increase plasma potassium (such as potassium-sparing diuretics and angiotensin-converting enzyme [ACE] inhibitors; see Table 2.2, and Chapters 12 and 16). Potassium levels should be monitored before starting heparin in patients at risk and regularly throughout treatment, particularly if the treatment period is >7 days.

Drug interactions

Potentiation

Warfarin shows a notoriously wide range of drug interactions, which are of clinical importance because of its narrow therapeutic index. The most common interactions usually result in the enhancement of anticoagulant activity, and this appears largely to result from competition or inhibition of hepatic metabolism, although it is sometimes through displacement from protein-binding sites. The enhancement may lead to increased bleeding. Inhibitors of metabolism are likely to have rapid effects on the levels of warfarin. However, this alteration will take several days to have an effect on the INR and these effects will reverse on stopping the inhibitor, although, in the case of drugs with long half-lives, such as amiodarone, they may persist for some time. The dose of warfarin may then need to be altered.

In choosing drugs for patients who are taking warfarin the ideal is to select drugs that do not interact. When starting drugs known to interact with warfarin the British Society for Haematology (1998) recommends the following:

- For drug changes lasting fewer than 5 days with a known potentiating drug: no change, minor dose reduction for warfarin or omit one dose of warfarin.
- For longer drug changes: monitor INR after 1 week and alter warfarin dose accordingly.

In addition, when warfarin is initiated in a patient who is already taking a known interacting drug, the loading dose may need to be altered.

Some important drugs that may enhance the actions of warfarin (D indicates that a dose reduction of warfarin is likely) include:

- allopurinol
- amiodarone – may persist after discontinuation of amiodarone due to its long half-life (D)
- azapropazone (contraindicated)
- azoles – fluconazole, ketoconazole, miconazole
- clarithromycin
- co-trimoxazole (D)
- cytotoxic agents (carboplatin, mustine, cyclophosphamide, doxorubicin, etoposide, 5-fluorouracil, ifosfamide/mesna, methotrexate, procarbazine, vincristine and vindesine)
- disulfiram (D)
- erythromycin
- fibrates (D)
- H_2-receptor antagonists, cimetidine (famotidine, nizatidine and ranitidine are less likely to interact)
- hydrocodone (rarely)
- interferon
- isoniazid (rarely)
- lansoprazole (rarely)
- levothyroxine (D)
- metronidazole (D)
- non-steroidal anti-inflammatory drugs (NSAIDs) – diclofenac and flurbiprofen may increase INR
- omeprazole

- paracetamol – monitoring is required if taken regularly, but safer than aspirin
- penicillins (occasionally)
- quinolones (e.g. ciprofloxacin)
- selective serotonin reuptake inhibitors (SSRIs): fluoxetine (rarely)
- statins
- sulfinpyrazone (D)
- sulphonamides (D)
- tamoxifen (D)
- tetracyclines (rarely)
- tricyclic antidepressants
- zafirlukast (D).

In addition the anticoagulant effects of warfarin may lead to enhanced bleeding with antiplatelet drugs (aspirin, clopidogrel, dipyridamole) or drugs that lead to gastric bleeding. Aspirin may be combined with warfarin but there is an increase in bleeding tendency, although this is less marked with low doses. Warfarin may also lead to gastric bleeding with aspirin and other NSAIDs. Patients should be advised to use paracetamol for pain relief.

Reduced activity

Less frequently agents will reduce the activity of warfarin and this appears to be due to induction of its metabolism. In dealing with inducers, they take several days to alter the concentrations of warfarin and longer to alter the INR, and these effects are likely to persist for some time after an inducer is stopped. The dose of warfarin may then need to be altered.

Some important drugs that may reduce the actions of warfarin include:

- barbiturates
- carbamazepine – oxacarbazepine appears safe
- colestyramine – separate doses
- cytotoxic agents (azathioprine, cyclophosphamide, mercaptopurine and mitotane)
- disopyramide
- griseofulvin
- phenytoin – monitoring of both warfarin and phenytoin is required (see Chapter 24)
- rifampicin – the dose of warfarin may need to be increased (two- to threefold) several days after rifampicin is started

- St John's wort (avoid)
- vitamin K supplements and diet (including spinach, Brussels sprouts, broccoli, liver, lettuce)
- oral contraceptives – contraindicated in thromboembolic disorders.

The above lists have largely been compiled from *Stockley's Drug Interactions* by Baxter (2013). The list gives some important examples but more complete information should be sought from more detailed sources, including *Stockley's Drug Interactions*.

Over-the-counter considerations

Health professionals should be aware of products containing vitamin K, which may antagonise the effect of warfarin, e.g. multivitamin supplements and liquid dietary supplements. Herbal drugs also have the potential to interact with warfarin (see Chapter 4), e.g. close monitoring is required with garlic supplements. The dose of warfarin may need to be adjusted.

General counselling

In talking to patients, warfarin is usually referred to as 'thinning the blood'. It should be made absolutely clear to patients that they must stick to their dosage regimen and take it at the same time of day, conventionally at 6pm. If they miss a dose they should not take two doses together and they should inform their doctor at the next blood test.

- Patients should be informed that they must tell any doctor, dentist or pharmacist who treats them that they are receiving warfarin. The need to mention their treatment is essential when purchasing over-the-counter (OTC) medicines (including creams and gels, e.g. antifungal imidazoles) and supplements. Preparations containing vitamin K should be avoided.
- Females of childbearing age should be advised not to become pregnant while taking warfarin.
- Alcohol may be consumed in moderation but not in excess.
- Patients should avoid cranberry juice as this may interact with warfarin.

- Patients should avoid excessive consumption of green vegetables (particularly spinach, Brussels sprouts, lettuce, broccoli) and beetroot and liver. Changes to diets rich in vitamin K should be discussed with a healthcare professional, because a dose change of warfarin may be required. Warfarin therapy may also be altered after the consumption of regular or large quantities of foods such as avocado, ice cream, soya bean protein and the sweetener aspartame.

  Patients should report:

- haemoptysis
- blood in faeces
- blood in urine
- nosebleeds
- easy bruising
- skin changes (necrosis) and consult their doctor if they have diarrhoea or vomiting for 2 days or more.

Self-assessment

For the following questions concerning the prevention of thrombosis, choose the most appropriate answer:

1   *The oral anticoagulant warfarin is best described by which one of the following?*

    A   Thrombin antagonist
    B   Vitamin K antagonist
    C   Vitamin B_{12} antagonist
    D   Fibrinogen antagonist
    E   ADP receptor antagonist

2   *Following the administration of warfarin, which one of the following best describes its effects?*

    A   It takes several days for an effect
    B   Its effects occur immediately
    C   It requires extensive metabolism to have an effect
    D   It will cause a decrease in the patient's INR
    E   It reduces platelet aggregation

3   *Which one of the following is an important indication for warfarin?*

    A   Ischaemic heart disease

    B   Carotid artery disease
    C   Heart failure
    D   Atrial fibrillation
    E   Ventricular fibrillation

4   *Which one of the following does not pose a significant interaction with warfarin?*

    A   Cranberry juice
    B   Aspirin
    C   Erythromycin
    D   Amiodarone
    E   Digoxin

5   *The concurrent use of an enzyme inducer (e.g. rifampicin) is likely to lead to which one of the following in a patient taking warfarin?*

    A   Increased bleeding
    B   Increased INR
    C   Therapeutic failure
    D   The need for a lower dose of warfarin
    E   None of the above

6   *Which one of the following is a reason to use a low-molecular-weight heparin in preference to unfractionated heparin?*

    A   They are cheaper
    B   Fewer drug interactions
    C   Faster onset of action
    D   Do not require extensive monitoring
    E   Less likely to affect platelet counts

7   *Following the administration of unfractionated heparin, which one of the following best describes its effects?*

    A   They are delayed for several days
    B   INR will rise
    C   APTT will rise
    D   Platelet count will rise
    E   Platelet aggregation will decrease

8   *Atrial fibrillation is a risk factor for which one of the following?*

    A   Deep vein thrombosis
    B   Transient ischaemic attacks
    C   Cerebral haemorrhage
    D   Pulmonary embolism
    E   Unstable angina

Practice points

- Patients require extensive counselling to ensure compliance.
- Newer oral anticoagulants are increasingly being used

- Warfarin interacts with many drugs and the pharmacist should be vigilant of this and look for signs of enhanced actions of warfarin.
- Consider all requests for OTC medicines (especially NSAIDs) as a potential for drug interactions.

CASE STUDY

A 60-year-old woman who was taking warfarin (3 mg daily as a maintenance dose) for atrial fibrillation was prescribed erythromycin (500 mg q.d.s.) for a community-acquired chest infection. Five days into her course of erythromycin, she had passed blood in her urine and her INR was measured as 5.6.

Explain what appears to have happened to this patient.

- There is a well-recognised interaction between erythromycin and warfarin. It is likely that erythromycin has inhibited the metabolism of warfarin at the level of CYP450, leading to increased plasma concentrations of warfarin.

How should this situation be managed?

- Stop warfarin until the INR is back in range. If there is a major bleed it would be appropriate to give vitamin K or coagulation factors. A decision should be made around either stopping erythromycin or completing the course. But in any event, the INR should be monitored.

How might this situation have been prevented?

- This could have been prevented by choosing an appropriate non-interacting antibiotic such as tetracycline.
- Alternativley, as the interaction is not inevitable, erythromycin could have been prescribed with close monitoring of INR and adjusting the dose of warfarin as appropriate.

Several months later, her doctor would like to introduce statin therapy.

What advice would you give her doctor?

- There is a risk of interaction but this should be fine with INR monitoring. It appears that fluvastatin and rosuvastatin are affected most with pravastatin and simvastatin only having a minor interaction (Baxter 2013).

References

Baxter K, ed. (2013). *Stockley's Drug Interaction*, 8th edn. London: Pharmaceutical Press.

British National Formulary, latest edition. London: British Medical Association and Royal Pharmaceutical Society of Great Britain.

British Society for Haematology (1998). Guidelines on oral anticoagulation. *Br J Haematol* 101: 374–387. Updated in 2005, *Br J Haematol* 132: 277–285.

Department of Health (2001). *Advice on Travel-related Deep Vein Thrombosis*. London: Department of Health.

National Institute for Health and Care Excellence (2014). *Atrial Fibrillation: the management of atrial fibrillation*. Clinical Guideline 180. London: NICE.

RELY trial (2009). Dabigatran versus warfarin in patients with atrial fibrillation. *New Eng J Med* 361: 1139–1151.

Thomson R, Parkin D, Eccles M *et al.* (2000). Decision analysis and guidelines for anticoagulant therapy to prevent stroke in patients with atrial fibrillation. *Lancet* 355: 956–962. pmid: 10768433.

18

Anaemias

As with several medical specialities, haematology encompasses both minor and serious conditions. Of relevance to the pharmacist are the anaemias, because these are important conditions that are encountered on a regular basis: simple iron-deficiency anaemia is of particular importance.

Anaemias are characterised by reduced levels of haemoglobin and occur when the haemoglobin is <13.5 g/dL in males and <11.5 g/dL in females. The signs and symptoms depend on the severity but are related to impaired oxygen transport and delivery due to reduced levels of haemoglobin. Key symptoms include:

- weakness
- lethargy
- impaired exercise tolerance
- shortness of breath

although cardiovascular adaptations, coupled to reduced blood viscosity, may result in tachycardia. In severe anaemia, particularly in more elderly people, there may be angina due to impaired delivery of oxygen to the cardiac muscle, and anaemia may also lead to heart failure. Skin colour is not a reliable sign, because this is determined by blood flow, but pale nail beds and conjunctiva may be present. In haemolytic anaemias, jaundice may be present.

Iron-deficiency anaemia

As the name implies, it is due to impaired iron balance and for this to occur the bone marrow's iron stores must be depleted. The deficiency in iron leads to impaired synthesis of haemoglobin and the production of smaller red cells, which have a reduced mean corpuscular volume (MCV <75 fL; see Appendix 2), and this is referred to as microcytic anaemia. In addition to the above features, the patient may also have:

- spoon nails (koilonychia)
- sores on the corner of the mouth (angular stomatitis)
- painful, red tongue (glossitis)
- unusual food cravings.

As commented above, for iron-deficiency anaemia to develop the iron stores must be depleted. As the diet normally provides the body's requirement for iron, coupled with the fact that iron is efficiently recycled from destroyed red cells, iron-deficiency anaemia is a chronic condition that occurs when input is impaired, output is increased or there are increased demands.

Input is reduced with:

- poor diet (in infants)
- surgical removal of stomach
- malabsorption (coeliac disease, Crohn's disease).

Clinically the main cause is when there is chronic and excessive blood loss through:

- gastrointestinal bleeding (often from ulcers and chronic non-steroidal anti-inflammatory drug [NSAID]-induced damage, but also from colitis, carcinoma, haemorrhoids)
- chronic heavy menstruation (menorrhagia); hence iron-deficiency anaemia is more common in women due to a more precarious iron balance.

Demand is increased in pregnancy due to the fetal requirements and the expansion in the maternal circulating volume, and anaemia, to varying degrees, is very common. Pregnancy tends to increase corpuscular volume and any iron deficiency tends to reduce the volume; these opposing factors may cancel out, leading to normocytic anaemia.

Goals of treatment

These are twofold: to identify and treat the underlying cause and to restore both the iron stores and the level of haemoglobin.

Pharmacological management

The most straightforward approach to restoring iron stores is to give ferrous iron. This is generally in the simple and inexpensive form of oral ferrous sulphate, although this may be poorly tolerated due to gastric irritation and other forms may be used, such as ferrous fumarate. Slow-release preparations have lower bioavailability, as the iron is released in the lower small intestine, where it is not absorbed. The ferrous sulphate is given as 200 mg up to three times daily (once or twice daily in less severe anaemia) with a view to building up the iron stores and increasing the haemoglobin at a rate of approximately 1 g/dL per week. The first response that may be measured is an increase in the reticulocyte count, due to newly formed maturing red blood cells. Once the haemoglobin has returned to normal, iron therapy should be continued for 3 months to build up the iron stores. In prophylaxis of anaemia in pregnancy, the iron may be combined with low doses of folic acid, to ensure an adequate supply of folate.

Interactions with iron therapy

Iron preparations exhibit a range of interactions, largely related to the reduced absorption of the iron or the interacting drug from the gastrointestinal tract. Some important examples are detailed in Table 18.1.

Table 18.1 Clinically significant interactions of iron preparations with other drugs

Interacting drugs	Consequences	Comments
Ferrous salts with antacids	Antacids reduce the absorption of ferrous salts	Their administration should be separated. H_2-receptor antagonists do not significantly affect the absorption of ferrous salts
Ferrous salts with colestyramine	Colestyramine binds ferrous salts and may reduce their absorption	Their administration should be separated
Ferrous salts with neomycin	Neomycin may increase or decrease the absorption of ferrous salts	
Ferrous salts with quinolones	Ferrous salts decrease the absorption of quinolones	The quinolone should be taken at least 2 hours before the ferrous salt
Ferrous salts with tetracyclines	Concomitant administration of these agents reduces the plasma concentrations of both iron and tetracyclines	Their doses should be separated
Ferrous salts with levodopa or carbidopa	Ferrous sulphate reduces the bioavailability of these anti-Parkinsonian drugs	Their doses should be separated and the control of Parkinson's disease monitored
Ferrous sulphate with levothyroxine	Ferrous sulphate reduces the effects of levothyroxine	Their doses should be separated

Counselling

The patient should be counselled that the anaemia is likely to be a symptom of another condition, which should be identified and treated. If patients request iron tablets without a diagnosis, they should be referred to their GP for a blood test and, if appropriate, identification of the underlying cause.

Iron

Clearly, counselling should be directed towards ensuring compliance and completing the course of iron until stores are replenished. The doses should be evenly spaced or at least 6 hours apart because absorption may be reduced by the previous dose. Patients should also be alerted to any important interactions and advised not to take over-the-counter antacids at the same time as the iron salt. The patient should also be made aware of the side effects of iron; these largely affect the gastrointestinal tract and include:

- gastric irritation, which may be reduced by taking the iron with food; however, this may reduce its absorption (although foods rich in vitamin C may actually enhance absorption)
- nausea
- altered bowel habits with constipation or diarrhoea
- the stools will be darkly coloured
- excessive iron is toxic in children.

Foods rich in iron include (Webster-Gandy *et al.*, 2006):

- Meat (especially liver)
- Eggs
- Fish
- Dark-green leafy vegetables and pulses
- Bread and flour
- Yeast extract
- Breakfast cereals (especially bran flakes).

Megaloblastic anaemia

This is a rarer form of anaemia due to abnormal red blood cell maturation as a result of defective DNA synthesis, and the bone marrow contains megaloblasts, abnormal precursor cells in which nuclear maturation is impaired in relation to that of the cytoplasm. The abnormal production of red cells results in increased cell volume and is referred to as macrocytic anaemia (MCV >95 fL); there is also a reduced level of haemoglobin. An increased MCV without anaemia may be due to alcohol misuse – a common cause of macrocytosis, which is unrelated to megaloblastic anaemia. However, in severe alcoholism, the toxic effects of alcohol on the bone marrow may lead to megaloblastic anaemia.

In megaloblastic anaemia the symptoms are those of mild anaemia and may also include jaundice, because the enlarged red cells are more likely to undergo haemolysis, raising the level of bilirubin. Megaloblastic anaemia is due to a deficiency of either vitamin B_{12} or folate, and this may be associated with a painful red tongue (glossitis), sores at the corner of the mouth (angular stomatitis) and neuropathy (in vitamin B_{12} deficiency).

Vitamin B_{12} (as a cofactor) and folate (as component) are essential for DNA synthesis, and a deficiency of either impairs synthesis. As there is a substantial rate of red blood cell production with a high requirement for DNA synthesis, impaired DNA synthesis results in the formation of megaloblasts in the bone marrow. In severe forms impaired DNA synthesis may lead to reduced production of white blood cells and/or platelets.

Deficiencies of vitamin B_{12} can be due to:

- vegan diet
- Crohn's disease, which leads to impaired absorption of vitamin B_{12}
- gastrectomy, which leads to the loss of the intrinsic factor for the absorption of vitamin B_{12}
- metformin, which may reduce the absorption of vitamin B_{12}.

In addition, pernicious anaemia is a special subset and is due to an autoimmune destruction of the intrinsic factor, which is released by the stomach to facilitate the absorption of vitamin B_{12}.

Folate deficiency may be due to:

- dietary deficiency in people with alcohol problems

- pregnancy due to increased demand
- malabsorption in coeliac disease
- chronic inflammatory conditions such as Crohn's disease, rheumatoid arthritis, tuberculosis
- drug induced: methotrexate and trimethoprim are folate antagonists by inhibition of dihydrofolate reductase; phenytoin and phenobarbital may also cause deficiency, possibly due to enzyme induction increasing the requirement for folate.

Pharmacological management

This clearly depends on the cause. If a deficiency of vitamin B_{12} is identified as the cause then hydroxocobalamin is given intramuscularly, which avoids the need for absorption from the gastrointestinal tract, because this may be impaired. Oral vitamin B_{12} may of course be used in otherwise healthy vegans. Once the stores have been replaced, maintenance treatment may need to be continued for life. Intramuscular hydroxocobalamin is also appropriate as prophylaxis in patients who have had gastrectomy or ileal resection.

Folate deficiency is simply treated by oral folic acid (5–15 mg daily) and this, depending on the cause, may need to be lifelong.

Drug interactions

The drugs used to treat megaloblastic anaemia have a limited number of interactions (Table 18.2).

Other anaemias

There is a range of other anaemias that are beyond the scope of this book. However, a brief description of some of them may be appropriate.

Renal anaemia

The kidney is the source of the hormone erythropoietin, which is released in hypoxia (secondary to anaemia, climbing to altitude and chronic obstructive pulmonary disease, for example) and acts on the bone marrow to increase the production of red blood cells. Renal failure is associated with reduced levels of erythropoietin, which leads to normocytic anaemia. Patients with renal failure and those on dialysis accordingly receive erythropoietin. They may also receive prophylactic iron and folic acid (see Chapter 19).

Haemolytic anaemias

This is a class of anaemia and is due to excessive destruction of red cells, which leads to reduced haemoglobin levels. The increased breakdown of red blood cells leads to raised bilirubin levels and this results in jaundice. This may occur in megaloblastic anaemia. The increased erythropoiesis required to replace the cells may actually lead to folate deficiency. Examples of this include:

Table 18.2 Clinically significant interactions of folic acid or vitamin B_{12} with other drugs		
Interacting drugs	**Consequences**	**Comments**
Folic acid with phenytoin, phenobarbital	As commented above, these anticonvulsants may lead to folate deficiency	In patients treated with folate, the concentrations of the anticonvulsants may fall, leading to impaired seizure control. Monitoring and dose adjustment may be required
Folic acid with trimethoprim, co-trimoxazole	The weak antifolate actions of trimethoprim may substantially reduce the effectiveness of folic acid	They should not be used together
Folic acid with magnesium trisilicate	The absorption of folic acid is reduced	
Folic acid with sulfasalazine	The absorption of folic acid is reduced	
Vitamin B_{12} with H_2-receptor antagonists	H_2-receptor antagonists reduce the absorption of oral vitamin B_{12}	Analogues given by injection are not affected

- spherocytosis: a genetic and abnormal reduction in the red blood cell membrane protein, spectrin, which leads to fragile cells
- sickle cell anaemia: due to the haemolysis of the sickle-shaped cells
- in glucose-6-phosphate dehydrogenase (G6PD) deficiency, where certain drugs may cause red cell damage (see Chapter 6)
- infections such as malaria.

Aplastic anaemia

This is a serious condition in which there is insufficient production of red blood cells, white blood cells and platelets (pancytopenia). The patient has decreased resistance to infections, increased bleeding and the symptoms of anaemia. Most cases are acquired due to viral infection, radiation or drugs (including cytotoxic agents, chloramphenicol, sulphonamides and insecticides). Treatment is via antilymphocyte globulin to prevent suppressor killer T cells from damaging the stem cells, ciclosporin and sometimes bone marrow transplantation for cure.

Drug-induced haematological changes

See Chapter 6.

Self-assessment

For the following questions concerning anaemias, choose the most appropriate answer.

Case: A 25-year-old woman is 6 months pregnant and expecting her first child. A blood test revealed the following:

Haematological parameter	Value	Reference range
Haemoglobin	7.5 g/dl	13.5–17.5 g/dl
Mean corpuscular volume	79 fl	76–99 fl
Neutrophil count	3×10^9/L	$2–7.5 \times 10^9$/L
Platelet count	150×10^9/L	$140–400 \times 10^9$/L
Blood group	O Rhesus negative	

1 *Which one of the following best describes this patient?*

a Microcytic anaemia
b Macrocytic anaemia
c Normocytic anaemia
d Anaemia due to a recent haemorrhage
e Pancytopenia

2 *Which one of the following groups of clinical features is she likely to have?*

a Increased risk of infection and fatigue
b Breathlessness and fatigue
c Increased bruising and swollen ankles
d Jaundice and increased bruising
e Haemolysis and increased coagulation

3 *Which one of the following treatments is appropriate?*

a Vitamin K
b Vitamin B_{12} and folic acid
c Ferrous sulphate
d Blood transfusion with O Rhesus positive blood
e Erythropoeitin

Practice points

- Iron-deficiency anaemia is a common occurrence and its underlying cause should be identified and treated.
- Iron-deficiency anaemia may be a presenting feature of NSAID-induced gastric damage.
- Iron preparations have a range of drug interactions.

References

Webster-Gandy J, Madden A, Holdsworth M, eds (2006). *Oxford Handbook of Nutrition and Dietetics*. Oxford: Oxford University Press.

Further reading

Hoffbrand AV, Moss PAH (2001). *Hoffbrand's Essential Haematology*, 7th edn. Oxford: Blackwell Science.

19

The renal patient

This chapter deals specifically with the management issues surrounding patients with renal impairment, which may be associated with other conditions such as diabetes mellitus, hypertension or chronic heart failure. Renal failure has important implications for drug treatment but is a condition in its own right, which must be managed with a view to preserving renal function and dealing with its complications such as anaemia, bone disease, hypertension and uraemia. The focus of this chapter is on renal impairment and chronic renal failure, which are likely to be encountered in primary care, whereas acute renal failure is largely beyond the scope of this book.

Renal function is reflected by the glomerular filtration rate (GFR), which may be estimated from plasma creatinine levels (see Chapter 2) or estimated GFR (eGFR). In terms of renal function, the following classes are used to classify chronic kidney disease (CKD):

eGFR: >90 mL/minute per 1.73 m^2 with signs of kidney damage (CKD stage 1)

eGFR: 89–60 mL/minute per 1.73 m^2 – mild renal impairment (CKD stage 2)

eGFR: 59–30 mL/minute per 1.73 m^2 – moderate renal impairment (CKD stage 3)

eGFR: 29–15 mL/minute per 1.73 m^2 – severe renal impairment (CKD stage 4)

eGFR: <15 mL/minute per 1.73 m^2 or dialysis – renal failure (CKD stage 5).

Renal failure may be acute or chronic and is classified according to cause:

- Prerenal: this involves reduced renal perfusion, as occurs acutely in hypovolaemia, and secondary to heart failure or renal artery stenosis.
- Intrinsic: this represents pathological damage to the tubular, interstitial or glomerular regions that occurs in the kidney itself and may be due to diabetic nephropathy, hypertension, glomerulonephritis (which is largely an immunological disease), pyelonephritis (associated with infection) or nephrotoxic damage, e.g. caused by drugs (see Chapter 6).
- Postrenal: this is secondary to impaired renal outflow as occurs with renal stones, tumours and prostatism.

Acute renal failure

Management of acute kidney injury

This topic is beyond the scope of this book but the mainstays of therapy are diuretics and the use of dopamine as a renal vasodilator, coupled with the correction of potassium levels.

Chronic renal failure

Chronic failure represents a long-term deterioration in renal function with the progressive loss of nephrons and impaired renal function over many years. The most common causes are glomerulonephritis, diabetic nephropathy and hypertension. The consequences of chronic renal failure are related to the extent of impairment. Characteristically there is protein loss in the urine (proteinuria), which leads to less protein in the plasma (hypoalbuminaemia). This resulting reduction in colloidal osmotic pressure in the plasma, coupled with reduced water excretion, leads to tissue oedema. Impaired excretion of toxins leads to uraemia which represents the build-up of urea, phosphate, guanidines, phenols and organic acids in the blood, and leads to the following clinical features:

- skin coloration (lemon tinge)
- itching
- nausea and vomiting
- constipation
- pericarditis
- neurological changes, which may include personality changes and cognitive impairment
- fatigue, which is an important presenting complaint.

The impaired renal function leads to significant changes in blood biochemistry which may include:

- increased creatinine and urea
- hyperkalaemia
- hyponatraemia or normal sodium levels
- hypocalcaemia
- hyperphosphataemia
- acidosis.

In addition, chronic renal failure is associated with the following complications.

Complications

Anaemia

Normocytic anaemia occurs secondary to chronic renal failure, as the kidneys produce erythropoietin (EPO) which regulates red cell production (see Chapter 18) and its absence will reduce red cell synthesis. In addition, the uraemic toxins may cause bone marrow suppression and further depress red cell synthesis.

Renal bone disease (renal osteodystrophy)

The kidneys play a major role in calcium balance and renal failure also has consequences for bone mineralisation. In this respect the kidney is involved in the activation of vitamin D_3 (colecalciferol). Specifically, dietary and endogenously synthesised colecalciferol is converted by the liver to 25-hydroxycolecalciferol, which is then converted by renal 1α-hydroxylase to 1,25-hydroxycholecalciferol. This more active derivative is involved in promoting calcium uptake from the gastrointestinal tract, and is consequently impaired in renal failure. This reduction in calcium absorption leads to less calcium for bone mineralization. Furthermore, the reduced levels of 1,25-hydroxycholecalciferol lead to an increase in the release of parathyroid hormone (PTH) from the parathyroid gland as a negative feedback in response to reduced levels of 1,25-hydroxycholecalciferol. In addition, low calcium also stimulates the release of PTH and this results in hyperparathydroidism, which is associated with increased osteoclastic resorption of bone and calcium release. The calcium may be deposited at sites other than skeletal muscle such as blood vessels. In addition, phosphate excretion is impaired in renal failure, leading to increased phosphate in the plasma, which also promotes calcium loss from the bones. Consequently, renal failure is associated with impaired bone mineralisation, which carries the risk of fractures.

Hypertension

Hypertension is associated with renal failure because renal ischaemia leads to activation of the renin–angiotensin–aldosterone system, resulting in salt and fluid retention together with vasoconstriction. These in turn lead to hypertension and an ensuing vicious circle, which causes further renal damage. Both the hypertension and fluid overload may precipitate heart failure.

Renal failure and impaired drug excretion

Many drugs and/or their metabolites are excreted by the kidneys, especially via the weak acid and base transporters in the proximal tubule.

Consequently, in renal impairment and chronic renal failure, drugs may accumulate and reach toxic levels. Therefore, for renally excreted drugs, impairment should be determined by measuring plasma creatinine levels and estimating the GFR. The *British National Formulary* contains an extensive section dealing with the use of drugs in renal impairment. More specialist and detailed literature includes *Renal Drug Handbook* (Ashley and Dunleavy 2014) which details how specific regimens should be altered. Generally, the approaches to renal impairment are dose reduction of the maintenance dose, increasing the dosing interval or choosing an alternative drug that is not extensively cleared by the kidneys, e.g. digoxin is largely renally excreted and plasma levels will rise in renal impairment. This is dealt with by either reducing the maintenance dose of digoxin or using digitoxin as an alternative that largely undergoes hepatic elimination. When a loading dose is required, and the patient has a 'normal' extracellular volume, then the initial dose is unaffected (see Chapter 7), but it may need to be increased if the volume is increased due to oedema or ascites.

Patients with impaired renal function may be more sensitive to the pharmacological actions and side effects of certain drugs, e.g. in the volume-depleted state, α blockers such as prazosin have enhanced hypotensive effects.

Although impaired renal function may lead to drug toxicity through impaired excretion, this may reduce the effectiveness of drugs that require renal excretion for their actions. Examples of these include thiazide diuretics, drugs used in urinary tract infections that require excretion into the bladder to act (e.g. nalidixic acid, nitrofurantoin) and uricosuric agents that promote excretion of uric acid (e.g. probenecid).

Goals of treatment

These are to reduce the progressive loss of renal function, to limit or reverse complications such as anaemia, hypertension and renal bone disease, to reduce uraemia and provide symptomatic relief, and to normalise the electrolytic balance of the body.

Management of chronic renal failure

The degree of intervention required is governed by the degree of renal impairment. Detailed guidance is produced by the Renal Association (www.renal.org) and should be consulted.

Management of early chronic renal failure

Early chronic renal failure may be managed with diuretics (see Chapters 12 and 16) and a diet that is low in sodium, potassium and protein. In choosing a diuretic, attention must be paid to renal function, as thiazides and thiazide-like agents (except metolazone) are ineffective in moderate renal failure because are themselves renally excreted to enable them to act at their site of action, the distal tubule. Loop diuretics may be used in moderate and severe renal impairment but high doses may be required. The object of the low-protein diet is to slow down the accumulation of nitrogenous end-products of protein metabolism. A low-protein diet is, however, associated with malnutrition and the loss of muscle mass and reduced immune responses that are adverse to health.

Management of itching due to uraemia

Chlorphenamine may be used to relieve itching associated with uraemia.

Management of nausea

See Chapter 9.

Management of hypertension

As commented above, hypertension may lead to renal damage and may also be induced in renal damage as a consequence of activation of the renin–angiotensin–aldosterone system. What is clear is that reducing blood pressure with antihypertensive drugs will reduce the rate of loss of renal function, as assessed by a reduction in the rate of decline of GFR and protein excretion. A target blood pressure of 130/80 mmHg or less is aimed for in patients with stable renal failure and a target of 125/75 mmHg in patients with progressive disease with proteinuria.

The Ramipril Efficacy In Nephropathy (REIN) trial by the GISEN Group (1997) reported that ramipril was more effective than blood pressure lowering alone at reducing proteinuria and the rate of decline in GFR in non-diabetic nephropathy. The implication from this is that ramipril, and other angiotensin-converting enzyme (ACE) inhibitors, may be renally protective in renal failure and that ACE inhibitors should therefore be used to treat the hypertension associated with renal failure. Although it should be noted that ACE inhibitors may themselves lead to renal impairment (especially in renovascular disease) and renal function should be monitored, ACE inhibitors may increase potassium and this may enhance hyperkalaemia associated with renal failure. ACE inhibitors may also reduce the release of EPO which may compound the associated anaemia. Angiotensin receptor antagonists can substitute for ACE inhibitors in type 2 diabetes for renal protection (see Chapter 37), but whether this is the case for patients who are not diabetic remains to be determined.

Generally speaking, ACE inhibitors have a significant role in the management of hypertension in renal disease, especially when there is proteinuria. Calcium-channel blockers are also widely used.

Hyperlipidaemia

There is an association of hypercholesterolaemia and hypertriglyceridaemia with renal failure and statins are often prescribed (see Chapter 13) to lower plasma cholesterol and reduce the cardiovascular risk. The dose of statin should take account of the level of renal impairment with appropriate reductions, and fluvastatin should be avoided in severe renal impairment.

Management of renal anaemia

Oral iron is often given initially to build up iron levels before treatment with EPO. EPO may then be given subcutaneously or intravenously, with the dose adjusted to restore haemoglobin levels to a target of >10 g/dL. The treatment of anaemia should improve exercise tolerance and reduce the risk of precipitating heart failure. EPO is, however, associated with an increase in blood pressure in a number of patients. There are also rare reports of pure red cell aplasia (failure of red cell production) in patients receiving EPO-α by the subcutaneous route. This is believed to be due to the production of antibodies to EPO and treatment with EPO should be stopped.

Management of renal bone disease

1α-Hydroxycholecalciferol (alfacalcidol) and calcitriol are hydroxylated derivatives of vitamin D and are given in renal failure to compensate for impaired endogenous production. Patients taking these agents should have their calcium levels measured to avoid hypercalcaemia and the dose is chosen to correct the increased parathyroid hormone levels.

The additional problem contributing to renal bone disease is phosphate, because its elimination is impaired in renal failure. To reduce this problem, phosphate binders are taken with meals to bind phosphate in the gastrointestinal tract and prevent its absorption. Foods rich in phosphate include protein-rich foods, dairy products, cereals, nuts, chocolate and cola drinks. Phosphate binders used are calcium salts (carbonate or acetate) and the polymer, Sevelamer.

Calcium-based phosphate binders show a range of interactions by increasing gastric pH and altering the absorption of certain drugs (see Chapters 6 and 8 dealing with antacid interactions). For agents affected in this way, the dose should be separated in time from the phosphate binder.

Hyperkalaemia

Increased plasma levels of potassium occur in renal failure and are potentially life threatening if they rise too high. Hyperkalaemia may be prevented by polystyrene sulphonate ion exchange resins such as calcium polystyrene sulphonate, which is given orally or rectally. Sodium polystyrene sulphonate exchanges sodium for potassium in the gastrointestinal tract and is excreted rectally. Sodium polystyrene sulphonate may lead to sodium overload, which should be avoided. These resins are also constipating and a laxative should be given.

Severe hyperkalaemia is treated with insulin (given with glucose to prevent hypoglycaemia), which promotes cellular uptake of potassium.

Dialysis

Once renal function is substantially impaired and pharmacological and dietary means alone do not control the condition, renal function must be replaced by artificial means, involving either peritoneal dialysis or haemodialysis, before transplantation.

Continuous ambulatory peritoneal dialysis

A permanent indwelling catheter is implanted through the abdominal wall. Sterile salt solution (2–3 L), similar to plasma but with no protein or potassium, is repeatedly run into the peritoneal cavity where it lies next to the mesenteric blood vessels. Uraemic substances accumulating in the blood enter the fluid and approach equilibrium. The solution is then discarded and replaced, and this crudely performs the main functions of the kidney. As the dialysate has zero potassium, it equilibrates with plasma and so draws potassium off down its diffusion gradient, e.g. if the plasma potassium concentration is 4 mmol/L then 10 L of dialysate fluid per day transfers 40 mmol of potassium per day. Therefore, dietary potassium must not exceed this or hyperkalaemia will occur. Adding osmotic solute (glucose) to the peritoneal dialysate can produce 1–1.5 L/day of peritoneal water loss by osmosis and the intake must be controlled to match this. This method of dialysis carries a significant risk of peritoneal infection.

Haemodialysis

This involves the exchange of substances from the blood with dialysate across an artificial semipermeable membrane outside the body using a machine. Once again, substances diffuse into the dialysate and altering potassium and glucose concentrations may enable regulation of potassium and circulating volume. Patients receiving haemodialysis are usually anticoagulated with heparin to prevent activation of clotting triggered by the foreign surfaces of the machine.

Drug choice and dialysis

Both continuous ambulatory peritoneal dialysis (CAPD) and haemodialysis provide routes for drug elimination and certain drugs may be efficiently removed from the body via these routes. The elimination will be determined by their permeability across the natural or artificial membranes, protein binding (drugs with high binding are less likely to be eliminated), the degree of hepatic elimination and water solubility. Hence in choosing drugs for patients on dialysis it is important to establish how the particular form of dialysis (as they may handle drugs differently) will affect drug elimination. In addition, antihypertensive drugs may be omitted or delayed on the day of haemodialysis to prevent hypotension. Accordingly, specialist advice and literature should be consulted when prescribing for patients on dialysis. Specialist books that detail how regimens for an extensive range of drugs should be altered in dialysis include *Renal Drug Handbook* (Ashley and Dunleavy 2014).

Renal transplantation

Renal transplantation of kidneys from a living donor or cadaveric donor represents the best chance of a cure in end-stage renal failure. Replacement of the kidney will restore renal function, including vitamin D_3 activation and the production of EPO, and their replacement will no longer be required. However, to prevent an immunological rejection of the transplanted kidney, lifelong immunosuppression will be required (except in donations from an identical twin).

Immunosuppression

A range of immunosuppressants are used in various combinations: triple therapy of ciclosporin, prednisolone and azathioprine is commonly used. The immunosuppressants are summarised in Table 19.1.

Over-the-counter considerations

Renal impairment and failure represent an important consideration for providing over-the-counter (OTC) medicines as certain products may not be suitable. Important examples of this are the non-steroidal anti-inflammatory drugs (NSAIDs) which are available OTC (aspirin and ibuprofen as either tablets or topical preparations) because they may cause sodium retention and also a deterioration in renal function, and should be avoided. Paracetamol is considered a safe alternative. Similarly, effervescent products should not be used due to their appreciable content of sodium, which may lead to fluid overload in renal impairment.

Other considerations include avoiding oral rehydration therapy for diarrhoea, which will also increase the salt load; antidiarrhoeal agents such as loperamide would be a better alternative. The load of electrolytes should also be considered when using antacids, and OTC H_2-receptor antagonists are suitable alternatives for dyspepsia. Also aluminium and calcium salts used as phosphate binders will provide relief.

Herbal medicines

It is especially important that renal patients report their usage of herbal medicines, because some herbal preparations such as cat's claw and juniper berries

Table 19.1 Summary of actions and adverse effects of some immunosuppressant agents

Immunosuppressant	Mechanism of action	Comments
Azathioprine	Inhibits nucleic acid synthesis and prevents lymphocyte production	May lead to bone marrow suppression with reductions in red cell, platelet and white blood cell production
Ciclosporin	Prevents activation of T lymphocytes	Ciclosporin has many drug interactions; its metabolism may be inhibited by cytochrome P450 inhibitors such as macrolides, imidazoles, diltiazem, verapamil and cimetidine. Its metabolism may be induced by antiepileptic drugs, rifampicin and St John's wort. It is nephrotoxic and may cause hypertension
Corticosteroids	A range of immunosuppressant actions	Widespread steroid side effects
Tacrolimus	Prevents the activation of T lymphocytes	
Mycophenolate mofetil	Is converted to mycophenolic acid which has a more selective action than azathioprine and inhibits DNA synthesis	May cause gastrointestinal side effects such as diarrhoea and vomiting. It is less likely than azathioprine to cause leukopenia

may cause renal damage. Furthermore, herbal remedies may interact with prescribed medicines, e.g. St John's wort induces the metabolism of ciclosporin, and could of course render the immunosuppressant less effective and potentially lead to rejection of a transplanted kidney.

Counselling

Phosphate binders

- These should be taken 10–15 minutes before meals.
- They should also be taken with snacks containing protein.
- Renagel and Phosex should be swallowed whole; Calcichew may be chewed.
- They should not be taken with antacids which contain aluminium or calcium.
- Phosphate binders should not be taken at the same time as iron tablets.

Immunosuppressants

- These must be taken continuously or the transplanted kidney may be rejected; patients should stop taking them only if advised by their doctor.
- Patients should ensure that they have adequate supplies.
- Patients taking immunosuppressants should not receive live immunisations.

- Patients taking steroids should consult their general practitioner (GP) if they come into contact with chickenpox.
- Patients taking immunosuppressants are more susceptible to infections and are regarded as a 'special group', who should have a lower threshold for referral.
- Patients taking tacrolimus, sirolimus or ciclosporin should avoid grapefruit and grapefruit juice for 1 hour before taking the drug.
- Patients taking tacrolimus may develop headaches, nausea and trembling, and should consult their GP.
- Patients taking azathioprine or mycophenolate mofetil should consult their GP if there is easy bruising or signs of infection that may be due to bone marrow suppression.
- Patients should always take the same brand of ciclosporin.
- The administration of ciclosporin and sirolimus requires counselling (see *British National Formulary*).
- Tacrolimus has been associated with cardiomyopathy, which should be monitored.
- Immunosuppressants (except corticosteroids) are associated with an increased risk of skin cancer and patients taking them should wear sunblock in sunny weather.
- Tacrolimus has been reported to interact with ibuprofen (and this may also occur with other NSAIDs), leading to renal impairment.

Practice points

- Many patients with chronic renal failure also have diabetes mellitus and the treatment of these conditions should occur in tandem. *Metformin should be avoided.*
- Blood pressure should be at or below the target levels.
- ACE inhibitors play a major role in the management of hypertension in patients with chronic renal disease.
- Renal patients are likely to be taking many different drugs, which should be reviewed regularly.
- Patient compliance may be improved by producing a list of drugs to take and when.
- Patients with chronic renal failure should be considered for the management of anaemia, renal bone disease (involving phosphate binders and vitamin D) and hypertension.
- Renal impairment and failure and also dialysis have implications for the use of many prescription and OTC drugs.
- *Renal Drug Handbook* (Ashley and Dunleavy 2014) is an essential resource.

Self-assessment

Consider whether the following statements are true or false. In a patient with chronic renal disease:

1 Creatinine levels will be lower.
2 There is a risk of normocytic anaemia.

3 Renal bone disease may be prevented by adding phosphate to the diet.
4 Tight management of blood pressure is essential.
5 ACE inhibitors are effective at preventing diabetic nephropathy.

References

Ashley C, Dunleavy A, eds (2014). *Renal Drug Handbook*. 4th edn. London: Radcliffe.

British National Formulary, latest edition. London: British Medical Association and Royal Pharmaceutical Society of Great Britain.

GISEN Group (1997). Randomised placebo-controlled trial of the effect of ramipril on decline of glomerular filtration rate and risk of terminal renal failure in proteinuric, non-diabetic nephropathy. *Lancet* 349: 1857–1863.

Further reading

Ashley C, Morlidge C, eds (2008). *Introduction to Renal Therapeutics*. London: Pharmaceutical Press.

Online resources

www.renal.org
The website of the Renal Association, which produces clinical guidelines on the management of renal disease (accessed October 2015).

www.kidney.org
The website of UK National Kidney Foundation, which provides patient information (accessed October 2015).

www.renalpharmacy.org.uk
The website of the UK Renal Pharmacy Group (accessed October 2015).

PART **E**

Respiratory diseases

20

Coughs and colds

This is clearly a key topic in community practice, with many patients having consultations for a range of related illnesses. Nevertheless, this can be a controversial area as some commonly used remedies are of questionable value.

Colds or acute coryza

This is a very common occurrence, usually resulting from either rhino- or adenovirus infections, which produce symptoms of a runny nose (rhinorrhoea), sneezing and pyrexia. The common cold is often referred to as a 'flu-like' illness but it should be noted that influenza is an entirely different and more serious infection. Infants may have around 12 colds per year and adults can expect to have 1–2 per year. Colds are self-limiting with a typical course of 1 week. However, there are a number of complications, including sinusitis, otitis media and secondary chest infections.

Treatment of a cold

Treatment of the cold is generally directed at symptomatic relief. The mainstay of treatment should be regular ibuprofen and/or paracetamol to reduce the increased temperature. Additional simple measures include steam inhalation, which appears to hydrate the airways and promote the removal of mucus. Zinc lozenges have been advocated for reducing the length of colds but there is no evidence to support this.

Nasal decongestants

Topical nasal decongestants are also effective at reducing the symptoms of excessive mucus production. Topical decongestants, such as xylometazoline and oxymetazoline, are α-adrenoceptor agonists which cause nasal vasoconstriction and so reduce the flow of mucus. The only major problem is that prolonged use (5–7 days) may lead to rebound congestion (rhinitis medicamentosa).

Systemic decongestants are also widely used but are probably less effective than topical agents and their systemic administration may be associated with side effects. Systemic agents include phenylephrine, which has direct sympathomimetic activity, whereas pseudoephedrine and phenylpropanolamine both have direct and indirect sympathomimetic vasoconstrictor actions, leading to nasal vasoconstriction. Their sympathomimetic activity also means that they are unsuitable for patients with:

- severe ischaemic heart disease
- uncontrolled hypertension
- hyperthyroidism
- diabetes.

Indeed, phenylpropanolamine, when used at higher doses than those in the UK, has been implicated in causing stroke in patients in the USA. The Commission on Human Medicines (CHM, formerly the Committee on Safety of Medicines) has now indicated that the daily dose of phenylpropanolamine should not exceed 100 mg. In theory, pseudoephedrine should cause bronchodilation via activation of β_2-adrenoceptors on the bronchial smooth muscle, which may be of benefit in infections that involve the airways. Sympathomimetics show a range of interactions and in particular will be potentiated by monoamine oxidase inhibitors (MAOIs), which precludes their concurrent use. Some important interactions are detailed in Table 20.1.

Cough mixtures

Although a cough is a symptom and not an illness, it is appropriate to consider cough mixtures here because they are widely used in colds. Cough mixtures are divided into antitussives (cough suppressants) such as codeine, dextromethorphan and pholcodine, and expectorants, e.g. guaifenesin, ipecacuanha and ammonium chloride. In general, cough mixtures are of doubtful medicinal value, but do provide an appreciable placebo effect, from which patients may derive benefit. Antitussives contain opioids that act on the

Table 20.1 Some interactions of drugs with oral sympathomimetic agents

Drugs	Consequences	Comments
Phenylephrine with MAOIs	The pressor activity of phenylephrine is substantially enhanced by MAOIs	This is largely because phenylephrine is normally metabolised by MAO and only small amounts enter the circulation. In the presence of an MAOI, this may lead to a fatal hypertensive crisis. Their concurrent use should be avoided
Indirectly acting sympathomimetic agents (e.g. phenylpropanolamine, pseudoephedrine) with MAOIs	This combination may lead to a fatal hypertensive crisis	Their concurrent use should be avoided
Indirectly acting sympathomimetic agents (e.g. phenylpropanolamine, pseudoephedrine) with tricyclic antidepressants	The actions of indirectly acting sympathomimetic agents would be expected to be reduced by tricyclic antidepressants	This is not believed to be significant
Phenylephrine with tricyclic antidepressants	The pressor actions of phenylephrine would be expected to be increased by tricyclic antidepressants	This is not believed to be significant
Phenylephrine/phenylpropanolamine with β blockers	No significant interaction between OTC phenylephrine and β blockers occurs	• Phenylpropanolamine has been shown to cause a pressor effect in patients taking β blockers but this is not regarded as clinically significant. • Phenylpropanolamine should not be taken by patients with hypertension, heart disease or hyperthyroidism
Phenylpropanolamine with caffeine	The pressor effects of phenylpropanolamine are enhanced by caffeine and this may result in hypertension in susceptible patients	

MAOIs, monoamine oxidase inhibitors; OTC, over-the-counter.

cough centres in the brain to suppress the cough. Codeine in particular has the potential for dependence and pronounced opioid side effects such as constipation. These agents will suppress the cough and remove the symptoms. However, the cough serves the purpose of clearing the lungs and cough suppression may be inappropriate. Indeed, retention of sputum means that they are harmful in chronic obstructive pulmonary disease (COPD) and asthma, and may also mask worsening symptoms. Expectorants are intended to facilitate mucus removal but there is no convincing evidence to support this occurring at the doses used.

Given the apparent lack of efficacy of cough mixtures, a simple linctus may be beneficial by a soothing action and a placebo effect.

Compound preparations

Many proprietary compound preparations are available and typically contain some of the following: an antitussive, an antipyretic (paracetamol or ibuprofen), a systemic decongestant and an antihistamine. The effectiveness of each agent has been considered above, except antihistamines. Sedating (or old) antihistamines such as promethazine will promote sleep (which could be disturbed by the cough) and their antimuscarinic side effects will help dry up the secretions.

Over-the-counter medicines and young children with colds

Many cold preparations contain powerful opioids, sympathomimetics and antihistamines and there is a significant risk of overdose, particularly in young children. It is for this reason that they should not be sold for children under the age of 6 years. Once again, ibuprofen or paracetamol should be the mainstay of therapy.

Echinacea

Echinacea is widely used to shorten the duration and reduce the severity of cold symptoms. To date, there have been trials that both confirm and question its efficacy. There is currently no evidence to support its effectiveness in colds.

Influenza

As commented above, this must be distinguished from flu-like illnesses. Influenza is an upper respiratory tract infection that has a more severe course and is associated with more complications and significant mortality. Indeed, more people died in the epidemic of Spanish flu (1918–19) than were killed in the First World War. It is caused by influenza viruses A, B and C. The associated symptoms include pyrexia, chills, headache, muscle aches, backache, sore throat, cough and runny nose, and it is followed by post-viral debilitation which may persist for several weeks after the infection.

Treatment of uncomplicated influenza is directed towards symptomatic relief, including ibuprofen and/or paracetamol for pain relief and reduction of pyrexia. A recent development has been the introduction of viral neuramidase inhibitors, such as zanamivir and oseltamivir, which prevent the entry and release of viral particles from host cells. These drugs are effective against influenza A and B. Zanamivir is given by inhalation and this has occasionally been associated with bronchospasm and so should be used with caution in asthma (a bronchodilator should be available) and avoided in severe asthma. In 2002, the National Institute for Health and Care Excellence (NICE) released guidance recommending that zanamivir was not for use in normally healthy patients but was appropriate for:

- patients >65 years of age
- patients with chronic respiratory diseases
- patients with cardiovascular disease (but not hypertension)
- immunocompromised patients
- patients with diabetes mellitus.

It is now extended to chronic renal disease and must be started within 48 hours of the start of symptoms.

Amantadine (an anti-Parkinsonian drug) also has a limited role in the prevention of influenza A and acts by inhibiting viral DNA replication. It is best used as prophylaxis in patients who are at risk but who cannot be immunised or while immunisation takes effect (2 weeks).

Immunisation now plays an important role in the prevention of influenza in vulnerable patients and annual immunisation is recommended for:

- patients >65 years of age
- people in residential care homes
- patients with:

– chronic respiratory conditions
– chronic heart disease
– chronic renal failure
– diabetes mellitus
– immunosuppression due to drugs, disease or following a splenectomy.

Acute bronchitis

A potential complication of an upper respiratory infection is acute bronchitis, which may be viral or bacterial. A viral infection may give rise to a dry cough, whereas a secondary bacterial infection is more often associated with the production of thick green sputum. Additional symptoms may include a wheeze and breathlessness.

In healthy patients acute bronchitis usually resolves spontaneously in 1–2 weeks but may exacerbate asthma and COPD (see Chapter 22) and there is a risk of bronchopneumonia. As mentioned in Chapter 22, patients with COPD may be given prophylactic antibiotics to take at the start of an exacerbation, and if appropriate may receive a steroid. In normally healthy patients symptomatic relief may be all that is required. Elderly patients or those with concurrent illnesses such as heart disease or diabetes may be treated with amoxicillin; in patients who are penicillin allergic, tetracycline or erythromycin may be prescribed. Failure of initial treatment with amoxicillin may be followed by the use of co-amoxiclav, tetracycline or a macrolide.

Pneumonia

Pneumonia involves infection of the alveoli as opposed to the bronchi. This may lead to sputum (which may be bloodstained, and is often rusty in appearance), breathlessness, pleuritic chest pains and fever. In pneumonia acquired in the community (as opposed to hospital) the principal causative agents are *Streptococcus pneumoniae* (most), *Haemophilus influenzae* and *Chlamydia pneumoniae,* while *C. psittaci* is associated with contact with birds. Given the potential seriousness of pneumonia, antibacterial treatment is appropriate with amoxicillin (or erythromycin if penicillin allergic) being used first line

for mild, community-acquired infections. Depending on response and the strain of bacteria, other agents that may be used include: tetracycline, flucloxacillin, erythromycin, clarithromycin, cefuroxime, cefotaxime and gentamicin, alone or in various combinations; *C. psittaci* and *C. pneumoniae* are treated with a macrolide or tetracycline, and *H. influenzae* with cefaclor (see Chapter 34). As a preventive measure immunisation against *Streptococcus pneumoniae* is recommended for patients aged >65 years and patients at risk (including those with chronic respiratory, cardiac, renal and hepatic diseases), and patients with diabetes mellitus.

Acute sinusitis

This is infection of the facial sinuses, and is usually bacterial, with *S. pneumoniae, H. influenzae* and *Staphylococcus aureus* being the common causative organisms. Sinusitis is associated with discomfort and purulent discharge. Treatment may include nasal decongestants and analgesics to provide symptomatic relief. Sinusitis should normally resolve spontaneously but, in severe or poorly resolving cases, systemic antibiotics (amoxicillin, co-amoxiclav, erythromycin or doxycycline) are appropriate. There is no evidence that topical antibacterial agents are effective.

Otitis media

This is earache due to middle-ear infection and is very common in children, often after a cold or sore throat. On examination the eardrum is bulging and inflamed. The cause is often viral but may also be bacterial (mostly due to *S. pneumoniae, H. influenzae, Moraxella catarrhalis* and, less commonly, *S. pyogenes)* and there is no way of identifying the causative agent unless the eardrum is perforated and a swab taken for culture.

The initial management is for pain relief with either paracetamol and/or ibuprofen, and this is certainly appropriate for the first day or so because most cases will resolve spontaneously. Further treatment with antibiotics is controversial as many cases are viral. Some practitioners prescribe antibiotics blind and amoxicillin is used, but 15% of *H. influenzae* are resistant due to β-lactamase production and so co-amoxiclav or cephalosporins may be more appropriate; macrolides may also be considered. However, evidence indicates that antibiotics shorten the course of the infection by only a couple of days, and then only in about 15% of patients, so their empirical use is often unnecessary (Damoiscaux *et al.* 2000). Furthermore, the use of antibiotics is associated with side effects (such as diarrhoea and nausea) and overuse has been implicated in secretory otitis media ('glue ear').

Sore throats – pharyngitis and tonsillitis

Pharyngitis, other than that due to irritation (e.g. smoke), is mostly viral in origin and thus requires symptomatic relief. This typically involves paracetamol or ibuprofen. Interestingly, antibacterial lozenges are of no value and may in fact irritate the inflamed mucosa, whereas local anaesthetic lozenges may sensitise the mucosa. Indeed, simple sugar-free boiled sweets may provide relief.

Some sore throats are caused by bacteria, generally due to infection with group A β-haemolytic streptococci. It is particularly difficult to distinguish a bacterial sore throat from a viral infection. Some features that may point to a bacterial infection are an inflamed pharynx with yellow/white exudates on the tonsils, enlarged, tender cervical lymph nodes, and a sore throat in isolation not accompanied by upper respiratory tract infection. Bacterial sore throats may be treated with antibiotics when there is proven streptococcal infection, they fail to resolve spontaneously, the symptoms are severe and may involve systemic symptoms such as scarlet fever, or in children with diabetes mellitus. Currently phenoxymethylpenicillin for 10 days is the standard first-line drug treatment for infections by β-haemolytic streptococci but cephalosporins and macrolides are also effective. Amoxicillin and ampicillin should not be used blind, because in glandular fever they frequently lead to a maculopapular rash.

Previously rheumatic fever and glomerulonephritis were occasional complications of streptococcal throat infections. This is because *S. pyogenes* antigens cross-react with human connective tissue. Group A streptococci share antigenic properties with heart valve glycoprotein leading to damage, nephritis and also arthritis. This complication is very rare nowadays but patients who have previously had endocarditis, a history of nephritis or artificial heart valves should receive antibiotics during throat infections.

Sore throats are a common occurrence in patients with drug-induced neutropenia and patients who are taking:

- carbamazepine
- phenytoin
- clozapine
- mianserin
- gold salts
- carbimazole
- 5-aminosalicylates
- azathioprine.

These patients should be counselled to report sore throats because this may indicate neutropenia and a white blood cell count is required. Inhaled steroids may also promote candidal infections of the throat (see Chapter 22).

Cough

A cough is not an illness but a symptom of a range of other conditions, from trivial to serious (see Chapter 1).

Self-assessment

Consider whether the following statements are true or false concerning coughs and colds:

1 Uncomplicated otitis media in a child is usually managed by using simple analgesia.
2 Prolonged use of nasal decongestants can lead to long-term inhibition of mucus production.
3 A sore throat can indicate neutropenia.
4 Coughing up blood (or haemoptysis) is a serious alerting symptom.
5 Amoxicillin is commonly prescribed for simple chest infections.

Counselling and practice points

It is impossible to provide generic counselling for the infections described above; however, there are several important points that should be borne in mind:

- Simple analgesia and antipyretic treatment with paracetamol and/or ibuprofen has a major role in many of these conditions. Paracetamol tends to be used first line in pyrexia and is favoured because it has limited adverse drug reactions (ADRs) and interactions; ibuprofen may be added in resistance.
- Symptomatic relief has a major role in colds, sore throats, otitis media and sinusitis. Reassurance of parents plays an important role with children.
- Cough mixtures generally lack efficacy but have an appreciable placebo effect.
- Antitussive agents may cause sputum retention that is potentially harmful in COPD and asthma.
- Sympathomimetic agents are best administered via the topical route; with the oral route there is the potential for systemic effects and life-threatening interactions with concurrent MAOIs.
- Over-the-counter (OTC) cold remedies containing opioids, sympathomimetics and antihistamines should not be used in children aged <6 years.

- In pharyngitis and otitis media, most cases are viral and it is difficult to identify bacterial infections. Antibiotic treatment is appropriate on the suspicion of a bacterial infection, in a poorly resolving infection or in patients who are at risk.
- Be alert for pharyngitis – as a symptom of neutropenia – as an ADR.
- Be alert for cough as a symptom of a range of diseases (see Chapter 1).
- When a course of antibiotics is prescribed, the importance of completing the course should be emphasised and instructions given about when to take the agent in relation to food.
- In influenza, zanamivir has been recommended for use in vulnerable patients, but must be started within 48 hours of the appearance of symptoms. It carries the risk of bronchospasm and patients with asthma should have a bronchodilator available.
- Given the need for prompt initiation of zanamivir, systems should be in place to ensure that it is available for immediate dispensing.
- Immunisation against influenza and *Streptococcus pneumoniae* are recommended for patients at a high risk of complications.

CASE STUDIES

Case 1

Mr NC (35 years old), who has previously been in good health, visits his general practitioner complaining of a 'nasty, painful and irritating cough'. On questioning, the GP establishes that the patient has retrosternal pain on coughing and that the cough is non-productive. The GP recommends paracetamol if there is any fever.

The GP's next patient is Mr CC (65 years), who has previously been in good health and is complaining of a 'nasty cough', is slightly breathless and has been coughing up thick green sputum for 5 days. On auscultation the GP hears wheezing in a previously healthy chest. The GP prescribes amoxicillin 500 mg three times daily to be taken for 1 week and recommends paracetamol if required.

Why has the GP treated these patients differently?

- Mr NC probably has a viral infection leading to a non-productive painful cough, whereas Mr CC appears to have acute bronchitis, which may well be secondary to a recent bout of viral tracheitis – the bacterial infection is indicated by a cough productive of green sputum. Antibiotics may be appropriate, although less so in a previously healthy chest.

How would you counsel Mr CC?

- He should complete the course, even if the cough clears up, because there may still be bacteria present (especially the more resistant strains), so the complete course is required for full eradication.
- He should take the antibiotic three times a day: breakfast, lunch and bedtime is a traditional and convenient spacing.
- As a common side effect of antibiotic treatment, he might get diarrhoea.

Case 2

Mrs PT visits the above GP complaining of a sore throat and a raised temperature. Following an examination, the GP recommends that she take either paracetamol or ibuprofen, rest and take plenty of fluids.

Mrs SP is the next patient and complains of the same symptoms. Following a throat examination the GP observes pus exudates and enlarged cervical lymph nodes. Phenoxymethylpenicillin 500 mg four times daily was prescribed for 10 days.

Why has the GP treated these patients differently?

- Most cases of pharyngitis are viral and thus require symptomatic relief. Some infections are bacterial (streptococcal) and present with similar symptoms. On examination, the bacterial infection may be suggested by an inflamed pharynx with yellow/white exudates visible on the tonsils. The patient may have enlarged, tender cervical lymph nodes. Mrs PT has a viral infection and Mrs SP a presumed bacterial infection.

Comment on the choice of antibiotic.

- Phenoxymethylpenicillin is recommended first line. Amoxicillin and ampicillin should not be used blind in a sore throat because in glandular fever they generally lead to a maculopapular rash.

Case 3

An 18-year-old female student visits her GP complaining of a sore throat and general tiredness. Following a limited consultation the GP gives her a prescription for amoxicillin 500 mg three times daily. The following day, the student develops a maculopapular rash and seeks your advice.

How might you respond to the rash?

- She should stop taking the amoxicillin. She should take an antihistamine (loratadine 10 mg daily or chlorphenamine 4 mg four times daily, but sedation may be a problem) for relief of the rash.

(continued)

(continued)

What are the likely causes of the rash?

- Penicillin allergy.
- Glandular fever; amoxicillin should not be given blind for a sore throat as 90% of patients with glandular fever develop a rash. This does not mean a lifelong allergy to penicillins.

What further tests and treatment may be appropriate for this patient?

- A blood test (Monospot or Paul–Bunnell test) for glandular fever. If she has glandular fever then symptomatic relief is required and she should avoid alcohol.
- If she has a penicillin allergy, she should be prescribed a non-penicillin, non-cephalosporin such as erythromycin (250 mg four times daily) and the allergy documented on her medical records.

References

Damoiseaux RAMJ, van Balen FAM, Hoes AW *et al.* (2000). Primary care based randomised, double blind trial of amoxicillin versus placebo for acute otitis media in children aged under 2 years. *BMJ*, 320: 350–354. pmid: 10657332.

National Institute for Health and Care Excellence (2002). *Guidance of the use of zanamivir (Relenza) in the treatment of influenza.* Technology Appraisal Guidance no. 15. London: NICE.

21

Allergy

Allergy may be viewed as an inappropriate immune response provoked by a foreign agent, the allergen, which leads to a troublesome pathophysiological response; in the extreme there may be life-threatening anaphylaxis.

In an allergic response an antigen (allergen) leads to increased immunoglobulin E (IgE) synthesis. The IgE becomes attached to mast cell surfaces and the cross-linking of IgE by the allergen leads to calcium entry. This is followed by mast cell degranulation and the release of inflammatory mediators (including histamine and leukotrienes) leading to increased vascular permeability, chemotaxis, and increased production of mucus and oedema (due to increased vascular permeability and vasodilatation in response to histamine).

There are a number of conditions associated with allergic responses and these include allergic rhinitis, allergic asthma, contact dermatitis (see Chapter 36), drug-induced skin reactions (see Chapter 6) and anaphylaxis.

Allergic rhinitis

Disease characteristics

Allergic rhinitis may be perennial (throughout the year), seasonal (as in hayfever) or occupational, resulting from exposure to chemicals, dusts, and animal dander and urine. The clinical features include:

- nasal itching
- rhinorrhoea
- sneezing
- itchy throat
- wheezing
- conjunctival symptoms, which involve itchiness and bilateral red eye, worsened by irritants such as smoke.

The precise balance of symptoms may vary between the causes, with the perennial disease having less prominent eye symptoms.

In response to allergen exposure, mast cells and T lymphocytes are activated with tissue recruitment of basophils and eosinophils. Histamine is the primary mediator from mast cells and basophils and acts largely on H_1-receptors to evoke the characteristic symptoms, whereas actions at H_2- and H_3-receptors also occur, leading to nasal obstruction. In addition, leukotrienes, prostaglandins and kinins also contribute to the inflammatory response.

Goals of treatment

These are to provide symptomatic relief with the minimum of side effects.

Management

The first approach is to minimise exposure to allergens such as grass pollen in the spring, tree pollen at other times and house-dust mites; simple measures such as vacuuming the house, washing bed clothes at 60°C and freezing pillows may help.

Antihistamines

Initial pharmacological treatment is directed against histamine and involves H_1-receptor antagonists or antihistamines. These agents remove the symptoms of rhinorrhoea, itching, conjunctivitis and sneezing but not nasal obstruction. Older sedating agents include:

- chlorphenamine (Piriton)
- promethazine (Phenergan)
- alimemazine (Vallergan).

Some antihistamines (especially promethazine) have prominent antimuscarinic effects, which may limit their use. More recently, non-sedating agents have been introduced that have a better side-effect profile, which favours their use. Examples of non-sedating antihistamines include:

- acrivastine (Benadryl)
- cetirizine (Zirtek)
- fexofenadine (Telfast)
- loratadine (Clarityn)
- desloratadine (Neoclarityn), which is a metabolite of loratadine and all, except acrivastine, can be used once daily.

Topical antihistamines

Antihistamines such as azelastine are available as topical nasal and eye drops for the rapid relief of nasal and eye symptoms. Patients are probably better maintained on oral antihistamines but topical antihistamines may have a limited role as 'on demand' treatment against a background of continuous oral drug treatment. In addition, ocular antihistamines may be of use for the relief of occasional symptoms. Some ocular preparations may also contain sympathomimetic vasoconstrictors such as xylometazoline to reduce red eye.

Topical intranasal corticosteroids, e.g. beclometasone, budesonide, fluticasone and triamcinolone

Corticosteroids reduce the production of cytokines and chemokines, and the infiltration of antigen-presenting cells, T cells, eosinophils in the tissue and mast cells in epithelial mucosa. Clinical trials have shown that they are superior to oral or topical antihistamines for nasal symptoms but take several days for an effect, during which time an oral antihistamine is appropriate.

Administration via the nasal route reduces the side effects associated with corticosteroids, such as the risk of hypothalamic–pituitary–adrenal axis suppression, but in children their height should be monitored for height suppression. Patients with allergic rhinitis may also be asthmatic and, although the topical nasal steroids may be used in addition to inhaled steroids, there is an increased risk of side effects. Intranasal steroids should be avoided during nasal infection.

Oral steroids are not recommended as first-line treatment but can be used for short periods (<2 weeks) in severe disease or when control of symptoms is essential, e.g. during examination times. Indeed, by reducing mucus production in severe disease, they may enable topical agents to penetrate more easily.

Topical cromones: sodium cromoglicate and nedocromil sodium

The action of cromones is poorly defined but they may inhibit cytokine release from mast cells, possibly by blocking calcium channels. They may also inhibit sensory nerve activity and suppress local reflexes. Their effects are weak but they are devoid of side effects and are largely for seasonal disease. Eye drops containing cromones may also be effective for conjunctival symptoms. In both cases it may take several days for cromones to exert an effect.

Muscarinic antagonists: ipratropium

The muscarinic antagonist ipratropium is available as a nasal spray and will reduce the rhinorrhoea but will not affect other nasal symptoms such as itchiness. The older antihistamines also have appreciable antimuscarinic activity, which will contribute to their actions.

Decongestants, e.g. oxymetazoline, xylometazoline

These sympathomimetic agents are dealt with in Chapter 20. In the context of allergic rhinitis, these are applied topically and provide relief from nasal obstruction but once again their use should be limited to a week due to rebound congestion.

Hyposensitisation

This involves desensitisation of a patient towards an allergen but is very rarely carried out these days. To achieve this the patient is challenged with increasing subcutaneous doses of the allergen over time, starting with a very low dose, and this is believed to reduce the IgE response. This may be effective for severe allergic rhinitis when the allergen is identified and conventional treatment has failed, and may also be appropriate for wasp and bee venom stings. However, the process carries a significant risk of anaphylaxis and so hyposensitisation for allergic rhinitis is contraindicated in people with asthma, although, in the case of bee and wasp stings, the allergic response may be fatal and so asthma is not an absolute contraindication.

A introduction has been Grazax, which is a sublingual tablet containing an extract of Timothy grass to cause desensitisation. It is appropriate for patients with a proven grass allergy and who fail to respond to standard treatment. For it to be effective it should also be given for 16 weeks before and during the grass pollen hayfever season. At the moment its place in therapy remains to be established.

Choice of drugs (Figure 21.1)

Oral antihistamines and/or intranasal steroids seem to be the mainstay of therapy, with other agents being added to treatment in response to symptoms. Oral antihistamines tend to be used for mild or intermittent disease, whereas intranasal steroids are perhaps best used for persistent, moderate and severe disease, especially with nasal symptoms. Combining oral antihistamines and regular intranasal steroids would probably be the best approach in more severe disease. Other considerations are detailed in Table 21.1.

Drug interactions

The most significant interactions in the past have resulted from the increase in plasma concentrations of terfenadine due to various inhibitors of cytochrome P450, including macrolides. Inhibition of cytochrome P450-dependent metabolism prevents the breakdown of terfenadine to its active metabolite (fexofenadine), and the augmentation of terfenadine levels is associated with Q–T prolongation and fatal arrhythmias. In 1997 this resulted in terfenadine being changed from an over-the-counter (OTC) medicine

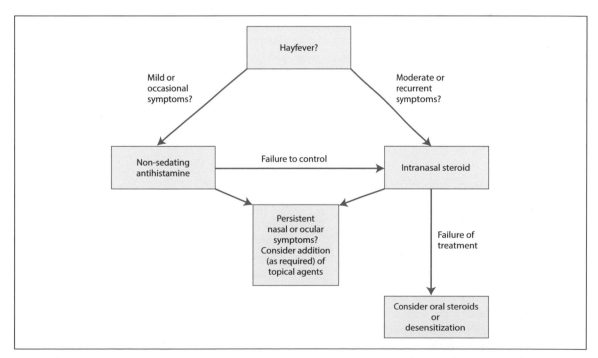

Figure 21.1 Typical management of allergic rhinitis. The scheme indicates the central role of either oral antihistamines or intranasal corticosteroids with 'add ons' of topical agents.

Table 21.1 The effects of concurrent conditions on drug choice in allergy

Condition	Effect on drug choice	Comments
Symptoms affecting sleep	This would favour the use of a sedating antihistamine	
Patient must be alert (e.g. driving, exams)	• This would preclude the use of a sedating antihistamine • Non-sedating antihistamines would be appropriate or nasal or, rarely, oral steroids	• The sedating effects are enhanced by alcohol • There is no evidence that alcohol enhances the effects of the newer, non-sedating antihistamines but patients should exercise caution
Glaucoma, prostatic hypertrophy, urinary retention	• Ipratropium is best avoided • Antimuscarinic side effects of certain older antihistamines mean that they should be used with caution in these conditions. Nasal steroids may rarely affect glaucoma. Vasoconstrictors, such as xylometazoline, should be avoided in angle-closure glaucoma	• Newer, non-sedating antihistamines are generally devoid of antimuscarinic actions and would be appropriate • The use of other drugs with antimuscarinic effects should be taken into account
Q–T prolongation	Avoid mizolastine	Mizolastine is associated with Q–T prolongation, leading to arrhythmias
Epilepsy	Antihistamines may occasionally lead to convulsions	Caution should be exercised
Porphyria	Avoid certain antihistamines	Cetirizine, chlorphenamine, cyclizine, doxylamine, loratadine and alimemazine are considered safe. Refer to the *British National Formulary*
Asthma	Steroids and leukotriene receptor antagonists are also used for asthma	Intranasal steroids may be used concurrently with inhaled steroids taken for asthma, but this may increase the chances of an ADR
	Antihistamines are of no clear benefit in asthma	Leukotriene receptor antagonists reduce the symptoms of allergic rhinitis and this may be a reason to choose them in concurrent asthma
Risk of anaphylaxis	This may be a reason to avoid continuous use of antihistamines	Antihistamines may mask the early warning symptoms
Renal impairment	• Avoid acrivastine in moderate impairment • Chlorphenamine is used for pruritus associated with renal failure	

ADR, adverse drug reaction.

to a prescription-only medicine (POM) and, since the introduction of fexofenadine, it has been discontinued. Other specific interactions are detailed in Table 21.2.

Counselling

General counselling may be directed at avoiding contact with allergens and limiting them in the home. Patients with hayfever may benefit from wearing sunglasses and should avoid going outdoors and keep the windows closed when the pollen count is high. For occupation-related allergies the patient should be advised to wear suitable protective clothing.

Antihistamines

• Patients taking sedating antihistamines should be advised that their ability to drive or operate machinery may be impaired. The sedation will be enhanced by alcohol.
• Non-sedating antihistamines rarely affect skilled tasks in this way but patients should be advised to exercise caution.

Topical antihistamines

Nasal antihistamines would be best used as an add-on to oral treatment with worsening symptoms.

Table 21.2 Examples of interactions with antihistamines

Drugs	Consequences	Comments
Alcohol with sedating antihistamines	The sedating effects are enhanced by alcohol	There is no evidence that alcohol enhances the effects of the newer non-sedating antihistamines but patients should exercise caution
Mizolastine with erythromycin, ketoconazole or antiarrhythmics (class I and III) which prolong Q–T interval	Concomitant use should be avoided due to the risk of potentially fatal torsade de pointes arrhythmias	Caution with cimetidine, ciclosporin and nifedipine
Older antihistamines with antimuscarinic agents (e.g. tricyclic antidepressants, certain antipsychotics)	Potentiation of antimuscarinic side effects	These will also oppose the actions of acetylcholinesterase inhibitors used in dementia

Decongestants

These should only be used for 5–7 days due to the risk of rebound congestion.

Ocular agents

- Ocular antihistamines are best used for occasional eye symptoms.
- Long-term use of eye drops containing xylometazoline should be avoided due to vasoconstrictor effects on the eye.
- Contact lenses should not be worn during conjunctival symptoms or after the application of drugs.

Topical corticosteroids

- In seasonal rhinitis treatment should be started a week or two before the appearance of pollen.
- These drugs will take several days to act and in the meantime an oral antihistamine may be used for relief.
- They should be used continuously, even if the patient feels better.

Cromones

- They will take a few days for an effect to occur.
- They should be used continuously, even if symptoms resolve.

Intranasal agents

Correct application is important. The patient should shake the container, close the other nostril with a finger, bend forward, spray and inhale, but avoid sniffing.

Allergy and anaphylaxis

Many foreign substances can elicit an allergic response, affecting many systems, including the skin and airways. Examples of important allergens include:

- drugs (especially penicillins, streptokinase, non-steroidal anti-inflammatory drugs [NSAIDs] including aspirin, monoclonal antibodies, vaccines, radiological contrast media)
- food (particularly nuts and seafood) but should be distinguished from food intolerance
- insect bites
- snake venom
- latex
- household chemicals or pollutants.

Drug-induced allergy

This is a serious Type B adverse drug reaction and affects a minority of patients on second exposure to the drug, even to minute doses, and manifests as an allergic response. Allergic drug reactions are dealt with in more detail in Chapter 6.

Management of allergic reaction

Regardless of the cause, the first measure is to remove the patient from exposure to the allergen or prevent exposure. In an allergic reaction leading to a maculopapular rash or urticaria, an oral antihistamine should be considered the mainstay of treatment. In local allergic responses to insect stings, an oral antihistamine should be given and topical hydro-cortisone may be applied. In both cases, topical anti-histamines such as mepyramine should be avoided because they may irritate the tissue. As a secondary measure for more severe reactions, an oral steroid may be appropriate.

Prophylaxis

When it is anticipated that medical treatment, such as the use of radiological contrast media or monoclonal antibodies, may lead to an allergic response, patients may receive a prophylactic oral antihistamine and possibly a corticosteroid.

Anaphylaxis

Anaphylactic shock is a serious life-threatening aller-gic reaction due to production of IgE and involves high yields of mediators, especially histamine. Anaphylactoid shock is related to anaphylaxis but does not involve IgE. Anaphylaxis may manifest within 30 minutes of exposure and symptoms include:

- angioedema (including swollen lips, eyelids and tongue)
- shortness of breath
- wheezing
- generalised itch
- hypotension.

Oedema is an important feature, with extrava-sation of fluid from the circulation leading to hypo-tension and airway obstruction. Antihistamines may mask the early symptoms of anaphylaxis and so they should be avoided as continuous treatment in patients at risk.

Treatment of anaphylaxis

Basic life support measures are essential and involve maintaining airways and laying the patient flat. Treatment is aimed at bronchodilation, supporting the circulation and suppressing the immune response. To this end 'shock boxes' containing adrenaline (epinephrine), chlorphenamine and hydrocortisone are available.

Initially adrenaline is given intramuscularly and this may be repeated at 10-minute intervals accord-ing to blood pressure and respiration. The purpose of administering adrenaline is to restore blood pres-sure by increasing cardiac output, via activation of cardiac β_1-adrenoceptors, and vasoconstriction via α-adrenoceptors. The adrenaline will also act on bronchial β_2-adrenoceptors to oppose the bronchos-pasm. In patients who are receiving non-selective β blockers, the effects of adrenaline will be reduced and so intravenous salbutamol should also be considered. Further measures include oxygen, an inhaled β_2 ago-nist if there is a wheeze, a saline infusion to restore circulating volume in hypotension and intravenous antihistamine (e.g. chlorphenamine) to oppose the effects of histamine.

As a secondary measure to suppress the immune response, hydrocortisone may be given intravenously.

Adrenaline for self-administration

Patients at risk of anaphylaxis may be given adren-aline for self-administration via intramuscular injec-tion as required, e.g. after a bee sting. These patients require instructions in the use of the adrenaline administration devices and should be advised to wear a Medic Alert bracelet.

Drug interactions with adrenaline

As commented above, adrenaline may be less effec-tive in patients taking β blockers and higher doses of adrenaline or intravenous salbutamol should be used. The interaction between non-selective β block-ers (such as propranolol) and adrenaline in normo-tensive patients is discussed in Chapter 6. Topical β blockers such as timolol eye drops for glaucoma may also interact with adrenaline. In patients who are at risk of anaphylaxis it may be sensible, if possible, to swap from β blockers to alternative drugs.

The effects of adrenaline are enhanced by tricyclic antidepressants which prevent the uptake of adren-aline and so increase its concentration. Accordingly, lower doses of adrenaline should be used in patients who are taking tricyclic antidepressants. Alterna-tively, the antidepressant may be changed to a selec-tive serotonin reuptake inhibitor, which should not interact with adrenaline.

Practice points
- Oral antihistamines and/or nasal steroids should be regarded as the mainstay of therapy for allergic rhinitis.

- Prompt recognition of the symptoms of anaphylaxis is essential.
- Patients at risk of anaphylaxis should be counselled on how to use an adrenaline autoinjector.

CASE STUDY

A 40-year-old lorry driver visits his community pharmacy complaining of hayfever, which he had as a child but remembers the drugs that he took as being 'awful' as they made him feel worse than the hayfever.

Past medical history: asthma
Drugs:
salbutamol 200 micrograms as required
beclometasone 200 micrograms twice daily

What symptoms is the patient likely to have?
- Nasal itching, rhinorrhoea, sneezing and conjunctival symptoms, which are worsened by irritants

He would like something that will clear up his hayfever; what do you suggest?

- A non-sedating H_1-receptor antagonist such as loratadine or acrivastine may be recommended. These are available OTC and should not interfere with his ability to drive. Several weeks later he complains that, although he is much better, his nose is still blocked and his eyes are still watery.

What OTC medication might you prescribe?
- Possibilities include:

  - a topical nasal steroid such as beclometasone for prophylaxis and treatment; it may be added to the inhaled steroid
  - sodium cromoglicate nasal spray or eye drops, but these will take several days to act; he should not drive immediately after the drops if his vision is blurred
  - antihistamine eye drops for fast relief.

References

British National Formulary, latest edition. London: British Medical Association and Royal Pharmaceutical Society of Great Britain.

22

Asthma and chronic obstructive pulmonary disease

Asthma

Disease characteristics

Asthma is a common clinical condition affecting 5–10% of the population and appears to be on the increase. It is especially prevalent in children but also has a high incidence in more elderly patients. Asthma is defined as reversible increases in airway resistance, involving both bronchoconstriction and inflammation.

Underlying pathology

In order to appreciate the causes and treatment of asthma, it is important to understand the control of bronchial calibre, and hence airway resistance. Parasympathetic innervation results in acetylcholine acting on bronchial muscarinic M_3-receptors, which cause bronchoconstriction and increased mucus secretion. The bronchial smooth-muscle cells also contain β_2-adrenoceptors, which are linked via adenosine cyclic 3':5'-monophosphate (cAMP) to bronchodilation. The β_2-adrenoceptors have no direct innervation but are responsive to circulating adrenaline (epinephrine), which stimulates bronchodilation (Figure 22.1). In addition, the mucous glands contain β_2-adrenoceptors,

which inhibit mucus secretion. There are also a limited number of sympathetic fibres that release noradrenaline (norepinephrine), acting on β_2-adrenoceptors at parasympathetic ganglia to inhibit transmission. Non-adrenergic non-cholinergic fibres also play a role in which nitric oxide and vasoactive intestinal polypeptide are inhibitory transmitters and substance P is an

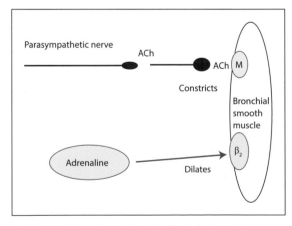

Figure 22.1 Autonomic control of bronchial smooth muscle with direct parasympathetic innervation (leading to bronchoconstriction) and circulating adrenaline (leading to bronchodilation). ACh, acetylcholine; M, muscarinic.

excitatory transmitter. These sensory nerve fibres are thought to play a role in local reflex responses to irritant stimuli.

An asthma attack may comprise an early (immediate) phase with bronchospasm which may be followed by a late phase (Figure 22.2), characterised by both increased airway resistance and inflammation. Other variations include an immediate phase alone, a late phase without an immediate phase and recurrent late phases.

An asthma attack is often provoked by allergens, cold air, viral infections, smoking, certain foods or exercise. It should also be noted that asthma has a genetic component and is associated with atopy. The immediate phase of the attack is associated with the release of spasmogens (histamine, prostaglandin D_2, leukotrienes LTC_4 and LTD_4, and platelet-activating factor [PAF]) from mast cells and mononuclear cells, which lead to rapid bronchospasm (Figure 22.3). Chemotaxins (including LTB_4 and PAF) then attract leukocytes (especially eosinophils and mononuclear cells), which lead to inflammation and airway hyperactivity, associated with the late phase. This second phase occurs some 3–6 hours after the initial release of the mediators.

Long-term growth changes in the bronchial smooth muscle in asthma lead to hyperplasia, with associated increases in airway responsiveness. This is referred to as remodelling.

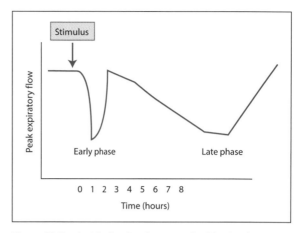

Figure 22.3 An idealised asthma attack with stimulus leading to the early phase with this being followed several hours later by a late phase. The attack is shown by the decreases in peak expiratory flow, indicating an increase in airway resistance.

Drug-induced asthma

Non-steroidal anti-inflammatory drugs (NSAIDs) may provoke asthma in a number of sensitive individuals (about 15% of people with asthma). This is achieved by inhibition of cyclo-oxygenase, and is thought to lead to more arachidonic acid being available as a substrate, resulting in increased leukotriene production.

β blockers may also induce bronchospasm, by blocking the $β_2$-adrenoceptors on the bronchial smooth muscle. It is for this reason that β blockers (even in eye drops for glaucoma) are contraindicated in asthma (and often, but not always, avoided in chronic obstructive pulmonary disease [COPD]). $β_1$-adrenoceptor antagonists should be used only in *extreme* circumstances in patients with asthma and under supervision.

Clinical features

The leading clinical features are wheezing, breathlessness, a tight chest and cough, which are intermittent and may be worse at night or on exercise.

Asthma is due to reversible increases in airway resistance, characterised by reversible decreases in the ratio of forced expiratory volume in the first second (FEV_1) to the forced vital capacity (FVC). A value of less than 70% suggests increased airway resistance

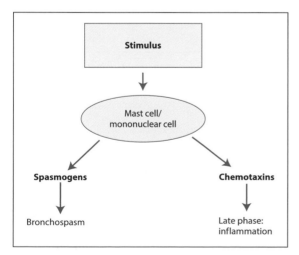

Figure 22.2 Phases of an asthmatic attack with early bronchospasm and the late inflammatory phase.

and in asthma the change should be reversed by a β_2-adrenoceptor agonist. In diagnosis, a reduction of peak expiratory flow (PEF) or FVC which improves with therapy (β_2-adrenoceptor agonist or a trial of steroids) is consistent with asthma.

In people with asthma the airway resistance may also show variations throughout the day and typically increases in the morning; this is termed 'morning dipping'. In children, the diagnosis is often based on a history that may include wheezing, cough (a persistent dry nocturnal cough may be the only feature), exacerbations on infection and a family association. Asthma is associated with atopy and individuals are likely to have a history of eczema and/or hayfever.

Asthma is divided further into episodic asthma and chronic asthma. Episodic asthma tends to occur in atopic individuals who have periods of attacks associated with provoking factors such as viral infection, allergens or exercise. The attacks include wheezing and breathlessness but the patient shows no symptoms between attacks. Chronic asthma runs a course of prolonged periods of breathlessness and wheezing, with a cough and wheezing at night. The cough is often productive of mucoid sputum. Severe acute asthma (status asthmaticus) is a serious and potentially life-threatening occurrence that involves severe bronchospasm: its management is considered later.

Goals of treatment

Given the two key phases of an asthmatic attack, treatment is divided into relief of symptoms, which is achieved by bronchodilators (relievers) and may reverse the early phase, and prevention using anti-inflammatory agents (preventers).

Pharmacological basis of management

β-adrenoceptor agonists, e.g. salbutamol, terbutaline

These are the agents of first choice and act on β_2-adrenoceptors on the bronchial smooth muscle to increase cAMP, leading to rapid bronchodilation and reversal of the bronchospasm associated with the early phase (Figure 22.4). Prolonged use is associated with receptor down-regulation, making them less effective. However, there is some evidence that

concomitant treatment with corticosteroids may reduce receptor down-regulation.

Long-acting β-adrenoceptor agonists, e.g. formoterol (eformoterol), salmeterol

Although these are also β_2-adrenoceptor agonists, which cause bronchodilation, the rate of onset of long-acting β_2-adrenoceptor agonist is slow and, more importantly, through its lipophilic properties the molecule is retained near the receptor for a prolonged period, which means that its action persists. Accordingly, they are not used to reverse an attack but cause prolonged bronchodilation, which is preventive. Following initial safety concerns, they should not be used as sole therapy and should always be prescribed alongside an inhaled steroid. They are more effective than xanthines or cromones.

Xanthines: aminophylline, theophylline

These are also bronchodilators, but are not as effective as β_2-adrenoceptor agonists and are given orally (theophylline or aminophylline, which is theophylline with ethylenediamine) or occasionally intravenously (aminophylline with improved solubility). Pharmacologically, their actions are less clear; they are phosphodiesterase III and IV inhibitors and so will potentiate cAMP by preventing its breakdown, which leads to bronchodilation. Additional therapeutic actions may include blockade of adenosine receptors, which leads to bronchial smooth-muscle relaxation, and anti-inflammatory actions through a

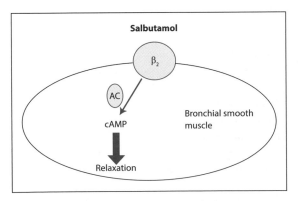

Figure 22.4 The mechanism of bronchodilation in response to a β_2-agonist. This leads to G-protein-dependent activation of adenylyl cyclase (AC) and an increase in intracellular adenosine cyclic 3′:5′-monophosphate (cAMP).

reduction in mediator release. Xanthines show a narrow therapeutic window (see Chapter 7), with toxic concentrations leading to nausea and central nervous system (CNS) stimulation as side effects.

Corticosteroids: inhalation (beclometasone, budesonide, fluticasone) and oral (prednisolone)

These agents have an anti-inflammatory action via activation of intracellular receptors, leading to altered gene transcription. This results in decreased cytokine production and the synthesis of annexin (also known as lipocortin), which inhibits phospholipase A_2, and the production of prostaglandins and leukotrienes.

Fungal oral infections occur as a common side effect with inhalation, due to local immunosuppression. Laryngeal myopathy may also lead to hoarseness. Systemic steroid effects, including adrenal suppression and bone resorption, occur with high-dose inhalation or oral dosing.

Leukotriene receptor antagonists: montelukast, zafirlukast

This class of orally active drugs block leukotriene receptors and so will oppose the bronchoconstrictor and inflammatory actions of leukotrienes. They should be used as a 'preventer' therapy. Given their actions against the leukotrienes they are of particular use in atoptic asthma and montelukast is also used in seasonal rhinitis.

Cromones: nedocromil sodium, sodium cromoglicate

Sodium cromoglicate is thought to prevent both the early and late phases of an attack. Its action is uncertain but may include a reduction in sensory nerve reflexes, stabilisation of mast cells, and a reduction in the release of PAF and cytokines. Cromones are effective only in a few patients: prevention of bronchoconstriction is an early effect and prevention of the late phase may require up to a month of treatment to occur. There is also some evidence that cromones may be effective in exercise-induced asthma.

Immunoglobulin E antibodies: omalizumab

This novel agent has a role in treatment-resistant asthma. It is a monoclonal antibody that is directed against free immunoglobulin E (IgE), but not bound IgE, and prevents IgE from binding to immune cells that would otherwise lead to allergen-induced mediator release in allergic asthma.

Choice of drugs

The initial approach is to educate the patient to recognise and avoid trigger factors such as dust, animals, smoke and cold air. Lifestyle advice regarding weight reduction may be beneficial in overweight patients. Breastfeeding of infants is also recommended because it protects against the development of asthma.

Drugs have a major role in the management of asthma but two major problems limit their effectiveness: undertreatment and poor patient compliance, largely due to poor inhaler technique. The pharmacological basis of the treatment of asthma is well established and described in the British Thoracic Society (BTS) and Scottish Intercollegiate Guidelines Network (SIGN) joint British guidelines (2014) and has a stepped-care approach (Figure 22.5), with treatment being stepped up if the patient requires a β_2-agonist more than twice a week. These guidelines recommend favouring the use of alternative drugs before increasing the dose of inhaled steroids. Another important feature is the emphasis that inhaled steroid dosages should be the minimum required for control.

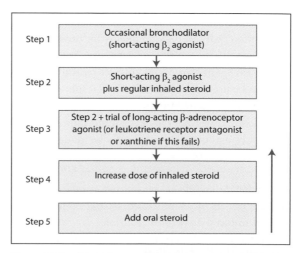

Figure 22.5 Stepped-care approach to the management of asthma in adults according to British Thoracic Society (BTS) and Scottish Intercollegiate Guidelines Network (SIGN) joint British guidelines (2014).

The treatment should be reviewed regularly (3 months) and a step-down considered in patients who are stabilised. If a reduction in the dose of the inhaled drug is appropriate then it should be reduced by 25–50%, with further reductions considered thereafter at 3-monthly intervals.

The role of leukotriene receptor antagonists has now been established in the BTS/SIGN guidelines. In addition, their pharmacological action suggests that they would oppose NSAID-induced asthma, by blocking the actions of leukotrienes, which are implicated in this adverse drug reaction.

Long-acting β_2-adrenoceptor agonists have a valuable role in addition to, and not in place of, inhaled steroids. Their prolonged action means that they are of particular benefit in nocturnal asthma but it is important that their effectiveness does not lead to reduced compliance with inhaled steroids. Indeed, combined preparations of long-acting β_2-adrenoceptor agonists and corticosteroids may help improve compliance.

Immunisations against pneumococcal infection and influenza are appropriate for patients with asthma.

In severe disease, and to reduce the need for steroids ('steroid sparing'), immunosuppression with ciclosporin or methotrexate is used in some patients. In asthma that proves to be mediated by IgE and not controlled by full optimum therapy (stage 5 of BTS guidelines), omalizumab may be added.

Children

In children there is also a stepped-care approach with different BTS/SIGN guidelines for those aged <5 years. Essentially steps 1 and 2 are similar to those in adults, except at step 2 a leukotriene receptor antagonist can be used if an inhaled steroid is inappropriate, while at step 3 a leukotriene receptor antagonist can be added to a steroid. However, if this fails to control the child's asthma, referral should be made to a respiratory physician.

During treatment, it is recommended that the child's height should be monitored in relation to the adverse effects of uncontrolled asthma on height and steroid-induced growth retardation.

Exercise-induced asthma

The BTS/SIGN guidelines indicate that β_2-adrenoceptor agonists (long and short acting), inhaled steroids, xanthines, leukotriene receptor antagonists and cromones protect against exercise-induced asthma whereas antimuscarinic agents do not. The guidelines also suggest that exercise-induced asthma may indicate poor management of asthma and that treatment should be reviewed.

Pregnancy

During pregnancy control of asthma is important. β_2-adrenoceptor agonists and inhaled steroids are used as normal and oral steroids may be used as normal in severe asthma. Leukotriene receptor antagonists may be continued if they were essential for control before pregnancy but should not be introduced.

Choice of inhaler

The choice of an inhaler device is crucial for effective delivery of the drugs. Metered dose inhalers (MDIs) are the most commonly used; however, it should be recognised that many patients have a poor inhaler technique and require counselling in their use. To overcome problems of coordination of breathing with administration, a spacer may be used in which the drug is distributed for inhalation. This may also reduce steroid-induced oral candidiasis.

In addition, in the selection of an inhaler the following should be taken into account:

- The age of the patient: for children under 5 years of age, the NICE (2000) recommends that inhaled therapy should be via a pressurised MDI and spacer, with a mask if required. When this is not possible or effective, then nebulised therapy is appropriate; a dry powder inhaler may also be considered for 3 to 5 year olds. NICE guidelines (2002) recommend that, for children aged 5–15 years, a pressurised MDI and spacer be used for regular corticosteroid therapy, unless adherence is problematic. For other inhaled therapy, especially bronchodilators, the device that best allows spontaneous use should be chosen. The inhaler requirements should be reviewed at least annually.
- Impaired respiratory function: this may make a breath-activated device impossible to use.
- The lifestyle of the patient: can the inhaler be used at school or work?
- The physical ability of the patient, e.g. patients with arthritis may not be able to activate the

pressurised inhalers or refill devices. Patients with poor eyesight may be unable to read the dose counters.

Adverse drug reactions and interactions

Asthma therapy largely involves inhalation, which limits systemic effects. Having said that, over-administration or absorption may of course lead to side effects. Systemic effects of β_2-adrenoceptor agonists include tremor and tachycardia, due to activation of peripheral β_2-adrenoceptors and cardiac β-adrenoceptors, respectively. The sympathomimetic actions of β_2-adrenoceptor agonists mean that they should be used with caution in conditions where increased sympathetic activity would be undesirable, such as in hyperthyroidism, arrhythmias, hypertension and diabetes mellitus. Prolonged overuse of β_2-adrenoceptor agonists is also associated with hypokalaemia, caused by activation of the sodium pump, leading to cellular uptake of potassium.

Systemic side effects of ipratropium are antimuscarinic in nature but are limited. When using nebulised ipratropium, the drug should not come into contact with the eyes because this may lead to glaucoma.

Xanthines are given either orally or intravenously and will of course have systemic effects. This is important because xanthines have a narrow therapeutic window and toxicity may lead to gastrointestinal and CNS side effects. Accordingly, monitoring of plasma levels and side effects is important.

Side effects of inhaled corticosteroids are dose related and are more pronounced at the higher doses (>800 micrograms of beclometasone dipropionate equivalent in adults and 400 micrograms of beclometasone dipropionate equivalent in children). These include height suppression in children (which should be monitored), adrenal suppression, osteoporosis, skin thinning, cataracts and anti-insulin effects leading to diabetes. Inhalation of the steroid may lead to impaction on the throat, which may promote local candidiasis. Adrenal suppression is a recognised adverse effect of inhaled steroids and may present as non-specific symptoms such as weight loss, nausea, hypoglycaemia and reduced consciousness. To avoid these problems, the maximum licensed doses should not be exceeded and the lowest effective dose should

be used. Oral corticosteroids are more likely to lead to systemic effects and are associated with gastric damage (see Chapter 8).

Leukotriene receptor antagonists have been associated with Churg–Strauss syndrome (lung vasculitis), which may be accompanied by a rash. This may be more likely to occur when oral steroid therapy is reduced or stopped.

In terms of drug interactions, there are no obvious intergroup interactions that would have a significant bearing on therapy. However, xanthines, by preventing the breakdown of cAMP, will potentiate the actions of β_2-adrenoceptor agonists. This is generally considered desirable but the side effects of β_2-adrenoceptor agonists (including risk of hypokalaemia) may also be enhanced. The hypokalaemic effect of β_2-adrenoceptor agonists and xanthines will also be potentiated by concomitant corticosteroids and potassium-losing diuretics (loop diuretics and thiazides). Plasma potassium levels should be monitored in patients with severe asthma.

Theophylline, in particular, has a number of significant interactions. These interactions are largely at the level of cytochrome P450, with some inducers of cytochrome P450 reducing the concentrations of theophylline, whereas some inhibitors may augment the plasma levels. In view of its narrow therapeutic window, theophylline should be used with caution and monitored appropriately and the dosage altered if necessary. Some drugs that may influence plasma levels of theophylline are summarised in Table 22.1.

In addition, theophylline may enhance renal excretion of concomitant lithium therapy, leading to reductions in its plasma concentrations, which should be monitored and the dosage increased if necessary.

β_2-adrenoceptor agonists and corticosteroids used in combination are particularly effective in the control of asthma. A laboratory-based study by Roth *et al.* (2002) demonstrated that β_2-adrenoceptor agonists and corticosteroids interact at the cellular level to enhance gene transcription. It was proposed that this might contribute to their antiproliferative effects on the bronchial smooth muscle.

Over-the-counter considerations

Respiratory complaints form a large proportion of requests for over-the-counter (OTC) medicines such as cough mixtures and sympathomimetics (see Chapter 20). This raises issues for patients with asthma or COPD. In both conditions a cough may suggest poor control or an exacerbation and review of inhaler technique or a referral is appropriate. Furthermore, as commented above, a nocturnal cough in a child may arouse the suspicion of asthma. Of particular importance, antitussive agents are contraindicated in COPD because they may lead to sputum retention.

Despite many people's perceptions, asthma alone is not a sound reason to avoid sympathomimetics. However, on theoretical grounds they would be expected to enhance the sympathetic actions and side effects in patients taking β_2-adrenoceptor agonists and should be used with caution. Topical agents are less likely to have systemic effects and are preferred to oral ones (see Chapter 20), although, once again, the request for a sympathomimetic may indicate an inter-current infection.

Counselling

Counselling has a major role in ensuring patient compliance and correct inhaler technique. General counselling should include advice to avoid precipitating factors, including caution with NSAIDs and avoidance in patients with a known sensitivity to them. Smoking and smoky atmospheres must be avoided. Patients should always have a short-acting β_2-adrenoceptor agonist inhaler available and should ensure that they do not run out of supplies. Attention should be paid to inhaler technique because a significant number of patients are incapable of using a pressurised inhaler or have a poor technique leading to failure of treatment. Patients should monitor their own PEF and may require counselling in the use of peak flow meters. Specific advice is as follows.

Spacers

● The device should be washed out monthly and left to air dry after use to prevent static electricity from causing the drug particles to stick to it.
● They should be replaced every 6–12 months.

Short-acting β_2-adrenoceptor agonists

● They should be used as required to relieve an attack.
● They may be used before an event that may trigger asthma such as exercise.
● If they are required more than once a day, patients should consult their general practitioner (GP) with a view to moving up the ladder of care.

Table 22.1 Some drugs that may influence plasma levels of theophylline	
Drugs that may increase plasma levels of theophylline	**Drugs that may decrease plasma levels of theophylline**
Aciclovir	Barbiturates
Amiodarone (rare)	Carbamazepine
Oral contraceptives (but not thought to lead to toxicity)	Rifampicin
Disulfiram	Ritonavir
Erythromycin: this is much less of a problem with clarithromycin	Tobacco smoke
	Levothyroxine
Fluvoxamine	Ketoconazole (isolated reports)
Cimetidine	
Phenylpropanolamine	
Ciprofloxacin	
Carbimazole	
Nifedipine, verapamil and fluconazole (isolated reports)	

- Patients should not exceed the maximum dose or frequency in 24 hours.
- CFC-free inhalers may taste and feel different to CFC-containing preparations.

Long-acting β₂-adrenoceptor agonists

These will not relieve an attack but are used to prevent an attack.

Inhaled corticosteroids

- The judicious use of steroids outweighs any adverse effects, even in children.
- Inhalation limits their systemic effects.
- These will take several days to have an effect.
- If taking with a β₂-adrenoceptor agonist, the β₂ agonist should be taken first to dilate the airways, which will aid deposition of the steroid.
- They may cause a sore throat: to reduce the chances of this occurring, patients should rinse their mouth or gargle after use.
- High-dose steroids from an MDI should be administered with a spacer device, to prevent impaction on the throat.
- These are preventive and should be taken even when the patient is stabilised with few or no attacks.
- Steroid cards should be issued to those with high-dose inhalers.
- With doses exceeding 800 micrograms beclometasone (or equivalent) per day, there is a risk of osteoporosis. Measures to avoid this should be encouraged, such as exercise, adequate calcium and vitamin D intake, smoking cessation and hormone replacement therapy, if appropriate.

Oral steroids

- These may have an important role in poorly controlled asthma.
- They should be taken in the morning.
- Any indigestion should be reported.
- The patient should not stop taking the steroid suddenly if the course is longer than 3 weeks.
- If patients have never had chickenpox, they should avoid contact with the virus and consult their GP if they are exposed to it.

Xanthines

- Patients should be vigilant for signs of toxicity such as tremor, palpitations, nausea and CNS stimulation.
- Patients should avoid excess caffeine.
- Patients should not change from brands on which they are stabilised.

Cromones

They may themselves cause wheezing due to the irritant effects of the powder on the airways.

Leukotriene receptor antagonists

- These should not be used for an acute attack.
- They may cause a headache.
- Any rash while taking them should be reported.
- Patients taking zafirlukast should report nausea, jaundice or other signs of liver damage.

Acute severe asthma

Although acute asthma attacks are largely beyond the scope of this book, a brief description of their features and management is appropriate. It should be recognised that asthma may be life threatening and prompt recognition of clinical features is important. In a severe attack the following may be present:

- The patient is unable to complete a sentence.
- There may be tachycardia (>110 beats/minute; greater in children).
- There may be tachypnoea (>25 breaths/minute; greater in children).
- Peak flow >35 to <50% of predicted.

Signs and symptoms of life-threatening attacks include:

- a silent chest
- cyanosis
- bradycardia
- exhaustion
- peak flow <35% of predicted.

In a severe acute attack the treatment is:

- oxygen (40–60%)
- nebulised β₂-adrenoceptor agonist (e.g. salbutamol or terbutaline) as soon as possible

- oral prednisolone or intravenous hydrocortisone; prednisolone 40–50 mg daily should be continued for at least 5 days.

In a life-threatening attack the following may be added:

- nebulised ipratropium
- intravenous magnesium sulphate
- intravenous aminophylline, provided that the patient is not already receiving a xanthine.

Chronic obstructive pulmonary disease

Disease characteristics

COPD encompasses both chronic bronchitis and emphysema, and is typically a disease of late onset with a very close association with a history of smoking. Some smokers are more susceptible to developing COPD than others, while a smoker's cough may be an early manifestation of the disease. COPD may also appear in former smokers decades after they have stopped smoking. In most patients, COPD is generally a combination, to varying degrees, of both chronic bronchitis and emphysema.

In the past chronic bronchitis was defined as sputum production for 3 months of the year for two consecutive years. A more helpful definition of COPD is a chronic reduction in the predicted FEV_1 (<80%), with the following grades:

- Mild COPD: FEV_1 is 80–50% of predicted.
- Moderate COPD: FEV_1 is 49–30% of predicted.
- Severe COPD: FEV_1 is <30% of predicted.

The FEV_1/FVC ratio is likely to be <0.7 and, unlike asthma, there is little variation in PEF. Absolute PEF measurements tend to underestimate the extent of COPD, and FEV_1 is the measurement recommended by the BTS for diagnosis and monitoring.

Chronic bronchitis is an inflammatory response (usually following many years of smoking), leading to proliferation of goblet cells with excess mucus production, which leads to airway obstruction. The chronic inflammation, oedema and fibrosis also lead to increases in airway tissue thickness. These changes

lead to the symptoms of a productive cough, wheeze, dyspnoea and acute exacerbations with infections. In more severe disease, the dyspnoea is disabling, there may be secondary polycythaemia and pulmonary hypertension may lead to right-sided heart failure (cor pulmonale). Emphysema is similarly linked to smoking, although in a very small proportion of patients it is due to a genetic deficiency of α_1-antitrypsin. There is marked destruction of the alveoli, leading to dilatation, with reduced elastic recoil of the airways, so the airways are held open during expiration.

Goals of treatment

The prognosis of COPD depends on severity but is generally poor with progressive deterioration. The key goal of treatment is to improve respiratory function.

Pharmacological basis of therapy

Bronchodilators including the short and long-acting β_2-agonists (see above) play a major role in the management of COPD.

Muscarinic M-receptor antagonists: short acting (ipratropium) and long acting (tiotropium)

These agents are given by inhalation and block parasympathetically-mediated bronchoconstriction with only limited systemic side effects. Tiotropium bromide is a new long-acting member and may be given once a day. The bronchodilator effects of muscarinic antagonists are less than those of β_2-adrenoceptor agonists and they are of little or no value in the treatment of asthma but play an important role on COPD.

Management (Figure 22.6)

The treatment of COPD was reviewed by NICE in 2010 and their guidelines should be consulted. In the first instance, smoking cessation must be emphasised, because this may lead to a slowing of the disease process and a reduction of carboxyhaemoglobin. The pharmacological management is based on the drugs used in asthma, described above.

Bronchodilators

In general, patients with COPD are less responsive to bronchodilators because bronchospasm is not a feature of COPD. However, some patients do benefit from β₂-adrenoceptor agonists and they are widely prescribed for the relief of symptoms and for use before exercise. Traditionally, muscarinic antagonists such as ipratropium have also been used to oppose vagally mediated bronchoconstriction and appear to be as effective as β₂-adrenoceptor agonists, but have a slower rate of onset and so are less effective as relievers. More recently the longer-acting muscarinic antagonist, tiotropium, has been introduced. The combination of a β₂-adrenoceptor agonist and muscarinic antagonist may give an even better response.

The BTS guidelines suggest that all patients with COPD should receive a bronchodilator reversibility test. Here a positive response is defined as >200 mL increase in FEV$_1$ and >15% increase of the baseline value in response to inhaled bronchodilators. This should identify patients who would benefit most from bronchodilator therapy. Responses with >500 mL increase in FEV$_1$ may, in fact, reveal asthma.

The role of long-acting β₂-adrenoceptor agonists in COPD has now been established and they are of benefit in addition to short-acting β₂-adrenoceptor agonists and muscarinic antagonists.

Xanthines have less of a role in COPD due to their narrow therapeutic window and offer no advantages over β₂-adrenoceptor agonists or muscarinic antagonists. However, some patients may empirically show an improvement with xanthines.

The role of corticosteroids

Despite the inflammatory nature of COPD, corticosteroids are relatively ineffective in most patients; indeed the disease process may make the patients less responsive to steroids. However, approximately 15% of patients respond to corticosteroids and this is often due to undiagnosed asthma as opposed to COPD. NICE (2010) recommends that an inhaled steroid in combination with a long-acting β₂-adrenoceptor agonist or long-acting muscarinic antagonist should be used in patients with FEV$_1$ that is 50% or less than predicted.

Other considerations

The BTS and NICE recommend that patients with COPD should be immunised against influenza and pneumococcal infection, although evidence for the effectiveness of the latter is yet to be fully established. Depression should be identified and treated.

Long-term oxygen therapy is the only treatment known to improve the outlook in patients with severe COPD. By providing 24–28% oxygen for at least

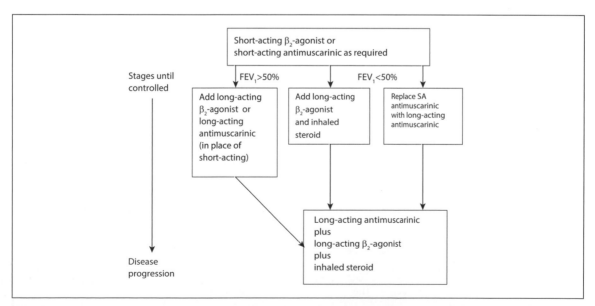

Figure 22.6 Summary of the NICE guidance (2010) on the management of chronic obstructive pulmonary disease. SA, short acting.

15 hours a day the consequences of hypoxia (e.g. pulmonary hypertension, cor pulmonale and polycythaemia) are reduced. The oxygen concentration should not exceed 28%, because higher concentrations will lead to carbon dioxide trapping.

In the presence of cor pulmonale, leading to peripheral oedema, the administration of diuretics is appropriate. Venesection (bleeding the patient) should be considered for polycythaemia.

In an acute exacerbation, the use of bronchodilators may be increased. Oral steroids may also be added for 7–14 days. Antibiotics may be of benefit in acute exacerbations and may be given to motivated patients who would be able to initiate treatment at the start of an exacerbation. The BTS recommends that antibiotics are of value only if at least two of the following are present: purulent sputum, increased breathlessness and increased volume of sputum.

Counselling

Smoking cessation must be emphasised because this will slow the progression of the disease. Exercise should be encouraged to improve exercise tolerance and weight loss encouraged in overweight patients.

For drug-specific counselling, see the comments above for the drugs used in asthma.

Self-assessment

For the following questions concerning asthma and COPD, choose the most appropriate answer:

1 *Which one of the following classes of drugs is contraindicated in asthma?*

   A Antimuscarinic drugs
   B ACE inhibitors
   C β_1-adrenoceptor antagonists
   D Clopidogrel
   E Nitrates

2 *NSAID-induced asthma is thought to be due to which one of the following?*

   A Diversion of arachidonic acid to the lipoxygenase pathway
   B Inhibition of lipoxygenase pathway

   C Reduced production of bronchodilator prostaglandins
   D Release of acetylcholine
   E Increased levels of bradykinin

3 *Long-acting β_2-adrenceptor agonists (such as salmeterol) are best used under which one of the following conditions?*

   A When a short-acting β_2-adrenceptor agonists (such as salbutamol) alone is insufficient
   B To relieve attacks
   C As first-line therapy
   D When an inhaled steroid (such as beclometasone) is insufficient
   E When the patient also has hypertension

4 *Which one of the following is an important counselling point for an inhaled steroid (such as beclometasone)?*

   A It will relieve an attack
   B Do not take if you have a cold
   C Stopping taking when you notice an improvement in control
   D It may cause constipation
   E It will take several days to work

5 *When are cromone inhalers best used?*

   A In children
   B For NSAID-induced asthma
   C With concurrent hayfever
   D In COPD
   E They are of little or no benefit

6 *Which one of the following is a target of anti-asthma therapy?*

   A Leukotriene receptors
   B Histamine H_1-receptors
   C Histamine H_2-receptors
   D β_1-adrenoceptors
   E α_2-adrenoceptors

7 *What is the second messenger associated with β_2-adrenceptor activation?*

   A Tyrosine kinase
   B IP_3
   C PPAR-γ
   D cAMP
   E AMP kinase

8 *COPD is usually caused by?*

A *H. pylori* infection
B Smoking
C Untreated asthma
D Asbestos
E Left sided heart failure

9 *Which one of the following forms the mainstay of therapy for most cases of COPD?*

A Inhaled steroids
B Antimuscarinic drugs
C Broad spectrum antibiotics
D Theophylline
E 100% oxygen

10 *COPD predisposes towards which one of the following?*

A Anaemia
B Right-sided heart failure
C Angina
D Pulmonary embolism
E Atrial fibrillation

Practice points

- Asthma can kill.
- Many patients with asthma may be undertreated.
- Be alert for the overuse of bronchodilators. In asthma, if a short-acting β_2-agonist is required for relief more than twice a week, the patient should be reviewed with a view to stepping up treatment.
- Poor inhaler technique is a major cause of undertreatment.
- In both cases, smoking cessation is essential.
- In asthma a written action plan improves health outcome.
- Some patients with COPD demonstrate a positive response to steroids and these patients should be identified and treated.
- Patients with COPD are often maintained on a number of drugs and it may be difficult to deduce rationally which agents confer the most benefit.

CASE STUDY

Mr SM (aged 65) has COPD with an FEV_1 of 55% predicted. He is a current smoker with a 50 pack-year history (i.e. he has smoked the equivalent of one packet of cigarettes per day for 50 years). He has been prescribed:

salbutamol MDI 200 micrograms as needed
tiotropium MDI 18 micrograms once daily.

How should you counsel this patient?

- He should be advised that giving up smoking will slow down the progression of COPD.
- He should take salbutamol as required, and before activities that may provoke shortness of breath. Taking salbutamol before ipratropium may help more ipratropium get into the lungs.

Several months later Mr SM is still taking salbutamol and tiotropium but now with beclometasone 500 micrograms twice daily (as his FEV_1 have deteriorated). However, he is short of breath and has thick green sputum, which is occasionally streaked with blood.

What is the likely cause of this exacerbation?

- The symptoms may point to a chest infection.

(continued)

(continued)

What treatment may be appropriate?

- An antibacterial such as amoxicillin 500 mg three times daily or erythromycin or tetracycline. He should also be advised to increase his use of the bronchodilators and may be prescribed a short course of oral steroids.

Several weeks later the patient's condition has not improved.

What tests may be appropriate?

- Further investigations are appropriate. As he is a smoker this may point to other serious pathologies (e.g. lung cancer, tuberculosis) and a chest X-ray is appropriate.

References

British National Formulary, latest edition. London: British Medical Association and Royal Pharmaceutical Society of Great Britain.

British Thoracic Society (BTS) and Scottish Intercollegiate Guidelines Network (SIGN) (2014). *British guidelines on the management of asthma.* www.brit-thoracic.org.uk

National Institute for Health and Care Excellence (2000). *Guidance of the use of inhaler systems (devices) in children under the age of 5 years with chronic asthma.* Technology Appraisal Guidance no. 10. London: NICE.

National Institute for Health and Care Excellence (2002). *Inhaler devices for routine treatment of chronic asthma in older children (aged 5–15 years).* Technology Appraisal Guidance no. 38. London: NICE.

National Institute for Health and Care Excellence (2010). *Chronic obstructive pulmonary disease: Management of chronic obstructive pulmonary disease in adults in primary and secondary care.* Clinical Guideline no 101. London: NICE.

Roth M, Johnson PRA, Rudiger JJ *et al.* (2002). Interaction between glucocorticoids and β_2 agonists on bronchial airway smooth muscle cells through synchronised cellular signalling. *Lancet* 360: 1293–1299. pmid: 12414205.

Further reading

Tattersfield AE, Knox AJ, Britton JR *et al.* (2002). Asthma. *Lancet* 360: 1313–1322. pmid: 12414223.

Online resources

www.asthma.org.uk
The website of the UK National Asthma Campaign (accessed June 2016).

www.brit-thoracic.org.uk
The website of the British Thoracic Society and provides professional information, including clinical guidance (accessed June 2016).

Central nervous system disorders

23

Migraine

This is a common and often debilitating condition, which is frequently undertreated. It is characterised by a severe headache, which may be unilateral and throbbing, and lasts for 4–72 hours. There may also be vomiting, photophobia, phonophobia and sensitivity to movement. Migraine is more common in women. In 10–25% of patients with migraine (migraineurs) the headache is preceded, by approximately 1 hour, by an aura with visual (flashing and zigzag lines) and other sensory disturbances, and this is referred to as 'classic migraine'. Most cases of migraine are, however, without an aura and termed 'common migraine'. In terms of diagnosis, migraine must be differentiated from cluster and tension headaches and other causes of headache.

Pathophysiology

Migraine is a neurovascular disease and is thought to be due to an abnormal neuronal discharge, which initiates a train of further neurological activations. The precise mechanisms underlying an attack are not fully understood and this is an area of much controversy. There is thought to be 'cortical spreading depression', a wave of depolarisation across the cortex, which depresses neuronal activity, and this may lead to an aura. There is also activation of serotonergic (5-hydroxytryptamine/serotonin or 5HT) neurons, leading to perivascular inflammation and the release of vasodilator and pain mediators, namely prostanoids, calcitonin gene-related peptide (CGRP) and kinins, resulting in vasodilatation and pain. In summary, there is a humoral response, which leads to a vascular response with disturbed brain function and pain.

Although the precise causes are unclear, migraine may be triggered by a range of influences including emotions (e.g. anxiety, depression and fatigue), hormonal influences (e.g. menstrual cycle, puberty, oral contraceptives, pregnancy and menopause), vision, sound, smoking, smell, unaccustomed exercise, and too much or too little sleep. The role of foods such as cheese, red wine, chocolate, citrus fruits and coffee is unclear.

Goals of treatment

These are twofold: prevention and relief of attacks. In the first instance therapy is directed at relief but, in recurrent attacks, prophylaxis is introduced.

Pharmacological basis of management

Analgesics, e.g. aspirin, diclofenac, ibuprofen, paracetamol, tolfenamic acid

These may be used in an acute attack to inhibit the production of the noxious and vasodilator prostanoids. As discussed in Chapter 30, preference for paracetamol or a non-steroidal anti-inflammatory drug (NSAID) will be determined by side effects and concurrent illness. In addition to the analgesics, antiemetics such as metoclopramide, or prochlorperazine may be given, because these will reduce any associated nausea. In the case of metoclopramide, its prokinetic actions will also increase gastric emptying and accelerate the uptake of the analgesics given at the same time. This is particularly important, because migraine is associated with gastrointestinal disturbances, which may reduce transit. Diclofenac may be given as suppositories or intramuscularly when there is vomiting, because absorption via the oral route will be limited.

The use of low doses of codeine in over-the-counter (OTC) preparations may be inappropriate because the doses present have only weak analgesic effects but have marked opioid side effects (e.g. constipation), and may lead to analgesic or overuse headache with persistent use (see Chapter 30). Opioids are not recommended as therapy for migraine.

Triptans, e.g. almotriptan, eletriptan, naratriptan, rizatriptan, sumatriptan, zolmitriptan

Sumatriptan, the prototypical member of this group, was developed to revolutionise the management of migraine. Triptans are $5HT_{1D}$ full agonists but they also activate $5HT_{1B}$- and $5HT_{1F}$-receptors; these actions cause cerebral vasoconstriction to abort an attack. Triptans may also act presynaptically to inhibit neuronal release of CGRP and Substance P, which are associated with inflammation and vasodilatation. In addition, they may act directly on neuronal cells to reduce excitability. The use of 5HT-receptor agonists to manage migraine may seem counterintuitive, given the role of 5HT in migraine, but it should be noted that these agonists are selective for subtypes of $5HT_1$-receptor and are used to abort an attack after its initiation (which is thought to involve 5HT acting at $5HT_2$-receptors). They should be taken when there is mild pain and not during any aura.

The vasoconstrictor action of triptans means that they may cause chest pain and are therefore contraindicated in patients with ischaemic heart disease, peripheral vascular disease or a history of cerebrovascular accident. Sumatriptan tablets have poor bioavailability but may also be given by a nasal spray or subcutaneously by an auto-injector. The newer agents may be given as tablets or in some cases (rizatriptan and zolmitriptan) as wafers that dissolve on the tongue. If a patient fails to respond to the first triptan used, switching to an alternative triptan may be effective.

Ergotamine

This is an ergot alkaloid with $5HT_{1D}$ partial agonist activity, so it acts in a similar manner to the triptans but its use is limited by widespread side effects including nausea, vomiting and gastrointestinal disturbances and is no longer recommended.

Prophylactic drugs

A number of diverse drugs have been used for prophylaxis of migraine over the years and include pizotifen, an antagonist of both $5HT_2$- and histamine H_1-receptors; certain β blockers (principally propranolol) are also widely used for prophylaxis. In addition, tricyclic antidepressants (amitriptyline), sodium valproate, calcium-channel blockers (verapamil) and the $α_2$-adrenoceptor agonist clonidine are also used for prophylaxis. The therapeutic action of these diverse agents in preventing migraine is unclear. The National Institute for Health and Care Excellence guidance (NICE 2012) supports the use of propranolol or the antiepileptic drug topiramate (Chapter 24) for use in prophylaxis.

Drug choice

Migraine management should be reviewed regularly with a stepped-care approach and some key points are summarised here:

- Step 1: for mild and occasional attacks simple analgesia (paracetamol, aspirin or ibuprofen) with or without an antiemetic, taken as soon as possible. The inclusion of metoclopramide as an antiemetics will enhance absorption.
- Alternatively a triptan should be used, with choice being governed by cost. Some patients may not respond to a particular triptan and may benefit from swapping to another triptan.
- Step 2: combinations, e.g. triptan plus an NSAID.

One recognised complication of therapy is that analgesics and triptan are associated with medication overuse headaches and so their prolonged use should be monitored.

For severe or frequent attacks (more than two per month), prophylaxis may be added and NICE (2012) recommend topiramate or propranolol. Despite the addition of prophylaxis, many patients are resistant to this and also find the associated side effects unacceptable.

Drug choice will be influenced by concurrent illness and conditions; migraine may also influence other drug choices such as oral contraceptives and some considerations are summarised in Table 23.1.

Drug interactions

The interactions of triptans and other antimigraine drugs are complex. Although certain drugs are predicted to

Table 23.1 Some considerations for the choice of drugs in migraine		
Condition	**Drugs affected**	**Comments**
Vomiting	Sumatriptan	If vomiting occurs then the subcutaneous route should be used. The nasal spray is not appropriate because ingestion is also involved
Ischaemic heart disease	Triptans and ergotamine	Contraindicated in ischaemic heart disease because these agents may cause coronary vasoconstriction
Ischaemic heart disease or hypertension	β blockers	These would be reasons to choose β blockers for prophylaxis
Peripheral vascular disease	Triptans and ergotamine	These should be avoided due to vasoconstriction
Cerebrovascular accidents	Triptans and ergotamine	These should be avoided due to vasoconstriction
Age	Triptans	Triptans are not recommended in patients aged >65 years
Wolff–Parkinson–White syndrome	Zolmitriptan	This is contraindicated
Asthma or peptic ulceration	NSAIDs should be used with caution or avoided	See Chapters 8 and 22
Contraception	Combined oral contraceptives	• Migraine is associated with an increased risk of ischaemic stroke. As combined oral contraceptives may compound this risk they should be avoided in patients with migraine with aura, in severe migraine and in migraine without aura but with at least one other risk factor (aged >35 years, smoking, diabetes mellitus, hypertension, hyperlipidaemia, obesity, family history). They should be used with caution in patients with migraine without aura, who do not have any of these risk factors • Patients who develop migraine or who have increased incidences or severity after starting combined oral contraceptives should stop taking them • Progesterone-only contraceptive pills may be used with caution • A current focal migraine attack is a contraindication to emergency hormonal contraception • Migraine is not a contraindication to hormone replacement therapy

(continued)

Table 23.1 *(continued)*

Condition	Drugs affected	Comments
Menstrual migraine		This is migraine without aura around the time of menstruation. It may be managed by mefenamic acid or transdermal oestrogen for 3 days before menstruation and for 7 days afterwards
Conception	Topiramate	Topiramate is associated with an increased risk of teratogenesis
Depression	Amitriptyline	This would be a reason to choose amitriptyline as a prophylactic agent. Similarly, amitriptyline would be appropriate if there are sleep problems
Depression	Clonidine, β blockers	This would be a reason to avoid β blockers and clonidine because they may aggravate depression

NSAIDs, non-steroidal anti-inflammatory drugs.

interact with triptans, evidence for these adverse effects is often lacking or incomplete. The reader is therefore referred to specialised literature such as *Stockley's Drug Interactions* (Baxter 2013). Some important interactions are summarised in Table 23.2.

Over-the-counter medicines and dietary supplements

Sumatriptan is available as an OTC medicine for the acute treatment of migraine attacks with or without aura in adults aged 18–65 years. As outlined above, sumatriptan is recommended when appropriate use of analgesics with or without antiemetics has been ineffective. Important considerations for OTC supply:

- It is not suitable for a first attack or for patients who have had fewer than five previous attacks.
- The first attack should have occurred more than 12 months previously.
- The occurrence of four or more attacks per month or requests for four or more packs per month warrant referral.
- Pharmacists should be alert for the increased risk of stroke with sumatriptan in women taking combined oral contraceptives. Worsening symptoms and migraine with aura should be referred.

In addition, patients with three or more risk factors for cardiovascular disease should not be supplied with OTC sumatriptan. These include:

- obesity (body mass index or BMI >30 kg/m^2)
- diabetes
- men >40 years and postmenopausal women
- hypercholesterolaemia
- smoker (10 or more a day)
- family history of heart disease <55 years for men and <65 for women.

Alternative therapies

Supplements requested in the pharmacy for the treatment of migraine include feverfew, riboflavin (vitamin B$_2$) and magnesium. Feverfew is a herbal preparation, riboflavin a water-soluble vitamin and magnesium an essential mineral. In the case of feverfew a systematic Cochrane review (Pittler *et al.* 2002) concluded that there was a lack of evidence to support the effectiveness of feverfew in the treatment of migraine. There is some recent evidence which demonstrates the effectiveness of acupuncture in migraine and this is now incorporated into NICE (2012) clinical guidelines.

Counselling

The first general advice, which may be effective in some patients, is the identification and avoidance of trigger factors as mentioned above (certain foods, emotional stress, changes in sleep patterns and hormonal changes, including oral contraceptives). Indeed, a trigger diary may be helpful in identifying

Table 23.2 Some important interactions of antimigraine drugs

Interacting drugs	Consequences	Comments
Triptans with nitrates or β blockers	Triptans should not be taken with either nitrates or β blockers in ischaemic heart disease because of the risk of coronary vasoconstriction	
Triptans with antidepressants	The combination of an SSRI and sumatriptan is contraindicated by the manufacturers owing to the possible potentiation of 5HT	This only occasionally leads to adverse effects
Ergotamine with triptans	These combinations are contraindicated due to enhanced vasoconstrictor effects	Concurrent ergot derivatives and rizatriptan are contraindicated by the manufacturers, who recommend that ergot derivatives should be taken at least 6 hours after rizatriptan and that rizatriptan should be taken 24 hours after ergots. The manufacturers advise that zolmitriptan and ergotamine should be taken at least 6 hours apart
Sumatriptan with lithium	This combination is contraindicated	
Sumatriptan, rizatriptan with MAOIs	MAOs metabolise sumatriptan and rizatriptan and so MAOIs may increase their concentrations	These combinations are contraindicated
Rizatriptan with propranolol	Propranolol doubles the plasma levels of rizatriptan	The dose of rizatriptan should be halved to 5 mg and the doses separated by 2 hours
Tolfenamic acid with magnesium hydroxide or aluminium hydroxide	Magnesium hydroxide accelerates the rate of absorption of tolfenamic acid (this will enhance the onset of action) whereas aluminium hydroxide may slow the rate of absorption	Aluminium hydroxide should be given separately
Ergotamine with erythromycin	Erythromycin may inhibit the metabolism of ergotamine, leading to severe side effects such as peripheral vasoconstriction	Their concurrent use should be avoided
Ergotamine with tetracycline	Risk of ergotism	Concurrent use should be monitored
Pizotifen with triptans	There is no evidence that pizotifen interacts with sumatriptan and zolmitriptan	

5HT, 5-hydroxytryptamine or serotonin; MAOIs, monoamine oxidase inhibitors; SSRI, selective serotonin reuptake inhibitor.

and avoiding stimuli. Rest and sleep may provide some relief from an attack. Specific counselling points are described below.

NSAIDs and paracetamol

See Chapter 30.

- These should be taken at the start of an attack, even before the headache develops.
- The use of diclofenac suppositories does not avoid side effects, including gastrointestinal toxicity or hypersensitivity.

Triptans

- Triptans should be taken at the onset of a headache and not during the aura because they will not stop the aura and not all auras lead to a headache.
- Side effects of triptans include nausea, dizziness, dry mouth, warm sensations and tingling, and transient increases in blood pressure.
- Some patients experience chest symptoms of tightness, shortness of breath and occasionally pain. If there is chest pain, patients should consult their GP.

- Wafers should be placed on the tongue and allowed to dissolve.
- Triptans may cause drowsiness.
- In a high proportion of patients taking a triptan, the migraine may recur within 12 hours.
- Frequent use may lead to chronic daily headache or exacerbation of migraine.

Prophylactic agents

Some of these are covered in Chapters 12 (β blockers, clonidine, calcium-channel blockers), 24 (topiramate) and 25 (tricyclic antidepressants).

Pizotifen

- Pizotifen may cause drowsiness and weight gain.
- Pizotifen is best taken at night due to its sedating actions.

Self-assessment

For the following statements concerning migraine, choose the most appropriate answer:

1 *Triptans are best described as:*

a 5HT$_3$ receptor antagonists
b Serotonin-selective reuptake inhibitors
c 5HT$_{1D}$ full agonists and 5HT$_{1B}$- and 5HT$_{1F}$-receptor partial agonists
d 5HT$_2$ receptor antagonists
e Prophylactic agents

2 *Triptans lead to:*

a Vasodilatation
b Vasoconstriction
c Inhibition of prostanglandin production
d Antiemetic effects
e Release of neuropepetides such as CGRP

3 *Which one of the following drugs is advocated for prophylaxis in migraine?*

A Phenytoin
B Lithium
C Fluoxetine
D Topiramate
E Diazepam

Practice points

- Pharmacological treatment is initially simple analgesia and /or triptan.
- Soluble preparations are preferred due to delayed gastric emptying during migraine.
- Triptans are recommended when treatment with simple analgesia with or without antiemetics has failed.
- Nausea and vomiting may make the oral route ineffective.

CASE STUDY

A 35-year-old woman who has a history of migraine since the age of 15 years now requires further medication, as ibuprofen is ineffective at managing her condition.

Her current medication is:

sertraline 50 mg once daily
Microgynon.

Comment on her current medication.

- It should be noted that combined oral contraceptives may lead to increases in migraine. Instead, progesterone-only contraceptives pills may be used. Her age and obesity (revealed later on) would also favour the use of progesterone-only contraceptives pills (with caution) or alternative contraceptive measures.

- Sertraline is a selective serotonin reuptake inhibitor (SSRI) that may lead to headaches and nausea, and so one needs to be certain that her symptoms are not related to the SSRI.

What antimigraine treatment would be appropriate in her case?

- The next likely step would be simple analgesic with an antiemetic plus a triptan (sumatriptan, zolmitriptan or rizatriptan as first-line). If she is maintained on the sertraline then the use of a triptan is contraindicated by manufacturers of sumatriptan due to the possibility of central nervous system toxicity through potentiation of the effects of 5HT. However, *Stockley's Drug Interactions* (Baxter 2013) points out that the combination of sumatriptan and an SSRI only occasionally leads to adverse effects and suggests that they may be used together with caution.
- Her depression is compounded by her obesity (BMI = 35) but she has shown motivation in losing weight and her general practitioner is prepared to prescribe an antiobesity drug.

What advice would you give her GP in drug choice?

- Orlistat, which acts on pancreatic lipases, would be a safer choice. In terms of future antimigraine treatment, pizotifen should be avoided because this may cause weight gain. She should be encouraged to take regular exercise and maintain a healthy diet.

References

Baxter K, ed. (2013). *Stockley's Drug Interaction*, 10th edn. London: Pharmaceutical Press.

National Institute for Health and Care Excellence (2012). *Headaches: Diagnosis and management of headaches in young people and adults*. Clinical Guideline 150. London: NICE.

Pittler MH, Vogler BK, Ernst E (2002). Feverfew for preventing migraine (Cochrane review). In: *The Cochrane Library* issue 2. Oxford: Update Software.

Further reading

Goadsby PJ, Olesen J (1996). Fortnightly review: diagnosis and management of migraine. *BMJ* 312: 1279–1283. pmid: 8634619.

Online resources

www.migrainetrust.org
The website of the Migraine Trust, with professional and patient information on migraine (accessed April 2015).

24

Epilepsy

Disease characteristics

This is the most common serious neurological condition, with 3–5% of the population experiencing some form during their lifetime. There are several forms, ranging from temporary loss of concentration (absences) to full-blown seizures with convulsions and loss of consciousness. The seizures are divided into partial and generalised seizures and the major forms are described below.

Generalised seizures

In generalised seizures, abnormal electrical activity spreads simultaneously throughout the cerebral cortex and there are several forms:

- Tonic–clonic convulsions (or previously 'grand mal' seizures) involve sudden loss of consciousness; the limbs may stiffen (tonic) and then jerk (clonic). There is often tongue biting and incontinence. On regaining consciousness, the patient is often drowsy and confused.
- Tonic seizures involve going stiff but without loss of consciousness.
- Atonic seizures involve loss of tone and becoming limp.
- Absences (or petit mal epilepsy) often occur in children who go blank and stare for

approximately 10–30 s: this may be mistaken for daydreaming.
- Myoclonic epilepsy is characterised by abrupt jerks, which may affect the whole body, arms or legs.

Partial seizures

These are focal seizures that are localised to a brain region and produce simple symptoms such as muscle contractions and abnormal sensory changes without collapsing. Simple partial seizures involve changes in activity whereas complex partial seizures involve changes in awareness. In secondary generalised seizures activity starts in one area and then spreads, which may lead to a full seizure.

Causes

In general, epilepsy is due to abnormal neuronal discharges, which may or may not spread across the brain. The cause may be the result of a structural lesion, secondary to trauma, or caused by some unidentified change. Biochemical changes such as hypoglycaemia, hyperglycaemia, hyponatraemia or alcohol abuse may also lead to seizures, and infections such as meningitis may cause seizures. In some cases, particularly those appearing later in life, they may be due to lesions such as brain tumours, which should be excluded. Therapeutic drugs, particularly when used in combination, may induce seizures in patients with or without a history of epilepsy and important examples are:

- quinolones
- tricyclic antidepressants
- selective serotonin reuptake inhibitors (SSRIs)
- antihistamines
- bupropion
- donepezil
- baclofen
- lithium
- mefloquine
- theophylline
- tramadol.

In addition, withdrawal from alcohol, benzodiazepines and barbiturates is associated with seizures.

Goals of treatment

These are to control seizures with the lowest possible dose, and with fewest side effects.

Pharmacological management

For a first seizure it is important to exclude other pathologies that may have caused the seizure, important examples of which are detailed above. In the absence of any obvious cause, a first or isolated seizure may go untreated, because in a high proportion of patients (up to 50%) they may not recur. However, once a patient has a subsequent seizure, epilepsy may be diagnosed and antiepileptic drugs (AEDs) are prescribed to prevent further seizures. In general, AEDs either reduce neuronal excitability, and so prevent the spread of neuronal discharges or potentiate inhibitory transmitters such as γ-aminobutyric acid (GABA). Given these depressant actions on the brain, AEDs are associated with a wide range of central side effects, which are summarised together with their modes of action in Table 24.1.

Vagal nerve stimulation

This involves insertion of a generator into the chest, with electrodes connected to the vagus nerve. The stimulator provides electrical impulses every 3–5 minutes and, during an aura or the early stages of a seizure, the patient or an observer can activate the stimulator to stimulate the vagus, which is thought to disrupt attacks. The mechanism by which this occurs is unclear.

Drug choice

The aim of pharmacological therapy is to control seizures and this is ideally achieved by using one drug at an effective dose. If the first drug fails to control epilepsy at its maximum dose, a second drug is often tried as the first drug is withdrawn slowly. Only after failure of monotherapy is combined therapy used. Currently, sodium valproate and carbamazepine are widely used, with lamotrigine having a much increased role, and phenytoin and phenobarbital being less widely used. Some choices of AEDs are summarised in Table 24.2.

In some cases, seizures increase around menstruation and this is termed 'catamenial epilepsy'. In these patients the benzodiazepine clobazam may be used around that time.

In status epilepticus, a prolonged seizure lasting more than 30 minutes, benzodiazepines such as diazepam, lorazepam or clonazepam may be given to stop the attack. The rectal route may be more practical during a seizure. If this fails to control the seizure, intravenous phenytoin or phenobarbital may be used or even general anaesthetics.

Other considerations include concurrent diseases or conditions and some important examples are depression and pregnancy.

Affective disorders

Depression is an important consideration, and this may well occur secondary to patients developing epilepsy. The use of antidepressants is associated with decreasing the seizure threshold, which may lead to episodes of epilepsy, and so antidepressants should be used with caution in epilepsy. In concurrent bipolar affective disorder carbamazepine may be considered as a compelling choice because it is effective in this condition. It should be noted that carbamazepine may be used effectively with lithium, but there have been instances of increased neurotoxicity with this combination.

Table 24.1 Summary of the pharmacological actions and adverse effects of antiepileptic drugs

Antiepileptic drug	Mechanism of action	Adverse effects and comments
Sodium valproate	Acts weakly by potentiating GABA and causing use-dependent blockade of Na$^+$ channels	• Sedation, ataxia, diplopia, nystagmus, weight gain, nausea, hair loss and tremor • May rarely cause thrombocytopenia and agranulocytosis • Liver dysfunction and failure have occurred • Pancreatitis may also occur • Associated with high incidence of birth defects
Carbamazepine	Use-dependent blockade of Na$^+$ channels	• Induces its own metabolism and so the dosage is increased gradually • It is associated with sedation, erythematous rashes, dizziness, and diplopia (double vision) • It is also associated with hyponatraemia, which itself may reduce seizure threshold • May cause agranulocytosis and thrombocytopenia • It is an important enzyme inducer
Oxcarbazepine	Derivative of carbamazepine	As for carbamazepine but causes less enzyme induction and skin rashes. Hyponatraemia is more problematic than with carbamazepine
Phenytoin	Use-dependent blockade of Na$^+$ channels	• It shows zero-order pharmacokinetics (Chapter 7), so achieving therapeutic concentrations is difficult and side effects such as nystagmus are indicative of toxic effects • It frequently causes adverse effects, including gingival hypertrophy, hair growth, coarsening of facial features, diplopia, sedation and ataxia. It may cause agranulocytosis • Risk of folate deficiency leading to megaloblastic anaemia • It is an important enzyme inducer
Lamotrigine	Use-dependent blockade of Na$^+$ channels and decreased release of the excitatory transmitter, glutamate	• Less sedating than the older agents but there may be dizziness and ataxia • It is associated with skin reactions, including toxic epidermal necrolysis and Stevens–Johnson syndrome
Gabapentin	Inhibition of voltage-operated calcium channels.	Associated with dizziness, ataxia, somnolence, diplopia, nystagmus and nausea
Pregabalin	Inhibition of voltage-operated calcium channels, reducing exocytosis of neurotransmitters	Associated with dizziness, drowsiness, diplopia and increased appetite
Vigabatrin	Potentiates GABA by inhibiting its metabolism via the GABA transaminase enzyme	Associated with drowsiness and fatigue. It may cause irreversible visual field defects
Topiramate	Uncertain, but it may act via blockade of sodium channels and/or enhancing the actions of GABA by binding to a modulatory site	CNS side effects such as confusion, dizziness, fatigue and memory impairment
Ethosuximide	Inhibition of T-type calcium channels	Associated with gastrointestinal side effects, drowsiness and dizziness
Phenobarbital	Enhances the effects of GABA at opening the GABA receptor associated chloride channel	• Sedation is a major problem and it is rarely used • It is an important enzyme inducer • Tolerance is a problem • Rebound seizures on withdrawal are common

Table 24.1 *(continued)*

Antiepileptic drug	Mechanism of action	Adverse effects and comments
Primidone	Metabolised to phenobarbital	As for phenobarbital
Benzodiazepines, e.g. clonazepam, clobazam diazepam	Enhance the actions of GABA via the benzodiazepine receptor	Sedation and dependence
Levetiracetam	Uncertain	Dizziness, somnolence, diplopia, tremor, depression and headaches
Tiagabine	Inhibitor of GABA reuptake	Dizziness, somnolence, nervousness and tremor

CNS, central nervous system; GABA, γ-aminobutyric acid.

Table 24.2 Summary of drug choices in the different forms of epilepsy

Form of epilepsy	First-line	Second-line	Antiepileptic drugs to avoid
Absence	• Sodium valproate • Lamotrigine	Ethosuximide	Carbamazepine
Generalised tonic–clonic	• Sodium valproate • Lamotrigine • Carbamazepine	Levetiracetam	Vigabatrin
Myoclonic	• Sodium valproate • Topiramate • Levetiracetam	• Clonazepam • Ethosuximide • Lamotrigine	Carbamazepine
Partial seizures	• Sodium valproate • Carbamazepine • Lamotrigine	• Phenytoin • Gabapentin • Vigabatrin • Clonazepam	

Pregnancy

Pregnancy is a major issue in patients with epilepsy because the associated physiological changes may increase the incidence of seizures. Furthermore, AEDs are associated with a range of birth defects, e.g. carbamazepine and sodium valproate are associated with increased risks of neural tube defects and phenytoin and phenobarbital are associated with cleft palates. Other adverse effects may include impaired psychomotor development in the child, cardiac defects and facial abnormalities. Some patients who are seizure-free for some time may have their AED withdrawn before conception. However, if this is not the case, continuing AEDs during pregnancy is considered important because seizures during pregnancy may have serious consequences for both the mother and the fetus. Pharmacokinetic changes in pregnancy may also reduce the effectiveness of some AEDs.

The management of epilepsy during pregnancy is usually under specialist care. There has been much debate around the safety of AEDs in pregnancy, with lamotrigine and carbamazepine being favoured in females of childbearing age and sodium valproate being associated with a high incidence of birth defects. Sodium valproate and older agents such as phenobarbital and phenytoin should be avoided in women of childbearing age if possible, due to the increased risk of birth defects. To reduce the chances of neural tube defect, patients often receive 5 mg folic acid daily before conception and for at least the first 12 weeks of pregnancy. Carbamazepine, phenytoin and phenobarbital are also associated with increased neonatal bleeding (including intracranial bleeds) and vitamin K is given to the mother from week 36 of pregnancy before delivery and to the baby at birth.

Breastfeeding

Breastfeeding is considered safe for mothers taking carbamazepine, phenytoin and sodium valproate.

Breastfeeding while taking phenobarbital, primidone, vigabatrin (risk of visual defects) and ethosuximide should be avoided. Breastfeeding is considered safe with newer agents such as lamotrigine, and gabapentin if taken during pregnancy. Non-hormonal methods of contraception may be required during breastfeeding by patients prescribed enzyme-inducing drugs because progestogen-only contraceptives may be less effective.

Contraception

Compounding the issue of pregnancy is the established interaction of the enzyme-inducing AEDs (carbamazepine, oxcarbazepine, phenytoin, phenobarbital and topiramate) with oral contraceptives; they accelerate their metabolism, which may lead to contraceptive failure. To overcome this problem alternative contraception such as barrier methods or intrauterine devices should be used. Although lamotrigine does not interact to affect the effectiveness of oral contraceptives, the plasma concentration of lamotrigine can be reduced by oral contraceptives and also by sex hormones in pregnancy. In both cases the effectiveness of lamotrigine may be decreased and this may require an increase in dosage.

Young children

It should be noted that young children may require higher doses per kilogram of body weight of antiepileptics, with more frequent doses due to more rapid metabolism of these drugs.

Drug interactions

AEDs show a wide range of interactions and the reader is referred to specialised literature such as *Stockley's Drug Interactions* (Baxter 2013). However, a few important points to note are that carbamazepine (oxcarbazepine to a lesser extent), phenytoin and phenobarbital induce cytochrome P450, and accelerate the metabolism of other drugs. Indeed, one reason to favour monotherapy is that many of the AEDs interact with each other, often increasing each other's metabolism. By contrast, sodium valproate inhibits the metabolism of lamotrigine, thus increasing its plasma half-life. Some important examples of

other interactions due to induction of metabolism are as follows.

Carbamazepine, phenytoin and phenobarbital may significantly accelerate the metabolism of:

- doxycycline but not other tetracyclines
- warfarin (phenytoin may also potentiate the actions of warfarin)
- indinavir, nelfinavir, saquinavir
- dihydropyridines
- corticosteroids
- oestrogens and progestogens
- theophylline
- levothyroxine
- certain other AEDs.

In addition, given the hepatic route of metabolism of some AEDs, there is scope for inhibitors of these pathways to interact with AEDs, resulting in increased concentrations and promoting toxicity. Important examples of this are the interactions of carbamazepine with erythromycin, clarithromycin, diltiazem, verapamil, certain selective serotonin reuptake inhibitors (SSRIs, e.g. fluoxetine and fluvoxamine) and cimetidine (transiently). St John's wort may induce the metabolism of carbamazepine, making it less effective. Having commented on the extensive range of drug interactions with AEDs, it should also be noted that gabapentin is not known to have any significant interactions.

Monitoring

AEDs are associated with a range of serious adverse drug reactions (ADRs) affecting the liver (see Chapter 6) and haematological system (see Chapter 6), so monitoring is appropriate. Baseline monitoring of haematology and biochemistry is often carried out before starting treatment. Liver function tests (LFTs) are essential with sodium valproate before treatment and during the first 6 months, including a determination of the international normalised ratio (INR). Some of the inducing AEDs may alter LFTs (see Chapter 2) via enzyme induction (e.g. increased levels of γ-glutamyl transferase [GGT]), and may also promote damage due to the enhancement of drug metabolism, which may give rise to toxic metabolites.

Blood counts should be determined if there are signs of reduced white cell counts (leukopenia due to agranulocytosis) such as increased infections (e.g. sore throats, fevers, mouth ulcers) or thrombocytopenia (increased bruising), which may occur with carbamazepine, ethosuximide, lamotrigine, phenytoin (the manufacturer recommends monitoring of blood counts) and sodium valproate (principally thrombocytopenia). If serious blood disorders such as leukopenia or thrombocytopenia are identified then the AED should be withdrawn under the cover of another agent.

Visual fields should also be measured every 6 months with vigabatrin.

Withdrawing antiepileptic drugs

In many patients it is undesirable that they are maintained indefinitely on AEDs; indeed, the condition that may have led to their seizures may have resolved. Therefore, after a suitable seizure-free period, the patient and doctor may consider withdrawal of therapy. Typically, patients who are seizure-free for 2–4 years are considered, because a substantial proportion will remain seizure-free on withdrawal. Withdrawal of AEDs may itself decrease the seizure threshold, so this should be gradual with a dose reduction over time. Typical reducing regimens are dose reductions (e.g. carbamazepine by 100 mg, sodium valproate by 200 mg) every 4 weeks. Benzodiazepines and phenobarbital should be withdrawn over several months. During the withdrawal period, and for 6 months afterwards, patients should not drive, because the withdrawal may precipitate seizures or the patient's epilepsy may return. When changing medication, the original drug should be withdrawn only once the new drug is established.

Over-the-counter medication and supplements

Over-the-counter (OTC) issues in epilepsy involve screening for ADRs and drug interactions and providing support to patients to aid compliance. Drugs such as cimetidine, a cytochrome P450 inhibitor, should be avoided (see earlier). Female patients should be advised to consult their doctor before planning a pregnancy,

for counselling and prescription of folic acid together with a medication review. Patients with epilepsy should not take evening primrose oil or ginkgo biloba due to a risk of seizures with these agents.

Counselling

To achieve adequate control of epilepsy, patients should be informed of the importance of compliance, because omitting doses or abrupt withdrawal may cause a rebound increase in the occurrence of seizures.

Informing family and colleagues about their condition and what to do in the event of a seizure may help as seizures can appear frightening.

Haematological and hepatic adverse effects

Patients taking carbamazepine, oxcarbazepine, ethosuximide, gabapentin, lamotrigine, phenytoin and sodium valproate should be counselled to report promptly signs of blood disorders such as sore throats, mouth ulcers, fevers or easy bruising. In the case of lamotrigine, patients should also report rashes or flu-like illnesses. Patients taking carbamazepine, oxcarbazepine and sodium valproate should report symptoms that may indicate liver damage such as jaundice, itching, nausea and vomiting.

Skin reactions

Many of the AEDs may cause skin reactions (see Chapter 6). Although many of these are harmless, some may be serious, so patients should consult their doctor.

Sedation

Many of the AEDs may cause sedation, so patients should be warned of this possibility. When taking carbamazepine, gabapentin, vigabatrin, topiramate, barbiturates and benzodiazepines, patients should be specifically advised that sedation may affect their ability to operate machinery.

Driving

This is subject to clear regulations of the driving licensing authorities (see the *British National Formulary*) and the onus is on patients to report their condition. Patients should also stop driving for 6 months on withdrawal of AEDs. In addition, all of the AEDs may impair driving and so patients should be alerted to this.

Alcohol

Alcohol may enhance central nervous system (CNS) side effects such as sedation in some AEDs such as carbamazepine. Excessive fluid intake may also predispose patients taking carbamazepine and oxcarbazepine to hyponatraemia, which itself may lead to seizure. Hence patients should be cautioned against excessive alcohol intake.

Drug interactions

Patients should inform all healthcare professionals that they are taking AEDs.

Pregnancy

Female patients should be advised to discuss with their GP the issues surrounding pregnancy and epilepsy (see above) before stopping contraception. Advice should be given on the interaction of antiepileptics and oral contraceptives, the risks associated with unplanned pregnancy and the risks/benefits of AED use during pregnancy.

Bone

The enzyme-inducing AEDs (carbamazepine, phenytoin and phenobarbital) have been associated with accelerated metabolism of vitamin D, leading to impaired calcium levels. These effects have been associated with rickets and osteomalacia, so the importance of a balanced diet should be stressed. This may be particularly important in the presence of additional risk factors such as early menopause and use of corticosteroids.

Side effects

In addition to the extensive range of side effects reported above, some other drug-specific counselling points are as follows.

Phenytoin

This may cause increased growth of the gums.

Vigabatrin

This may cause irreversible changes in vision, which should be reported.

Practice points

- Epilepsy is a common condition, which is usually managed by drugs.
- Monotherapy is preferred.
- Pharmacists have an important role in ensuring adherence to AEDs.
- AEDs have a wide range of interactions and the enzyme inducers may cause a failure of oral contraception.
- AEDs are associated with a range of side effects and may cause birth defects.
- Lamotrigine and carbamazepine are favoured in females of childbearing age.
- In treatment failure, check that the dose has been increased to an appropriate maintenance dose, and/or check blood levels before a new prescription, e.g. carbamazepine induces its own metabolism, requiring a gradual dose increase.

Self-assessment

For the following questions concerning epilepsy, choose the most appropriate answer:

1 *Absence epilepsy may present as which one of the following?*

A A simple faint
B A seizure
C Temporary loss of attention
D The absence of EEG activity
E Narcolepsy

2 *Which one of the following antiepileptic drugs is a potent enzyme inducer?*

A Topiramate
B Sodium valproate
C Carbamazepine
D Ethosuximide
E Lamotrigine

3 *Which one of the following antiepileptic drugs is preferred in females of childbearing age?*

A Lamotrigine
B Sodium valproate
C Phenytoin
D Phenobarbital
E None of the above

4 *Phenytoin shows zero-order kinetics which leads to which one of the following?*

A Many drug interactions through enzyme inhibition
B Its dose is dependent only on renal function
C Its effects wear off over time
D Small dosage changes lead to disproportionate changes in plasma concentration
E Its interaction with its receptor is independent of the plasma concentration

---

CASE STUDY

Mrs FT is a 35 year-old woman and had been in general good health but while out walking has some form of collapse with loss of consciousness. Although she regained consciousness, she was admitted to the local Emergency Department by ambulance. On admission, the doctor took a full history (including use of prescription and recreational drugs) and bloods for routine biochemistry. She was discharged with no further action but was told that she must inform the vehicle licensing authorities and was made an appointment for an MRI scan.

What questions should the doctor have asked in relation to the 'funny turn'?

- Was there loss of consciousness?
- Was there injury? *Tongue biting would be consistent with epilepsy.*
- Were there any unusual movements? *This might implicate epilepsy.*
- Was there incontinence? *Incontinence of urine is common in epilepsy.*
- What colour did the patient go? *Extreme pallor during the episode and flushing after the attack might suggest a cardiac cause.*
- What provokes an attack? *e.g. Flashing lights in certain forms of epilepsy.*
- Were there any prodromal symptoms? *e.g. An aura in epilepsy.*
- How did the patient recover? *With neurological causes there may be confusion.*
- How long did it last?
- Does the patient have a current illness or are they receiving any drugs?

Why were biochemical tests performed?

- To exclude hypo/hyperglycaemia, hyponatraemia as causes.

Why was no action taken?

- The seizure might be a 'one off'; common practice not to start drug treatment until further fits. A brain scan was arranged to exclude pathology such as a tumour.

Before she had her scan, she was readmitted having had a further attack (stopped by lorazepam followed by intravenous phenytoin, 15mg/kg). This time the doctor arranged an immediate MRI scan, an EEG and a chest radiograph. Once these tests were carried out it was decided to start drug treatment with either carbamazepine, sodium valproate or lamotrigine.

(continued)

(continued)

Which drug would you recommend? Why?

- Lamotrigine and carbamazepine have the best safety records in pregnancy. Valproate is more teratogenic and should be avoided in females of childbearing age.

What monitoring and counselling is appropriate for your suggested regimen?

- To achieve adequate control of epilepsy, patients should be informed of the importance of compliance, as omitting doses or abrupt withdrawal may cause a rebound increase in the occurrence of seizures.
- Pregnancy: Female patients should be advised to discuss with their general practitioner the issues surrounding pregnancy and epilepsy before stopping contraception. Advice should be given on the risks associated with unplanned pregnancy and the risks/benefits of antiepileptic drug use during pregnancy.
- Many of the antiepileptic drugs may cause skin reactions. Although many of these are harmless, some may be serious and so the patient should consult their doctor.
- Driving: This is subject to clear regulations of the driving licensing authorities and the onus is on the patient to report their condition.
- In addition, all of the antiepileptic drugs may impair driving and so patients should be alerted to this.

Lamotrigine

- Report immediately signs of blood disorders such as sore throats, mouth ulcers, fevers or easy bruising.
- Report any flu-like illnesses immediately.
- Report any rashes immediately.

Carbamazepine

- Sedating, caution in operating machines.
- Effects of alcohol enhanced.
- Report immediately signs of blood disorders such as sore throats, mouth ulcers, fevers or easy bruising.
- Report symptoms which might be due to liver damage such as jaundice, itching, nausea and vomiting.
- Inducing agent – range of interactions including failure of oral contraceptives.
- If of Han/Hong Kong Chinese or Thai origin screen for HLA-B* 1502 allele owing to risk of Stevens–Johnson syndrome.
- Monitoring should include a full blood count and liver function test

  After 3 years without further seizures the GP would like to stop the antiepileptic treatment.

What advice should you give the GP?

- In many patients it is undesirable that they are maintained indefinitely on antiepileptic drugs; indeed the condition which may have led to their seizures may have resolved. Withdrawal of antiepileptic drugs may itself decrease the seizure threshold so this should be gradual with a dose reduction over time.

What driving advice is appropriate?

- Patients should also stop driving for 6 months on withdrawal of antiepileptic drugs.

References

Baxter K, ed. (2013). *Stockley's Drug Interactions,* 10th edn. London: Pharmaceutical Press.

British National Formulary, latest edition. London: British Medical Association and Royal Pharmaceutical Society of Great Britain.

National Institute for Health and Care Excellence (2012). *The epilepsies: diagnosis and the management of the epilepsies in adults in primary and secondary care.* Clinical Guideline 137. London: NICE.

Online resources

www.epilepsy.org.uk
The website of Epilepsy Action (British Epilepsy Association), a very useful resource for information on epilepsy, with excellent patient information (accessed July 2015).

http://www.epilepsysociety.org.uk/
The website of Epilepsy Society, a very useful resource for information on epilepsy with excellent patient information (accessed July 2015).

25

Affective disorders

Disease characteristics

Affective (emotional) disorders consist of changes in mood, with the most common manifestation being depressed mood. Typically this is a long-standing condition that may be associated with feelings of low self-esteem, a lack of motivation and an inability to derive pleasure, and sleep may be disturbed, often with early waking. The cause is often difficult to identify and may be multifactorial with risk factors including creative, perfectionist and neurotic personality types, stressful life events, history of abuse in childhood, the later stages of pregnancy, after childbirth and with a hereditary link, particularly in bipolar disorder. There is also a close association with chronic illnesses (such as multiple sclerosis, myocardial infarction, stroke, Parkinson's disease, cancer, human immunodeficiency virus [HIV]), and may be precipitated by major events such as bereavement and divorce. Depression may complicate or worsen pre-existing diseases. In addition certain drugs may lead to or exacerbate depression, e.g. isotretinoin, corticosteroids, mefloquine, varenicline, benzodiazepines and alcohol. Substance misuse is also a significant cause. For detailed guidance on the management of depression the reader is referred to guidance of the National Institute for Health and Care Excellence (NICE).

Underlying pathology

The underlying pathology of affective disorders is poorly understood and the diverse causes may result in a spectrum of conditions. The classic explanation comes from the monoamine theory, which is now over half a century old, but does not, however, satisfactorily account for all of the pathology. This theory links reduction in the monoamine neurotransmitters noradrenaline (norepinephrine) and 5-hydroxytryptamine (5HT, serotonin) as the main biochemical changes linked to clinical symptoms of depression. The theory was developed after the observation that drug-induced changes in monoamine neurotransmitters either caused or improved symptoms of depression, e.g. the antihypertensive reserpine was withdrawn due to side effects of depression, which were thought to be caused by a reduction in noradrenaline and 5HT-mediated transmission in the brain. By contrast the anti-tuberculosis drug isoniazid, which increased levels of catecholamines, enhanced mood. Antidepressant drugs were, therefore, designed to increase the availability of noradrenaline and 5HT in the brain, leading to a clinical response.

Anomalies exist in the theory in that some drugs affect noradrenaline and/or 5HT activity without evoking changes in mood, e.g. methysergide, a 5HT antagonist, does not produce a depressed mood, as might be predicted. A further discrepancy in the monoamine theory is the delayed onset of antidepressant action despite a rapid change in monoamine levels detectable by analysis of noradrenaline and 5HT metabolite concentrations in cerebrospinal fluid or urine. A change in receptor numbers has therefore been proposed as an important mechanism because a common and delayed down-regulation of β-adrenoceptors and $5HT_2$-receptors is observed after prolonged antidepressant treatment.

Additional theories to the monoamine hypothesis are changes in dopaminergic and also glutametergic function, altered brain development with reduced levels in brain-derived neurotrophic factor and dysregulation of the hypothalamic–pituitary–adrenal axis (Hasler 2010).

Despite the anomalies in the monoamine theory, increased availability of monoamines in the brain remains the most effective biochemical manipulation used in the treatment of depression, being common to all antidepressant drugs.

Classification and clinical features

Depressive illness is classified according to the criteria of the *Diagnostic and Statistical Manual of Mental Disorders,* 5th edition (DSM-V: American Psychiatric Association 2012) and the *International Statistical Classification of Diseases and Related Health Problems* 10th revision (ICD-10: World Health Organization 1992). These classifications are intended to differentiate between normal and pathological states through assessment of behavioural, psychological and biological dysfunction, with the aim of classifying disorders, not people.

Postnatal depression

The diagnosis of postnatal depression is made if any of the criteria below are met and symptoms occur within 4 weeks of childbirth.

Seasonal affective disorder

It is increasingly recognised that affective disorders may follow a seasonal pattern, with onset during the winter months. Accordingly, seasonal affective disorder (SAD) is when a regular and recurrent temporal relationship is observed and seasonal psychosocial stressors are excluded (e.g. unemployment every winter). In addition, two major depressive episodes will have been present in 2 years. Full remission or a switch from depression to mania or hypomania also follows a temporal relationship, such as occurs in springtime. Major depressive episodes should also be absent outside the seasonal episodes. Finally, major depressive episodes with a seasonal onset should outnumber those without seasonal onset during the patient's life.

Dysthymic disorder

Dysthymic disorder include depressed mood for most of the day for most days for at least 2 years. The symptoms cause significant distress or reduced social or occupational functioning. At least two or more of the following symptoms are present with no more than 2 months without symptoms:

- poor appetite or overeating
- altered sleep requirements
- reduced energy or fatigue
- low self-esteem
- poor concentration or indecisiveness
- feelings of hopelessness.

In addition, the criteria require that no major depressive episodes have been diagnosed within the first 2 years. This excludes the possibility of partial remission after a major depressive episode. Full remission would include being symptom free for 2 months. Diagnosis is made after the exclusion of other mental disorders, drug abuse, medication (see Chapter 6) or underlying disease such as hypothyroidism.

Children

Dysthymic disorder may present as irritable mood in children and adolescents, with duration of at least 1 year.

Unipolar affective disorder (major depression)

Unipolar depression is the most common disorder, affecting one in six people. As many as one in three is likely to suffer an episode of unipolar depression in his or her lifetime. Diagnosis of a major depressive episode is currently considered when typically five or more of the following symptoms have been present on most days or nearly every day for 2 weeks and are causing clinically significant distress or impaired functioning. In addition, one of the symptoms must be one of the first two symptoms listed below. Major depressive disorder is diagnosed following one or more major depressive episodes, including:

- depressed mood
- loss of interest or pleasure in all or most activities
- increased or decreased appetite, particularly associated with significant weight change (more than 5% in a month and not dieting)
- altered sleep
- psychomotor agitation or retardation
- fatigue
- worthlessness or excessive or inappropriate guilt
- reduced ability to think or concentrate or indecisiveness
- recurrent thoughts of death or suicide

and not explained by substance abuse, or general medical conditions such as hypothyroidism.

Children

In children and adolescents, the symptom of depressed mood (first point above) may present as irritable mood. In addition, weight changes may present as a failure to make expected weight gains (see below).

Psychotic depression

A depressive episode may also present with additional psychotic symptoms. The term 'psychosis' is used to describe severe mental illness with loss of contact with reality. Thought processes are often altered and patients suffer hallucinations and delusions (see Chapter 28). Psychosis is a component of severe schizophrenia, depression and bipolar affective disorder. For a discussion of the psychotic symptoms associated with antimuscarinic drugs, see Chapter 28.

Severity

The severity of a depressive episode may be mild, moderate or severe. An episode is described as mild if the number of symptoms required for a positive diagnosis is exceeded only marginally. A severe episode

will present with numerous additional symptoms to those required to make a diagnosis, and a marked disruption to normal functioning occurs. Moderate illness falls between the two extremes. It is also recognised that some patients may have sub-threshold depression, which itself can be responsible for significant symptoms.

Children

Depression in children and adolescents is now increasingly recognised, often presenting as self-criticism, pessimism about the future, lack of energy, sleep disturbance, stomach-ache, headache, indecision and difficulty concentrating. Children may lack interest in activities that they previously enjoyed. Risk factors include a family history of affective disorders, stress, viral infections and a history of abuse. There is sparse information relating to the treatment of childhood depression but this may involve cognitive-behavioural therapy (CBT) and possibly the selective serotonin reuptake inhibitor (SSRI) fluoxetine, according to clinical trial data. It is generally recognised that the risks of other SSRIs such as citalopram, paroxetine and sertraline generally outweigh the benefits in children under 18 years of age. There is no good evidence for the use of tricyclic antidepressants (TCAs) for depression in children. Recent NICE guidance has reminded practitioners that, in prescribing antidepressants for patients under 18, the advantages must outweigh the disadvantages and, when treatment is indicated, fluoxetine should be used and paroxetine avoided. Monitoring for behavioural changes and suicidal thoughts is essential, particularly during the early stages of treatment.

Goals of treatment

Treatment aims are to improve the quality of life, including the ability to work and function socially, together with the prevention of suicide. This should of course be achieved with the minimum of side effects. Drug treatment should ideally be used with appropriate CBT or psychotherapy, which may hasten recovery and prevent recurrence. Detailed guidance for the provision of psychological interventions is given by NICE (2009).

Pharmacological basis of management

Serotonin-selective reuptake inhibitors 'SSRIs', e.g. citalopram, escitalopram (active isomer of citalopram), fluoxetine, fluvoxamine, paroxetine, sertraline

As the name implies, SSRIs selectively inhibit the neuronal reuptake of 5HT, thus enhancing synaptic concentrations of 5HT and down-regulating presynaptic 5HT-receptors. SSRIs have a different side effect profile to TCAs, including nausea, diarrhoea, constipation, dizziness, headache, altered platelet function, anorexia, insomnia, loss of libido, and delay or failure of orgasm. Some SSRIs are also licensed for the treatment of anxiety, panic and obsessive–compulsive disorders (see Chapter 26).

Tricyclic antidepressants (TCAs), e.g. amitriptyline, lofepramine, nortriptyline

TCAs are similar in structure to phenothiazines (prochlorperazine, thioridazine) and inhibit the neuronal uptake of noradrenaline and 5HT, leading to augmented concentrations in the synaptic cleft. The increase in catecholamines may lead to down-regulation of presynaptic α_2-adrenoceptors and 5HT receptors and postsynaptic β-adrenoceptors. In addition, TCAs exhibit binding at a range of receptors, including muscarinic receptors, histamine, α_1-adrenoceptors and 5HT-receptors. The inhibition of muscarinic receptors results in side effects such as dry mouth, blurred vision, constipation and urinary retention. TCAs vary in the degree of sedation that they cause (with amitriptyline and dosulepin having significant effects and lofepramine being less sedating) and this may have a bearing on their use where sedation may be an advantage or unwanted. TCAs may cause cardiac effects such as Q–T interval prolongation and the potentiation of catecholamines also predisposes to heart block and arrhythmias. The cardiac effects of TCAs (except lofepramine), together with increased effects of alcohol, including respiratory depression, mean that these agents are dangerous in overdose. They are not suitable for patients with ischaemic heart disease, aged >70 years or those patients who are thought to be at high risk of attempting suicide.

Monoamine oxidase inhibitors: isocarboxazid, moclobemide, phenelzine, tranylcypromine

Monoamine oxidase inhibitors (MAOIs) are very rarely used because of their widespread side effects and drug interactions, including those with tyramine-containing foods. Their use is now only in a specialist setting. They were the first antidepressants used after the observation that treatment with isoniazid for tuberculosis improved mood. MAOs metabolise catecholamines so, once again, the action of MAOIs is to increase the concentration of these neurotransmitters. As a result, MAOIs also prevent the breakdown of tyramine, the indirectly acting sympathomimetic amine which is present in the diet. By preventing the breakdown of tyramine, this amine causes the release of catecholamines and leads to a hypertensive response. Tyramine is present in certain foods such as yeast extracts (including Bovril and Marmite), some wines and beers, avocado, banana, pickled herring and cheese, and this response is known as the 'cheese reaction'. As most MAOIs inhibit MAO irreversibly, these reactions may persist for 2–3 weeks after the cessation of treatment until a new MAO is synthesised.

MAO exists as either MAO-A, which metabolises predominantly noradrenaline and 5HT, or MAO-B, for which phenylethylamine is a substrate. Tyramine and dopamine are metabolised by both subtypes. In an attempt to reduce side effects and interactions, selective inhibitors of MAO have been developed, e.g. moclobemide, a selective reversible inhibitor of MAO-A (RIMA), reduces interactions with food because tyramine is metabolised by MAO-B. The MAO-B inhibitor selegeline is used to treat Parkinson's disease.

Noradrenaline reuptake inhibitors: reboxetine

Reboxetine is one of the newer noradrenaline reuptake inhibitors. It selectively inhibits noradrenaline reuptake, providing an option for patients who cannot take TCAs (Table 25.1) but who are resistant to the effects of SSRIs.

Table 25.1 Some considerations when choosing the most appropriate antidepressant

Condition	Cautions and contraindications	Compelling drug choices
Cardiovascular disease	All antidepressants, including lithium, should be used with caution due to increased effects of sympathetic and serotonergic systems. Venlafaxine has been associated with dose-related hypertension	SSRIs are preferred
Recent MI	TCAs are contraindicated	SSRIs considered safe, particularly sertraline (Glassman *et al.* 2002)
Arrhythmias	TCAs are contraindicated. Venlafaxine and antipsychotics may cause Q–T interval prolongation. Atypical antipsychotics have not been associated with this but caution is needed if co-prescribed with drugs known to prolong the Q–T interval (Chapter 6)	• SSRIs (not fluoxetine) • Avoid fluoxetine and trazodone, which can cause atrial fibrillation
Stroke	Avoid MAOIs due to the risk of a hypertensive episode. Use venlafaxine with caution due to dose-related hypertension (see above)	
Insomnia	SSRIs may occasionally cause insomnia. Lofepramine is a less-sedating TCA	Sedating TCAs (e.g. amitriptyline, dosulepin), maprotiline, mianserin or trazodone
Risk of deliberate self-harm or suicide attempt	See text	
Epilepsy	All antidepressants have the potential to lower the convulsive threshold and should be used with caution and avoided in poorly controlled epilepsy	• Carbamazepine and lamotrigine (unlicensed indication) may be considered in bipolar affective disorder • Additional risk factors include diabetes mellitus or concurrent treatment with drugs known to lower the convulsive threshold (Chapter 24)
Bipolar affective disorder – manic phase	TCAs, MAOIs and SSRIs are contraindicated. Antidepressants may trigger bipolar disorder, particularly in patients with hypomania and/or a family history	Mood stabilisers (lithium, neuroleptics, carbamazepine and valproate – see text). Combining SSRI treatment (avoiding long-acting preparations, e.g. fluoxetine) with a mood stabiliser may reduce the risk of switching to mania (Grunze *et al.* 2002)
Anxiety disorders	Long-term use of propranolol and/or benzodiazepines should be avoided because these drugs may aggravate depression	For depression with associated anxiety symptoms, refer to Chapter 26
Migraine	SSRIs may cause headache (Chapter 6)	TCAs may be appropriate (Chapter 23)
Neuropathic pain		TCAs or carbamazepine
Alcoholism	Sedative effects of TCAs enhanced	
Eating disorders		High-dose fluoxetine is indicated for bulimia nervosa
Parkinson's disease treated with co-beneldopa, co-careldopa, levodopa	Irreversible MAOIs should be avoided with drugs used to increase dopamine	
Peptic ulcer disease	Increased risk of GI bleeds, so caution with SSRIs. Consider high-risk patients such as those with a history of previous GI bleed and/or aged over 80 years (Chapter 8)	

Table 25.1 *(continued)*

Condition	Cautions and contraindications	Compelling drug choices
Urinary problems (prostatism), glaucoma and constipation	Caution with TCAs and maprotiline and mirtazapine due to antimuscarinic side effects	
Hyperthyroidism	Caution with TCAs due to augmentation of sympathetic nervous system. Lithium should be used with caution and initiated when patients are euthyroid. Regular monitoring of thyroid function is essential (Chapter 2)	

GI, gastrointestinal; MAOIs, monoamine oxidase inhibitors; MI, myocardial infarction; SSRIs, selective serotonin reuptake inhibitors; TCAs, tricyclic antidepressants.

Serotonin–noradrenaline reuptake inhibitors: venlafaxine

A relatively new reuptake inhibitor is venlafaxine. The mechanism of action involves the inhibition of both serotonin and noradrenaline reuptake, as with TCAs. Serotonin–noradrenaline reuptake inhibitors (SNRIs), however, fail to bind to additional receptors and therefore demonstrate fewer side effects compared with TCAs, including a lack of sedative and antimuscarinic side effects, but do cause gastrointestinal side effects. In addition, an analysis of fatal toxicity of antidepressants in the UK reported that venlafaxine toxicity is greater than for other serotonergic agents and similar to some TCAs (Buckley and McManus 2002). The MHRA (Medicines and Healthcare products Regulatory Agency) has highlighted problems of serious cardiac arrhythmias and cardiotoxicity in overdose with venlafaxine.

Noradrenergic and specific serotonergic antidepressants: mirtazapine

Observations of the pharmacological activity of mianserin have been exploited in the development of mirtazapine. This agent exhibits α_2-adrenocepter antagonist activity, inhibiting negative feedback by these presynaptic receptors and thus producing an increase in noradrenaline and 5HT transmission. Mirtazapine also inhibits $5HT_2$- and $5HT_3$-receptors, preventing sexual dysfunction and nausea, respectively. Sedation predominates in early treatment but antimuscarinic side effects are limited.

Serotonin receptor modulators: nefazodone and trazodone

Nefazodone and trazodone are similar in structure and exhibit mixed serotonergic activity, including both inhibition of serotonin reuptake and the selective inhibition of postsynaptic 5HT-receptors. Trazodone also acts at adrenoceptors, with nefazodone exhibiting less activity at these receptors.

TCA-related antidepressants: bupropion, maprotiline, mianserin, nomifensine

In the ongoing search for antidepressants with fewer side effects, reduced toxicity in overdose and no delayed onset of action, a number of agents have been developed that do not fit the above classes of MAOI, SSRI or TCA, e.g. some agents possess a non-TCA structure but exhibit similar modes of action. The mechanisms thought to be involved in the antidepressant effects of these TCA-related agents include:

- the inhibition of noradrenaline uptake (nomifensine and maprotiline)
- a small reduction of 5HT uptake and possibly inhibition of dopamine uptake (nomifensine)
- agents that do not affect amine uptake (mianserin, bupropion)
- inhibition of 5HT- and α_2-adrenoceptors, thereby inhibiting negative feedback and increasing release of noradrenaline without the conventional effects on the reuptake of noradrenaline and serotonin (mianserin)

- unknown mechanisms – bupropion is efficacious but fails to demonstrate biochemistry in common with conventional antidepressant activity.

Benzodiazepines (e.g. clonazepam, lorazepam) and β blockers

These are used on a temporary basis in depression with a component of severe anxiety or hyperactivity (see Chapter 26), e.g. a short-acting benzodiazepine such as lorazepam may be used when antidepressants are initiated, before the onset of efficacy. Long-term use may worsen depression and lead to addiction to benzodiazepines and apparent worsening anxiety (withdrawal reactions, see Chapter 6).

Flupentixol

Lower doses of flupentixol compared with those used in schizophrenia are indicated for the treatment of depressive illness.

L-Tryptophan

L-Tryptophan, a precursor for 5HT, is an amino acid found in food. It has a mild antidepressant effect but use is limited to prescribing by hospital specialists for patients with chronic severe depression who are already taking other antidepressants. This is mainly due to the risk of eosinophilia–myalgia syndrome (increased eosinophils in blood, with muscle pain) and close monitoring of the eosinophil count and muscle symptoms is required.

Electroconvulsive therapy

Electroconvulsive therapy (ECT) is reserved for severe and suicidal depression, with greatest efficacy in depression with psychomotor retardation (literally, a slowing of muscular and mental activity), such as depressive stupor. This is a condition of near unconsciousness, apparent mental inactivity and a reduced response to stimulation. The procedure is carried out under general anaesthesia and a convulsion is induced by passing an electric current through the brain. The main side effects are temporary confusion and memory loss. This treatment should therefore be used with caution in elderly patients with cognitive impairment.

Other risks to be considered are those associated with general anaesthesia and the use of ECT during pregnancy. These risks are considered alongside the benefits and potential risks of withholding treatment. The mechanism involved remains unclear but ECT is an effective treatment with rapid onset.

Lithium

Lithium is a useful adjunct in the treatment of resistant depression. It may be added to TCA or SSRI treatment under specialist supervision. The use of TCAs and SSRIs is associated with a risk of switching patients into mania, a particular problem when treating the depressive phase of bipolar disorder. The highest risk is associated with the use of TCAs.

Non-pharmacological therapy

Structured counselling based on theoretical models includes psychotherapy or CBT. Psychotherapy may be of particular benefit to patients with a history of abuse or social history such as stressful life events. CBT has been shown to be effective in mild depression and in combination with antidepressants in moderate depression (Scott *et al.* 1997). This would seem logical because neurotic, perfectionist, obsessional or anxious personality types may be linked to depression. The negative thought patterns associated with these personality types are identified and addressed during CBT. In addition, increased insight and the avoidance of overly stressful situations contribute to successful treatment. The reader is referred to *Mind over Mood* (Greenberger and Padesky 1995) for an excellent CBT-based workbook for motivated patients. Computerised CBT is also recommended for the treatment of mild depression (NICE 2009). In addition, a meditation-based approach to CBT known as mindfulness-based CBT has been developed and is recommended by NICE for patients with recurrent depression. This is not widely available at the moment but workbooks such as *The Mindful Way through Depression* (Williams *et al.* 2007) and *Mindfulness-Based Cognitive Therapy for Depression: A new approach to preventing relapse* (Segal *et al.* 2002) are available for patients and therapists, respectively. Patients with SAD may benefit from light therapy (Levitt *et al.* 2002).

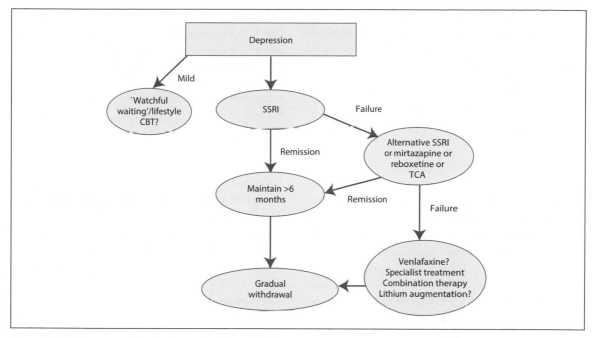

Figure 25.1 Summary of the management of unipolar depression, which incorporates NICE (2009) guidance. CBT, cognitive-behavioural therapy; SSRI, serotonin-selective reuptake inhibitor; TCA, tricyclic antidepressant.

Choice of drugs in unipolar affective disorder

NICE guidance recommends that, before drug treatment in mild depression, a 2-week period of 'watchful waiting' is appropriate with advice on exercise, sleep and anxiety management. CBT is also recommended. When drug treatment is appropriate the choice is between an SSRI and a TCA, with the most appropriate drug class being selected, according to:

- sedative properties
- side effect profile
- previous response
- potential for toxicity in overdose
- concurrent disease (see Table 25.1).

Although SSRIs and TCAs are generally regarded as equally effective, SSRIs have a superior side effect profile and are safer in overdose and so should be regarded as first-line agents. Current guidance indicates that antidepressants should not be used in mild depression and that they are really effective only in moderate-to-severe cases. Generally fluoxetine or citalopram are regarded as appropriate for first-line

usage. TCAs should be used only if SSRIs fail to control the condition or are contraindicated. In cases where sedation is required TCAs such as amitriptyline might be chosen in preference to SSRIs.

Treatment should be continued for at least 6 months after symptoms resolve to prevent relapse and recurrence. The recommended length of treatment varies according to the severity of symptoms and the number of episodes suffered. The duration of treatment of a second episode should be at least 12 months. For recurrent depression antidepressant treatment is usually continued for at least 2 years after two or more depressive episodes in the recent past and associated with significant functional impairment. The need for ongoing maintenance treatment is assessed according to age, concurrent conditions and other risk factors.

Risk of suicide

TCAs are avoided in patients considered to be at risk of committing suicide, such as those with a history of contemplating or attempting suicide. This is due to the toxic effects of TCAs (except lofepramine) in overdose. SSRIs are preferred due to relative safety in overdose, although patients should be monitored closely during early treatment with all antidepressants and particularly SSRIs, due to a possible increased risk of suicide attempts. Alternative treatment includes the use of mirtazapine, nefazodone and reboxetine, which are considered to be relatively safe in overdose. For a discussion of the use of venlafaxine, see SNRIs above.

Treatment failure

Failure of treatment (typically after 4 weeks) may lead to a different class being used. It should be noted that a failure of TCAs may reflect too low a dosage being prescribed, because it has been found that older TCAs are more effective in the 125–150 mg dose range than at lower doses. A subsequent failure with TCAs or SSRIs may be a reason to consider using venlafaxine, or in some specialist settings combination therapy may be used. Specialists may also use lithium augmentation.

Effectiveness of antidepressants

The effectiveness of antidepressants has been established over many years by numerous clinical trials, analyses and clinical experience. However, one meta-analysis has indicated that certain agents (fluoxetine, venlafaxine, nefazodone and paroxetine) lack or have limited efficacy beyond a placebo effect (Kirsch *et al.* 2008). This analysis is clearly controversial but current opinion and guidance certainly support their use in moderate-to-severe depression.

Bipolar affective disorder

Bipolar depression is characterised by cycling between depression and mania and has a strong hereditary link, although no specific gene(s) has been identified to date. It is less common than unipolar depression, affecting 1 in 100 of the population.

Manic episode

By contrast to the symptoms of depression outlined above, the manic phase of bipolar affective disorder presents as abnormally and persistently elevated expansive or irritable mood. The diagnostic criteria classify a manic episode when three or more of the following symptoms are significant and present for at least 1 week and/or require hospital admission:

- inflated self-esteem or grandiosity
- reduced requirement for sleep
- rapid speech with pressure to keep talking
- flight of ideas
- distractibility
- increased goal-directed activity or psychomotor agitation (compare psychomotor retardation in depressive symptoms)
- reduced inhibitions such as sexual indiscretion and uncontrolled spending.

In addition, the criteria state that a diagnosis is made when the above symptoms are sufficient to impair normal occupational and social activities and relationships with others, require hospital treatment to prevent self-harm or harm to others, or psychotic features are present. Again, additional causes such as medication, ECT, light therapy, drug abuse or hyperthyroidism should be excluded.

Hypomania

Hypomania is diagnosed when mood becomes persistently elevated, expansive or irritable compared with normal mood and persistent throughout the day for at least 4 days. The significant presence of three or more of the symptoms listed for a manic episode or four if the mood is irritable may result in a diagnosis of hypomania. Additional requirements are that others observe an uncharacteristic change in mood and functioning. A hypomanic episode differs from mania in that there is minimal effect on social or occupational function, hospital admission is not required and psychotic symptoms are absent. Additional causes such as medication should be excluded, as stated previously.

Rapid cycling

The diagnosis of rapid cycling is made when four episodes of mood disturbance occur, according to the above criteria, during a 12-month period. Partial or full remission occurs for at least 2 months between episodes. Alternatively a switch between a depressive and manic episode may occur.

Treatment

Lithium remains the first-line agent for both acute treatment and prophylaxis of bipolar disorder, although a delay in the onset of action necessitates the concurrent use of neuroleptics (see Chapter 28) in acute mania. Lithium is a monovalent cation that mimics the role of sodium ions by permeating fast voltage-sensitive channels responsible for generating action potentials in excitable tissue.

Lithium exerts many effects on neurotransmission and its relatively selective action on the brain and kidney has not been elucidated fully. The main site of action is the inhibition of recycling by hydrolysis of the intracellular second messenger inositol triphosphate (IP_3) to phosphatidyl inositol in cell membranes. This reduces the effects of substances that activate receptors (e.g. α_1-adrenoceptors) linked to IP_3 generation and subsequent Ca^{2+} release from intracellular stores. The extensive distribution of such receptor systems throughout the body suggests many potential effects of lithium. The apparent selectivity has been suggested to result from selective uptake of lithium dependent on sodium channel activity.

Toxic effects of lithium may result from reduced hormone responses involving the second messenger, adenosine cyclic 3′:5′-monophosphate (cAMP), e.g. the inhibition of cAMP-mediated antidiuretic hormone (ADH) activity in the kidney results in polyuria and polydipsia. Sodium ions are retained, leading to increased ADH secretion and possible damage of renal tubules. The failure of the thyroid gland to respond to thyroid-stimulating hormone (TSH) may result in an enlarged thyroid gland and hypothyroidism.

Anticonvulsants, e.g. carbamazepine and valproate

Carbamazepine and valproate are used second line as prophylactic mood stabilisers in bipolar disorder and lack the extrapyramidal effects of the antipsychotic drugs. The mechanism of action has not yet been elucidated fully but is thought to involve effects on ion channels, increasing the release of the inhibitory and excitatory neurotransmitters, γ-aminobutyric acid (GABA) and glutamate, respectively. The anticonvulsants lamotrigine and gabapentin have an unlicensed role in bipolar affective disorder when other treatments have failed.

Antipsychotics, e.g. haloperidol and chlorpromazine

Antipsychotics such as haloperidol and chlorpromazine may be used to control psychotic symptoms, which may be associated with depression and particularly during the manic phase of bipolar disorder. They have a rapid rate of onset and so may be initiated together with lithium, controlling the manic phase until the lithium begins to exert its effects in patients with bipolar disorder. The blockade of dopamine D_2-receptors is thought to be the predominant mode of action. Haloperidol is often preferred due to reduced sedative and cardiovascular effects compared with chlorpromazine. The atypical antipsychotic olanzapine has been licensed for use in bipolar disorder and is less likely to cause extrapyramidal effects compared with the older agents (see Chapter 28).

Drug choice in bipolar affective disorder

The acute (manic) phase of bipolar affective disorder is often associated with psychosis and therefore treated with antipsychotics such as haloperidol and/or benzodiazepines such as lorazepam for severe cases. These drugs are used for a few days until the effects of lithium are achieved. The atypical antipsychotic olanzapine is also used to treat moderate-to-severe manic episodes. However, lithium remains the treatment of choice for both acute and long-term prophylaxis; olanzapine may be added to lithium for patients with residual symptoms. Maintenance treatment is given under specialist supervision according to the risk of withdrawing the drug compared with its benefit. The need for continued treatment is assessed regularly and maintenance is recommended beyond 3–5 years only when the benefit of continuing the drug is apparent, e.g. the presence of symptoms during a trial of gradual dose reduction.

Other agents such as the anticonvulsants valproate and carbamazepine may be considered when treatment with lithium has failed. Carbamazepine is indicated for the prophylaxis of manic-depressive psychoses for patients unresponsive to lithium therapy. Valproic acid in the form semisodium valproate is licensed for acute mania whereas sodium valproate remains unlicensed for this use. Carbamazepine may particularly benefit patients with rapid cycling between mania and depression (four or more episodes per year). Both carbamazepine and valproate are currently considered to be second choice for prophylaxis due to an inferior efficacy compared with lithium. The anticonvulsants lamotrigine and gabapentin are unlicensed for bipolar disorder and should be initiated only by specialists. Lamotrigine may be considered for the treatment of the depressive phase of bipolar depression when TCA- or SSRI-induced 'switching' to the manic phase is problematic (Calabrese *et al.* 1999). Guidelines published by the World Federation of Societies of Biological Psychiatry suggest that combining SSRIs (or bupropion) with a mood stabiliser (lithium or lamotrigine) reduces the risk of switching, to a level observed when mood stabilisers are used alone (Grunze *et al.* 2002). It was noted that lithium might also possess anti-suicide properties.

Concurrent conditions: additional considerations when prescribing in affective disorders

Some considerations for choosing a suitable antidepressant are summarised in Table 25.1.

Diabetes mellitus

MAOIs should be used with caution due to an increased risk of hypoglycaemia. Lithium ions may impair glucose tolerance and may cause diabetes mellitus. There is no evidence, however, for loss of glycaemic control of existing diabetes but careful monitoring is recommended. Olanzapine has been associated with hyperglycaemia or exacerbation of pre-existing diabetes mellitus and should be used with caution in these patients. Monitoring of patients with risk factors for type 2 diabetes, particularly obesity, is important when prescribing olanzapine, which may also cause weight gain.

Renal impairment

- Lithium should be avoided in renal impairment. For patients with mild renal impairment, a dose reduction and close monitoring are advised.

- SSRIs should be generally avoided in severe renal impairment. In moderate impairment, dose reduction may be needed.
- The dose of venlafaxine also requires reduction in moderate renal impairment.
- Small doses of antipsychotics are used in severe renal impairment. Lower doses of risperidone or olanzapine may be required.

Liver function

TCAs and MAOIs are contraindicated in severe liver disease. TCAs are preferable to MAOIs but sedative effects are increased. Lofepramine is associated with hepatic toxicity. MAOIs are implicated in the development of idiosyncratic hepatotoxicity. Reduced doses of SSRIs are advised with avoidance in severe liver disease. Antipsychotics can precipitate coma and phenothiazines are hepatotoxic. Atypical antipsychotics such as risperidone and olanzapine may be used at reduced doses.

Pregnancy and breastfeeding

TCAs are preferred if necessary for the treatment of unipolar depression during pregnancy and breastfeeding. This is due to greater experience of their use in pregnancy compared with SSRIs, and lower known risks, with the exception of toxicity in overdose. There is also evidence for a small risk of congenital cardiac defects with certain SSRIs and so TCAs are now preferred in pregnancy..

Drugs used for bipolar disorders are often associated with fetal abnormalities and therefore preconception counselling is important. In view of the teratogenic risk associated with lithium in the first trimester, it is recommended that pregnancy be excluded before the initiation of lithium therapy. Ideally, all treatment is withdrawn for at least the first trimester. Alternatively, reducing the dose, particularly of lithium, is considered. For patients taking carbamazepine, folic acid 5 mg supplements are recommended before conception and up to week 12 of pregnancy (see Chapters 3 and 24).

Miscellaneous

Lithium is not recommended for patients with Addison's disease, because disturbances in sodium homeostasis may result. Blood pressure monitoring is recommended if doses of venlafaxine exceed 200 mg/day.

Drug interactions

Drug interactions involving antidepressants may result from: altered drug levels due to effects on drug absorption, metabolism or excretion; overstimulation of monoamine neurotransmission; an increased risk of cardiac arrhythmias due to prolongation of the Q–T interval and the risk of convulsions due to a lowering of the convulsive threshold. The following section highlights some examples.

Antidepressant combinations

Co-prescribing two or more antidepressants is not recommended due to the risk of toxicity, e.g. co-prescribing MAOIs, particularly irreversible MAOIs, increases the risk of hypertensive crises and stroke (see above). Despite this, the combinations of some antidepressants such as MAOIs or SSRIs with TCAs or atypical agents may be beneficial but only under expert supervision. Monitoring for adverse drug reactions is advised with all combinations. Examples of problems requiring particular awareness are given in Table 25.2.

Serotonergic syndrome

The Sternbach diagnostic criteria indicate that three or more of the following symptoms should be present before differentiating serotonin syndrome from neuroleptic malignant syndrome (see Chapter 6): confusion, hypomania, incoordination, tremor, agitation, diaphoresis (sweating), shivering, fever, myoclonus (muscle spasms) and hyperreflexia (Sternbach 1991).

Lithium and olanzapine

It should be noted that there is no evidence for an interaction between lithium and olanzapine. Table 25.3 provides examples of drug interactions involving antidepressants.

Monitoring

Renal function and electrolytes (creatinine and sodium)

Hyponatraemia may occur with high doses of TCAs or SSRIs or in elderly patients, and particularly with either co-prescribed diuretics, laxatives or concurrent

Table 25.2 Problems associated with the co-prescribing of antidepressants

Interacting antidepressants	Consequences	Comments
Fluoxetine with TCAs (amitriptyline, clomipramine, imipramine and nortriptyline) or trazodone	• Increased levels of TCAs • Increased risk of sedation due to trazodone	• Dose adjustment is required during concurrent use • Trazodone and fluoxetine are effective when co-prescribed but patients may develop increased side effects such as sedation • The long half-life of fluoxetine means that this interaction may persist after the drug is stopped
Fluvoxamine with TCAs (amitriptyline, clomipramine, imipramine and trimipramine) or maprotiline	Increased serum levels of the TCA or maprotiline	• Dose adjustment is required to prevent toxicity • There is no evidence for the same interaction with desipramine
Lithium with TCAs or SSRIs	An unpredictable risk of serious effects such as serotonin or neuroleptic malignant syndromes (see text)	Lithium is occasionally used successfully with TCAs or SSRIs but monitoring for ADRs is important
Paroxetine with TCAs (desipramine, imipramine and trimipramine)	Increased serum levels of the TCA	Patients should therefore be monitored closely for ADRs and the dose reduced if necessary

ADRs, adverse drug reactions; SSRIs, selective serotonin reuptake inhibitors; TCAs, tricyclic antidepressants.

Table 25.3 Examples of drug interactions involving antidepressants

Drug	Consequences	Comments
Antidepressants with alcohol	• Increased side effects such as drowsiness and reduced alertness • Increased risk of accidents when driving or operating machinery	• Possible antagonism of antidepressant effect with chronic alcohol intake • Temporary mood-enhancing effect may contribute to a vicious cycle of alcohol abuse
Induction of hepatic enzymes		
Carbamazepine with haloperidol, oral contraceptives or phenytoin	Reduced effects of the latter	Increased doses may be required
SSRI-mediated inhibition of hepatic enzymes		
Fluvoxamine with theophylline	Risk of a rapid and potentially toxic increase in theophylline levels	• This combination should be avoided • Alternatively, the theophylline dose should be reduced to about half • Limited evidence suggests that a similar interaction does not occur between fluoxetine and theophylline
Fluoxetine, fluvoxamine, sertraline and paroxetine with anticoagulants, MAOIs, alcohol, selegiline, antipsychotics, lithium, phenytoin, carbamazepine and omeprazole	Increased effects	• Evidence suggests that the SSRI citalopram does not interact with warfarin • Note that SSRIs differ in their profile of cytochrome P450 inhibition
Lithium levels increased		
ACE inhibitors, diuretics (particularly thiazides) and analgesics	Reduced excretion of lithium	• Consider impairment of renal function as a risk factor • Monitoring is required with a possible reduction in lithium dose • Aspirin and paracetamol are considered safe to use with lithium
Lithium with theophylline or metronidazole	Increased plasma concentrations of lithium	Close monitoring is required
Lithium levels reduced		
Lithium with ispaghula husk	Serum levels of lithium may be reduced	• Monitoring with appropriate dose adjustment is recommended • The mechanism involved may be due in part to the sodium content of effervescent granules
Lithium with methyldopa or clonazepam	Enhanced neurotoxicity	Avoid concurrent use
Lithium with haloperidol	Risk of rare but serious neurotoxic reaction, particularly in patients with a history of extrapyramidal effects with antipsychotics or if high doses of haloperidol are used	• Symptoms include fever, tremor, confusion and extrapyramidal effects • Patients should be monitored closely for ADRs, with prompt withdrawal due to a risk of brain damage • The co-prescribing of haloperidol with lithium in acute mania is extremely beneficial

Table 25.3 *(continued)*		
Drug	**Consequences**	**Comments**
Lithium with baclofen	Increased risk of baclofen induced hyperkinetic activity	Patients should be monitored closely
MAOIs with pethidine	Risk of a potentially life threatening reaction	Pethidine should not be given with MAOIs unless a lack of sensitivity is confirmed
Paroxetine or sertraline with tramadol	The combination of two or more serotonergic drugs may lead to a potentially fatal condition resulting from overstimulation of 5HT receptors	Monitoring for symptoms of serotonin syndrome is advised (see text)
SSRIs or MAOIs with 5HT agonists (sumatriptan)	Risk of serotonin syndrome (see text)	Avoid concurrent use
TCAs and some atypical antidepressants (venlafaxine) *with* other drugs known to prolong the Q–T interval	Q–T interval prolongation and risk of potentially fatal arrhythmias	• The CHM warns against the use of more than one drug known to prolong the Q–T interval • If concurrent use is unavoidable, patients should report irregular heartbeat, palpitations and dizziness immediately
TCAs or SSRIs with other drugs which lower the convulsive threshold	Increased risk of convulsions	

5HT, 5-hydroxytryptamine or serotonin; ACE, angiotensin-converting enzyme; ADRs, adverse drug reactions; CHM, Commission on Human Medicines; GI, gastrointestinal; MAOIs, monoamine oxidase inhibitors; NSAIDs, non-steroidal anti-inflammatory drugs; SSRIs, selective serotonin reuptake inhibitors; TCAs, tricyclic antidepressants.

illness leading to dehydration. The CHM warns that hyponatraemia should be considered in patients developing confusion, drowsiness or convulsions while taking antidepressants.

Lithium (see Appendix 2)

Urea and electrolytes and full blood count

Baseline measurements of blood urea and electrolytes (U&Es), serum creatinine, thyroid function, a full blood count (FBC) and the exclusion of pregnancy are required before the initiation of lithium therapy. Concurrent diseases such as cardiac disease are also considered (see Table 25.1).

During maintenance therapy, the following monitoring is recommended:

- serum creatinine every 6 months
- thyroid function tests every 6–12 months with counselling to report warning symptoms (4–6 weeks if TSH is elevated)
- an FBC annually
- serum lithium levels at least 3-monthly (see Chapter 7)
- U&Es every 6 months.

Ischaemic heart disease

An electrocardiogram is recommended before the initiation of lithium treatment for patients with a history of cardiac problems.

Liver function

Liver function should be assessed before and during the first 6 months of treatment with sodium valproate or valproic acid (see Chapter 24). Raised liver enzymes may be transient and a clinical assessment of clinical features and liver function tests (see Chapter 2), including prothrombin time, should be continued until the levels return to normal. Risk factors include children <3 years of age, metabolic or degenerative disease, organic brain disease or severe seizures with learning disability.

Blood counts

Patients taking mianserin should have blood counts checked every 4 weeks for the first 3 months of treatment. Blood monitoring should be performed for patients taking mianserin or carbamazepine who develop fever, sore throat, stomatitis or other signs of infection. Mirtazapine treatment warrants blood counts and immediate cessation of treatment if blood dyscrasias are suspected.

Withdrawal

Once a patient has been in remission, withdrawal of the antidepressant should be considered after a sufficient period of sustained remission. Withdrawal may precipitate a reaction (e.g. depression, sensory and balance problems, mood changes and gastro-intestinal disturbances) in any patient (particularly with paroxetine and venlafaxine) and should involve a dose reduction over at least 4 weeks or up to 6 months in patients who have been on long-term maintenance therapy. Abrupt withdrawal of lithium should be avoided because this may increase the frequency of manic episodes and shorten the time to relapse.

Over-the-counter considerations

An important role of the pharmacist is to recognise and refer patients with symptoms of depression, advise patients about drug interactions associated with antidepressant medication, and provide advice and reassurance relating to side effects and the need for prolonged treatment. Table 25.4 highlights important issues and drug interactions associated with antidepressants and over-the-counter (OTC) prescribing.

Alcohol

TCAs, fluvoxamine, isoniazid, maprotiline, mianserin and trazodone may enhance the effects of alcohol. In patients who are taking MAOIs, the hypotensive effects may be enhanced by alcohol and the tyramine content of certain beers and red wines should also be considered. It should also be noted that alcohol misuse may be related to depression. The central nervous system (CNS)-depressant effect of alcohol

Table 25.4 Antidepressants and over-the-counter (OTC) prescribing

OTC medicines	Comments
Sedative antihistamines such as diphenhydramine, promethazine are licensed for the treatment of insomnia	• Use is limited to 2 weeks. Repeated requests may point to depression • They should not be used together with TCAs due to enhanced antimuscarinic effects and sedation
Indirectly acting sympathomimetic decongestants (phenylpropanolamine, pseudoephedrine, ephedrine)	• The action of indirectly acting sympathomimetics is likely to be blocked by TCAs • There is, however, limited evidence for this interaction (Chapter 20) • Avoid with MAOIs (Chapter 20)
Directly acting sympathomimetic decongestants (phenylephrine)	These should not be taken by patients prescribed MAOIs or within 14 days of cessation of MAOIs because there is a substantial risk of enhanced pressor activity (i.e. increased blood pressure) (Chapter 20)
Antacids and sodium-containing preparations (cystitis and effervescent products)	These should be avoided with lithium
Cough preparations containing dextromethorphan	A rare but serious interaction (serotonin syndrome) with paroxetine contraindicates concurrent use
Fybogel	May reduce lithium levels
Cimetidine	• This inhibits the metabolism of amitriptyline, doxepin, imipramine, moclobemide, nortriptyline, sertraline • Use ranitidine as an alternative
NSAIDs	Ibuprofen increases plasma concentrations of lithium. Aspirin or paracetamol are appropriate alternatives

MAOIs, monoamine oxidase inhibitors; NSAIDs, non-steroidal anti-inflammatory drugs; TCAs, tricyclic antidepressants.

may cause or exacerbate depression, with the temporary mood-enhancing properties contributing to a 'vicious circle'.

Caffeine

Lithium levels may be reduced by excess caffeine intake. Levels may increase following abrupt withdrawal of caffeine intake (e.g. Pro Plus and some analgesic preparations). The effects of caffeine may also be deleterious in depression associated with anxiety (see Chapter 26).

Herbal medicines

The herbal medicine, St John's wort is widely advocated for depression but should not be recommended. Although St John's wort has been shown to be better than placebo as an antidepressant for the short-term treatment of mild-to-moderate depression it is associated with significant side effects and drug interactions (see Chapters 4 and 6). In the context of depression, it inhibits the reuptake of 5HT, and may potentiate the action of SSRIs, and so should not be used with conventional antidepressants. A Cochrane systematic review concluded that there is evidence that some preparations of St John's wort demonstrate similar efficacy compared with conventional antidepressants for mild-to-moderate depression (Linde *et al.* 2005). However, results cannot be extrapolated to all preparations because content varies.

General counselling

General counselling points might include:

- To ensure continued treatment, according to the advice of the prescriber, for 6–24 months after recovery to prevent relapse. The analogy between a broken bone healing while in plaster is a useful explanation for the need to continue treatment even when well.
- Not to stop taking medication suddenly or without the advice of the prescriber, but reassure that antidepressants are not addictive.
- Be prepared for a delayed effect of 2–4 weeks and a possible worsening of symptoms in the first week. Sleep improvement may be an early beneficial effect in those receiving sedative TCAs for this purpose.

- The side effects of antidepressants, particularly nausea, should subside after the first week.
- Patients taking any antidepressant should be cautious when driving due to the risk of drowsiness and impaired reaction times.
- The return of insomnia may provide the first signs of relapse, particularly in bipolar disorder. Patients should be taught to recognise and report early warning symptoms. Short-term treatment with hypnotics may be appropriate. The maximum benefit of antidepressants is obtained when symptoms are recognised early.
- Women should be advised about adequate contraception and to discuss the issues of antidepressant treatment before planning a pregnancy. This enables the prescriber and patient to discuss the risk versus benefit of antidepressant treatment during pregnancy, the possibility of a trial without treatment or changing to an alternative drug associated with lower risk. This is particularly important for women taking lithium salts and SSRIs.
- In view of the stigma still associated with depression, it may help to reassure patients that depression is common.
- Lifestyle changes such as increasing exercise and reducing alcohol and/or caffeine intake may be beneficial.
- A structured approach to exercise comprising up to three sessions per week of moderate duration.
- Diet is important for mental health (see Chapter 3) and the Mental Health Foundation has provided a useful booklet for patients with depression (see Online resources at end of chapter).
- Counselling may help the patient to make appropriate lifestyle changes when possible to prevent recurrence. It may also be useful to explain the importance of the duration of symptoms, comparing depression with normal 'low mood'. It may help to eliminate fear of relapse if the patient is reminded that experiencing occasional low mood is normal.

SSRIs

- Side effects include gastrointestinal disturbances (nausea, abdominal pain, diarrhoea, constipation, indigestion), postural hypotension, palpitations, increased sweating and sexual dysfunction (impotence, delay or failure of orgasm). There is an increased risk of extrapyramidal effects with paroxetine.

- Sexual dysfunction is a common cause of noncompliance with SSRIs, affecting up to 60% of patients. Sensitive counselling is therefore important when treatment is initiated.
- Reaction times may be impaired and patients should therefore be cautious, particularly when driving.
- Report any rash, particularly with fluoxetine, as treatment may need to be stopped.
- Treatment should not usually be stopped abruptly, particularly paroxetine, because withdrawal symptoms may occur. Patients should be advised to continue their treatment according to the advice of the prescriber, even when feeling better. This prevents the risk of relapse on cessation of treatment, which is withdrawn gradually over at least 4 weeks, or slower if withdrawal symptoms occur.

TCAs

- TCAs may cause drowsiness, so advise caution if driving (less with imipramine and lofepramine). Drowsiness may be enhanced by alcohol.
- The dose should be taken at night if sedation is required and also to limit daytime sedation.
- Side effects of TCAs include dry mouth, blurred vision and constipation. Initial sedation, confusion and motor incoordination should improve after 1–2 weeks of treatment.

Newer antidepressants

- Trazodone, nefazodone, reboxetine and venlafaxine may cause drowsiness and therefore patients should be advised to exercise caution if driving. Drowsiness may be increased by alcohol.
- Patients taking venlafaxine should report any palpitations or rashes, urticaria or related allergic reactions.

MAOIs

- These may cause drowsiness, so advise caution if driving. Drowsiness may be increased by alcohol.
- Patients should avoid tyramine-containing food such as cheese, red wine, yeast extracts (e.g. Marmite), chicken and beef liver, salami, soy sauce and avocado. Only fresh food should be eaten and stale food avoided.

- A warning card should be given.
- Side effects of MAOIs include overexcitement, insomnia, weight gain, dry mouth, blurred vision, constipation and postural hypotension (increased by alcohol). An early warning of food interactions may be a throbbing headache indicating a rapid increase in blood pressure.

Others (mianserin, mirtazapine, flupentixol)

- Patients taking mianserin or mirtazapine should report signs of infection such as fever or sore throat.
- Flupentixol may cause drowsiness but can also be alerting and therefore should not be taken in the evening.

Lithium

- Patients should maintain adequate fluid intake and avoid dietary changes leading to a change in sodium intake (including use of salt substitute) or the sudden introduction or discontinuation of caffeine (see Table 25.3).
- Alcohol intake should not exceed the recommended limits (see Chapter 3 and Table 25.3).
- Treatment information is available for patients from the National Patient Safety Agency (http://www.nrls.npsa.nhs.uk).
- Preparations may vary widely in bioavailability. Monitoring may be required if patients change brand.
- Symptoms of drowsiness are usually transient.
- Signs of toxicity, including nausea, vomiting, tremor, lack of coordination, extreme thirst, diarrhoea and excessive urination, should be reported urgently.
- Symptoms of hypothyroidism should prompt referral. These include lethargy, feeling cold and weight gain.
- Fluid loss due to diarrhoea, vomiting and intercurrent infection (particularly with profuse sweating) may necessitate discontinuation of treatment. The prescriber should be contacted.
- Patients should not take ibuprofen.
- Inform patients of the importance of regular blood tests and the need to leave 12 hours after the last dose (see Chapter 7).
- Patients should inform health professionals that they take lithium.

Antipsychotics

See Chapter 28.

Anticonvulsants

See Chapter 24.

Benzodiazepines

For short-term use only (see also Chapter 27).

Self-assessment

For the following questions concerning the treatment of affective disorders, choose the most appropriate answer:

1 *Which one of the following is a common initial side effect of treatment with an SSRI?*

A Sedation
B Dry mouth
C Constipation
D Nausea
E Urinary retention

2 *The beneficial effects of antidepressant occur when?*

A On the first day of treatment
B Within 2–3 days of treatment
C Within the first week of treatment
D Within 2–4 weeks of treatment
E After 6 months

3 *SSRIs are preferred to tricyclic antidepressants because:*

A SSRIs are less addictive
B SSRIs are more effective
C SSRIs are faster acting
D SSRIs have fewer side effects
E SSRIs are cheaper

4 *In a patient with cardiovascular disease and depression, which is the most appropriate treatment?*

A A mono-oxidase inhibitor
B A tricyclic antidepressant
C An SSRI
D A benzodiazepine
E A β blocker

5 *In mild depression which one of the following do NICE advocate as first-line treatment?*

A Low dose SSRIs
B Benzodiazepines
C Dietary modifications
D Cognitive-behavioural therapy
E L-Tryptophan supplementation

6 *Which significant problem does St John's wort pose?*

A Addiction
B Dangerous in overdose
C It has no pharmacological effects
D It is a potent inducer of drug metabolism
E It is associated with renal toxicity

7 *The pharmacokinetics of lithium are influenced most by which one of the following?*

A Renal function
B Hepatic function
C Gender
D Genetics
E Rate of gastrointestinal absorption

8 *Which one of the following is thought to explain the mode of action of lithium in bipolar affective disorder?*

A It acts via PPAR-γ
B It acts via nitric oxide
C It increases cGMP
D It interferes with IP_3 recycling
E It is a dopamine receptor antagonist

Practice points

- Be alert for signs of depression in patients because stigma may still prevent patients from volunteering symptoms. Depression remains underdiagnosed (particularly in men) in primary care, and undiagnosed or undertreated depression is a significant cause of suicide. Pharmacists may identify patients requesting OTC hypnotics or herbal preparations for stress.

(continued)

(continued)

- Mild depression does not warrant the use of antidepressants.
- NICE guidance recommends that an SSRI should be considered as first-line treatment in moderate-to-severe depression.
- Close monitoring for signs of suicide is important during early treatment with all antidepressants. Consider also the danger of TCAs when taken in overdose.
- In patients who are at risk of suicide, only small quantities of drugs should be supplied.
- Compliance with treatment may be improved by warning patients of side effects and worsening of symptoms in the first week of treatment, together with the delayed onset of action.
- In treatment failure, consider compliance and encourage the patient to report troublesome side effects.
- Avoid abrupt withdrawal of antidepressant treatment.
- Most MAOIs inhibit MAO irreversibly, so the potential for drug interactions may persist for 2–3 weeks after the cessation of treatment. The SSRI fluoxetine also has a long half-life.
- Adequate doses, particularly of older TCAs, should be used to obtain a therapeutic effect.

- TCAs should not be prescribed to people aged >70 years because of the increased risk of adverse drug reactions in this age group.
- CBT has been shown to be as effective as antidepressants in mild depression and in combination with antidepressants for moderate depression. Beneficial effects include improved compliance, reduction of negative thought patterns and reduced exposure to stress.
- Regular use of propranolol for anxiety associated with depression may worsen depression. SSRIs should be considered (see Chapter 26).
- Be alert for the use of alcohol for temporary mood elevation, leading to a worsening of symptoms and risk of alcohol misuse.
- Hyponatraemia should be considered in patients developing confusion, drowsiness or convulsions while taking antidepressants.
- Prescriptions for lithium should be written using the brand name.
- It may be useful to repeat patient counselling at least annually during long-term treatment, particularly with lithium, and check that the patient retains the appropriate warning card.

CASE STUDIES

Case 1

A female patient complains to her pharmacist of anxiety, dizziness, tremor and headache and asks to sit down. She asks if it could be due to stopping her antidepressant treatment. She has been prescribed paroxetine 20 mg daily. How do you reply?

- Patients taking all antidepressants, but particularly paroxetine, may experience a withdrawal syndrome if treatment is stopped suddenly. The patient should be advised to take a paroxetine tablet as soon as possible and return to her general practitioner for a discussion about her treatment. You could enquire about the duration of treatment and, if appropriate, reinforce the importance of continuing to take the tablets after remission. Antidepressants should be withdrawn gradually over at least 4 weeks and up to 6 months after long-term maintenance therapy.

Case 2

A female patient requests Nytol tablets for insomnia. Her patient medication record (PMR) reveals that she takes diazepam 2 mg as needed. She admits to feeling awful due to a hangover and has been feeling depressed for the last few weeks. Do you sell the Nytol?

- No! She may be suffering from depression and should be referred to her GP for assessment because she may require an antidepressant. Depression may be exacerbated by benzodiazepine treatment. If appropriate, you could educate her regarding the risk of dependence with benzodiazepines.
- You could advise her that alcohol causes insomnia and depression and recommend that she should discuss this with her GP.
- She may have depression associated with anxiety, for which an SSRI may be appropriate (see earlier).
- An additive effect of Nytol with benzodiazepines (and alcohol) may cause increased drowsiness.

Case 3

A 24-year-old male patient presents a prescription for fluoxetine 20 mg daily and trazodone capsules 100 mg per day. Are you happy to dispense this prescription?

- Yes. An interaction between the two drugs may result in elevated plasma concentrations of the trazodone, but concurrent use may be beneficial.
- Co-prescribing antidepressants is not recommended, but in this case a specialist had prescribed the combination. Advise the patient to report side effects and particularly excessive sedation.

Case 4

A National Health Service FP10 prescription is presented for 20 mL/day of fluoxetine liquid 20 mg/5 mL for postnatal depression. The drug was originally prescribed by the hospital. Are you happy to dispense the prescription?

- No. The dose is greater than the maximum daily dose for fluoxetine. This prescription should have been for paroxetine 10 mg/5 mL.

Case 5

A patient presents with a prescription for EpiPen (adrenaline injection). You see from his PMR that he is also prescribed lofepramine. Do you dispense the prescription?

- Interaction between adrenaline and lofepramine may lead to a life-threatening hypertensive crisis.
- If adrenaline is required, an SSRI would be a more appropriate antidepressant.

Case 6

A 55-year-old man known to you for poor compliance with lithium for his bipolar affective disorder complains of tremor. He has difficulty signing his name. He is also taking amitriptyline and tells you that he only needs this. He's going to stop his lithium because of the tremor. What advice should this patient receive?

(continued)

(continued)

- Poor compliance is common in patients with bipolar affective disorder because they may fail to recognise their symptoms as abnormal. It is imperative that the patient be encouraged to continue with his lithium.

What is the most likely cause of his tremor?

- Lithium and amitriptyline may interact, causing tremor. The patient should be referred to his GP. The combination of lithium and TCAs can be beneficial but also produces serious and unpredictable problems such as convulsions, serotonin syndrome and neuroleptic malignant syndrome. Patients should be monitored closely. Tremor is a side effect of lithium and severe tremor may also be a sign of lithium toxicity.

References

American Psychiatric Association (2013). *Diagnostic and Statistical Manual of Mental Disorders,* 5th edn (DSM-IV). Washington, DC: American Psychiatric Press.

British National Formulary, latest edition. London: British Medical Association and Royal Pharmaceutical Society of Great Britain.

Buckley NA, McManus PR (2002). Fatal toxicity of serotonergic and other antidepressant drugs: analysis of United Kingdom mortality data. *BMJ* 325: 1332–1333. pmid: 12468481.

Calabrese JR, Bowden CL, Sachs GS *et al.* (1999). A double-blind placebo-controlled study of lamotrigine monotherapy in outpatients with bipolar I depression. Lamitcal 602 Study Group. *J Clin Psychiatry* 60: 79–88. pmid: 10084633.

Glassman AH, O'Connor CM, Califf RM *et al.* (2002). Sertraline treatment of major depression in patients with acute MI or unstable angina. *JAMA,* 288: 701–709. pmid: 12169073.

Greenberger D, Padesky CA (1995). *Mind Over Mood.* New York: Guilford Press.

Grunze H, Kasper S, Goodwin G *et al.* (2002). World Federation of Societies of Biological Psychiatry (WFSBP) guidelines for biological treatment of bipolar disorders, part 1: Treatment of bipolar depression. *World J Biol Psychiatry,* 3: 115–124. pmid: 12478876.

Hasler G (2010). Pathophysiology of depression: do we have any solid evidence of interest to clinicians? *World Psychiatry* 9: 155–161.

Kirsch I, Deacon B J, Huedo-Medina TB *et al.* (2008). Initial severity and antidepressant benefits: a meta-analysis of the data submitted to the Food and Drug Administration. *Pub Lib Science Medicine* 5: 260–268 (accessed online at www.plosmedicine.org).

Levitt AJ, Lam RW, Levitan R (2002). A comparison of open treatment of seasonal major and minor depression with light therapy. *J Affective Disord* 71: 243–248.

Linde K, Mulrow CD, Berner M *et al.* (2005). St. John's wort for depression. *Cochrane Database System Rev* issue 1: CD000448.

National Institute for Health and Care Excellence (2009). *Depression: The treatment and management of depression in adults.* Clinical Guideline 90. London: NICE.

Scott C, Tacchi M, Jones R *et al.* (1997). Acute and one-year outcome of a randomised controlled trial of brief cognitive therapy for major depressive disorder in primary care. *Br J Psychiatry* 171: 289–292.

Segal Z, Williams M, Teasdale J (2002). *Mindfulness-Based Cognitive Therapy: A new approach to preventing relapse.* New York: Guildford Press.

Sternbach H (1991). The serotonin syndrome. *Am J Psychiatry* 148: 705–713. pmid: 2035713.

Williams M, Teasdale J, Segal Z *et al.* (2007). *The Mindful Way through Depression: Freeing yourself from chronic unhappiness.* New York: Guilford Press.

World Health Organization (1992). *The International Statistical Classification of Diseases and Related Health Problems,* 10th revision (ICD-10). Geneva: WHO.

Online resources

www.apni.org
The website for the Association for Post Natal Illness (accessed October 2015).

www.mentalhealth.org.uk
For information about mental health including useful booklets such as *Healthy eating and depression,* for patients (accessed October 2015).

www.mind.org.uk
The website for the mental health charity, MIND (accessed October 2015).

www.sada.org.uk
The website for the Seasonal Affective Disorders Association (accessed October 2015).

www.sane.org.uk
The website of the mental health charity, SANE (accessed October 2015).

26

Anxiety disorders

Anxiety is a disabling condition, often associated with depression. It is more common in women and displays a peak onset in the early 20s. The term 'anxiety' is applied to a disproportionate response to fearful triggers such as flying and many social situations, and encompasses panic, phobic, obsessive–compulsive and general anxiety disorders. There is a significant impact on quality of life and personal achievement and, in extreme cases, patients are unable to leave their home. There is a hereditary component of vulnerability to anxiety, which may be triggered by adverse life events. There is also a link to certain personality traits and anxiety experienced in childhood. Drug-induced causes include:

- caffeine
- initial treatment with selective serotonin reuptake inhibitors (SSRIs)
- sympathomimetics
- nicotine
- overuse of β-adrenoceptor agonists, alcohol, amphetamines, cocaine
- withdrawal from alcohol, amphetamines, cocaine, benzodiazepines or antidepressants.

Disease characteristics

Before considering the characteristics of anxiety, terms in common use are defined:

- Fear: an emotional reaction to danger accompanied by physiological (mainly autonomic) and behavioural changes such as avoidance of fear-producing situations. Short-term fear such as fear of flying may be managed by single doses of benzodiazepines such as diazepam.
- Anxiety: generalised and often pathological fear, which may be unpredictable and often uncontrollable. It differs from fear in that there is not always an identifiable trigger.
- Phobia: a disabling or pathological fear of an object or situation such as social phobia or arachnophobia (a fear of spiders or arachnids).

Underlying pathology

Anxiety is considered to be pathological when a persistent or distressing response is triggered by non-threatening events and causes significant impairment of normal social or occupational functioning. The underlying pathology remains to be elucidated fully but is thought to involve disrupted serotonergic, glutametergic, GABA-ergic (GABA is γ-aminobutyric acid) and noradrenergic systems together with the involvement of corticotrophin-releasing factor, particularly in the complex interactions of the limbic system, a group of brain regions involved in the physiology of emotion.

Clinical features

Patients present with heightened autonomic symptoms including palpitations, tachycardia, difficulty breathing, dizziness, sweating, tremor, facial flushing and general feelings of panic. Patients may occasionally appear pale. There may also be profound fear of experiencing a heart attack or severe asthma attack. These symptoms may be caused or exacerbated by a number of other medical conditions. The diagnosis may therefore involve ruling out conditions such as asthma, heart disease, hyperthyroidism, vestibular disorders, menopause, hypoglycaemia, epilepsy and phaeochromocytoma (vascular tumour of the adrenal gland). Questioning patients about the frequency and nature of attacks, together with the presence of any fear or phobias, may point to a diagnosis of anxiety. Symptoms of depression may also be present and may form the primary diagnosis (see Chapter 25).

Classification

The following section considers the more common disorders presented to health professionals. These include panic attacks, phobias, obsessive–compulsive disorder (OCD) and general anxiety disorder (GAD). When considering the symptoms suggestive of these disorders, additional causes such as drug abuse, medication or medical conditions including hyperthyroidism are investigated and first excluded. In addition, as the symptoms of mental disorders often overlap, the criteria for similar disorders are considered before confirming a diagnosis, e.g. patients presenting with anxiety may fulfil the criteria for major depression, with the latter being diagnosed and treated.

General anxiety disorder

GAD differs from panic disorder, phobias and OCD in that it is persistent rather than short-lived and tends not to demonstrate situation-specific triggers. It may occasionally remain after unsuccessful treatment of panic or depressive disorders. Symptoms include a more general description of feeling 'on edge', irritable and tense most of the time. Diagnosis of GAD is made in the presence of the following symptoms:

- excessive anxiety and worry for more than 6 months and occurring on most days

- the patient cannot easily control the worry
- three or more of the following are present for more than 6 months and occur most days:

  - restless or 'on edge'
  - easily fatigued
  - difficult concentrating
  - irritability
  - muscle tension
  - sleep disturbance.

Panic disorder: panic attacks

Panic attacks commonly develop from phobic or hypochondriac symptoms and may progress to agoraphobia. A panic attack is defined by an intense period of fear with four or more of the following symptoms present, having developed abruptly and reaching a peak within 10 minutes:

- palpitations and/or increased heart rate
- sweating
- tremor
- shortness of breath or sensation of smothering
- choking feeling
- chest pain or discomfort
- nausea or abdominal symptoms
- dizzy or faint feeling
- feeling of depersonalisation or unreality
- fear of losing control
- fear of dying
- paraesthesia ('pins and needles')
- chills or hot flushes.

A diagnosis of panic disorder is made when patients suffer recurrent panic attacks according to the following:

- Recurrent panic attacks, some of which may occur spontaneously. These may be unpredictable and often unrelated to specific situations
- At least one of the attacks has been followed 1 month or more later by at least one of the following:

  - worry about future attacks
  - worry about the consequences of an attack such as losing control, suffering an asthma or heart attack
  - a significant change in behaviour due to the attack such as avoidance behaviour.

Agoraphobia

Agoraphobia is indicated by anxiety associated with places or situations and a fear of embarrassment or that it is difficult to escape or that help is not available. These include being alone outside the home, in a crowd, standing in a line, on a bridge, and travelling by bus, train or car. Avoidance behaviour or severe distress occurs in relation to these triggers. Social or specific phobias are considered if avoidance behaviour relates to a limited number of situations such as social situations.

Specific phobias

The sufferer describes excessive fear occurring in response to an object or situation such as flying, animals, heights or the sight of blood. Exposure to the trigger often produces anxiety symptoms and may fulfil the criteria for a panic attack. Avoidance behaviour may be present. Normal social and occupational functioning is adversely affected as a result of the phobia. Again, diagnosis is made after the exclusion of other mental disorders, or disease- or drug-related causes.

Children

Symptoms in children may present as tantrums, crying, freezing or clinging, particularly described as a variant of normal behaviour.

Social phobia

Social phobia is diagnosed in the presence of symptoms described for specific phobias. However, the trigger relates to social situations or performance, during which sufferers worry that they will be humiliated or embarrassed.

Children

Social phobia is identified after an assessment of age-related social relationships with familiar people and the anxiety must occur during interaction with peers and not just with adults. Symptoms are the same as for specific phobias but with a social trigger.

Obsessive–compulsive disorder

OCD comprises a continuous and difficult-to-control preoccupation with an object, activity or recurrent thoughts. With the exception of children, the patient tends to be aware that the behaviour is unnecessary or unreasonable. Again, a diagnosis is also dependent on the duration (e.g. more than 1 hour a day) and/or the impact on the patient's quality of life. The diagnosis of OCD is made in the presence of obsessions or compulsions as follows.

Obsessions

- The presence of inappropriate recurrent and persistent thoughts, impulses or images causing distress or anxiety.
- The above cannot be explained as excessive worries triggered by adverse life events.
- Patients attempt to ignore or substitute the thoughts, impulses or images and recognise them as produced by their own mind.

Compulsions

- The patient feels driven to repetitive behaviour such as hand washing, checking that a door is locked, counting or praying. This occurs in response to an obsession or strict rules, e.g. not stepping on the cracks in the pavement.
- The behaviour is intended to prevent the occurrence of an adverse situation such as injury but is not a realistic method of avoiding such occurrences, e.g. believing that avoiding the cracks in the pavement will prevent a serious illness.

Post-traumatic stress disorder

This involves a reaction to a traumatic event that carries the threat of death or serious injury to the patient or other. There is also a significant level of continued experience in dreams, because 'flashbacks' or feelings associated with the incident are triggered by stimuli reminiscent of the scene, e.g. getting into a car may trigger the distress of a previous car accident. Avoidance behaviour may also be present. Additional symptoms not present before the event and with a duration of at least 1 month include two or more of:

- insomnia
- irritability or outbursts of anger
- poor concentration
- increased vigilance
- exaggerated response to non-threatening stimuli.

Children

The effect of post-traumatic stress in children may present as agitated or disorganised behaviour. The event may be revisited through play or in dreams.

Acute stress disorder

The presentation of acute stress disorder is similar to that for post-traumatic stress disorder but with the exception that the duration is at least 2 days but not more than 4 weeks. Acute stress disorder occurs within 4 weeks of the traumatic event and three or more symptoms of dissociation are present in a positive diagnosis:

- numbness, detachment or lack of an emotional response
- reduced awareness of surroundings or being 'in a daze'
- the situation does not feel real to the patient (derealisation)
- the patient feels 'unreal', as in depersonalisation
- the patient has incomplete recollection of important aspects of the event (dissociative amnesia).

Goals of treatment

Treatment is initiated when symptoms meet the criteria detailed above together with a significant impairment of social and/or occupational functioning and relationships with others. The goals of treatment are to alleviate the symptoms of panic and anxiety, improve the quality of life, and prevent relapse and recurrence. Initially, this may include identifying and dealing with causes such as associated depression and substance abuse.

Pharmacological management

The use of antidepressants with behavioural therapy combined with lifestyle advice, including the importance of regular exercise and the avoidance of drugs causing anxiety such as caffeine, may improve the long-term outcome.

Antidepressants

If drug therapy is required or chosen then many antidepressants have been shown to be effective anxiolytics. Many of the SSRIs are indicated for anxiety-related disorders; for example, citalopram is indicated for panic disorder, and paroxetine for panic disorder, social anxiety, generalised anxiety disorder and post-traumatic stress disorder. Based on cost and effectiveness, NICE (2011) recommend sertraline as first line for GAD followed by another SSRI or a serotonin–noradrenaline reuptake inhibitor.

Pregabalin

The antiepileptic drug pregabalin is now used in GAD and is used when antidepressants have not provided benefit.

β-adrenoceptor antagonists (propranolol)

Propranolol is the most commonly used β blocker for treating the physical symptoms of anxiety associated with the effects of adrenaline (epinephrine)-mediated activation of β-adrenoceptors. These include palpitations, tremor and tachycardia.

Benzodiazepines

Although benzodiazepines have been used in anxiety, their use is no longer advocated due to issues over dependency, and they should only be considered for short-term usage if considered essential.

Buspirone

Buspirone is rarely used. Buspirone activates serotonin $5HT_{1A}$-receptors, binds to dopamine receptors, and may also target noradrenergic and dopaminergic transmission in the brain. The effects on 5HT are thought to be the main mechanism by which buspirone exerts its anxiolytic effects. Side effects include dizziness, nausea and headache, as occur with selective serotonin reuptake inhibitor (SSRI) antidepressants. There is also a delay of 2–3 weeks before an anxiolytic effect. Buspirone differs from the benzodiazepines in that it does not cause sedation.

Drug choice in anxiety

The treatment of anxiety usually involves a combination of psychological therapy with the use of SSRIs.

Long-term pharmacological intervention

According to severity, SSRIs may be used, particularly if the anxiety is associated with underlying depression (see Chapter 25) or chronic symptoms of more than 4 weeks, or when benzodiazepine treatment has failed (Table 26.1). A delay of 2–4 weeks may precede the onset of efficacy of antidepressants in anxiety disorders. However, symptoms may persist for 4–8 weeks in panic disorder and up to 10 weeks in OCD. Treatment is continued for at least 6 months on cessation of symptoms, as for depression, and maintenance treatment may be indicated for recurrent episodes. The treatment of OCD may be continued for a year or more. Table 26.1 summarises the use of antidepressants for anxiety disorders.

It is important to note that antidepressants and particularly paroxetine are associated with an initial worsening of panic symptoms when used to treat panic disorder. The most common adverse effects reported by patients taking SSRIs long term include tiredness, weight gain and sexual dysfunction.

Non-pharmacological intervention

Counselling such as cognitive-behavioural therapy (CBT) may be used to help the patient overcome fear and phobias, thereby aiding recovery and reducing the risk of relapse as many anxiety disorders follow a chronic course. Patients may also benefit from relaxation techniques such as progressive muscle relaxation. Behavioural therapy may include a gradual exposure to feared situations.

Concurrent disease

Prescribing decisions in treating anxiety in the presence of concurrent diseases include the following.

β blockers (propranolol)

β blockers are a compelling choice for anxious patients with ischaemic heart disease, hypertension or migraine, but should be avoided in asthma and used with caution in chronic obstructive pulmonary disease (COPD). It should be noted that long-term use may cause or exacerbate depression (see also Chapter 6).

Benzodiazepines

See Chapter 27.

Antidepressants

See Chapter 25.

Buspirone

Buspirone is contraindicated in epilepsy, severe hepatic or renal impairment, pregnancy and breastfeeding.

Drug interactions

These are largely dealt with elsewhere (β-adrenoceptor antagonists, see Chapter 12; benzodiazepines, see Chapter 27; antidepressants, SSRIs, see Chapter 25).

Table 26.1 The use of antidepressants in anxiety disorders

Anxiety disorder	Drugs indicated
General anxiety disorder	SSRIs (initially sertraline), serotonin–noradrenaline reuptake inhibitor (SNRI; venlafaxine, duolexetine) and pregabalin (if other treatments are not tolerated or failed)
Obsessive–compulsive disorder	Fluoxetine (initial choice), fluvoxamine, paroxetine, sertraline, or escitalopram. Clomipramine might be appropriate after an initial failure with an SSRI.
Panic disorder	Antidepressants, particularly citalopram or escitalopram, paroxetine, imipramine (unlicensed) or clomipramine (unlicensed)
Phobias	Antidepressants generally, particularly clomipramine
Social phobia	Paroxetine or escitalopram
Post-traumatic stress disorder	Paroxetine

SNRI, serotonin–noradrenaline reuptake inhibitor; SSRI, selective serotonin reuptake inhibitor.

Buspirone

- Contraindicated with monoamine oxidase inhibitors (MAOIs).
- Increased drowsiness and weakness when combined with alcohol.
- Risk of serotonin syndrome with citalopram and possibly fluoxetine and other SSRIs. Fluvoxamine may reduce the effects of buspirone.
- Cytochrome P450 enzyme inhibitors such as erythromycin and itraconazole increase buspirone levels, requiring a dose reduction. Diltiazem, verapamil and possibly ketoconazole may interact by the same mechanism.
- Rifampicin induces cytochrome P450 and may therefore reduce levels of buspirone and necessitate an increased dose.

Herbal medicines

Patients may request or take damiana, cowslip, hops, lady's slipper and St John's wort for anxiety (see Chapter 4). These products cannot be recommended by healthcare professionals on the basis of a lack of clinical evidence for safe and efficacious use, and should be avoided with conventional treatment for anxiety. Of particular note is kava, a herbal preparation for anxiety that has been withdrawn after reports of hepatotoxicity. There was also a case reported in which a patient developed a semi-comatose state after concurrent ingestion of kava and alprazolam.

Patients with anxiety should particularly avoid herbs with sympathomimetic activity (see Chapter 4) and stimulants such as ginseng. Herbs with sedative properties include valerian, St John's wort and possibly ginseng, and should not be taken with benzodiazepines (see Chapters 4 and 27). Other herbs associated with causing anxiety include cola and mate.

Counselling

Patients benefit from an empathic approach together with education to increase their understanding of their symptoms. General counselling may include lifestyle advice, as outlined in Chapter 3. Particular emphasis should be placed on smoking cessation and the avoidance of excessive caffeine intake. Motivation for regular exercise may be gained by an explanation of the 'fright or flight' response as occurs when faced with threatening situations. Anxiety is a magnified reaction to situations that may not actually be threatening but invoke a 'fright or flight' response in the patient. A summary of counselling about non-pharmacological interventions includes the following:

- Avoid excess intake of caffeine, alcohol, nicotine and decongestants. It should be noted that caffeine is present in many over-the-counter (OTC) products, including analgesics, tonics and some products marketed to increase energy.
- Patients may be at risk of abusing alcohol due to a temporary relief of symptoms. A vicious circle may result, as described in Chapter 25, and therefore it is useful to highlight this to patients considered at risk.
- Relaxation tapes may help to alleviate anxiety symptoms.
- Practise relaxation techniques, including:
  - progressive muscle relaxation, involving progressive tensing and relaxing of major muscle groups
  - yoga: a Hindu tradition consisting of a series of exercises encompassing stretching, balance and muscle toning, with a focus on controlled breathing throughout
  - meditation: a method of relaxation of the mind involving repetitive methods such as internal or vocal chanting of a word, phrase or sound.

A diary of symptoms together with situations that provoke or alleviate symptoms may help the patient to feel in control and serves to highlight progress. It also helps health professionals to determine the severity of the disorder.

Specific counselling

Specific counselling for SSRIs, tricyclic antidepressants, β-adrenoceptor antagonists and benzodiazepines is given in Chapters 12, 25 and 27. Points particularly relevant in the treatment of anxiety include the following.

Antidepressants

Patients may be confused by the use of antidepressants for anxiety. It may therefore be helpful to inform patients that antidepressants are used to treat anxiety disorders even in the absence of depression.

SSRIs

- In the treatment of panic disorder with paroxetine, panic symptoms may worsen during initial treatment. Patients should be reassured that this is normal and not a reason to stop treatment.
- Treatment should not be stopped abruptly and should be continued for at least 6 months or up to 12 months or longer.

Benzodiazepines

These are only recommended for short-term (2–4 weeks) symptomatic relief. Use is restricted due to the risk of tolerance and dependence.

β blockers (propranolol)

β blockers treat the symptoms of anxiety and tend to be used on a 'when required' basis. If they are taken regularly, they should not be stopped suddenly because rebound anxiety will occur, with the risk of developing a 'vicious circle' and subsequent psychological dependence on β blockers.

Buspirone

- A response may not be observed for up to 2 weeks.
- This is indicated for short-term use, although the risk of dependence and abuse is low.
- Side effects include dizziness, headache, nervousness, light-headedness, excitement and nausea. These tend to be transient, occurring at the start of treatment.
- Buspirone rarely causes sedation but patients should be advised not to drive until they have established that they do not suffer any sedative effects with buspirone.

Self-assessment

For the following questions concerning anxiety, choose the most appropriate answer:

1 *General anxiety disorder is best managed by which one of the following drugs?*

   a Diazepam
   b Caffeine
   c Sertraline
   d Zopiclone
   e Lithium

2 *Which one of the following drugs is indicated in the British National Formulary for obsessive–compulsive disorder?*

   a Fluvoxamine
   b Citalopram
   c Lofepramine
   d Haloperidol
   e Lithium

Practice points

- Psychological therapy plays a major role
- Some antidepressants are indicated for anxiety disorders.
- Benzodiazepines are not recommended and are only reserved for the short-term treatment of severe anxiety.
- Lifestyle advice is important to prevent long-term psychological dependence on drugs.
- Underlying depression should be identified and treated.
- Patients often present with physical symptoms, thereby delaying a diagnosis.

CASE STUDY

A 26-year-old man reports sporadic difficulty with breathing, which usually occurs when he is sitting in an office full of people at work. He is concerned that he may have asthma but has no history of asthma, although he does suffer from hayfever. He is not taking any medication at the moment. Should this patient receive a salbutamol inhaler?

(continued)

(continued)

- This is an interesting case, with vague symptoms that may point to asthma, particularly as he has a history of hayfever. On further questioning, however, the patient also reported an increase in heart rate, sweating, facial flushing and feelings of panic about his breathing. Salbutamol was therefore not appropriate and could have exacerbated his symptoms. He admitted to regular consumption of alcohol and caffeine, although he regularly visited a gym. A diagnosis of panic attacks was made; the patient was advised to cut down on alcohol and particularly caffeine, and continue with his exercise. He was given a prescription for 60 propranolol 10 mg tablets three times daily when required.

What are possible alternative causes of these symptoms?

- Underlying conditions such as hyperthyroidism and asthma may produce the above symptoms and these should be excluded. The exclusion of asthma is particularly important when prescribing propranolol, which would otherwise be contraindicated. The measurement of lung function may be considered (see Chapter 22). Cardiac causes are perhaps unlikely in view of his age. Substance abuse should also be excluded.

What advice should be given about propranolol?

- Propranolol may help with the symptoms of anxiety but regular use may lead to rebound anxiety on withdrawal, and without appropriate advice this may progress to chronic use of propranolol. The patient should be advised to use the propranolol occasionally for the temporary relief of symptoms, e.g. propranolol may be taken before difficult situations known to trigger an attack with a view to breaking the association between the situation and an attack (conditioned anxiety). The importance of lifestyle changes with or without CBT should be stressed.
- The patient should be advised to report symptoms of wheeze and return if his symptoms do not improve. He could also be warned that propranolol will decrease exercise tolerance. Anxiety may be associated with depression, so chronic use of propranolol may not be appropriate because it may cause or exacerbate depression. An SSRI and/or CBT may be indicated. This case was resolved with lifestyle changes and intermittent use of propranolol. The patient identified an association with drinking caffeine and excess alcohol.

References

National Institute of Health and Care Excellence (2011). *Generalised anxiety disorder and panic disorder (with or without agoraphobia) in adults: Management in primary, secondary and community care*. Clinical Guideline 113. London: NICE.

World Health Organization (1992). *The International Statistical Classification of Diseases and Related Health Problems*, 10th revision (ICD-10). Geneva: WHO.

Online resources

www.adaa.org
The Anxiety Disorders Association of America, a comprehensive educational site, provides up-to-date information for patients and healthcare professionals on the nature and treatment of anxiety disorders (accessed October 2015).

www.phobics-society.org.uk
The Anxiety Disorders Charity providing help and advice for patients and carers of phobics, including access to literature, counselling and support groups (accessed October 2015).

www.anxiety.org.uk
Is the website of Anxiety UK and provides patient information and support (accessed October 2015).

27

Insomnia

Characteristics

Insomnia is an extremely common complaint, affecting 1 in 10 people, particularly elderly patients, and may have multiple causes such as stress, chronic illness, pain and depression. The effects on quality of life are extensive, and insomnia and its treatment are also risk factors for accidents.

Causes of insomnia

There are numerous causes of insomnia, which if addressed may resolve the problem without the requirement for treatment with hypnotic drugs. Causes of insomnia include:

- environmental factors: noise, extremes of temperature, poor ventilation
- lifestyle factors: stress, shift work, jet lag
- disease: poorly controlled asthma or chronic obstructive pulmonary disease, heart failure, chronic pain, hyperthyroidism, dementia, schizophrenia, anxiety and depression, or menopausal symptoms
- drugs, including sympathomimetics, selective serotonin reuptake inhibitors, β blockers, thyroid hormones, corticosteroids, caffeine, statins, theophylline and alcohol
- indirect drug causes: diuretics if taken at night, hypoglycaemia after insulin administration or a persistent cough caused by angiotensin-converting enzyme inhibitors
- withdrawal from drugs including nicotine, alcohol, antidepressants, hypnotics, opioids, cannabis, amphetamines, and MDMA (3,4-methylenedioxymethamfetamine) or ecstasy.

Clinical features

Symptoms of insomnia include a delay in falling asleep, failure to maintain sleep or early morning wakening. The result is often permanent tiredness. The most common presentation is a delay in falling asleep, which is particularly associated with stress, shift work, noise or drugs. Insomnia is classified according to the duration of the problem, as shown in Table 27.1.

Goals of treatment

Initially, potential causes of insomnia should be identified and any underlying problems such as pain or

Table 27.1 Classification of insomnia according to the duration of symptoms

Description of insomnia	Duration	Common causes
Transient	2–3 days	Noise, shift work, jet lag
Short term	3–4 weeks	Stress, depression, drugs such as caffeine or decongestants
Chronic	Most nights for 3 weeks or longer	Severe disease, drug abuse, including alcohol and mild hypnotic dependence

depression treated. There is an important role for patient education and non-pharmacological methods such as counselling and relaxation techniques. The aim is to establish a normal sleep pattern without the use of long-term hypnotics. Patients dependent on hypnotics, including over-the-counter (OTC) preparations, should be supported during gradual withdrawal from these drugs. Referral for cognitive-behavioural therapy or specific abuse counselling may be required for chronic insomnia. Sleep clinic referrals are reserved for sleep apnoea, epilepsy during sleep, longstanding insomnia resistant to treatment or after suspicion of exaggeration by the patient.

Pharmacological basis of management

Benzodiazepines, e.g. flurazepam, loprazolam, lormetazepam, nitrazepam, temazepam

Benzodiazepines reduce anxiety and aggression, induce sleep, reduce muscle tone and coordination, and produce an anticonvulsant effect. The main mechanism of action involves increased activity of the inhibitory neurotransmitter, γ-aminobutyric acid (GABA), in the brain. This occurs after binding of the drug to a regulatory site, the benzodiazepine receptor, on $GABA_A$-receptor complexes. Differences in the sensitivity of numerous subtypes of $GABA_A$-receptors to benzodiazepines account for some of their different clinical uses, e.g. clonazepam and diazepam exhibit greater anticonvulsant activity. Short-acting benzodiazepines such as temazepam, lormetazepam or loprazolam are reserved for the treatment of insomnia to reduce the risk of a hangover effect persisting the following day. Tolerance and dependence are also problematic with benzodiazepines.

Related hypnotics: 'Z-drugs': zaleplon, zolpidem, zopiclone

These newer agents, which have a non-benzodiazepine structure, have been developed with the aim of reducing adverse effects such as hangover and dependence. These drugs exhibit a shorter duration of action and are thought to be selective for subtypes of benzodiazepine receptor and/or selectively target individual subunits of these receptors. In practice, however, the adverse effects appear to be similar to conventional benzodiazepines.

Sedating antihistamines, e.g diphenhydramine, promethazine

Sedating antihistamines are histamine H_1-receptor antagonists (see Chapter 21). They also exhibit antimuscarinic effects, resulting in side effects, including dry mouth, blurred vision, constipation and urinary retention. They are available in OTC preparations for the short-term relief of insomnia.

Drug choice

Treatment may often require non-pharmacological intervention such as lifestyle changes, or reviewing drug-related causes or treating underlying illness. Occasionally, pharmacological intervention with benzodiazepines is required but this should be short term due to the following problems:

- an increased risk of falls in elderly people
- a hangover effect the next morning
- confusion, amnesia, cognitive impairment and impaired coordination
- a risk of road traffic accidents associated with benzodiazepines with long half-lives and the short-acting hypnotic zopiclone

- the disruption of normal sleep patterns
- chronic use associated with anxiety and depression
- tolerance and therefore the requirement for higher doses
- the risk of dependence and abuse
- withdrawal effects, including rebound insomnia
- a risk of life-threatening respiratory depression if an overdose of benzodiazepines is taken with alcohol, although they are relatively safe if taken without alcohol or other substances of abuse.

Summary

Hypnotics are licensed for the short-term treatment of insomnia for no more than 3 weeks and ideally for only 1 week and using intermittent doses such as every third night. Agents with a short half-life should be given. These include temazepam, loprazolam and lormetazepam. Diazepam may be given as a single dose at night if the patient also has anxiety during the day.

Short-acting benzodiazepines (temazepam, loprazolam, lormetazepam)

These agents are preferred due to a reduced risk of hangover effect in the short-term treatment of insomnia. Loprazolam exhibits erratic absorption, which may increase its duration of action.

Long-acting benzodiazepines (diazepam, flurazepam, nitrazepam)

The longer-acting benzodiazepines are rarely used to treat insomnia due to residual side effects, particularly affecting elderly patients. The exception is diazepam used for insomnia associated with anxiety. It is also the preferred agent for withdrawal from chronic use of benzodiazepines because withdrawal effects are less pronounced.

Other hypnotics

'Z-drugs' are associated with withdrawal symptoms, tolerance and dependence. Current evidence suggests that they offer little advantage over benzodiazepines. Chloral hydrate is no longer recommended because there is no evidence of real benefit for elderly patients and the treatment of children is rarely justified. Clomethiazole is occasionally used for elderly patients due to reduced confusion and hangover effects. Short-term use is again indicated due to the risk of dependence.

Concurrent disease

Table 27.2 indicates disease states that may preclude the use of certain hypnotics.

Hepatic impairment

Hypnotics should be avoided in severe liver disease because they may precipitate coma. Reduced doses of some hypnotics may be used in milder hepatic disease and the *British National Formulary* and/or summary of product characteristics should be consulted.

Renal impairment

Small doses of hypnotics are recommended due to increased cerebral sensitivity associated with severe renal impairment.

Special groups

Pregnancy and breastfeeding

Non-pharmacological treatment is preferred during pregnancy and breastfeeding.

Elderly people

The requirement for sleep is reduced in elderly people and this group is likely to expect to sleep for longer than is actually required. Hypnotic use in this group should be avoided due to an increased risk of side effects, particularly drowsiness and confusion, which may increase the risk of falls. The enhanced effects are mainly due to an age-related reduction in hepatic metabolism. Reduced doses are indicated if treatment is necessary.

Children

Hypnotics should not be used in children, with the possible exception of night terrors and somnambulism (sleep walking). Alternatives for treating night terrors include waking the child 15 minutes before the time that a night terror usually occurs and then allowing him or her to go back to sleep. A bedtime routine is particularly important for children.

Drug interactions

Drug interactions with hypnotics generally result from an additive effect with other drugs with sedative properties such as alcohol, antihistamines, antidepressants and opioids.

Table 27.2 Concurrent disease states to be considered when prescribing hypnotics

Disease	Comments
Cardiac disease	Chloral hydrate is contraindicated
COPD	• Hypnotics should be used with caution, particularly in patients with hypoxia, due to reduced respiratory drive • Benzodiazepines may cause or worsen dementia. Avoid if possible, or use low doses of short-acting agents
Dementia	• Zolpidem has also been associated with memory impairment and vigilance is required for these effects with all 'Z-drugs' • Antimuscarinic effects of OTC older antihistamines oppose effects of acetylcholinesterase inhibitors used in dementia
Depression	• Hypnotics should not be used alone as long-term use may exacerbate depression • Sedating TCAs (e.g. amitriptyline, dosulepin), maprotiline, mianserin or trazodone may be appropriate • SSRIs may cause insomnia
Glaucoma, prostatic hypertrophy and urinary retention	Antimuscarinic side effects of sedative antihistamines mean that they should be used with caution in these conditions
Muscle weakness	Benzodiazepines should be used with caution
Osteoporosis	The risk of fractures may be increased in elderly patients due to falls associated with hypnotics
Porphyria	Some antihistamines, benzodiazepines and chloral hydrate may be unsuitable
Respiratory depression	All hypnotics should be avoided
Sleep apnoea	Benzodiazepines, zaleplon, zolpidem and zopiclone should be avoided

COPD, chronic obstructive pulmonary disease; SSRIs, selective serotonin reuptake inhibitors; TCAs, tricyclic antidepressants.

Over-the-counter considerations

Sedating antihistamines are available for the short-term relief of insomnia but patients should be advised to consult their general practitioner (GP) if symptoms persist after 2 weeks. However these drugs are associated with a hangover effect and may also lead to tolerance, headaches, psychomotor impairment (including impaired reaction times) and antimuscarinic effects.

Herbal medicines

Patients with insomnia may commonly take or request products containing valerian, camomile, hops, gentian, passionflower (*Passiflora*), wild lettuce and pulsatilla, e.g. combinations of these herbs are present in Kalms, HRI night and Nytol herbal. Until more information about the pharmacological activity, efficacy and safety of these products is available, the same precautions observed with conventional hypnotics may be appropriate, e.g. the potential for drug interactions and concurrent disease as outlined above should be considered. Advice about non-pharmacological intervention is also relevant. For a discussion on the recommendation of herbal preparations, the reader is referred to Chapter 4.

Patients who take herbal preparations for insomnia should avoid herbs with sympathomimetic activity (see Chapter 4) and stimulants such as ginseng. Herbs with sedative properties (see Chapter 4) should not be taken with hypnotics. Camomile and pulsatilla have been associated with hypersensitivity reactions and should be avoided by susceptible individuals such as people with asthma.

Dietary supplements

Melatonin is a hormone involved in the sleep–wake cycle, being secreted during the night. This is taken as a dietary supplement for jet lag and by shift workers, but reliable evidence for efficacy and long-term safety is lacking. People with depression, prescribed central nervous system depressants or women trying to conceive should avoid it.

Withdrawal from chronic benzodiazepine treatment

See Chapter 6.

Counselling

General counselling should focus on non-pharmacological options:

- Try to establish a routine of retiring to bed and rising at the same time each day.
- Avoid lying in bed worrying about being awake, because this may also contribute to conditioned insomnia and is more tiring than being awake and not worrying.
- Regular exercise may benefit insomnia but should be avoided a few hours before going to bed. A short walk in the evening may help.
- Alcohol should not be used to aid sleep because it is a diuretic, disturbing sleep in the latter part of the night, and also produces 'unrestful' sleep. Chronic use may itself cause insomnia.
- Avoid caffeine, nicotine (including 24-hour patches), thyroid hormones and decongestants, particularly after 4pm.
- Do not work, eat or watch television in the bedroom because conditioned insomnia may result whereby the bedroom is associated with being awake.
- Avoid napping during the day.
- Avoid intellectual activity before going to bed.
- Establish a routine each night such as reading, drinking warm milk or having a warm bath with lavender oil before retiring to bed.
- Eliminate environmental causes such as noise, light, extremes of temperature or poor air quality.
- Listen to relaxation tapes.
- Relaxation techniques are particularly useful for patients with stress-related insomnia who have difficulty in falling asleep. These include:
  - progressive muscle relaxation, involving progressive tensing and relaxing of major muscle groups

  - yoga, a Hindu tradition consisting of a series of exercises encompassing stretching, balance and muscle toning, with a focus on controlled breathing throughout
  - meditation, a method of relaxation of the mind involving methods such as repetitive internal or vocal chanting of a word, phrase or sound.

A sleep diary may be useful for identifying the cause, pattern and severity of insomnia. Patients may benefit from feeling more in control of the problem and from observing their progress. This method may also reveal patients with an unrealistic expectation of the duration and depth of sleep required. The following points may be recorded:

- the time of retiring to bed and approximate time taken to fall asleep
- the duration of sleep
- the number of times of waking during the night and the duration
- a score out of 10 of the feeling of tiredness each day
- a score out of 10 of the feeling of tension and irritability
- general comments such as alcohol or caffeine intake and other potential causes.

Counselling and the use of hypnotics

Generally, patients should be warned that hypnotics help only the symptoms and not the causes of insomnia. They are recommended only for short-term intermittent use. Informing patients that withdrawal from regular use of hypnotics causes rebound insomnia leading to the desire to continue taking the treatment may help prevent this road to dependence:

- Intermittent use, preferably every third night, is recommended to avoid tolerance. It may be useful to explain that this means that the sedative effect is lost if hypnotics are taken every night.
- Treatment is ideally restricted to no more than 1 week to prevent the development of dependence.
- Hypnotics may cause drowsiness, which may persist to the next day. Patients should therefore be cautious if driving or performing other skilled tasks. Alcohol adds to these effects and should be avoided.

- Following withdrawal from hypnotics, sleep may be disturbed for a few days and may feature vivid dreams due to increased rapid eye movement (REM) sleep for many weeks.

- Patient education relating to the risks and benefits of withdrawing from hypnotics may improve the outcome.

Practice points

- Reinforce non-pharmacological options for treating insomnia.
- Patients should be asked about the use of OTC hypnotics and frequent requests should lead to a referral to the general practitioner.
- Long-term users of benzodiazepines should be changed to the equivalent dose of diazepam before gradual withdrawal, with regular review and encouragement.

Self-assessment

Consider whether the following statements are true or false. In the management of insomnia:

1 Diuretics may be a cause.
2 Temazepam is a long-acting benzodiazepine.
3 Diet is often an important cause of insomnia.
4 Promethazine is a safe drug for regular treatment of insomnia.
5 Early morning wakening is often associated with depression.

CASE STUDIES

Case 1

A 45-year-old man with a history of bipolar affective disorder requests a sedative antihistamine from his pharmacist. He currently takes lithium and is away from home for a business meeting.

Should a supply be made?

- Insomnia may be an early sign of relapse in patients with bipolar affective disorder and therefore referral to the general practitioner is warranted. This patient was away from home and therefore could not see his GP until the following week and did not want to see a GP not familiar with his case. He was driving and therefore a sedating antihistamine was not the best choice due to the possibility of hangover effect the next morning. However, due to the risk of relapse of bipolar disorder, the problem of driving when tired and the absence of other symptoms, a supply was made with the recommendation that the patient take a tablet only every third night until he returned home. He was advised not to take them too late at night to prevent the residual effects next morning and to consult his GP if his symptoms did not improve within a week. He was also given advice and an information leaflet about non-pharmacological treatment of sleep problems, particularly the importance of avoiding alcohol and caffeine. He telephoned to thank the pharmacist on his return, saying that the advice and treatment helped him through a difficult week and he was now feeling much better.

Case 2

A 25-year-old woman with Crohn's disease presented to her GP complaining of insomnia mainly due to her painful condition. She was taking venlafaxine 75 mg twice daily in addition to her immunosuppressant therapy. She felt that her prednisolone treatment was aggravating her low mood and her Crohn's disease symptoms were still not controlled.

What course of action could the GP take?

- The patient should be referred back to her specialist to review her Crohn's disease medication, because this is likely to be the main cause of her insomnia. However, the GP may consider changing the antidepressant to a more sedating agent such as trazodone and reviewing her medication for pain. General counselling about sleep may also be beneficial, as outlined above.

Case 3

A 20-year-old female student presents with insomnia before her exams and asks for a prescription for sleeping tablets. She says that she 'has a few drinks' every night to help her unwind but wakes up in the night and cannot get back to sleep.

Would a short-term hypnotic help this patient?

- A short-term hypnotic may help depending on the amount of distress to the patient and the nature and duration of the exams. However, non-pharmacological intervention could be considered first, e.g. advising that alcohol is not an effective sedative due to disturbed sleep later in the night. She should be advised not to revise late in the evening and to try to revise somewhere other than where she sleeps. Further questioning of this patient revealed that she was taking Pro Plus, a caffeine-containing product, during the day. She was advised to reduce this gradually and was given a leaflet outlining general counselling for people with insomnia and to return if her problem did not improve.

References

British National Formulary, latest edition. London: British Medical Association and Royal Pharmaceutical Society of Great Britain.

28

Schizophrenia

Characteristics

Psychosis is defined as a disorder of thought and perception, of which schizophrenia is a key example. Schizophrenia presents with psychotic symptoms similar to the manic phase of bipolar affective disorder but differs in that deterioration of cognitive function is often observed over time. Many patients suffering from schizophrenia are unable to continue with their normal daily life. Approximately 1% of the population is affected: onset tends to be in the early 20s and has both genetic and environmental components. Patients may be reassured that one in five patients may suffer only a single acute episode, although seven in ten suffer at least two acute episodes. Drugs such as amphetamines may induce psychotic symptoms or worsen schizophrenia, mainly as a result of dopamine release. Recent evidence of cannabis use in young people has now been linked to the development of schizophrenia.

Clinical presentation

The symptoms of schizophrenia are grouped as positive or negative. Patients may describe positive symptoms as 'dreaming while awake'.

Positive symptoms

- Hallucinations: false perceptions of sounds, images, taste, smells or other sensory images that do not have a real stimulus.

- Delusions: these are irrational beliefs, which cannot be altered by logical reasoning, e.g. being controlled by others.
- Thought disorder and disorganised communication, e.g.:
  - thought broadcasting – thoughts are 'expressed freely' to others
  - thought insertion – thoughts are inserted by another person
  - thought withdrawal – thoughts are stolen by another person.

Negative symptoms

- Reduced activity with emotional flattening (psychomotor retardation, see Chapter 25).
- Withdrawal from society.
- Cognitive deficit and therefore unemployment.

Other: catatonic

A catatonic state encompasses motor (movement) abnormalities, including overactivity and violence or standing in strange positions.

Classification

The term 'schizophrenia' literally translates as 'split mind' and is often misinterpreted as a split personality. This is potentially an unhelpful label and the term 'a patient with psychotic symptoms' may be more appropriate. A diagnosis is made if two or more of the following symptoms are present for most of the time over a period of 1 month. The required time period is shorter if the symptoms are treated successfully with medication. Symptoms include:

- delusions
- hallucinations
- disorganised speech
- disorganised or catatonic behaviour
- negative symptoms: affective (emotional) flattening.

Schizophrenia results in considerable impairment of social and occupational functioning, including interpersonal relationships and self-care. A diagnosis may also be made on the basis of the presence of hallucinations alone if these comprise a voice giving a running commentary on the patient's behaviour or thoughts, or two or more voices communicating with each other. A longer period, 6 months or more, of milder symptoms may also result in a diagnosis of schizophrenia and may include milder manifestations of at least two of the above symptoms (such as strange beliefs) or only negative symptoms. Finally, substance abuse and concurrent disease are excluded as the cause before a positive diagnosis of schizophrenia can be made.

Pathophysiology

Schizophrenia is considered a neurodevelopmental rather than a neurodegenerative disease, mainly affecting the cerebral cortex, as predicted from the cognitive symptoms. The pathophysiology of schizophrenia remains elusive, although new and interesting theories are beginning to emerge. Historically, schizophrenia has been associated with overactivity of dopaminergic neurotransmission and conventional treatment has been with dopamine receptor antagonists such as chlorpromazine. This theory, however, does not provide a complete explanation, e.g. the efficacy of antipsychotics (chlorpromazine, clozapine, sulpiride, trifluoperazine) is delayed for 7–10 days or more, suggesting an additional mechanism to simple antagonism of receptors. Alternative mechanisms may include a change in the number of receptors expressed in cells or perhaps an effect on signal

transduction within cells. However, classically there is an excellent correlation between affinity of antipsychotic drugs at dopaminergic receptors and effectiveness of the drugs in treating schizophrenia.

The modulation of dopaminergic neurotransmission remains important in newer, atypical antipsychotics but the role of serotonin or 5-hydroxytryptamine (5HT) is also recognised and effective treatment such as with clozapine is thought to be due to a greater effect on serotonergic transmission compared with dopaminergic systems. This may partly explain the beneficial effect of clozapine on negative symptoms. Other systems targeted include glutametergic, GABAergic (GABA is γ-aminobutyric acid) and noradrenergic, which are involved in the modulation of dopaminergic neurotransmission, e.g. antagonism of the glutamate N-methyl-D-aspartate receptor by drugs such as phencyclidine and ketamine produces symptoms similar to those observed in schizophrenia.

Pharmacological basis of management

All antipsychotics are dopamine D_2-receptor antagonists, thereby inhibiting dopaminergic neurotransmission, and this remains an important target for effective antipsychotic activity. Extrapyramidal and endocrine symptoms are often troublesome, particularly at higher doses, e.g. hyperprolactinaemia may also follow the inhibition of dopamine transmission, resulting in increased prolactin secretion. The reverse occurs when the dopamine receptor agonist bromocriptine is used to suppress lactation. Most antipsychotics also act as antagonists at receptors for other monoamines, including α-adrenoceptors, muscarinic and 5HT-receptors (mainly $5HT_2$). The affinity for these receptors determines the side effect profile. Histamine receptors may also be modulated by antipsychotics, but this is not thought to result in antipsychotic activity.

Conventional antipsychotics

The conventional antipsychotics were previously termed 'major tranquillisers' but this term is no longer used because this is not the main effect exploited in the treatment of schizophrenia. The term 'antischizophrenic' is also inaccurate because these drugs are 'antipsychotic' and are also used to treat psychotic symptoms associated with major depression and bipolar disorder (see Chapter 25) and delusional disorders. The main groups of these typical antipsychotics include:

- phenothiazines comprising three further groups (see *British National Formulary*):
  - group 1 (aliphatic), e.g. chlorpromazine
  - group 2 (piperidine), e.g. pipotiazine
  - group 3 (piperazine), e.g. prochlorperazine and trifluoperazine.

The following groups resemble the structure of the group 3 phenothiazines:

- butyrophenones, e.g. haloperidol
- diphenylbutylpiperidines, e.g. pimozide
- thioxanthenes, e.g. flupentixol
- substituted benzamides: sulpiride (often grouped with 'atypical' antipsychotics due to its reduced extrapyramidal effects).

Atypical antipsychotics, e.g. clozapine, olanzapine, risperidone

Atypical antipsychotics have vastly improved the treatment of schizophrenia, mainly as a result of reduced extrapyramidal effects. In addition, clozapine is one of the only antipsychotics to benefit negative symptoms and has a central role in treatment-resistant schizophrenia. These drugs are now considered for first-line treatment and are also used in the treatment of bipolar affective disorder (see Chapter 25). They are not, however, devoid of adverse effects, e.g. weight gain and metabolic effects (hyperglycaemia and dyslipidaemia with a risk of diabetes mellitus) are significant adverse effects particularly associated with olanzapine and clozapine (Newcomer 2007), and sexual dysfunction is a major factor in reduced compliance. Clozapine is associated with agranulocytosis and is therefore restricted to patients who have failed to respond to at least two antipsychotics (see below).

Adverse effects of antipsychotics

With the introduction of atypical antipsychotics, frightening extrapyramidal effects are less common,

being associated with conventional antipsychotics and particularly the group 3 phenothiazines, the butyrophenones and especially depot preparations of these groups. Common adverse effects with atypical antipsychotics include weight gain, sexual dysfunction and the risk of diabetes mellitus.

Weight gain

Weight gain is common with antipsychotics and may be a factor in the cause or exacerbation of type 2 diabetes mellitus.

Sexual dysfunction

Sexual dysfunction often has a significant effect on personal relationships and quality of life but is not discussed due to embarrassment. Symptoms range from altered libido to impotence in men or reduced lubrication in women and failure of orgasm. Fertility may therefore be an important issue. Sexual dysfunction is an important cause of non-compliance with both conventional and atypical antipsychotics.

Galactorrhoea and amenorrhoea

Endocrine effects such as galactorrhoea occur due to increased prolactin secretion (with the exception of aripiparazole). This includes an enlargement of the breasts and milk production. Other effects include missed periods (amenorrhoea), reduced libido and therefore reduced fertility.

Movement disorders

As described above, many of the adverse effects of antipsychotics result from the blockade of dopamine receptors and therefore include disorders of movement or endocrine disorders. These include Parkinsonian symptoms such as tremor and rigidity. This is not surprising considering the use of levodopa to replenish dopamine levels, thereby improving the symptoms of Parkinson's disease. Antimuscarinic drugs such as procyclidine are prescribed 'when required' to counteract these effects but should be used with caution due to the risk of irreversible tardive dyskinesia. The following terms are used to describe movement disorders.

Extrapyramidal effects

Extrapyramidal neurons comprise a system of nerves connecting the cerebral cortex, basal ganglia, thalamus, cerebellum, reticular formation and spinal neurons in complex systems not included in the pyramidal system. Extrapyramidal motor disorders are those affecting movement, which is regulated by dopamine in the extrapyramidal system. These include the following:

- Akinesia: literally 'lacking movement', a loss of normal muscular tone or responsiveness.
- Parkinsonism: symptoms associated with Parkinson's disease, including tremor, rigidity, salivation (drooling) and akinesia of the face. These effects are reversible when they are drug induced.
- Acute dystonia: abnormal or impaired posture or muscle spasms due to altered muscle tone. This often involves sustained contractions of neck and facial muscles and is reversible.
- Akathisia: an unwanted effect of antipsychotics (phenothiazines) involving involuntary movements or restless overactivity of the legs and/or body, e.g. pacing up and down, constantly changing leg position or foot tapping. This may easily be confused with the agitation for which the drug was prescribed.
- Tardive dyskinesia: a chronic condition characterised by repetitive involuntary movements, usually of the tongue, face, fingers, hands, legs and trunk, and resulting in drooling and lip smacking. The concurrent use of drugs with antimuscarinic activity may aggravate the condition, which may be irreversible, and therefore careful monitoring is important.

Cardiovascular effects

Some of the antipsychotic drugs are associated with cardiac arrhythmias through Q–T interval prolongation. This has led to the withdrawal of some drugs and is a particular problem with phenophiazines, notably chlorpromazine. It may be appropriate to screen the patient's ECG and heart rate and raise caution with potential drug interactions with other drugs associated with Q–T interval prolongation, e.g. amiodarone.

Both olanzapine and risperidone are associated with an increased incidence of stroke in elderly patients and they should not be used for the management of behavioural symptoms associated with dementia. The increased incidence of stroke in elderly patients would be a reason to avoid these agents but if they are used then patient's cardiovascular risk should be assessed.

Severe postural hypotension may occur with chlorpromazine and other phenothiazines due to the antagonism of α-adrenoceptors (see Chapter 12).

Antimuscarinic effects

The antimuscarinic effects of drugs may be peripheral or central. Peripheral effects such as dry mouth, blurred vision, urinary retention and constipation are summarised in Chapter 6. This pharmacological activity also accounts in part for the use of phenothiazines as antiemetics (see Chapter 9). The following central effects may occur with antipsychotics as a result of antimuscarinic activity:

- confusion
- disorientation
- visual hallucinations
- agitation
- irritability
- delirium
- memory impairment
- aggression and possibly violent behaviour
- sedation.

Caution is required in identifying drug-related central antimuscarinic effects to prevent the co-prescribing of antipsychotics with additional antimuscarinic effects. The subsequent occurrence of extrapyramidal effects such as dystonia, akathisia, tremor or rigidity then becomes apparent, with a risk of further antimuscarinic drugs such as procyclidine being added to control these effects. The iatrogenic problem is then worsened, with the risk of causing serious adverse drug reactions such as irreversible tardive dyskinesia, heat stroke or paralytic ileus (see Chapter 6).

Idiosyncratic and hypersensitivity reactions

Type B adverse drug reactions are less predictable from the pharmacological activity of antipsychotics and include photosensitivity, particularly with chlorpromazine (and also contact sensitivity), agranulocytosis, jaundice and neuroleptic malignant syndrome (see Chapter 6). The risk of agranulocytosis with clozapine is significant and white blood cell counts are required on a regular basis throughout treatment.

Tables 28.1 and 28.2 include a comparison of side effects between different groups of phenothiazines and a consideration of the most prominent side effects, considering both conventional and atypical agents.

Drug choice

The aims of treatment are to manage the initial psychotic symptoms, improve the quality of life and reduce the risk of relapse but with minimum adverse effects (particularly frightening extrapyramidal effects). Drug therapy is used in conjunction with psychological interventions including cognitive-behavioural therapy (CBT). Atypical antipsychotics have been associated with fewer extrapyramidal side effects and are commonly used as first-line treatment for newly diagnosed schizophrenia. Specified agents include amisulpiride, olanzapine, quetiapine, risperidone and zotepine, and low doses should be used for the first episode. This recommendation excludes clozapine due to the risk of agranulocytosis. Olanzapine appears to be associated with a greater risk of metabolic adverse effects including weight gain and this may make it less suitable as a first-line agent. The most difficult symptoms to treat are negative symptoms, for which clozapine may be required. Additional recommendations for the appropriate use of atypical antipsychotics include the following:

- Patients taking conventional antipsychotics and experiencing intolerable side effects (usually extrapyramidal) may be switched to an atypical antipsychotic.

- Patients suffering relapse and symptoms who were previously poorly controlled by conventional agents may benefit from an atypical antipsychotic.

- Symptoms of schizophrenia poorly controlled following trials with two or more antipsychotics (including at least one atypical) for 6–8 weeks may benefit from clozapine but initiated only in a hospital inpatient setting. Patients are required to register with a centralised monitoring service for early detection of agranulocytosis. A second antipsychotic may be added if there is a poor response with clozapine.

- There is convincing evidence that clozapine is more effective than conventional antipsychotics for the treatment of schizophrenia and that agranulocytosis is more likely to occur in children, adolescents and elderly people (Wahlbeck et al. 1999).

- Changing to an atypical antipsychotic is not appropriate if symptoms are controlled and side effects are mild and acceptable.

- The choice of drugs takes into account the risk profile for adverse effects such as weight gain, diabetes and cardiac arrhythmias.

- As commented above, olanzapine and risperidone are associated with a greater risk of stroke in elderly patients.

Aggressive symptoms

Haloperidol is the common choice for violent or aggressive patients and often first choice for acute treatment of psychosis, prescribed 'when required' alongside other antipsychotics. Drugs such as lorazepam or haloperidol may be administered by intramuscular injection. It should be noted that haloperidol is often the choice for elderly patients because it has a lower incidence of hypotension.

Table 28.1 A comparison of severity of common side effects of phenothiazines			
Adverse effect	**Phenothiazines**		
	Group 1	**Group 2**	**Group 3**
Extrapyramidal effects	++	+	+++
Antimuscarinic effects	++	+++	+
Drowsiness	+++	++	+

+++ severe, ++ moderate and + fewer in comparison to the other phenothiazines. Information derived from *British National Formulary*.

Table 28.2 Examples of common side effects produced by antipsychotics		
Side effect	**Drugs implicated**	**Drugs least likely to cause the ADR**
Extrapyramidal effects	Haloperidol, phenothiazines (see Table 28.1 for comparison), depot preparations	Atypical antipsychotics, including amisulpiride, sulpiride and particularly clozapine, olanzapine, quetiapine and risperidone
Antimuscarinic effects	Phenothiazines (see Table 28.1), clozapine	Haloperidol, amisulpiride, olanzapine, quetiapine, risperidone, sulpiride
Cardiac arrhythmias	Phenothiazines, pimozide, clozapine	Amisulpiride, flupentixol, sulpiride, olanzapine, risperidone
Galactorrhoea	Sulpiride	Atypical antipsychotics
Parkinsonism	Fluphenazine, perphenazine, trifluoperazine, prochlorperazine	Atypical antipsychotics
Photosensitivity	Chlorpromazine	
Jaundice	Conventional antipsychotics, particularly phenothiazines (Chapter 6)	
Hypotension	Haloperidol, phenothiazines,	Amisulpiride, sulpiride, clozapine, risperidone, flupentixol, olanzapine, quetiapine
Drowsiness	Chlorpromazine (Table 28.1)	Amisulpiride, haloperidol, flupentixol, pimozide, quetiapine, sulpiride or zotepine
Sexual dysfunction (Chapter 8)	Phenothiazines, pimozide and sulpiride	
Weight gain	Chlorpromazine, risperidone, olanzapine, clozapine	Pimozide
Agranulocytosis	Clozapine	All antipsychotics, except clozapine

ADR, adverse drug reaction.

Depot preparations

Depot preparations may be used for maintenance therapy, given every 1–4 weeks, particularly when compliance is a problem, and may benefit people who exhibit considerable first-pass metabolism. A test dose may be given initially (see *British National Formulary* or summary of product characteristics). There may, however, be an increased risk of extrapyramidal side effects compared with oral agents. Problems include difficulty in titrating doses, pain on injection and variable pharmacokinetics according to muscle mass and rate of metabolism. Side effects may take weeks to dissipate following the last dose. A depot preparation of the atypical antipsychotic, risperidone, is now licensed and available and may be associated with fewer side effects, as discussed above.

Duration of maintenance treatment

Treatment with antipsychotics is often long term. However, patients who appear to be in remission may withdraw gradually from treatment with regular monitoring for signs of relapse for typically at least 2 years after the last acute episode. These patients include those who have suffered only one acute psychotic episode over 1–2 years of treatment and have responded well to treatment. Patients who have suffered two or more psychotic episodes are continued on medication for at least 5 years.

Non-pharmacological interventions

CBT is recommended alongside drug treatment, to help patients to understand their symptoms and develop coping mechanisms in order to control them.

It is particularly beneficial for persistent psychotic symptoms: longer courses of more than 6 months are recommended. Carers may also benefit from support in the form of CBT or counselling and supportive psychotherapy. These interventions are beneficial for the patient and aim to prevent relapse, reduce symptoms, increase insight and improve compliance with medication. It should therefore be possible for patients to live a fairly normal life and this should be emphasised at the start of treatment.

The effect of environmental factors on patients with schizophrenia is recognised and benefit may be gained from moving patients to a low-stress environment. Social, group and physical activities are also beneficial.

Concurrent disease

Table 28.3 summarises possible influences on the choice of antipsychotic drugs.

Drug interactions

Some of the older antipsychotic agents may cause Q–T interval prolongation and increase the risk of torsade de pointes arrhythmias. Accordingly, these drugs should be used with caution in elderly people, those with pre-existing arrhythmias and with other drugs that may prolong the Q–T interval. Atypical antipsychotics do not normally alter the Q–T interval but should be used with caution with drugs that do. Additional interactions are summarised in Table 28.4.

Monitoring

General

Monitoring for patients prescribed antipsychotics include a full blood count, liver function tests, blood pressure due to the risk of hypotension, electrocardiogram (ECG), weight, and temperature. Temperature

Table 28.3 Concurrent disease and the prescribing of antipsychotics

Disease	Comment
Cardiovascular disease, e.g. angina, arrhythmias, chronic heart failure, stroke	• Increased risk of arrhythmias with certain agents • Increased risk of hypotension in susceptible patients, e.g. elderly people or those prescribed antihypertensives. Reduced doses of antipsychotics may be recommended • Increased risk of stroke with olanzapine and risperidone in elderly patients
Closed-angle glaucoma	• Antimuscarinic drugs reduce drainage, therefore worsening this condition. Prochlorperazine and chlorpromazine use should be avoided • Patients at increased risk include those with diabetes mellitus and/or a family history of glaucoma
Prostatic hypertrophy	Antimuscarinic effects may lead to urinary retention
Depression	• There is currently no evidence for the benefit of antidepressants in patients with schizophrenia (Whitehead *et al.* 2002) • See also drug interactions (Table 28.4)
Diabetes mellitus	• Risk of type 2 diabetes due to weight gain with antipsychotics and particularly chlorpromazine, risperidone, clozapine and olanzapine • Risk of exacerbation or ketoacidosis (olanzapine)
Dementia and elderly people	• Drugs with antimuscarinic effects may cause or worsen dementia • Risperidone and olanzapine are associated with increased risk of stroke in elderly patients
Epilepsy	• The convulsive threshold is lowered by antipsychotics. Reduced doses may be indicated (e.g. clozapine) • Additional risk factors for convulsions are listed in Chapter 24
Parkinson's disease	Antipsychotics may exacerbate symptoms, mainly as a result of dopamine receptor antagonism
Severe respiratory disease	Use with caution, particularly in combination with other CNS depressants such as alcohol

CNS, central nervous system; NICE, National Institute for Health and Care Excellence.

Table 28.4 Examples of drug interactions involving antipsychotics

Drugs	Consequences	Comments
Clozapine with anticonvulsants (carbamazepine, phenytoin)	• Clozapine levels are reduced • Risk of additive bone marrow suppression (carbamazepine) • Risk of neuroleptic malignant syndrome (Chapter 6)	• Dose of clozapine may need to be doubled when used with carbamazepine or phenytoin • Monitor for signs of infection or neuroleptic malignant syndrome
Haloperidol and anticonvulsants (phenobarbital, carbamazepine, phenytoin) or rifampicin	Reduced levels of haloperidol	• Note that haloperidol may also increase carbamazepine levels • Sodium valproate appears not to interact • Isoniazid may increase haloperidol levels
Clozapine with benzodiazepines	Risk of severe hypotension and respiratory depression	• Monitor closely for signs of these adverse effects • Lorazepam may be prescribed 'when required' during acute schizophrenia
Clozapine with SSRIs (fluoxetine, fluvoxamine, paroxetine, sertraline)	Increased levels of clozapine and also increased risk of serotonin syndrome as both drugs increase serotonergic neurotransmission	• Dose of clozapine may require adjustment • This combination may be beneficial and is used commonly • Citalopram does not appear to interact
Haloperidol with fluvoxamine or quinidine	Risk of increased haloperidol levels	The dose of haloperidol may require adjustment
Haloperidol with indometacin	Severe drowsiness and confusion	Avoid combination or monitor closely
Haloperidol, phenothiazines, clozapine and olanzepine with tobacco (or cannabis smoke)	Reduced levels	Smokers may require an increased dosages or a reduced dose on cessation of smoking
Conventional antipsychotics (butyrophenones, phenothiazines and thioxanthenes) with antimuscarinics	Additive antimuscarinic effects (Chapter 6) with the risk of rare but serious effects including: • heat stroke • severe constipation • paralytic ileus • psychosis • reduced efficacy of antipsychotic treatment due to reduced plasma levels	• Concurrent use may be beneficial • Monitor for signs of antimuscarinic effects (see text) and consider risk factors such as exposure to hot and humid conditions, polypharmacy, high doses and/or impaired renal or hepatic function
Chlorpromazine and other antipsychotics with lithium	• Reduced levels of chlorpromazine • Risk of severe extrapyramidal effects and neurotoxicity	• Dose adjustment of chlorpromazine may be required • Severe side effects are rare but monitoring for these is important
Phenothiazines with trazodone	Severe hypotension	Additive hypotensive effects. Consider patients at increased risk such as those taking antihypertensive medication
Phenothiazines with TCAs	• Increased TCA levels and possibly phenothiazine levels • Increased risk of tardive dyskinesia, which may be caused and masked by elevated levels of either or both drugs	• This combination is often used but the safety of co-prescribing is not certain • For a discussion of effects on the Q–T interval, see text • Additional risk factors include high doses and polypharmacy
Pimozide with clarithromycin	Increased levels of pimozide	Increased risk of cardiotoxicity. Consider also use with other drugs known to prolong the Q–T interval (Chapter 6)

SSRIs, selective serotonin reuptake inhibitors; TCAs, tricyclic antidepressants.

monitoring is useful for the early diagnosis of neuroleptic malignant syndrome, although this is rare.

Cardiovascular

An ECG should be performed for patients at risk of cardiotoxicity such as those with pre-existing cardiovascular disease, elderly patients, those taking medication associated with prolongation of the Q–T interval and those prescribed high doses of antipsychotics.

Metabolic effects

Given the association with weight gain and the development of type 2 diabetes, NICE (2014) recommends that weight, fasting glucose, glycated haemoglobin (HbA_{1C}) and lipids are monitored during treatment.

Elderly

Drugs used in the treatment of schizophrenia may increase the risk of falls due to postural hypotension. Accordingly, lower doses are indicated. As commented above, olanzapine and risperidone are associated with an increased risk of stroke in elderly patients and should be avoided where possible.

Renal impairment

Lower doses of antipsychotics may be required in severe renal impairment, due to increased cerebral sensitivity. Lower doses of clozapine, quetiapine, risperidone or olanzapine are required in mild-to-moderate renal impairment with avoidance of clozapine in severe impairment. Sulpiride should be avoided in moderate renal impairment or lower doses used if essential.

Hepatic impairment

All antipsychotics have the potential to precipitate coma in patients with hepatic disease (see Chapter 11). Phenothiazines are hepatotoxic. Lower doses of clozapine, risperidone, quetiapine or olanzapine may be appropriate with regular monitoring of liver function.

Pregnancy and breastfeeding

Phenothiazines and butyrophenones tend to be preferred and in particular chlorpromazine, trifluoperazine or haloperidol, due to greater experience of use during pregnancy. Depot preparations are avoided unless compliance is a significant problem. Treatment is assessed according to risk versus benefit. There is

evidence of neonatal toxicity during the third trimester. Symptoms observed in the fetus include tremor, increased muscle tone, abnormal movements and feeding difficulties. Antipsychotics such as chlorpromazine, trifluoperazine, haloperidol or possibly flupentixol may be continued with caution during breastfeeding as necessary but the infant should be monitored for adverse effects such as oversedation.

Over-the-counter considerations

Patients may request supplements of polyunsaturated fatty acids for the symptoms of schizophrenia. There is not convincing evidence that the use of fish oil or evening primrose oil may improve symptoms in patients.

Counselling

Reassurance should be given that drug treatment is effective and, with adequate support, the patient should be given the opportunity to return to employment if desired. Pharmacists have key roles in empathic support and the provision of information relating to treatment as necessary.

General lifestyle advice (see Chapter 3) should be given due to the risk of weight gain, diabetes mellitus and cardiac effects with antipsychotics. Alcohol or drug misuse may exacerbate schizophrenia and should therefore be avoided, and patients referred for additional support if necessary.

Compliance with antipsychotic medication is a common problem due to side effects as described above and there may initially be a lack of insight, resulting in patients not recognising that they are ill. The importance of maintenance treatment in preventing relapse should be emphasised and patients or carers informed that intermittent therapy is not recommended. The side effects and particularly movement disorders should also be explained when treatment is initiated. Patients should be advised that treatment requires gradual withdrawal and should therefore not be stopped without the advice of their doctor.

Changing treatment

Patients should be warned about the risk of relapse and a transient worsening of side effects when changing to an alternative antipsychotic. It is important to reinforce that adherence to treatment should improve symptoms with fewer side effects over time. However, if symptoms persist, an alternative antipsychotic may be tried.

Blood dyscrasias

Patients should be advised to report symptoms of infection such as sore throat and pyrexia, particularly when prescribed clozapine.

Weight gain

Weight gain and the onset of type 2 diabetes should be monitored, particularly in patients prescribed olanzapine, clozapine, chlorpromazine, or risperidone, and also in patients at risk, such as those with obesity. When initiating treatment, it is useful to reinforce a healthy diet and exercise (see Chapter 3).

Sexual effects

Counselling at the onset of treatment may help reduce the effect on relationships and quality of life. The importance of compliance should be stressed due to the risk of relapse, and the patient encouraged to discuss problematic effects as they occur. Patients should also be advised to discuss a planned pregnancy.

Antimuscarinic effects

Patients should be warned of antimuscarinic effects, including dry mouth and eyes, blurred vision and constipation. Artificial saliva (e.g. Luborant) or sugar-free boiled sweets, artificial tears or laxatives should be prescribed as necessary. Co-prescribing with other drugs that have antimuscarinic activity may increase the risk of these effects and particularly severe constipation (risk of paralytic ileus and obstruction, particularly with clozapine), heat stroke (see Chapter 6) and psychosis. Patients should be advised of the importance of maintaining regular fluid intake, particularly in hot or humid conditions, due to the increased risk of heat stroke. There is also a risk of hypothermia during cold weather, due to poor temperature regulation.

Cardiovascular effects

Symptoms suggestive of arrhythmias should be explained and reporting encouraged, e.g. patients may become aware of palpitations and/or an altered pulse rate. Prescribers should monitor patients for these symptoms, particularly those at risk (discussed above). Blood pressure should be monitored as hypotension may occur, particularly when treatment is initiated. Also the risk of stroke should be taken into account when using olanzapine and risperidone.

Drowsiness (all antipsychotics and particularly chlorpromazine)

General counselling should be to warn the patient about drowsiness and the effect on driving and operating machinery. This may be particularly prevalent when treatment is initiated.

Photosensitivity

Photosensitivity may occur, particularly with chlorpromazine and therefore exposure to the sun or sunlamps should be avoided. High-factor sunscreen should be applied when exposure to ultraviolet light is unavoidable.

Extrapyramidal symptoms

Patients should be advised about the risk of extrapyramidal symptoms, because these can be frightening (see above).

Tardive dyskinesia

Patients should be advised to consult their doctor urgently if they develop fine involuntary movements of the tongue, because this adverse effect is often irreversible.

Self-assessment

For the following questions concerning the management of schizophrenia, choose the most appropriate answer:

1 *The antipsychotic drug, clozapine, is associated with which one of the following?*

   A Hypokalaemia
   B Its effectiveness decreases over several years
   C Preventing the patient from sleeping
   D Neutropenia
   E It is a potent enzyme inducer

2 *Which of the following best describes a key feature of antipsychotic drugs?*

A Dopamine receptor agonists
B Dopamine receptor antagonists
C Dopamine decarboxylase inhibitors
D They are dopamine precursors
E Inhibition of dopamine reuptake

Practice points

General

- Prompt diagnosis of patients with psychosis may improve the clinical outcome.
- Lifestyle changes are important in the management of schizophrenia (see Monitoring and Counselling sections).
- Regular screening for side effects and particularly weight gain, sexual dysfunction, drowsiness and extrapyramidal effects (e.g. tardive dyskinesia) is important.

Antipsychotics

- Starting treatment at a low dose and increasing gradually reduces side effects.
- Patients should be maintained on the lowest effective dose.
- Concurrent use of antipsychotics should be used only in the short term, e.g. when changing to an alternative antipsychotic.
- The dose for intramuscular injection is lower than the oral dose, due to the absence of first-pass metabolism by hepatic enzymes.
- Withdrawal should be gradual after long-term treatment with antipsychotics, because of the risk of withdrawal symptoms and possible relapse.
- Treatment should be withdrawn in the presence of early symptoms suggestive of tardive dyskinesia, because this is usually irreversible.
- When the patient is stabilised on an antipsychotic, the dosage interval may be reduced to once-daily administration because these drugs have a long half-life.

CASE STUDIES

Case 1

A 40-year-old male patient presents with worsening auditory hallucinations associated with messages he feels are being given to him by characters in a television soap opera. He recognises these symptoms and consults his general practitioner urgently according to previous advice. He is currently taking trifluoperazine 5 mg daily. He has been stable on this treatment for 20 years.

What action do you take?

- A short-term increase in his dose to 15 mg daily may control his symptoms until the period of stress has passed. Further increases (consider divided dosing) can be made at intervals of 3 days according to response. The dose can then be reviewed, particularly if side effects become troublesome. It may be useful to remind him about possible side effects and to discuss these if they become problematic. This case represents the benefits of education as the patient has control of his condition, helped by the support of his GP.

Case 2

The police arrest a 22-year-old man because of his involvement in a fight. He becomes uncommunicative and fails to cooperate. A friend at the scene comments that he has been concerned about his friend for some time as he recently lost his job and became uninterested in his appearance. He mentioned that aliens were laughing at him and told him that a group of men were planning to attack him before he started the fight. He was not provoked.

Which symptoms are typical of schizophrenia?

- This patient has negative symptoms, including lack of communication and loss of interest in his appearance. These may be the first symptoms to occur in schizophrenia and may also include a loss of interest in previous activities and relationships. Positive symptoms include hallucinations, paranoia and thought disorder.

What is the likely treatment for this patient?

- If the patient continues to be aggressive, he may be given haloperidol in the short term, possibly with an antimuscarinic agent 'when required' for the short-term prevention of extrapyramidal effects. He is likely to be prescribed an atypical antipsychotic. The misuse of drugs such as cocaine should be investigated because this may trigger schizophrenia.

References

British National Formulary, latest edition. London: British Medical Association and Royal Pharmaceutical Society of Great Britain.

Joy CB, Mumby-Croft R, Joy LA (2006). Polyunsaturated fatty acid supplementation for schizophrenia. *Cochrane Database System Rev* issue 2: CD001257.

National Institute for Health and Care Excellence (2014). *Psychosis and schizophrenia in adults: treatment and management.* Clinical guideline 178. London: NICE.

Wahlbeck K, Cheine M, Essali MA (1999). Clozapine versus typical neuroleptic medication for schizophrenia. *Cochrane Database System Rev* issue 3: CD000059.

Whitehead C, Moss S, Cardno A *et al.* (2002). Antidepressants for people with both schizophrenia and depression. *Cochrane Database System Rev* issue 2: CD002305.

29

Parkinson's disease

Characteristics

Parkinson's disease is a relatively common neurodegenerative disease often, but not always, associated with ageing. Parkinson's disease is a disease of movement and is associated with tremor, rigidity and poverty of movement. Terms used in Parkinson's disease include bradykinesia (slowness of movement), akinesia (lack of movement or rigidity) and dyskinesias (abnormal involuntary movements). The following may be associated with Parkinson's disease: an emotionless facial expression, stooping, autonomic dysfunction (including orthostatic hypotension, constipation and increased urinary frequency), depression, altered handwriting and sleep disturbances.

The underlying cause of the disease is uncertain but may have associations with environmental toxins, a weak genetic link, oxidative stress or, in early onset disease, a relationship with brain trauma as seen in boxers. The disease is characterised by degeneration of dopaminergic neurons in the nigrostriatal pathway in the basal ganglia, and current drug therapy is designed to replace or improve dopaminergic activity. The reduction in dopaminergic activity is also accompanied by increased activity of acetylcholine due to an imbalance. As indicated in Chapter 28, dopamine receptor antagonists (such as antipsychotic agents) may lead to drug-induced Parkinsonism, which involves rigidity and problems of movement but tremor is not an important feature.

The diagnosis of Parkinson's disease is generally made by a neurologist, based on symptoms and may involve brain imaging to exclude other pathologies.

Goals of treatment

The central goal of treatment is restoration of dopaminergic function and, ideally, prevention of neurological degeneration. Current therapies aim to restore dopamine but the effects are transient and so the achievable aim is symptomatic relief.

Pharmacological basis of management (Figure 29.1)

Levodopa (L-dopa)

In order to restore function to the dopaminergic system then the 'classic' treatment involves levodopa, which is the precursor of dopamine and so will increase levels of dopamine and provide some

Figure 29.1 Some of the principal sites of drug action in the management of Parkinson's disease. Principal drug classes shown in unshaded boxes. COMT, catechol-*O*-methyltransferase; MAO, monoamine oxidase.

relief from the symptoms. Administration of levodopa is associated with widespread side effects, notably nausea and hypotension due to the peripheral conversion of levodopa to dopamine. To reduce these problems, levodopa is given with an inhibitor of dopa decarboxylase such as carbidopa or benserazide and, as these agents do not penetrate the blood–brain barrier, peripheral conversion of levodopa is prevented although levodopa can still lead to central formation of dopamine.

Although levodopa is invaluable in the management of Parkinson's disease, patients often develop 'on–off' effects with rapid fluctuations between rigidity and involuntary movements. Levodopa is also associated with dose-related central nervous system side effects such as involuntary movements and psychiatric effects. Furthermore, its efficacy has a finite period and, after a number of years of usage, the patient may no longer derive benefit. Indeed, this is a reason to delay using levodopa in a patient with Parkinson's

disease and this is especially important in younger patients. Treatment with levodopa is also associated with an 'end-of-dose' effect, when its efficacy decreases towards the end of the dose and this is progressive with continued usage. This problem is partly related to the short plasma half-life of levodopa and shortening the dosage interval or using a modified-release preparation may help to overcome this problem. Previously patients were temporarily taken off levodopa as a 'dopamine holiday' but this is not advocated in the guidelines produced by the National Institute for Health and Care Excellence (NICE 2006).

Dopamine receptor agonists, e.g. bromocriptine, cabergoline, pergolide, ropinirole, rotigotine

These are dopamine D_2-receptor agonists (with variable activity at D_3-, D_4- and D_5-receptors) that increase dopaminergic activity in the basal ganglia and, as the principal peripheral receptor is the dopamine D_1-receptor, they have limited peripheral side effects. Their direct agonist activity circumvents the need for the nigrostriatal pathway to synthesise dopamine. However, they are generally less efficacious compared with levodopa but some practitioners prescribe dopamine receptor agonists, such as rotigotine, to younger patients or in early disease to delay starting levodopa, which has a finite usage (see above). They are also less likely to induce dyskinesias in patients. Dopamine receptor agonists also have a role as an adjunct to levodopa in patients who are inadequately controlled by levodopa alone.

Monoamine oxidase B inhibitors: rasagiline, selegiline

The isoenzyme monoamine oxidase B (MAO-B) is involved in the metabolism of dopamine and so inhibition of this enzyme will increase the concentrations of dopamine. Selegiline is given with levodopa to enhance its actions and may help to overcome the 'end-of-dose' effect. Rasagiline may also be used in this way or as monotherapy to augment endogenous levels of dopamine.

Unlike MAO inhibitors, which are occasionally used in depression, their selectivity for the B type means that their use is not complicated by the 'cheese' reaction with foods containing tyramine and so do not require dietary restrictions. Non-selective MAO inhibitors should not be given at the same time as levodopa because this may lead to a hypertensive crisis.

Catechol-*O*-methyltransferase inhibitors: entacapone, tolcapone

Catechol-O-methyltransferase (COMT) is also involved in the breakdown of dopamine, and inhibitors of this enzyme will also increase levels of dopamine, so enhancing dopaminergic function. They are used as adjuncts to levodopa therapy and may smooth out the 'end-of-dose effects'. Indeed, levodopa is also a substrate for COMT and its co-administration will prevent peripheral metabolism of levodopa, so optimising levels of levodopa for central conversion to dopamine. Some preparations of levodopa are formulated with entacapone in addition to dopa decarboxylase inhibitors.

Amantidine

This is also an antiviral agent, which is thought to act by increasing the release of dopamine.

Muscarinic receptor antagonists, e.g. procyclidine

As commented above, the decreased dopaminergic activity is accompanied by an imbalance of cholinergic activity and so muscarinic antagonists are useful to dampen down the cholinergic system. Muscarinic antagonists are often used where tremor is a leading feature, especially in younger patients. Interestingly, in the older antipsychotic drugs that were found to cause drug-induced Parkinson's disease, it was found that the agents with significant antimuscarinic binding were less likely to cause problems, due to reduced cholinergic activity (see Figure 29.1).

Drug choice

The most effective treatment for Parkinson's disease is levodopa in combination with dopa decarboxylase inhibitors and NICE guidance (2006) indicates that most patients will eventually require levodopa. However, as levodopa therapy has a finite period for its effectiveness, it may not always be used as first-line therapy, in which case dopaminergic agonists might be used. In choosing a dopamine agonist, the non-ergot agents (ropinirole, rotigotine) are preferred because they are not associated with fibrotic reactions (see later), which occur with ergot derivatives. MAO-B inhibitors may also be used as first-line therapy.

If a COMT inhibitor is added to therapy entacapone is the agent of choice as tolcapone is best avoided because it is associated with liver toxicity. The NICE (2006) have indicated that amantidine should be used to manage dyskinesia.

In the case of drug-induced Parkinsonism the approach is, where possible, to stop the causative agent. However, this may not be possible in all cases and, for example, in schizophrenia the approach might be to choose an agent less likely to cause the symptoms such as an atypical agent. As drug-induced Parkinsonism is essentially due to the agent blocking dopamine receptors, levodopa and dopamine receptor agonists are not appropriate for this condition and, where drug treatment is required, antimusarinic agents may be considered.

Neuroleptic malignant syndrome

This is a rare but severe reaction, usually to antipsychotics, but may occur with levodopa. Symptoms include fever, rigidity, altered mental status and autonomic dysfunction (e.g. loss of bladder and bowel control). It is usually managed by dose reduction of levodopa.

Fibrotic reactions

Ergot-derived dopamine receptor agonists (e.g. bromocriptine, cabergoline, lisuride, pergolide) are associated with causing fibrosis that may affect the lungs,

heart valves and retroperitoneum. If ergot derivatives are used it is advised that erythrocyte sedimentation rate (ESR), and electrolyte and creatinine levels should be monitored and a chest X-ray taken.

Depression

Parkinson's disease is associated with depression and, where antidepressant therapy is required, selective serotonin reuptake inhibitors (SSRIs) should be used although there are risks of interactions with selegiline (Table 29.1).

Drug interactions

In the context of drugs used in the management of Parkinson's disease, some interactions are summarised in Table 29.1. One key pharmacodynamic interaction

Table 29.1 Summary of important interactions with drugs used in the management of Parkinson's disease

Interacting drugs	Consequences	Comments
Levodopa or dopamine receptor agonists with antipsychotic agents and dopaminergic antiemetics (e.g. metoclopramide)	The dopamine receptor antagonists will oppose the actions and reduce the effectiveness of these anti-Parkinsonian drugs (and vice versa)	• This may lead to failure of treatment • Domperidone does not interact because it does not penetrate the blood–brain barrier
Levodopa or dopamine receptor agonists with antihypertensives	Increased hypotensive effects	This increases the risk of falls and may require dose reduction of the antihypertensive
Levodopa and benzodiazepines	Evidence of reduced effectiveness of levodopa	This has been reported for diazepam, chlordiazepoxide and nitrazepam
Levodopa and non-selective MAOIs	Risk of hypertensive crisis	• This combination should be avoided and levodopa should not be started until 2 weeks after stopping the MAO inhibitor • MAO-A-selective inhibitors (e.g. moclobemide) are safer and appear only to enhance the side effects of levodopa
SSRIs or TCAs with selegiline	Risk of serotonergic syndrome	Selegiline should be avoided with concurrent paroxetine or sertraline and only started after a significant washout time If TCAs are used the patient should be monitored for adverse events
Antimuscarinics with other drugs with antimuscarinic properties	Increased antimuscarinic side effects (e.g. dry mouth, blurred vision, urinary retention and constipation)	
Antacids with levodopa	Antacids might reduce the effectiveness of modified-release preparations of levodopa	This is a reason to separate the dose and antacid by 2–3 hours

SSRI, selective serotonin reuptake inhibitor; MAOI, monoamine oxidase inhibitor; TCA, tricyclic antidepressant.

is between dopamine receptor antagonists (e.g. antipsychotic agents) and levodopa and dopamine receptor agonists. The other issue, as commented above, is that many of the drug therapies for the management of Parkinson's disease involve positive drug interactions, e.g. levodopa and carbidopa.

Monitoring

In addition to the monitoring mentioned above for ergot derivates (ESR, electrolytes, creatinine levels and chest X-rays), liver function tests should be carried out for the COMT inhibitors (especially tolcapone) in view of the risk of liver dysfunction.

Counselling

Patients with Parkinson's disease should report their condition to the DVLA (Driver and Vehicle Licensing Agency). Levodopa-containing compounds and dopamine receptor agonists can cause the sudden onset of sleep and patients should be warned of this, especially in the context of skilled tasks such as driving. In all cases drug treatment should be adhered to and not stopped abruptly without medical advice.

Levodopa and dopamine receptor agonists

- The beneficial effects may take some time to become fully apparent.
- Levodopa and dopamine receptor agonists are also liable to cause orthostatic hypotension, so patients should be counselled about the possibility of a fall.
- Both levodopa and dopamine receptor agonists can cause abnormal involuntary movements.
- They may cause anxiety, hallucinations and vivid dreams.
- They are occasionally associated with behavioural changes, which may include abnormal gambling and hypersexuality.
- They may cause nausea and domperidone may help as it blocks their peripheral actions.

Levodopa

- If its effects start to wear off at the end of the dose or there are abnormal movements, the patient should consult their doctor.
- High protein diets may reduce the effectiveness of levodopa. This is due to competition of amino acids with levodopa for gastrointestinal absorption.

Dopamine receptor agonists

These are associated with dyspepsia.

Dopamine receptor agonists (ergot derivates)

Patients should be counselled to report cough, breathlessness and abdominal pain because these could indicate a fibrotic reaction.

Antimuscarinic agents

These are likely to cause dry mouth, blurred vision, constipation and urinary retention.

COMT inhibitors

- If patients are taking tolcapone they should be vigilant for signs of liver toxicity.
- These may discolour the urine.

Self-assessment

For the following questions concerning Parkinson's disease and its management, choose the most appropriate answer:

1 *Drug-induced Parkinson's disease is likely to be caused by which class of drugs?*

   A Antimuscarinic agents
   B Triptans
   C Dopamine receptor antagonists
   D SSRIs
   E Dopamine reuptake inhibitors

2 *Levodopa is best described by which one of the following?*

   A A dopamine agonist
   B A dopamine antagonist
   C A dopamine partial agonist
   D A dopamine precursor
   E A dopamine reuptake inhibitor

3 *DOPA decarboxylase inhibitors are often combined with levodopa to:*

   A Antagonise antimuscarinic side effects
   B Promote the passage of levodopa across the blood–brain barrier

C Reduce the chances of drug-induced
Parkinson's disease
D Prevent its renal elimination
E Reduce peripheral conversion to dopamine

4 *Levodopa therapy is limited by which one of the
following?*

A Hypokalaemia
B Its effectiveness decreases over several years
C Preventing the patient from sleeping
D Neutropenia
E It is a potent enzyme inducer

Practice points

- Parkinson's disease is a condition requiring specialist diagnosis and treatment.

- Treatment guidelines are set out by the NICE (2006) and should be consulted.
- Parkinson's UK provides a wealth of patient and professional advice.
- Levodopa (with a dopa decarboxylase inhibitor) is the classic treatment but is effective only for a finite period.
- Drugs (notably older antipsychotic agents) can lead to drug-induced Parkinsonism.
- Doses of co-careldopa should be checked carefully because confusion can occur between preparations. Note that a preparation should be stopped at least 12 hours before another levodopa/dopa decarboxylase inhibitor is started.

CASE STUDIES

Case 1

Mr AA, a 60-year-old man, gives a 6-month history of tremor in the right hand and has some difficulty in writing; he also complains of dyspepsia. On examination, one can see the tremor at rest and there is some slowness of finger movements. The general practitioner suspects Parkinson's disease and refers the patient to a neurologist. The neurologist is convinced that the initial diagnosis is correct and prescribes:

> rotigotine 2 mg patches (daily).

Would a CT or MRI scan help with diagnosis?

- No, there are no structural lesions but these may be used to exclude other pathologies.

Comment on the choice of drugs.

- This drug is often used as first line and is appropriate as monotherapy. Dopamine receptor agonists are also appropriate for relatively young patients with mild symptoms.

Why wasn't levodopa prescribed?

- The benefits of levodopa may be lost over time, so it might be wise to delay its use.

What are the driving implications for this man?

- He should inform the DVLA to judge his fitness to drive.
- Dopamine receptor agonists and levodopa are associated with a risk of the sudden onset of sleep and he requires counselling if he is driving.

(continued)

(continued)

After a year he still has significant symptoms and the following are prescribed:

Sinemet-Plus (levodopa and carbidopa)
domperidone 20 mg three times daily.

Why wasn't levodopa prescribed alone?

- Carbidopa prevents peripheral conversion of levodopa to dopamine and so limits peripheral side effects.

Comment on the choice of domperidone over metoclopramide.

- Domperidone has poor penetration of the blood–brain barrier, and so will not oppose central actions of dopamine. Metoclopramide penetrates the blood–brain barrier and will oppose the actions of dopamine and could cause drug-induced Parkinsonism.

The patient is severely depressed about having developed this condition.

Is drug treatment appropriate for his depression?

- Yes and an SSRI would be appropriate. TCAs may make the condition worse and the rarely used MAO inhibitors should be avoided with levodopa.

Case 2

Mr AB is a 60-year-old man who shows rigidity with slowness but no tremor. He has a history of hypertension, schizophrenia and vestibular disorder. His current medication is:

bendroflumethiazide 2.5 mg once daily
haloperidol 20 mg daily
temazepam 10 mg every night
cinnarizine 30 mg three times daily.

The GP makes a provisional diagnosis of drug-induced Parkinsonism.

What action would you recommend?

- Of the drugs that he is prescribed, haloperidol and cinnarizine are both associated with causing drug-induced Parkinsonism. The newer atypical antipsychotics (e.g. risperidone, olanzapine) are less likely to cause this and would a sensible alternative to use. If cinnarizine is essential to the management of this patient then it could be changed to betahistine (but not prochlorperazine, because this is also associated with drug-induced Parkinsonism).

References

National Institute for Health and Care Excellence (2006). *Parkinson's Disease: Diagnosis and management in adults in primary and secondary care.* Clinical Guideline 35. London: NICE.

Further reading

Clarke CE (2007). Parkinson's disease. *BMJ* 335: 441–445. pmid: 17762036.

Samili A, Nutt JG, Ranson BR (2004). Parkinson's disease. *Lancet* 363: 1783–1793. pmid: 15172778.

Online resources

www.parkinsons.org.uk
The website of the charity Parkinson's UK; provides a wealth of information for both patients and professionals (accessed July 2015).

PART G

Pain

30

Pain management

Pain is one of the most common complaints and impacts greatly on patients' quality of life, possibly leading to reduced mobility, insomnia and depression. Management of pain is complicated, particularly in elderly people, due to side effects such as constipation, and drowsiness with opioids and gastrointestinal bleeding with non-steroidal anti-inflammatory drugs (NSAIDs), and numerous drug interactions add to this prescribing challenge.

Acute pain is an important protective mechanism preventing or reducing injury by enabling rapid removal from harm. Chronic pain, lasting 6 months or longer, is not beneficial and is widely considered to be a disease.

Physiology of pain

The detection of pain occurs via nociceptive afferent neurons, mechanoreceptors and thermoreceptors, which transmit sensory information to the brain or dorsal horn of the spinal cord. Fast reflex actions involve direct transmission to the dorsal horn of the spinal cord without involving the brain, before the defence or motor response. A detailed description of pain physiology is beyond the scope of this book but terminology in common usage is defined as follows:

- noci: a prefix denoting pain or injury
- nociceptive: describes nerve fibres, endings or pathways concerned with pain

- nociceptors: any receptor that responds to stimuli resulting in the sensation of pain
- thermoreceptors: receptors activated by heat
- mechanoreceptors: receptors activated by light touch
- afferent (sensory) neurons transmit impulses from the sense organs and receptors to the brain or spinal cord
- efferent (motor) neurons transmit impulses from the brain or spinal cord (dorsal horn) to various tissues in response to stimulation by the sensory fibres, leading to defence responses such as muscle contraction to move away from the pain source
- nociceptive afferent (sensory) neurons: afferent fibres directly involved in the detection of pain. These are neurons with sensory endings in peripheral tissues. They are essentially bare nerve endings and are activated by mechanical, thermal or chemical stimuli. They may also set up local reflexes, such that stimulation may elicit a local response, e.g. vasodilatation
- Aδ-, Aβ- and C-fibres describe different types of nerve fibre involved in pain transmission.

Other transmitters of pain (inflammatory mediators, neurotransmitters and neuropeptides)

As described above, physical or chemical insults activate nociceptors resulting in neurotransmission to the brain and/or spinal cord. Inflammatory mediators, including bradykinin, histamine and 5-hydroxytryptamine/serotonin (5HT) produced by injured tissues, may modify the transmission of pain impulses. In addition, prostanoids, which do not produce pain directly, sensitise nociceptors.

Neuropeptides involved in pain transmission include the tachykinins: substance P (neurokinin-1), neurokinin A and calcitonin gene-related peptide (CGRP). These are released from sensory neurons and release inflammatory mediators such as histamine, 5HT, leukotrienes and prostaglandins from mast cells. This is known as neurogenic inflammation. These inflammatory mediators sensitise nociceptive nerve endings, lowering the trigger threshold of the nerve to produce hyperalgesia.

Ultimately, the perception of pain occurs in the cerebral cortex. An emotional component from the limbic system is also thought to contribute and explains the subjective response according to psychological characteristics such as anxiety and depression.

Excitatory and inhibitory neurotransmitters

Pharmacological targets include receptors for neurotransmitters involved in complex spinal neural activity. These include N-methyl-D-aspartate (NMDA) receptors for the endogenous excitatory amino acid, glutamate. Anaesthetic agents such as dizocilipine, and the less potent ketamine, are NMDA channel antagonists. The neurotransmitters γ-aminobutyric acid (GABA) and noradrenaline (norepinephrine) produce inhibitory effects. Adenosine is also thought to be involved, indicating a potential target for caffeine, a methylxanthine and adenosine receptor antagonist.

Opioids

Opioid receptors for the endogenous opioids (endorphins, enkephalins and dynorphins) are also involved in pain transmission and perception, affecting both the brain and the spinal cord. Activation of these receptors in the spinal cord leads to presynaptic inhibition and blockade of pain transmission.

Gate theory

The gate theory describes the modulation of pain signals either to prevent or to enhance the signal received by the brain. Noxious stimuli activate afferent neurons, invoking a neuronal impulse to the spinal cord. This signal may then be inhibited or enhanced before its transmission to the brain.

Types of pain

Pain is described as somatic, visceral or neuropathic according to its origin.

Somatic

Somatic pain is pain relating to the body wall but excluding the viscera. Pain tends to be localised and follows stimulation of peripheral pain receptors (nociceptors) in the skin and musculoskeletal system. Examples include osteo- or rheumatoid arthritis and myalgia.

Visceral

Visceral pain originates in the viscera, i.e. the internal organs of the body, particularly the abdominal and thorax organs. Visceral pain is usually poorly localised and often referred to peripheral sites, e.g. the pain associated with gallstones, myocardial infarction or appendicitis.

Neuropathic pain

As the name suggests, neuropathic pain results from nerve damage arising in the central or peripheral nerves. Neuropathic pain occurs as a result of disease affecting the sensory pathway and is independent of damage to peripheral tissue. This usually results from damage to neural tissue. Examples include postherpetic neuralgia, phantom limb, peripheral neuropathies (e.g. associated with diabetes), rheumatoid arthritis, trauma, central pain (following a stroke or in multiple sclerosis) and cancer pain due to the tumour impinging on nerves. Neuropathic pain occurs due to a lack of sensory input after sensory nerve damage and is often accompanied by allodynia, i.e. pain caused by non-noxious stimuli (e.g. touch).

The pathophysiology of neuropathic pain is not yet fully elucidated but is thought to involve spontaneous activity in the damaged sensory neurons. The pain is described as burning, shooting or scalding. Sensitivity to noradrenaline due to the expression of α-adrenoceptors may develop, resulting in sympathetically mediated pain.

Goals of treatment

The goals of treatment are to improve the quality of life and to delay disease progress by good pain control but with minimal side effects.

Pharmacological basis of management of NSAIDs, e.g. aspirin, diclofenac, diflusinal, flurbiprofen, ibuprofen, naproxen, piroxicam

NSAIDs are among the most widely used drugs for a number of conditions associated with inflammation. In addition to their anti-inflammatory effects, most NSAIDs possess analgesic and antipyretic effects.

Anti-inflammatory effects

When considering anti-inflammatory effects, it is useful to consider the process of inflammation. Important physiological mechanisms combine to produce vasodilatation, increased vascular permeability and cell accumulation. A number of mediators produce these effects to different extents depending on the nature of the inflammation. These mediators include nitric oxide, leukotrienes, prostaglandins and thromboxane; the prostaglandins PGE_2 and PGI_2 (prostacyclin) produce vasodilatation and oedema, in addition to sensitisation of nociceptors, as described above. Those mediators produced by cyclo-oxygenase (COX) activity, prostaglandins and thromboxane are the targets for NSAIDs. Production of the inflammatory mediators from membrane phospholipid and COX activity is detailed in Figure 30.1.

The inhibition of cyclo-oxygenase

The predominant mode of action of NSAIDs is inhibition of the COX enzymes, resulting in subsequent inhibition of prostaglandin and thromboxane production. Most NSAIDs are competitive inhibitors of COX, whereas aspirin irreversibly inactivates COX by acetylation. This action of aspirin is exploited for antiplatelet effects (see Chapter 15).

The anti-inflammatory effects vary between NSAIDs, with ibuprofen being the weakest and indometacin and piroxicam the most potent. Ibuprofen is therefore not considered suitable for the treatment of acute gout. Most NSAIDs are antipyretic due to

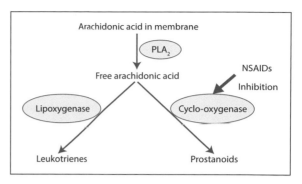

Figure 30.1 Production of the inflammatory mediators from membrane phospholipid, via phospholipase A_2 (PLA_2) and cyclo-oxygenase activity. NSAIDs, non-steroidal anti-inflammatory drugs.

inhibition of prostaglandin effects, which disrupt the hypothalamic regulation of temperature.

The difference in anti-inflammatory activity of NSAIDs is small compared with tolerability by patients. In the treatment of rheumatoid arthritis, therefore, larger doses of 1.6–2.4 g ibuprofen daily, which possesses only weak anti-inflammatory activity, are required. Longer-acting NSAIDs with more potent anti-inflammatory activity such as naproxen and piroxicam are useful in the treatment of chronic pain.

Analgesic effect

As described above, prostaglandins produced by inflamed tissue sensitise nociceptors to inflammatory mediators such as bradykinin and 5HT. NSAIDs therefore produce an analgesic effect in conditions associated with prostaglandin production. The beneficial effect in headache may result from inhibiting prostaglandin-mediated vasodilatation of the cerebral vasculature. Actions in the spinal cord may also contribute to the central effect.

Adverse effects

NSAIDs are associated with many adverse drug reactions (ADRs: see Chapter 6) but predominantly gastric toxicity with a risk of haemorrhage (see Chapter 8). Other ADRs include diarrhoea, nausea, rashes, urticaria, photosensitivity, sodium and water retention (with worsening of hypertension and chronic heart failure), and renal impairment. Renal toxicity may be due to inhibition of the effects of prostaglandins on renal blood flow or nephropathy. Some NSAIDs may precipitate asthma in certain individuals (see Chapter 22).

Adverse effects due to salicylates

In addition to the adverse effects caused by other NSAIDs, salicylates may also cause 'salicylism' including tinnitus, impaired hearing and vertigo. This usually occurs only after chronic use of larger doses, which may also lead to compensated respiratory alkalosis as a result of increased respiration. Aspirin may also cause encephalitis and liver problems, known as Reye's syndrome, in children aged <12 years and those <15 years with fever and/or viral illness. This advice is regarded as too complex in view of the wide availability of aspirin through general sale, and the Medicines Control Agency (now the Medicines and Healthcare products Regulatory Agency, MHRA) therefore recommended that aspirin should not be taken by any child under 16 years of age.

COX-2 inhibitors, e.g. celecoxib, etodolac, meloxicam

There are two subtypes of COX, COX-1 and COX-2, which show some variation in distribution and roles. COX-1 is the constitutive or 'physiological' isoform, found in most tissues and blood platelets. COX-2 is inducible and is produced in activated inflammatory cells; it is, therefore, the COX subtype involved in the production of prostaglandins and thromboxanes that are active in inflammation. The main anti-inflammatory activity of NSAIDs is therefore due to COX-2 inhibition. COX-1 inhibition is thought to produce toxic effects, including gastric irritation (see Chapter 8). Drugs selective for COX-2 have therefore been developed and are thought to be more selective for inhibition of prostanoids associated with inflammation, rather than those involved in physiological regulation. It is becoming apparent, however, that COX-2 inhibitors may not be as free from gastric toxicity as first thought (Jüni *et al.* 2002). A systematic review of the efficacy and safety of celecoxib compared with traditional NSAIDs for the treatment of osteoarthritis and rheumatoid arthritis reported similar efficacy for both treatments and an improvement in gastrointestinal safety and tolerability with celecoxib (Deeks *et al.* 2002).

Paracetamol

Paracetamol is the first-choice analgesic for conditions not associated with inflammation. It possesses analgesic and antipyretic activity with similar efficacy to aspirin, but is not thought to exhibit significant anti-inflammatory effects. Its mechanism of action is surprisingly unclear and proposed mechanisms include inhibition of COX-3, a novel COX variant, which is located in the brain; activation of transient receptor potential channels to modulate pain transmission; and augmentation of the endocannabinoid system.

In normal doses, paracetamol is well tolerated; however, hepatotoxicity occurs with doses only two to three times the maximum recommended dose due to saturation of metabolism involving conjugation with glutathione. Toxic metabolites are produced, causing liver necrosis and damage to renal tubules. Early administration (within 8 hours) of acetylcysteine increases glutathione formation and thereby prevents liver damage. As few as 20 tablets can produce severe hepatocellular necrosis in the absence of symptoms in the first few days. Nausea and vomiting subside within 24 hours but patients should be admitted to hospital urgently. Additional signs of liver toxicity include jaundice, abdominal tenderness (right upper quadrant) and hypoglycaemia. Patients at increased risk of liver damage include those taking concurrent enzyme inducers (carbamazepine, alcohol, phenytoin, rifampicin) and malnourished patients.

Nefopam

Nefopam is used for moderate pain resistant to treatment with non-opioid analgesics. Adverse sympathomimetic and antimuscarinic effects limit its use. These include nervousness, tachycardia, urinary retention, dry mouth and blurred vision.

Opioids

The term 'opioid' applies to morphine-like synthetic and endogenous compounds. Synthetic opioids are used to treat moderate-to-severe pain, often visceral in origin. They are reserved for more severe pain due to their unwanted effects of drowsiness, constipation, nausea and vomiting, tolerance and dependence. High doses may produce respiratory depression and hypotension.

Opioid receptors

The effects of opioids are mediated by opioid receptors. To date, three subtypes have been identified and termed μ-, κ- and δ-receptors. The main pharmacological effects are mediated by μ-receptors and include analgesia, respiratory depression, euphoria, miosis (pupil constriction), physical dependence, constipation and sedation. The κ-receptors are thought to produce dysphoria.

Most morphine-like drugs have a high affinity for μ-receptors with lower affinities for κ- and δ-receptors. The potency of agents such as codeine and methadone is lower than that of morphine, resulting in reduced pharmacological effects even at maximum doses.

Opioid receptors are distributed throughout the brain and spinal cord. The administration of morphine inhibits nociceptive pathways in the brain and dorsal horn of the spinal cord and from the peripheral terminals of nociceptive afferent neurons. Effects on the brain also contribute to the euphoric effect and subsequent reduction in the psychological component of pain.

Weak opioids, e.g. codeine, dihydrocodeine

Dihydrocodeine and codeine have similar moderate potencies. Weak opioids are most effective in combination with paracetamol (co-codamol, co-dydramol) but are associated with significant opioid side effects such as nausea and constipation.

Strong opioids, e.g. buprenorphine, diamorphine, fentanyl, morphine

Strong opioids form step 3 of the analgesic ladder (described below) and are prescribed for chronic non-malignant pain or in palliative care (see Chapter 33). It should be noted that the risk of psychological dependence is minimal when opioids are used for severe pain and this is not a reason to withhold treatment.

Adverse effects of opioids

The most common adverse effects of opioids are constipation, nausea and vomiting, and drowsiness. Respiratory depression is thought to result from reduced sensitivity of the respiratory centre (in the brain) to carbon dioxide, when higher doses of opioids are administered.

Nausea and vomiting

Nausea and vomiting occur due to the effects of opioids on the chemoreceptor trigger zone in the brain. This is fairly common but usually transient. Antiemetics (see Chapter 9) such as metoclopramide or prochlorperazine are often required when more potent opioids such as morphine are first prescribed. Dystonic (abnormal muscle tone, e.g. muscle spasms) reactions may occur, particularly in young and elderly people.

Constipation

Constipation is common with opioids (see Chapter 10) and co-prescribing of laxatives is required. Bulk-forming laxatives may not be appropriate due to the reduced motility of the colon and, therefore, the reduced reflex effect of increased bulk produced by these agents. Stool softeners combined with stimulants are often used (see Chapter 10). It should be noted that constipation occurs with low doses of codeine, including those used for cough suppression (see Chapter 20).

Tolerance and dependence

Chronic opioid use may result in tolerance, requiring an increase in dosage. Alternatively, another opioid may be administered. Tolerance to analgesia, emetic, euphoria and respiratory effects of opioids occurs but that to constipation and pupil constriction is much less marked. Dependence may be physical, involving a withdrawal syndrome, or psychological.

Other

Other adverse effects of opioids include bronchoconstriction (induced by morphine due to histamine release from mast cells), hypotension, bradycardia, pruritus and immunosuppression (after long-term opioid misuse). Table 30.1 summarises some important properties of opioids.

Tramadol

Tramadol exhibits opioid effects (μ receptor agonist) and also enhances the effects of 5HT and adrenergic pathways. The use of this drug for moderate-to-severe pain has increased due to reduced opioid side effects. Psychiatric reactions may, however, occur. The response of patients to tramadol varies considerably and the dose is therefore adjusted accordingly.

Table 30.1 A summary of some important properties of opioid analgesics

Opioid analgesic	Comments
Opioids for mild-to-moderate pain	
Codeine	• Constipating when used long term • Laxatives should be prescribed for all patients prescribed regular codeine
Dihydrocodeine	Nausea and vomiting increase with higher doses
Opioids for moderate-to-severe pain	
Alfentanil, fentanyl and remifentanil	• Injections used for intraoperative analgesia • Fentanyl patch used in palliative care (Chapter 33)
Buprenorphine	• Partial agonist at opioid receptors and therefore precipitates withdrawal symptoms in patients dependent on other opioids. This may result in breakthrough pain in patients changing from other opioids during treatment for pain • Longer duration of action, with the sublingual preparation producing analgesia for 6–8 hours
Dextromoramide (Palfium)	Shorter duration of action than morphine and less sedating
Diamorphine (heroin)	Less nausea and hypotension than with morphine
Dipipanone (Diconal)	• Contains cyclizine and therefore not recommended in palliative care (see Cyclimorph, Chapter 33) • Less sedating than morphine
Meptazinol (Meptid)	• Lower incidence of respiratory depression • Rapid onset of action, 15 minutes
Methadone	• Less sedating than morphine • Long half-life and may therefore accumulate with repeated doses
Oxycodone	• Similar to morphine • Used in palliative care (Chapter 33)
Pethidine	• Rapid onset of action but short acting and therefore not recommended for chronic pain • Less constipating than morphine but less potent analgesic
Tramadol	• Fewer opioid side effects, including reduced potential for addiction • May cause adverse psychiatric effects such as hallucinations and confusion • Risk of convulsions, especially when combined with other drugs known to reduce seizure threshold

Local anaesthetics, e.g. lidocaine, bupivacaine, levobupivacaine and prilocaine

Local anaesthetics inhibit reversibly the transmission of nerve impulses via blockade of voltage-sensitive sodium channels. Side effects include agitation, confusion, tremors, convulsions and respiratory depression. Cardiovascular side effects include myocardial depression, vasodilatation and subsequent hypotension. Local anaesthetics such as lidocaine are used in neuropathic pain.

Cannabinoids

There is good evidence that cannabinoids may exert analgesic effects through inhibition of synaptic transmission at both the spinal level and higher centres. Analogous to the opioid story, endogenous cannabinoids such as anandamide have been identified and may play a role in endogenous pain relief. Patients with certain chronic conditions such as multiple sclerosis appear to gain effective pain relief from cannabinoids. Sativex (Δ-9-tetrahydrocannabinol and cannabidiol) is now available as an oral spray for the relief of pain associated with spasticity in multiple sclerosis.

Tricyclic antidepressants

The pyschotropic effects of antidepressants may be of benefit for pain in patients with anxiety and depression. Tricyclic antidepressants (TCAs) also possess analgesic activity independent of these pyschotropic effects. Indeed, the analgesic effect tends to occur at lower doses than those used for depression. The mechanism is largely unclear but may involve inhibition of spinal neurons in pain pathways by increasing noradrenaline and 5HT concentrations in inhibitory pathways. TCAs may also block sodium channels and they are also NMDA-receptor antagonists.

Anticonvulsants

The anticonvulsants gabapentin and pregabalin have a role in the management of neuropathic pain but their mechanism of action is less clear and may involve altering GABAergic or inhibition of voltage-operated calcium channels in dorsal horn neurons.

Anticonvulsants such as carbamazepine, sodium valproate or phenytoin stabilise neuronal membranes. They are useful, therefore, to relieve neuropathic pain. Carbamazepine is widely used for neuropathic pain, including diabetic neuropathy. Its use may be limited by dose-related side effects (see Chapter 25). Phenytoin may be used as an alternative but consideration should be given to zero-order pharmacokinetics (see Chapter 7). It may take 3–4 weeks to reach steady state if loading doses are not used. Lamotrigine is also increasingly being used for neuropathic pain. Although the mechanism of action is unclear, the anticonvulsants are believed to block sodium channels, suppressing neuronal discharge at sites of injury.

Caffeine

Caffeine is added to a number of over-the-counter (OTC) preparations with the claim that it increases the analgesic effect of drugs such as paracetamol and aspirin. There is little evidence to support this and the regular use of these preparations may lead to chronic daily headache (see below) and be mildly habit forming. The alerting effect of caffeine may also be a disadvantage.

Counterirritants

Aδ- and C-fibres transmit pain signals to the dorsal horn of the spinal cord. These signals may be modulated by Aβ-fibres, thereby preventing transmission to the brain. This explains the effect of counterirritants such as menthol and capsaicin and/or rubbing, which activate Aβ-fibres and provide relief from pain caused by activation of C-fibres.

Chronic pain and central sensitisation

Dosing 'when required' is not appropriate in the treatment of chronic pain due to the principle of central sensitisation. This phenomenon also explains the benefit of administration of opioids before surgery. After damage to peripheral tissue, spinal neurons exhibit hyper-responsiveness to impulses from afferent neurons. This results in an increased perception of a similar intensity of pain. Therefore, if chronic pain recurs, it may be difficult to regain pain control due to the reduced threshold of the spinal neurons. Higher doses may be required to regain pain control. Maintenance treatment also removes the psychological component of fear and a dose reduction may then be possible.

Medication overuse headache

Medication overuse headache (MOH) is a common subtype of chronic daily headache. It may be caused by a withdrawal effect after the chronic use of analgesic preparations and results in a vicious circle, whereby analgesic administration is continued. It is becoming increasingly recognised as a problem associated with the overuse of analgesics in the treatment of headache. Inappropriate use of OTC analgesia is a particular problem due to the widespread availability of analgesics such as paracetamol, aspirin and ibuprofen from supermarkets and pharmacies.

MOH may follow the regular daily use of simple analgesics such as paracetamol, NSAIDs (more than four times a week), opioids or ergotamine more often than twice a week (Silberstein and Young 1995). Compound preparations containing caffeine or sympathomimetics may also contribute to MOH. Health professionals should be aware of the problem in patients presenting with chronic headache. The suspected causative drug should be withdrawn gradually and the patient monitored for improvement.

A study reported the occurrence of MOH due to excessive use of triptans. A critical number of dosages was reported as ten single doses per month, above which MOH included a migraine-like daily headache or an increase in frequency of migraine attacks. It was recommended that, on suspicion of triptan-induced MOH, the drug should be withdrawn temporarily (Limmroth *et al.* 2002).

Drug choice

The World Health Organization (1996) recommends that effective analgesia is given 'by the mouth, by the clock and by the ladder', i.e. the oral route is preferred for drug administration if possible and analgesia should be given regularly rather than 'when required'. The analgesic ladder starts with simple analgesics such as paracetamol or ibuprofen and progresses to mild and then strong opioids. Adjuncts including simple analgesics or pyschotropic agents may be added at any stage. Patients are then reviewed regularly and treatment stepped up or down as appropriate (Figure 30.2).

Paracetamol

Paracetamol is a common first-line agent, particularly for elderly patients, because of its reduced side effect profile and fewer drug interactions. The main problem of paracetamol use is life-threatening hepatotoxicity in overdose. Despite the widespread and recommended use of paracetamol, its effectiveness has been questioned under some circumstances. There is evidence that paracetamol is ineffective in back pain compared with placebo and has limited efficacy in osteoarthritis (Machado *et al.* 2014).

NSAIDs

Aspirin is indicated for the treatment of headache, transient muscle pain, dysmenorrhoea and pyrexia. For inflammatory conditions, safer alternatives include ibuprofen (see Chapter 8).

NSAIDs are indicated for inflammatory conditions such as back pain, soft-tissue inflammation and rheumatoid arthritis. High doses are required to achieve a full anti-inflammatory effect. NSAIDs may also be useful in the treatment of advanced osteoarthritis (see Chapter 31).

It is important to note that it may take up to a week to achieve the full analgesic effect of NSAIDs, while the full anti-inflammatory effect may take up to 3 weeks. A poor response after this time should be followed by an alternative NSAID as their responses vary.

Topical NSAID preparations are widely available but their efficacy is uncertain and the benefit of topical agents over oral preparations has not yet been demonstrated.

Opioids

Mild opioids include codeine and dihydrocodeine and may be prescribed in addition to simple analgesics

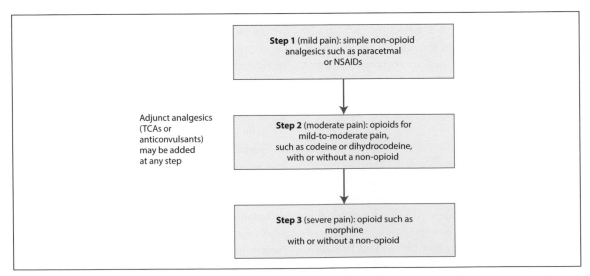

Figure 30.2 Stepped-pain management advocated by the World Health Organization. NSAIDs, non-steroidal anti-inflammatory drugs. TCAs, tricyclic antidepressants.

when these have failed to control pain in sole use. If this fails, more potent opioids may be introduced at step 3. This includes the treatment of chronic pain, which may not always be due to malignancy. For the use of opioids in palliative care see Chapter 32.

Compound preparations

The use of compound preparations containing paracetamol or aspirin with a low dose of opioid (8 mg codeine or 10 mg dihydrocodeine) is discouraged due to the lack of evidence, from single-dose studies, of efficacy compared with paracetamol or aspirin alone (Anon. 2000). Coupled to this is the difficulty of titrating individual drug doses and the risk of opioid side effects such as drowsiness and constipation, particularly in elderly patients. Initial prescribing of more than one agent should be for individual drugs, and then fixed doses of combination products should be used once control has been achieved if compliance is a problem. If regular use of higher doses is required, patients may be advised that tolerance to most side effects will develop, with the exception of constipation and pupillary effects. Elderly patients may require a lower dose of codeine such as 15–30 mg daily. The use of combination analgesics for chronic pain may be appropriate for these patients and may improve compliance.

An alternative regimen includes the use of regular paracetamol at 1 g up to four times a day, with a single dose of up to 60 mg codeine when required for more severe pain as a beneficial second step, although opioid side effects may be problematic. This type of regimen limits the development of tolerance to and dependence on opioids (Anon. 2000).

Topical preparations

Capsaicin is licensed for neuropathic pain but its use is limited due to an intense burning sensation, occurring when treatment is initiated. Capsaicin is a constituent of chilli powder and acts on vanilloid receptors to release and deplete neurotransmitters from sensory nerves, leading to counterirritation.

Nerve block

This involves the injection of local anaesthetics such as lidocaine close to a sensory nerve or plexus.

Steroids

Corticosteroids are used to treat pain associated with nerve compression, tissue swelling or raised intracranial pressure (see Chapter 33).

Relative effectiveness of analgesics in acute pain

The Oxford League Table of analgesic efficacy is an evidence-based comparison of analgesics in providing at least 50% pain relief for 4–6 hours in acute pain in placebo-controlled trials. The data assess effectiveness in terms of numbers needed to treat (NNT) and indicate that etoricoxib is the most effective compared with other analgesics:

Analgesic	Dosage	NNT
Etoricoxib	180–240 mg	1.5
Ibuprofen	600–800 mg	1.7
Paracetamol and codeine	1000 mg/60 mg	2.2
Ibuprofen	400 mg	2.6
Naproxen	400–440 mg	2.7
Morphine	10 mg i.m.	2.9
Paracetamol	1000 mg	3.8
Tramadol	75 mg	5.3
Codeine	60 mg	8.3

i.m., intramuscular; NNT, numbers needed to treat.

The data also reinforce a significant placebo effect with 18% of patients receiving greater than 50% pain relief (www.medicine.ac.uk/bandolier).

Non-pharmacological treatment

Non-pharmacological treatments used in pain management include simple measures such as rest, cooling, compression and elevation, the use of transcutaneous electrical nerve stimulation (TENS), warmth, physiotherapy and/or psychological support. Following a soft-tissue injury, rest, ice, compression and elevation (RICE) are recommended to reduce swelling and inflammation. Subsequent treatment may include the application of warmth, which aims to improve circulation of the affected area.

Transcutaneous electrical nerve stimulation

Current is applied to the painful area via two electrodes placed approximately 2 cm apart, until paraesthesia is experienced. Aβ-fibres are stimulated, closing the gating mechanism in the spinal cord and therefore inhibiting the transmission of A- and C-fibres. The release of endogenous opioids may also be stimulated. TENS machines are battery operated and portable, although not suitable for use while driving. They are used for chronic, postoperative and labour pain but their effectiveness remains to be fully established. Acupuncture is thought to work by a similar mechanism.

Physiotherapy

Physiotherapy may also include the use of warmth or electric currents. This physical technique also encompasses massage, exercises, infrared and ultraviolet rays, and manipulation of the affected joints or muscles.

Psychological support

Depression, insomnia, anxiety, fear, anger, boredom and social isolation all reduce the pain threshold. Conversely, sleep, rest, antidepressants, sympathy, diversion and understanding all raise the pain threshold. Consideration of psychological and lifestyle factors is an important part of pain management.

Specific conditions

The choice of analgesic is determined according to the cause and nature of the pain. The following section deals with specific conditions associated with pain.

Fever

Paracetamol is used first line due to its tolerability. Alternatively, ibuprofen may be used for pyrexia and is often added to paracetamol treatment when pyrexia is difficult to control.

Headache

Treatment should follow the analgesic ladder, with paracetamol being a suitable first-line choice. Diagnosis may include tension, cluster headaches, raised intracranial pressure, chronic daily headache, arteritis in patients aged >60 years or sinusitis. For a discussion of signs and symptoms and appropriate referral, see Chapters 1 and 23.

Migraine

See Chapter 23.

Dysmenorrhoea

Dysmenorrhoea or painful periods may be relieved by oral contraceptives and may resolve following a pregnancy. First-line analgesia is paracetamol and/or NSAIDs. Treatment is started a few days before a period to improve pain control of severe dysmenorrhoea (see Chronic pain and central sensitisation, above). More severe or secondary dysmenorrhoea, often associated with endometriosis, may also lead to vomiting and require treatment with an antiemetic.

The management of neuropathic pain

Strategies for the management of neuropathic pain involve the use of tricyclic antidepressants, anticonvulsants, opioids, local anaesthetics and capsaicin. A review of the literature and meta-analysis has provided good evidence to support the use of TCAs, serotonin–noradrenaline reuptake inhibitors (e.g. venlafaxine, duloxetine), pregabalin and gabapentin as first-line agents, with a weaker recommendation for the second-line use of lidocaine patches, tramadol or capsaicin (Finnerup et al., 2015). However, it was also recognised that the management of neuropathic pain is complex and an area in which pharmacotherapy could be improved.

Trigeminal neuralgia

Again, only a partial response is observed after treatment with opioids. Carbamazepine is used in acute trigeminal neuralgia and in extreme cases surgery may be required. Plasma levels of carbamazepine should be monitored at higher doses. Alternatives include oxcarbazepine, gabapentin, lamotrigine or phenytoin.

Postherpetic neuralgia

This results from acute herpes zoster (shingles) and is treated with amitriptyline or gabapentin (see Chapter 36). Capsaicin or topical local anaesthetic may be used.

Concurrent disease

The following section summarises the effect of concurrent disease on the prescribing of analgesics.

Gastrointestinal irritation and ulceration

See Chapter 8.

Cardiovascular disease

As discussed in Chapter 15, low-dose aspirin has a major role in the prevention of myocardial infarction and stroke. However, other COX inhibitors may not be used in place of aspirin for this role. Furthermore, the long-term use of high doses of certain NSAIDs (including ibuprofen and diclofenac, but not naproxen) have been associated with an increased risk of cardiovascular disease and caution should be exercised in patients at risk.

Table 30.2 summarises these and other considerations, including hypersensitivity reactions to NSAIDs. It should be noted that the cautions highlighted for opioids become less important in palliative care.

Drug interactions

Table 30.3 highlights some important drug interactions involving analgesics.

Pregnancy and breastfeeding

If possible, as with all drugs, analgesics should be avoided in the first trimester. If required for headache, pyrexia, musculoskeletal or dental pain, paracetamol is used first line. The use of analgesics during pregnancy and breastfeeding is summarised in Tables 30.4 and 30.5.

Over-the-counter considerations

Many analgesic preparations are available OTC and pharmacists are ideally placed to monitor pain control, identify drug interactions (see above) and refer conditions such as suspected rheumatoid arthritis for prompt assessment and prescription of higher doses of anti-inflammatory agents. Misuse and the risk of MOH may also be identified. The provision of lifestyle advice may benefit conditions such as gout, migraine and general painful conditions.

Simple analgesics such as ibuprofen and paracetamol are widely available from many outlets, including supermarkets. Accordingly, health professionals should always enquire about self-medication to ensure the correct use of medicines and avoidance of ADRs, e.g. worsening asthma associated with overuse of NSAIDs (and possibly paracetamol) or the risk of gastrointestinal toxicity with chronic NSAID use.

Table 30.2 Effects of concurrent conditions on drug choice		
Condition	**Drug implicated**	**Comments**
Chronic heart failure	NSAIDs, including COX-2 inhibitors	• May cause worsening CHF and fluid overload, due to sodium and water retention (Chapter 16) • An alternative such as paracetamol should be used if possible
Hypertension, oedema, renal failure, ischaemic heart disease and chronic heart failure	Effervescent preparations	• The sodium salt content of six effervescent co-codamol tablets is approximately equal to the recommended daily maximum intake of 6 g (2.4 g sodium). These preparations should be avoided, particularly by patients with renal failure or taking diuretics, as increased sodium intake may reduce the efficacy of these drugs • COX-2 inhibitors should not be used with low-dose aspirin, as any benefit of the former will be reduced • The combination of an NSAID and low-dose aspirin should be avoided if possible due to the increased risk of gastrointestinal toxicity
Hypotension	Opioids	Worsening of hypotension

(continued)

Table 30.2 *(continued)*

Condition	Drug implicated	Comments
Asthma	NSAIDs (chronic paracetamol), opioids	NSAIDs are contraindicated if there is a history of asthma, angio-oedema, urticaria or rhinitis induced by previous exposure (Chapter 22)
		• Preliminary evidence indicates that long-term, high-dose paracetamol use may worsen asthma (Shaheen *et al.* 2000). However, Levy and Volans (2001) concluded that any deterioration of asthma was short-lived but that practitioners should be alert to the possibility of worsening asthma • Opioids should not be used during an acute asthma attack, due to the risk of respiratory depression
Colitis	NSAIDs	May cause or exacerbate inflammatory bowel disease
Female infertility	NSAIDs	Female fertility may be reduced by long-term treatment
Hepatic impairment	Paracetamol, opioids, NSAIDs	• Dose-related toxicity, therefore larger doses of paracetamol should be avoided • Avoid or reduce doses of opioids, due to the risk of precipitating coma • Risk of fluid retention with NSAIDs, and increased gastrointestinal bleeding (secondary to impaired clotting). Avoid in severe liver disease
Prostatic hypertrophy	Opioids, nefopam	Increased risk of urinary retention
Renal impairment	NSAIDs (including topical preparations), opioids	• Use with caution, due to the risk of deterioration in renal function as a result of reduced renal perfusion, particularly in elderly patients and those with heart failure and cirrhosis. Additional risk factors include hypertension, diabetes and co-prescribing of drugs excreted renally, such as ACE inhibitors, digoxin and lithium • Use the lowest effective dose and monitor renal function (Chapter 2) • Avoid NSAIDs in moderate-to-severe renal failure • The effects of opioids may be increased and prolonged in moderate-to-severe renal failure, so they should be avoided or their doses reduced
Thyroid dysfunction	Opioids	Use with caution in hypothyroidism due to worsening of symptoms such as bradycardia and hypotension
Epilepsy	Tramadol, nefopam	• Tramadol should be avoided in patients with a history of epilepsy • Nefopam should not be used in patients with a history of convulsions

ACE, angiotensin-converting enzyme; CHF, chronic heart failure; COX-2, cyclo-oxygenase 2; NSAIDs, non-steroidal anti-inflammatory drugs.

Table 30.3 Some important interactions with analgesics

Interaction	Consequences	Comments
NSAIDs with ACE inhibitors	• Reduced antihypertensive effect due to effects on renal prostaglandins • Increased risk of renal damage	Monitor blood pressure and renal function
NSAIDs (except aspirin) with lithium	Increased levels of lithium and possible intoxication	Avoid unless lithium levels are closely monitored and the dose adjusted as necessary
NSAIDs with warfarin	Risk of bleeding due to increased anticoagulant effects and/or stomach irritation	• Normal doses of ibuprofen interact only rarely • Careful monitoring, particularly in elderly patients • Azapropazone is contraindicated
NSAIDs with alcohol	Possible increase in gastric irritation	

Table 30.3 *(continued)*

Interaction	Consequences	Comments
Paracetamol with warfarin	Paracetamol is the analgesic of choice for patients taking warfarin. However, long-term use of larger doses may increase the anticoagulant effect	
NSAIDs with alendronic acid	Risk of severe oesophagitis	Avoid concurrent use
NSAIDs with corticosteroids	Increased risk of gastrointestinal bleeding and ulceration	'Steroid-sparing effect' of indometacin and naproxen may allow dose reduction of corticosteroids
NSAIDs with SSRIs	Increased risk of gastrointestinal bleeding and ulceration	
NSAIDs with loop diuretics	Antihypertensive and diuretic effects reduced or abolished	• Ibuprofen, meloxicam and ketoprofen may not interact but monitoring is advised with all NSAIDs • Increased doses of diuretics may be required
NSAIDs with ciclosporin	Renal function may be reduced by some NSAIDs, resulting in nephrotoxicity and/or increased ciclosporin levels	Renal function should be monitored. Low doses of diclofenac should be used when newly prescribed
NSAIDs with methotrexate	Excretion of methotrexate may be reduced	Dose of methotrexate should be monitored closely
Colestyramine with diclofenac, ibuprofen, meloxicam, naproxen, piroxicam	• Reduced absorption of diclofenac and ibuprofen • Delayed absorption of naproxen (limited importance) • Increased clearance of meloxicam and piroxicam	• Doses should be separated by at least 2 hours • The separation of doses may reduce but not abolish the interaction involving piroxicam and meloxicam
Tramadol with SSRIs/TCAs	Small risk of serotonin syndrome	Monitor
Opioids with alcohol	Enhanced sedation	
Opioids with antibacterials	Rifampicin may reduce the plasma concentrations of methadone and possibly morphine	The dose of methadone or morphine may need to be increased
Opioids with antidepressants	The analgesic effects of morphine may be increased by clomipramine and possibly amitriptyline	This may be an advantageous interaction
Opioids with antiepilepetic drugs	Enzyme inducers may reduce the concentration of methadone	The dose of methadone may need to be increased
Pethidine with cimetidine	Reduced elimination of pethidine	Proton pump inhibitors or ranitidine are not known to interact
Morphine with metoclopramide	Increased absorption and enhanced effects of morphine	
Nefopam with anticonvulsants, TCAs and MAOIs	Nefopam may cause convulsions in susceptible patients. TCAs may reduce seizure threshold	• Nefopam should not be used in patients with a history of convulsions • Nefopam may have sympathomimetic activity and should not be given with MAOIs
Pethidine with phenothiazines	Increased analgesia and side effects	This may be used to advantage

ACE, angiotensin-converting enzyme; MAOIs, monoamine oxidase inhibitors; NSAIDs, non-steroidal anti-inflammatory drugs; SSRIs, selective serotonin reuptake inhibitors; TCAs, tricyclic antidepressants.

Table 30.4 The use of analgesic drugs in pregnancy

Drug	Trimester of risk	Comment
Paracetamol		• Not known to be harmful • Used first-line, avoiding high doses and chronic use as a precaution
Aspirin	3	• May delay or prolong labour due to COX inhibition • Impaired platelet function and risk of haemorrhage
NSAIDs	3	• Ketorolac is contraindicated • Avoid during pregnancy unless benefit outweighs risk • If necessary, use lowest effective dose (usually ibuprofen first-line) and avoid high-potency NSAIDs such as indometacin • Use in late pregnancy associated with risk of closure of the fetal ductus arteriosus while *in utero* and possibly pulmonary hypertension of the newborn • Delayed onset and increased duration of labour • NSAID use has been associated with increased risk of miscarriage (Nielsen *et al.* 2001) • Possible increased incidence and duration of bleeding in fetus and mother during delivery • No NSAID should be used after 32 weeks' gestation
Codeine, dihydrocodeine	3, particularly last few weeks	• Opioids may be used for moderate-to-severe pain • Long-term *in utero* exposure may result in neonatal withdrawal symptoms • Depression of neonatal respiration
Tramadol	Toxic in animal embryo studies	Manufacturer advises avoid in pregnancy

Information derived from the *British National Formulary* and *Therapeutics in Pregnancy and Lactation* by Lee *et al.* (2000). COX, cyclo-oxygenase; NSAIDs, non-steroidal anti-inflammatory drugs.

Table 30.5 Analgesic use during lactation

Drug	Comment
Paracetamol, codeine	Small quantities excreted into breast milk but they appear to be safe. Paracetamol is used first line. Codeine may cause constipation in the mother or baby and colic in the baby
NSAIDs (ibuprofen, naproxen, diclofenac)	Excreted into breast milk in small quantities but appear to be safe
Aspirin	Avoid, due to risk of Reye's syndrome

Information derived from the *British National Formulary* and *Therapeutics in Pregnancy and Lactation* by Lee *et al.* (2000). NSAIDs, non-steroidal anti-inflammatory drugs.

Counselling

General counselling should encourage patients to take analgesics if they are in pain. This may sound obvious but many patients are reluctant to take these drugs due to extensive publicity about side effects. Conversely, patients who take chronic analgesia, including OTC preparations, require regular review of treatment and the underlying cause of their pain, e.g. chronic use of co-codamol preparations for headache may be investigated for analgesia-induced headache or migraine.

Elderly patients may often report 'aches and pains' deemed to be an inevitable consequence of old age. Chronic pain is common in elderly people and may coexist with depression. Health professionals have an important role in identifying these patients and advising on appropriate treatment to enable pain control. Education, reassurance, support and patient counselling are particularly important in achieving good pain control. A pain diary outlining the influence of activity and analgesics may be useful in attaining good pain control. Pharmacists or carers may prepare monitored dosage systems as a memory aid for taking medication. These usually include four compartments per day so that all tablets are taken at the appropriate times.

Drug-specific counselling points are detailed below.

Paracetamol

- Paracetamol is one of the safest drugs at normal doses.
- Liver damage may occur after exceeding recommended doses and may take a few days or more to develop – help should be sought immediately.
- Take care not to exceed the maximum recommended dose by combining with other paracetamol-containing products such as OTC preparations for colds.
- Do not take more than two 500 mg tablets at a time.
- 4–6 hours should be left between doses.
- Do not take more than eight 500 mg tablets in 24 hours.

NSAIDs

- Patients should report symptoms of indigestion, wheezing or rashes immediately.
- NSAIDs are best taken with or after food and not on an empty stomach.
- Diclofenac and indometacin have a tendency to cause dizziness and patients should be warned that caution is advised when driving.
- Enteric-coated and slow-release preparations should be swallowed whole and not chewed.
- Enteric-coated tablets should not be taken at the same time of day as indigestion preparations.

Tiaprofenic acid

Report urinary symptoms, including increased frequency, nocturia, urgency, pain on urinating or blood in the urine, and stop taking medication immediately.

Indometacin

There is a high incidence of side effects with indometacin, including headache, dizziness and gastrointestinal disturbance.

Topical NSAIDs

- Avoid contact with the eyes, mucous membranes, or inflamed or broken skin.

- Discontinue taking if a rash develops.
- Wash hands immediately after application.
- Do not use with occlusive dressings.
- Avoid excess exposure of the treated area to sunlight as photosensitivity may increase.
- As absorption occurs, the same precautions with hypersensitivity to oral preparations should be observed, particularly when applying large amounts of topical NSAIDs.

Nefopam

- Urine may appear pink.
- Side effects include nervousness, palpitations, dry mouth, blurred vision and other sympathomimetic or antimuscarinic effects.

Gabapentin

See Chapter 24.

- Do not stop taking this medicine without the doctor's advice. Withdrawal should be gradual, over at least 1 week.
- Do not take indigestion remedies at the same time of day as this medicine.

Phenytoin and carbamazepine

See Chapter 24.

Opioids

- Opioids may cause drowsiness, so caution is needed when driving or operating machinery.
- Patients should avoid alcohol.
- Opioids may cause constipation. Laxatives are required with long-term treatment, preferably softeners and stimulants rather than bulk-forming agents.
- They may cause tolerance, requiring increasing doses during chronic treatment.
- Patients should avoid taking opioids regularly unless advised by a doctor or pharmacist, due to the risk of side effects, tolerance and dependence.

Self-assessment

Consider whether the following statements are true or false. In the management of pain:

1 Aspirin is the preferred NSAID.
2 Paracetamol is an effective analgesic but is not an NSAID.
3 Opioids are likely to cause constipation.
4 Amitriptyline is contraindicated in neuropathic pain.
5 Carbamazepine is used for acute pain.

Practice points

General

- Try paracetamol or ibuprofen first for mild-to-moderate pain. Patient counselling regarding the correct dose and effectiveness of paracetamol may help compliance.
- Analgesic combination products are not recommended because these products prevent the titration of individual drug doses. In addition, many combination products containing milder opioids with paracetamol or aspirin are no more effective than either drug alone when given as a single dose. Combination products may, however, be appropriate for the treatment of chronic pain and/or for patients with compliance problems.
- Chronic pain management should be managed 'by the mouth, by the clock and by the ladder', according to World Health Organization (1996) guidelines.

NSAIDs

- The use of two or more NSAIDs is not recommended and this includes low-dose aspirin. Low-dose aspirin should be combined with another NSAID only if absolutely necessary. Gastrointestinal protection with a proton pump inhibitor should be considered, particularly for elderly patients and when prescribing NSAIDs long term.
- Any benefits of COX-2 inhibitors are negated in combination with other NSAIDs, including low-dose aspirin.
- Allow up to a week to achieve the full analgesic effect of NSAIDs. The full anti-inflammatory effect may take up to 3 weeks at full doses.
- Aspirin should not be prescribed for children <16 years because of the risk of Reye's syndrome.
- The use of NSAIDs to treat postoperative pain may reduce the requirement for high doses of opioid analgesics.

Opioids

- Avoid regular use of opioids owing to tolerance, dependence, constipation and the risk of falls in elderly people. For severe pain, however, there is little risk of psychological dependence and the use of strong opioids is indicated (see Chapter 32).
- Regular opioid treatment should be accompanied by laxatives.

CASE STUDIES

Case 1

A patient complains that he is not having much pain relief with the co-codamol that you dispensed for him a week earlier for his osteoarthritis. He has been taking two tablets in the morning because he doesn't like to take too many. He has not tried paracetamol as he says 'it's not strong enough for this condition'.

How do you respond?

- A common misconception exists that paracetamol is effective to treat a headache or fever but little else. In fact, patients can be reassured that paracetamol is an extremely effective analgesic and relatively free from side effects. This is a suitable first choice in osteoarthritis and should be tried for at least a week of regular dosing. As this patient has not been taking regular co-codamol, it may be appropriate to try paracetamol 1 g four times a day alone for at least a week. He should be advised that he may need to take them regularly to control the pain.

Case 2

While performing a medication review, you come across the following record for an 80-year-old hypertensive female patient with 'painful knees':

dosulepin 75 mg twice daily
co-codamol 8/500 mg two up to four times daily
bendroflumethiazide 5 mg once daily.

How do you respond?

- The first consideration relates to the high risk of constipation with all three drugs. It is very likely that this patient will require treatment with laxatives such as a combination of lactulose solution (up to 15 mL twice daily) and senna tablets (1–2 at night as required). The dose of bendroflumethiazide is high for hypertension and may increase dehydration and subsequent electrolyte disturbances without a further reduction in blood pressure. Perhaps the addition of an alternative antihypertensive could be considered? The TCA may not be appropriate for this age group and a selective serotonin reuptake inhibitor (SSRI) may be more appropriate (see Chapter 25). Successful treatment of her depression is an important component of her pain management.
- Her analgesia should be reviewed, e.g. has she tried paracetamol alone at adequate doses?

Case 3

The following repeat prescription is for a 46-year-old woman:

diclofenac gel 1.16% apply three times daily 100 g
diclofenac sodium enteric-coated tablets 50 mg, take one three times daily
fluoxetine 20 mg capsules take one every morning

What should be the course of action?

- This patient is at risk of gastrotoxicity from the above prescription. SSRIs are associated with increased risk of bleeding events and using two NSAID preparations further increases this risk.
- The nature of her pain should be determined and pain control reviewed. Has paracetamol and/ or ibuprofen been used? A proton pump inhibitor should be considered if the diclofenac and fluoxetine are continued. Review the need for both diclofenac tablets and gel due to increased risk of side effects. Check for a history of peptic ulcer disease. Question the patient about signs and symptoms such as dyspepsia, gastric pain, dark stools and symptoms of anaemia.

References

Anon. (2000). The use of oral analgesics in primary care. *MeReC Bull* 11: 1–4.

British National Formulary, latest edition. London: British Medical Association and Royal Pharmaceutical Society of Great Britain.

Deeks JJ, Smith LA, Bradley MD (2002). Efficacy, tolerability, and upper gastrointestinal safety of celecoxib for treatment of osteoarthritis and rheumatoid arthritis: systematic review of randomised controlled trials. *BMJ* 325: 619–623. pmid: 12242171.

Finnerup NB, Attal N, Haroutounian S *et al.* (2015). Pharmacotherapy for neuropathic pain in adults: a systematic review and meta-analysis. *Lancet Neurol* 14(2): 162–173. pmid: 25575710.

Jüni P, Rutjes AWS, Dieppe PA (2002). Are selective COX 2 inhibitors superior to traditional non steroidal anti-inflammatory drugs? *BMJ* 324: 1287–1288. pmid: 12039807.

Lee A, Inch S, Finnigan D (2000). *Therapeutics in Pregnancy and Lactation*. Oxford: Radcliffe Medical Press.

Levy S, Volans G (2001). The use of analgesics in patients with asthma. *Drug Safety* 24: 829–841. pmid: 11665870.

Limmroth V, Katsarava Z, Fritsche G *et al.* (2002) Features of medication overuse headache following overuse of different headache drugs. *Neurology* 59: 1011–1014. pmid: 12370454.

Machado GC, Maher CG, Ferreira PH *et al.* (2014). Efficacy and safety of paracetamol for spinal pain and osteoarthritis: a systematic review and meta-analysis

of randomised placebo controlled trials. *BMJ* 350: 1225–1237.

Nielsen GL, Sorensen HT, Larsen H *et al.* (2001). Risk of adverse birth outcome and miscarriage in pregnant users of non-steroidal anti-inflammatory drugs: population based observational study and case–control study. *BMJ* 322: 266–270. pmid: 11157526.

Shaheen SO, Sterne JAC, Songhurst CE *et al.* (2000). Frequent paracetamol use and asthma in adults. *Thorax* 55: 266–270. pmid: 10722764.

Silberstein SD, Young WB (1995). Analgesic rebound headache. How great is the problem and what can be done? *Drug Safety* 13: 133–144. pmid: 7495500.

World Health Organization (1996). *Cancer Pain Relief, with a Guide to Opioid Availability*, 2nd edn. Geneva: WHO.

31

Musculoskeletal pain

Disorders of the muscles, joints and bones are a common cause of chronic illness and inability to work and have a considerable impact on quality of life. Musculoskeletal conditions include rheumatoid arthritis (RA), osteoarthritis, gout, muscle cramps and osteoporosis.

Disease characteristics and clinical features

Arthritis

Arthritis, literally inflammation of the joints, includes osteo- or rheumatoid types.

Osteoarthritis

Osteoarthritis is the most common form and is a degenerative disease of the joints due to wearing of articular cartilage with subsequent changes in the underlying bone. This may be secondary to obesity, fractures, dislocation, sports injuries, hyperparathyroidism, haemophilia, RA, gout or Paget's disease.

The pain of osteoarthritis differs from RA in that it usually occurs after exercise and at night. Any stiffness occurring in the morning tends to be transient. The pain may be present at rest and there is often tenderness. Joints of the feet (particularly the big toe), knees, hips, and cervical and lumbar spine are often affected. Diagnosis is usually by X-ray of painful joints, revealing a narrowing of the joint space due to loss of cartilage and the presence of osteosclerosis (increased bone density), osteocytes and cysts in the bone. There are no systemic (extra-articular) features.

Rheumatoid arthritis

RA is a chronic inflammatory condition affecting the synovial lining of the joints. Disease progression leads to ligament damage and erosion of bone: joints become deformed and tendons may rupture. RA tends to follow a relapsing–remitting course and is progressive.

The assessment of presenting symptoms of pain (see Chapter 30) includes the location of affected joints and timing of the pain, which is often worse in the morning and persists for an hour or more. The principal features include inflammation and swelling predominantly affecting the hands, wrists and knees. Symptoms progress to muscle wasting due to joint disuse, joint deformity and joint erosion. Extra-articular symptoms may also be present and include the following (Greene and Harris 2008):

- Non-specific: tiredness, depression and fever.
- Dermatological: nodules, palmar erythema (red palms), sweaty palms.

- Circulatory: Raynaud's syndrome, pericarditis, myocarditis, vasculitis, anaemia.
- Ophthalmic: keratoconjunctivitis sicca (dryness of the cornea and conjunctiva due to reduced production of tears), episcleritis (inflammation of the episclera resulting in painful red eyes sensitive to light) or scleritis (inflammation of the white of the eye).
- Neurological: trapped nerves, peripheral neuropathy.
- Pulmonary: lung nodules, pleurisy and pulmonary fibrosis.

RA is an autoimmune disease with rheumatoid factors (autoantibodies against immunoglobulin G) detected in serum. Radiological changes are also observed. The erythrocyte sedimentation rate (ESR) is elevated (see Chapter 2).

Gout

Gout occurs due to the overproduction of purines, resulting in acute arthritis. The metabolism of purines leads to the production of uric acid, which forms urate crystals in joints, particularly affecting the big toe (podagra). This triggers an inflammatory response. Gout may also occur as an adverse drug reaction (ADR; see Chapter 6), particularly due to thiazides, which impair the excretion of uric acid. Disorders such as heart failure, hypercalcaemia and hypertensive nephropathy are also associated with gout.

Gout presents with inflammation and joint pain affecting the big toe and may also affect the ankles, knees, elbows, wrists and fingers. The skin of the affected joint may flake after the initial onset of pain. The attack may resolve spontaneously after a few days or weeks. Laboratory tests reveal hyperuricaemia, although this is occasionally present with arthritic conditions.

Osteoporosis

Osteoporosis is a disorder of bone structure with a characteristic reduction of bone mass resulting in brittle bones at increased risk of fracture. Bone is constantly being absorbed by osteoclasts and new bone is formed by osteoblasts. In osteoporosis, absorption exceeds formation, with reductions in bone matrix and therefore strength. Causes include oestrogen deficiency, particularly after an early menopause, and age-related degeneration of bone, declining from a peak in the 20s. There are hereditary and lifestyle components and the most common drug cause is corticosteroids.

Osteoporosis may be asymptomatic, being diagnosed after fracture. Patients presenting with a fracture resulting from minimal trauma, also known as 'low trauma' fracture, are treated for osteoporosis and further investigations may not be necessary, because management is the same. Bone density scans (commonly dual energy X-ray absorptiometry or DEXA scans) are useful for early diagnosis and are increasingly performed for patients with risk factors for osteoporosis as follows:

- early menopause (<45 years of age); also prolonged secondary amenorrhoea
- aged >65 years
- family history of osteoporosis or low trauma fractures
- poor diet (lacking in calcium and vitamin D)
- low exposure to sunlight (reduced vitamin D)
- low body weight (body mass index or BMI <20)
- smoking
- excess alcohol intake
- low level of physical activity
- concurrent disease should be considered and treated (hyperthyroidism, hyperparathyroidism, osteomalacia or hypogonadism)
- drugs (corticosteroids: more than the equivalent of 7.5 mg of prednisolone daily for 3 months or more).

Pharmacological basis of management

The management of musculoskeletal conditions predominantly involves the relief of pain and the reduction of inflammation. In treating osteoporosis, lifestyle factors are also important and treatment may include the correction of calcium and vitamin D intake. Additional treatments target the mineralisation of bone using bisphosphonates, anti-oestrogens and oestrogens. Bisphosphonates reduce bone turnover and oestrogens and anti-oestrogens target and reduce the resorption of bone.

The pharmacology of analgesics, including non-steroidal anti-inflammatory drugs (NSAIDs), cyclo-oxygenase-2 (COX-2) inhibitors and topical counterirritants, together with non-pharmacological options, is discussed in Chapter 30.

Osteoarthritis

Osteoarthritis involves joint degeneration and may be improved by lifestyle measures such as weight reduction and increased exercise. Paracetamol is used first line, particularly in elderly people, followed by topical then oral NSAIDs with or without paracetamol. Topical capsaicin may provide relief. Advanced osteoarthritis may require full doses of NSAIDs. It should be noted, however, that NSAIDs do not alter the disease process and are mainly used for their analgesic effects. The benefits of NSAIDs are therefore compared with the risks, such as gastrointestinal toxicity (see Chapter 8), and alternative interventions such as lifestyle measures may be preferred (see Chapter 30).

Rheumatoid arthritis

NSAIDs are used for symptomatic treatment of pain associated with inflammation in RA and corticosteroids are occasionally injected locally into the affected joints, providing temporary relief. Disease-modifying antirheumatoid drugs (DMARDs) such as penicillamine, gold salts or antimalarials are used to suppress the disease process. These drugs are given for 4–6 months before a full response is observed. This may allow a subsequent reduction in the dose of NSAID. Sulfasalazine or methotrexate may be tolerated better than alternative DMARDs.

Disease-modifying antirheumatoid drugs

NSAIDs control the symptoms associated with RA but do not alter the disease progression and may even make it worse due to the increased availability of arachidonic acid as a substrate for lipoxygenase-mediated production of leukotrienes. DMARDs are therefore used to slow disease progression and include:

- gold compounds
- penicillamine

- sulfasalazine
- methotrexate
- chloroquine
- hydroxychloroquine.

Their mechanisms of action are complex and are yet to be fully elucidated. Immunosuppressants such as azathioprine, ciclosporin and corticosteroids are also used as DMARDs.

Corticosteroids

These drugs are used in the treatment of RA, e.g. when treatment with other anti-inflammatory drugs is unsuccessful. If long-term treatment is required, prophylaxis for the prevention of osteoporosis is required (see below). Courses of corticosteroids should use the lowest effective dose, e.g. 7.5 mg prednisolone. This is sufficient to reduce the rate of joint destruction in patients with moderate-to-severe disease that has been present for <2 years. Prednisolone treatment is required for 2–4 years for beneficial effects on joint destruction, before gradual dose reduction to prevent long-term adverse effects. It should also be noted that the effects of reduced joint destruction persist despite a possible reduction in symptom control, which may occur after 6–12 months, and this does not necessarily indicate a higher dose of prednisolone.

Cytokine modulators: etanercept, adalimumab and infliximab

These are newer immunomodulatory drugs, which have been introduced for severe refractory disease that has not responded to at least two other DMARDs, including methotrexate, and their use is restricted to rheumatologists. Etanercept is a fusion protein which binds to tumour necrosis factor α (TNF-α) and leads to its inactivation. Infliximab and adalimumab are monoclonal antibodies to TNF-α and so reduce its action in inflammation. These agents may be used alongside methotrexate or, in the case of etanercept and adalimumab, as monotherapy.

Osteoporosis

Agents used for the prevention or treatment of osteoporosis include bisphosphonates, vitamin D derivatives, hormone replacement therapy (HRT), calcitonin and selective oestrogen receptor modulators (SERMs).

It is also important that concurrent medication and other risk factors for falls are assessed in these patients and that preventive counselling includes advice about diet and exercise (see Counselling, below), e.g. concurrent diseases that may increase the risk of falls include hypothyroidism, epilepsy, diabetes mellitus, Ménière's disease and cardiovascular disease (particularly with a history of transient ischaemic attacks or arrhythmias). Drugs associated with an increased risk of falls, particularly in elderly patients, include:

- diuretics
- other antihypertensives, particularly α blockers, and the concurrent use of angiotensin-converting enzyme (ACE) inhibitors with diuretics
- antipsychotics
- benzodiazepines, sedating antihistamines and other drugs with sedative properties (see Chapter 6)
- alcohol.

Bisphosphonates (alendronic acid, etidronate, risedronate)

Bisphosphonates are now considered a first-line treatment for osteoporosis. They reduce the risk of vertebral fracture (alendronic acid and risedronate have been shown to reduce the risk of non-vertebral fractures) by reducing the turnover of bone. These drugs are enzyme-resistant analogues of pyrophosphate and, by binding to hydroxyapatite crystals, slow dissolution. They also inhibit osteoblast-mediated resorption.

Vitamin D and its derivatives

Vitamin D and derivatives, together with parathyroid hormone, cytokines and calcitonin, are involved in the metabolism and mineralisation of bone. Vitamin D requirements are met through diet, metabolism in the liver and kidney, and from reactions in the skin occurring in the presence of sunlight. The supplementation of vitamin D is partly dependent on the cause of deficiency, as follows:

- Poor diet or malabsorption is treated with supplements of vitamin D_2 (ergocalciferol), which is formed in plants, or vitamin D_3 (colecalciferol), formed in the skin in the presence of ultraviolet radiation. High doses (up to 1 mg or 40 000 units daily) of ergocalciferol are required by patients

with intestinal malabsorption or chronic liver disease.
- In renal failure, 1,25-dihydroxyvitamin D_3 (calcitriol) or 1α-hydroxycholecalciferol (alfacalcidol) is given. Deficiency would otherwise result because these hydroxylated compounds are usually formed in the kidney.

Hormone replacement therapy

Both HRT and bisphosphonates are indicated for the treatment of osteoporosis. Oestrogens have a protective effect on bone by preventing bone resorption. Postmenopausal women may benefit from HRT prophylaxis for osteoporosis, particularly after an early menopause. However, their use is limited due to increased cardiovascular risk (notably stroke) and certain cancers when used long term.

Tibolone

Tibolone possesses mixed oestrogenic, progestogenic and androgenic effects, and is used for the prevention of hot flushes and bone loss. This is given at least 1 year after the menopause because of problems with irregular bleeding. If the patient is to be changed from cyclical HRT, a withdrawal bleed is induced using progestogens, given until the withdrawal bleed has stopped. This minimises the risk of irregular bleeding during tibolone therapy.

Raloxifene

Raloxifene is an SERM used to treat osteoporosis. This is an analogue of tamoxifen, developed after the observation that, despite possessing anti-oestrogen activity, tamoxifen produces agonist-like oestrogenic activity in bone, because it is a partial agonist.

Prevention of osteoporosis

The first step in the prevention of osteoporosis is to identify patients who are at risk, as outlined above. Interventions such as lifestyle changes may then be addressed and the need for drug treatment considered, e.g. calcium and vitamin D intake is corrected by supplementation and HRT initiated for female patients, particularly after premature menopause. Treatment is continued for up to 5 years. This is a highly effective intervention for the prevention or treatment of osteoporosis. It should also be noted when prescribing HRT that:

- women with an intact uterus should be given HRT containing a progestogen to reduce the risk of endometrial cancer
- after a hysterectomy, a progestogen is not required
- oestrogens are contraindicated for patients with previous oestrogen-receptor-positive breast cancer.

When bisphosphonates are not appropriate (Table 31.1), HRT may be prescribed. It should be noted that disodium etidronate administration is alternated with calcium carbonate (Didronel PMO) because it can increase the risk of fractures due to reduced calcification of bone. Raloxifene is licensed for prophylaxis of postmenopausal osteoporosis. Further lifestyle interventions are outlined below (see Counselling).

Prevention of corticosteroid-induced osteoporosis

It is recognised that treatment with corticosteroids equivalent to more than 7.5 mg prednisolone daily for 3 months or more constitutes a risk factor for the development of osteoporosis. Such patients may benefit from a DEXA scan and may require treatment as indicated above, particularly in the presence of additional risk factors. Drugs with the best evidence to support their use for preventing corticosteroid-induced osteoporosis appear to be the bisphosphonates (Adachi and Papaioannou 2001). The American College of Rheumatism (Buckley et al. 2001) recommendations include the use of calcium and vitamin D supplements for all patients taking corticosteroids.

Current recommendations by the British Society for Rheumatology (see Online resources, below) are that patients prescribed a 3-month course (or longer) of the equivalent of 7.5 mg prednisolone daily should be offered treatment for the prevention of osteoporosis after the results of a DEXA scan. It is suggested that a DEXA scan revealing a T-score (number of standard deviations from the value of peak bone density of a 25- to 30-year-old woman) of −1.5 or less would indicate preventive treatment.

Gout

The treatment of gout involves the use of NSAIDs, with the exception of aspirin, which reduces urate excretion and ibuprofen due to its weak anti-inflammatory activity. Additional treatment may include allopurinol, colchicine, sulfinpyrazone and probenecid.

Table 31.1 Some considerations of the effects of concurrent conditions on drug choice in musculoskeletal conditions

Disease	Drug(s)	Comments
IHD	Colchicine, sulfinpyrazone, HRT	<ul><li>Sulfinpyrazone may cause salt and water retention and should therefore be used with caution</li><li>HRT is not indicated for the prevention of ischaemic heart disease (Chapter 15)</li></ul>
Upper gastrointestinal disorders: dysphagia, oesophagitis, gastritis, duodenitis or ulcers	Alendronic acid and risedronate sodium	May cause or exacerbate these disorders (Chapter 8)
Delayed gastric emptying	Alendronic acid and risedronate sodium	Contraindicated
Peptic ulcer disease	Sulfinpyrazone	Use with caution
Gastrointestinal disease	Colchicine	Use with caution since colchicine may exacerbate all gastrointestinal disease
Hypocalcaemia	Alendronic acid, risedronate sodium	Contraindicated
Venous thromboembolism	HRT, raloxifene	<ul><li>HRT is contraindicated in patients with a history of confirmed venous thromboembolism, active or recent arterial thromboembolic disease</li><li>Raloxifene also increases the risk of thromboembolism</li></ul>

HRT, hormone replacement therapy.

Acute gout

Acute gout is treated with high doses of NSAIDs including diclofenac, indometacin, ketoprofen, naproxen, piroxicam and sulindac. Allopurinol should not be initiated during or within 1 month of an acute attack because it may prolong the attack. The manufacturers recommend that prophylaxis with an NSAID or colchicine be given for the first month of treatment because allopurinol may precipitate a further attack. Patients already taking allopurinol when suffering an exacerbation should continue treatment.

Weight loss and dietary measures are also important (see Counselling below).

Chronic gout

The long-term management of gout includes prophylaxis with allopurinol or colchicine (short term only during initial treatment with allopurinol) and the reduction of inflammation by NSAIDs during an acute exacerbation.

Allopurinol

Allopurinol is a xanthine oxidase inhibitor and reduces the synthesis of uric acid.

Colchicine

The mechanism of action of colchicine in the treatment of gout involves inhibition of leukocyte migration into the joint by reducing the production of chemotaxins.

Sulfinpyrazone and probenecid

Sulfinpyrazone and probenecid inhibit uric acid reabsorption by the kidneys, thereby increasing excretion.

Nocturnal leg cramps

Quinine salts are used for nocturnal leg cramps but are effective only in a small proportion of patients, e.g. quinine sulphate or quinine bisulphate is given. It should be noted that quinine disulphate 300 mg contains less quinine than 300 mg quinine sulphate.

Concurrent disease

Some considerations are summarised in Table 31.1.

Drug interactions

Table 31.2 highlights some important drug interactions involving drugs used to treat musculoskeletal disorders. For interactions associated with NSAIDs, see Chapter 30.

Monitoring requirements

More detailed monitoring information is produced by the British Society for Rheumatology (see Online resources below).

Penicillamine

A full blood count (FBC) and urine (protein) should be monitored before the start of treatment, every 1–2 weeks for 2 months, every 4 weeks, and the week after a dose increase. In the presence of proteinuria, urea and electrolytes and 24-hour urine are tested (see Chapter 2).

Sulfasalazine

- Monitor differential white cell, red cell and platelet counts initially and at monthly intervals for the first 3 months.
- Liver function tests (LFTs) should be monitored monthly for the first 3 months.
- Renal function should be monitored at regular intervals.

Methotrexate

- Carry out an FBC, renal function tests and LFTs before starting treatment and repeat weekly until therapy is stabilised, then every 2–3 months. See also Counselling below.
- Treatment should not be started or should be discontinued if any abnormality of LFTs or liver biopsy is present or develops during treatment. Abnormalities return to normal after 2 weeks and treatment may be restarted if appropriate.
- Risk factors for haematopoietic suppression include advanced age, renal impairment and concomitant treatment with a second antifolate drug.

Gold

- Urine tests and FBCs (including total and differential white cell and platelet counts) should be performed before treatment is started and before each intramuscular injection.

Table 31.2 Some drug interactions involving drugs used in musculoskeletal conditions

Drugs	Consequences	Comments
Alendronic acid with antacids and calcium supplements	Reduced absorption	Separate the administration of alendronate from calcium supplements and antacids by at least 30 minutes
Penicillamine with aluminium or magnesium-containing antacids and iron salts		• Separate the administration of penicillamine by 2 hours • Caution if iron is withdrawn when patients are stabilised on penicillamine, due to risk of toxicity
Allopurinol with theophylline	Increased levels of theophylline	There is limited evidence for this interaction but monitoring for signs of theophylline toxicity is recommended
Alendronic acid with NSAIDs	Risk of severe oesophagitis	Avoid concurrent use
Allopurinol with warfarin	Increased bleeding	This interaction is reported to be uncommon but monitoring is prudent
Calcium and vitamin D supplements or corticosteroids with thiazide diuretics	Increased risk of hypercalcaemia or hypokalaemia	• Thiazides retain calcium and therefore monitoring of plasma calcium may be required (Chapter 2) • Increased risk of hypokalaemia if thiazides are given with corticosteroids (Chapter 2)
Quinine with digoxin	Small risk of increased levels of digoxin	Monitor for signs of digoxin toxicity
Methotrexate with NSAIDs	Reduced excretion and therefore increased risk of methotrexate toxicity	• Increased risk with higher doses of methotrexate and/or impaired renal function • Careful monitoring is recommended
Methotrexate with corticosteroids	• Increased risk of methotrexate toxicity • Possible steroid-sparing effect	Monitor for signs of methotrexate toxicity or reduced efficacy of corticosteroids
Methotrexate with co-trimoxazole or trimethoprim	Risk of severe bone marrow depression	Avoid concurrent use or monitor full blood count closely
Penicillamine with digoxin	Limited reports of reduced levels of digoxin	Monitor for signs of reduced efficacy (Chapter 16)

NSAIDs, non-steroidal anti-inflammatory drugs.

• During oral treatment, urine and blood tests are carried out monthly.
• The occurrence of blood disorders or proteinuria (repeatedly >300 mg/L and without urinary tract infection) necessitates withdrawal of treatment.

Antimalarials

• Measure renal and liver function before starting treatment.
• Monitor visual changes.

Corticosteroids

Monitoring during treatment with corticosteroids may include blood pressure, urinary glucose, weight gain, bone density, visual changes and lung function.

Sulfinpyrazone

Regular blood counts are recommended.

Etanercept, adalimumab and infliximab

Patients should be tested for tuberculosis before treatment.

Vitamin D supplements (e.g. ergocalciferol, calcitriol)

All patients receiving vitamin D supplements for the prevention and treatment of osteoporosis should have their plasma calcium levels monitored weekly when treatment is initiated, and then at regular intervals and when presenting with nausea and vomiting, which may suggest hypercalcaemia. Breast milk from mothers taking vitamin D supplements may also cause hypercalcaemia in the infant.

Disodium etidronate

Serum phosphate and alkaline phosphatase (and urinary hydroxyproline) should be measured before starting treatment and then every 3 months.

Alendronic acid and risedronate sodium

Hypocalcaemia and vitamin D deficiency should be corrected before initiating treatment.

Renal function

The following points are intended to highlight drugs to be used with caution in renal impairment:

- Allopurinol: dose adjustment is required in moderate-to-severe renal failure. There may be increased toxicity and rashes.
- Methotrexate: dose adjustment is required.
- Penicillamine is nephrotoxic and should be avoided if possible, or the dose reduced.
- Sulfasalazine should be avoided in severe renal failure. In moderate failure, there is an increased risk of toxicity, including crystalluria. A high fluid intake is therefore required.
- Antimalarials: use with caution.

- Alendronic acid or risedronate sodium is not recommended if creatinine clearance is <35 mL/minute.
- Disodium etidronate should be avoided in moderate-to-severe renal impairment or administered at a reduced dosage in mild impairment.

Hepatic function

The following points are intended to highlight drugs to be used with caution in hepatic disease:

- Methotrexate: dose-related toxicity, avoid in non-malignant conditions.
- Allopurinol: reduce dose.
- Gold: avoid in severe liver disease.
- Antimalarials: use with caution.

Pregnancy

Table 31.3 summarises examples of issues associated with drug use for musculoskeletal conditions during pregnancy. For information about NSAIDs, the reader is referred to Chapter 30.

Over-the-counter considerations

The availability of analgesic preparations over-the-counter is discussed in Chapter 30. In relation to musculoskeletal disorders, pharmacists are ideally placed to refer conditions such as suspected RA for prompt assessment and prescribing of higher doses of

Table 31.3 Some considerations of drug use in pregnancy		
Drug	**Trimester of risk**	**Comment**
DMARDs	3	Sulfasalazine is the DMARD of choice in pregnancy
Bisphosphonates	All	Contraindicated
Colchicine	All	Contraindicated
Corticosteroids		• Assess risk of not treating. Commonly used in asthma and inflammatory bowel disease during pregnancy • Risk of neonatal adrenal suppression with long-term high-dose treatment
Antimalarials	All	Hydroxychloroquine and chloroquine (except in malaria prophylaxis) should be avoided in pregnancy and breastfeeding

DMARDs, disease-modifying antirheumatic drugs.

anti-inflammatory agents and/or DMARDs. The provision of lifestyle advice may benefit conditions such as gout, migraine and general painful conditions. Pharmacists may also provide a screening service for osteoporosis as part of the multidisciplinary healthcare team.

Although widely used by patients with osteoarthritis, the supplements chondroitin and glucosamine are not recommended by the National Institute for Health and Care Excellence guidelines (NICE 2008).

Counselling

Patient counselling should comprise a combination of lifestyle factors, including advice about diet and exercise, together with information relating to drug treatment. Careful exercise is important to improve joint mobility, muscle strength, aerobic fitness and function, with the aim of promoting both physical and psychological health without worsening any fatigue or joint symptoms. This is also important in elderly people to prevent falls.

Osteoporosis

- Patients with risk factors for developing osteoporosis should maintain a high intake of calcium and vitamin D (milk, Cheddar cheese, Edam, yogurt, canned sardines and whitebait), e.g. half a litre (1 pint) of semi-skimmed milk or 100 g (4 oz) of Cheddar cheese contains 700–800 mg calcium. Supplements of calcium should be considered when a risk of deficiency is recognised, such as in strict vegetarians. Vitamin D should be included for the housebound and others with low exposure to sunlight.
- Recommended intakes of calcium and vitamin D are as follows:
  - calcium:
       males 11–18: 1000 mg daily
       females 11–18: 800 mg daily
       adults 19+ years: 700 mg daily
  - vitamin D: 400 iu daily.
- Weight-bearing exercise should be emphasised, particularly to women in their 20s, and immobility should be avoided. Exercise programmes are useful for patients with osteoporosis in building muscle strength, general wellbeing and improving posture, thereby reducing the risk of further fractures.

- Patients should stop smoking and avoid excess alcohol intake.
- Excess dieting and vigorous exercise routines, which result in amenorrhoea, should also be avoided by women of all ages.
- Hip protectors may help prevent hip fractures in elderly patients.

Bisphosphonates

- Bisphosphonates may cause gastrointestinal disturbance, oesophagitis (particularly alendronic acid) and occasionally bone pain.
- Premenopausal women initiated on bisphosphonates should be counselled about the appropriate use of contraception.

Alendronic acid

- Alendronic acid may be administered as a weekly dose.
- Patients should stop taking alendronate if they develop symptoms of oesophageal ulceration, e.g. dysphagia, dyspepsia, pain on swallowing or retrosternal pain.
- Tablets should be swallowed whole with a tumbler full of water while standing and not immediately before rising or retiring to bed.
- Tablets should be taken 30 minutes before breakfast (and other medication) and patients advised to remain standing or to sit upright for at least 30 minutes. Patients should not lie down until after breakfast.

Risedronate

- Food, particularly calcium-containing food (milk), iron and mineral supplements and antacids should be avoided for at least 2 hours before and after tablets are taken.
- Tablets are usually taken 30 minutes before breakfast (and other medication).
- Patient should remain standing or sit upright for at least 30 minutes. Patients should not take the tablets before rising or at bedtime.

Disodium etidronate

Food and milk should be avoided for at least 2 hours before and after tablets are taken.

Vitamin D

Excess intake may lead to hypercalcaemia, including symptoms of constipation, depression, nausea and vomiting, polyuria and polydipsia, weakness and fatigue. These symptoms should be reported to the prescriber.

NSAIDs

See Chapter 30.

Topical counterirritants (capsaicin)

See Chapter 30.

Quinine salts for nocturnal leg cramps

- Stretching the affected muscle regularly may reduce leg cramps.
- Take quinine salts for up to 4 weeks before improvement is observed.
- Reassess every 3 months.
- Caution is required because quinine is extremely toxic and has caused fatalities in children.

Allopurinol

- The affected joint should be rested.
- Avoid purine-rich food, including offal, anchovies, sardines, herring, mackerel, shrimps, crab, fish roes and meat extract.
- Reduce intake of protein.
- Maintain an adequate fluid intake of 2–3 L/day. This reduces plasma urate levels and prevents the formation of renal urate stones.
- Try to limit alcohol intake to 1 unit/day. Alcohol reduces the solubility of urate and beer contains high levels of purines.
- Gradual weight loss may improve symptoms. Avoid overeating.
- Take with or after food with plenty of water.
- Do not stop taking allopurinol unless advised by the prescriber.

Colchicine

- Dietary advice is as for allopurinol.
- Take until either pain is relieved or vomiting and diarrhoea occur, or a maximum dose of 6 mg has been reached (12 tablets of 500 micrograms).

Sulfinpyrazone

- Maintain an adequate fluid intake of 2–3 L/day.
- Take with or after food.
- Do not take with aspirin.

Penicillamine

- Penicillamine may cause nausea, so take 30–60 minutes before food or on retiring to bed.
- Do not take indigestion remedies or medicines containing iron or zinc at the same time of day as this medicine.
- The dose will be increased gradually.
- Penicillamine may cause loss of taste after 6 weeks' treatment, but taste will then return.
- Mineral supplements are not recommended during penicillamine treatment.
- Report sore throat, fever, infection, unexplained bleeding and bruising, purpura, mouth ulcers, metallic taste or rash to the doctor immediately.
- Penicillamine may cause rashes in the first few months of treatment. These should disappear when the drug is stopped, allowing reintroduction at a lower dose and gradually increasing. Later rashes may require cessation of treatment.
- Patients who are allergic to penicillin may also be hypersensitive to penicillamine, although this is rare.

Sulfasalazine

- Report unexplained bleeding, bruising or purpura, sore throat, fever or malaise. These symptoms are most likely to occur in the first 3–6 months of treatment.
- Sulfasalazine may cause rashes and gastrointestinal intolerance. Upper gastrointestinal intolerance is common at doses >4 g/day.
- Contact lenses may be stained.
- Urine may be coloured orange.

Methotrexate

- Treatment is taken weekly. This is an important safety issue and all prescriptions for methotrexate that are not for a weekly dose should be queried.
- Folic acid supplement 5 mg weekly will reduce side effects resulting from folic acid deficiency.

- Contact the doctor immediately with breathlessness or cough.
- Do not take over-the-counter (OTC) aspirin or ibuprofen without the prescriber's advice.
- Pregnancy: avoid conception (this applies to males and females) for at least 6 months after stopping treatment.

Gold

- Report sore throat, fever, infection, unexplained bleeding and bruising, purpura, mouth ulcers, metallic taste or rash to the doctor immediately.
- Also report breathlessness or cough immediately.
- Rashes with pruritus often occur after 2–6 months of intramuscular treatment and may require cessation of treatment.
- The most common side effect of oral therapy, diarrhoea, with or without nausea or abdominal pain, may respond to bulking agents or temporary dose reduction.
- Stop treatment at least 6 months before conception.

Antimalarials

- Report any visual disturbances.
- Do not take indigestion remedies at the same time of day.

Etanercept, adalimumab and infliximab (an alert card should be provided)

- Be vigilant for signs of serious infections (such as tuberculosis)

Etanercept

- Report any signs of infection or increased bleeding.

Infliximab

- Its use may be associated with a hypersensitivity reaction.
- Patients should always keep their alert card with them and be aware that hypersensitivity reactions may be delayed.

Corticosteroids

See Chapter 22.

Self-assessment

Consider whether the following statements are true or false. In the management of arthritis:

1 Paracetamol is considered as a first-line treatment for osteoarthritis.
2 Paracetamol should not be combined with NSAIDs.
3 Methotrexate is effective in osteoarthritis.
4 Patients taking methotrexate should be counselled to avoid self-medicating with OTC NSAIDs.
5 Infliximab is now recommended as first-line treatment for rheumatoid arthritis.

Practice points

- For NSAIDs, see Chapter 30.
- Methotrexate is given as a *weekly* dose.
- To reduce the risk of corticosteroid-induced osteoporosis, doses should be low and the course duration as short as possible. Long-term use of inhaled steroids may also reduce bone mineral density.
- Early intervention to prevent osteoporosis is important for patients prescribed corticosteroids because the greatest loss of bone occurs in the first 6–12 months.
- Prophylaxis for the prevention of osteoporosis should be considered alongside additional risk factors in patients prescribed the equivalent of 7.5 mg prednisolone or more daily for 3 months or more, and particularly in patients aged >65 years. Otherwise, a bone scan should be offered if treatment is likely to be continued for 6 months or longer.
- Patients suffering a fracture after relatively low trauma should be treated as for osteoporosis.
- Patients aged >65 years and those with low exposure to sunlight may be advised to take supplements of vitamin D (400 iu daily). Calcium supplements are indicated

(continued)

(continued)

if requirements are not met by the diet. Calcium and vitamin D supplements are recommended for all frail elderly people, including those at home, in hospital or in nursing or residential homes.

- The effects of calcium are less than HRT or other agents in the prevention and treatment of osteoporosis.
- Exclude vitamin D deficiency and secondary hyperparathyroidism in elderly patients with osteoporosis or osteomalacia.

CASE STUDY

A 45 year-woman has been diagnosed with rheumatoid arthritis and is initially managed on diclofenac (75 mg b.d.).

What are the clinical features of rheumatoid arthritis?

- RA is a chronic inflammatory condition affecting the synovial lining of the joints.
- Disease progression leads to ligament damage and erosion of bone: joints become deformed and tendons may rupture.
- RA tends to follow a relapsing, remitting course and is progressive.
- The principal features include inflammation and swelling predominantly affecting the hands, wrists and knees. Symptoms progress to muscle wasting due to joint disuse, joint deformity and joint erosion. Extra-articular symptoms may also be present.

Her doctor prescribes methotrexate (7.5 mg o.d.)

What tests are required before treatment is started?

- Full blood count
- Chest X-ray
- Renal function
- Liver function tests

How would you respond to this prescription?

- Methotrexate *must* always be prescribed a weekly dose.
- The prescriber should be contacted to ensure that it is changed to a weekly dose.
- NSAIDs such as diclofenac may interact with methotrexate, leading to increased plasma concentrations and toxicity. This interaction should be discussed with the doctor, as NSAIDs are commonly prescribed by rheumatologists alongside methotrexate but with caution and monitoring. A key problem occurs when patients self-medicate with NSAIDs and they should be counselled to avoid this.

A year later, her consultant would like to add infliximab to therapy.

What is the mechanism of action of infliximab?

- Monoclonal antibody to TNF-α

At her second infusion, she developed breathlessness and an itchy rash.

What appears to have happened and how should it be managed?

- Hypersensitivity reaction which should be managed by adrenaline, oxygen, an antihistamine and a steroid.

References

Adachi JD, Papaioannou A (2001). Corticosteroid-induced osteoporosis – detection and management. *Drug Safety* 24: 607–624. pmid: 11480493.

Greene RJ, Harris ND (2008). *Pathology and Therapeutics for Pharmacists*, 3rd edn London: Pharmaceutical Press.

National Institute for Health and Care Excellence (2008). *Osteoarthritis: The care and management of osteoarthritis in adults.* Clinical Guideline 59. London: NICE.

Online resources

www.nos.org.uk

The National Osteoporosis Society is a charity providing information for both patients and healthcare professionals. The main aims are to improve the diagnosis, prevention and treatment of osteoporosis (accessed October 2015).

www.rheumatology.org.uk

The website of the British Society for Rheumatology with access to latest guidelines, including recommendations for monitoring requirements (accessed October 2015).

PART **H**

Cancer

32

The cancer patient and chemotherapy

After cardiovascular disease, neoplastic disease or cancer represents the next largest cause of mortality, with more than one in three people developing cancer in their lifetime and one in four people dying as a result of it. The treatment of cancers is a highly specialised area and the aim of this chapter is to give an overview of cancer treatments.

Causes of cancer

Cancers involve the uncontrolled multiplication of cells with replication of altered or damaged DNA. There may be the loss of essential genes (including loss of tumour suppressors), the inactivation of cell cycle regulators and prevention of apoptosis leading to the uncontrolled proliferation of cells. This may lead to a primary tumour at the initial site but cancerous cells can invade locally, spread to the local lymph nodes and then to distant sites via metastasis. It is this latter event which is often associated with the terminal disease.

The causes of cancer are multifactorial and factors include DNA damage, environmental factors, genetic factors, smoking, alcohol, diet, obesity and viruses. Lifestyle factors have a clear association, for

example, approximately 90% of lung cancers are due to smoking.

Prevention, detection and screening

The primary aim is to reduce the risk of cancer by lifestyle changes such as smoking cessation and a healthy diet (see Chapter 3) and improved screening. Cancers may affect many organs and tissues within the body: cancers of the lungs, skin, breast and gastrointestinal tract are the most common. The outcome of cancer treatment varies between the sites affected and the stage at presentation, e.g. lung cancer has a very poor 5-year survival rate because it often presents at a late stage when it has spread via metastasis (in general this means spread to distant sites, including the liver, brain, lungs and bone). By contrast, treatment of testicular cancer often has a high cure rate if detected early. Healthcare professionals therefore have an important role in the education of patients to recognise and report serious symptoms early (see Chapter 1). This is particularly important for patients with additional risk factors such as a family history of breast or bowel cancer, and these patients should be encouraged to undertake regular screening. Interventions include the following:

- The provision of information relating to the importance of self-examination for lumps of the breast, testicles, neck or armpits.
- To alleviate fear and encourage early referral to improve outcome.
- To encourage patients to attend screening such as cervical smears and mammograms, and to discuss concerns with healthcare professionals.
- To educate patients about the risk of skin cancer and the importance of protecting skin from the sun, particularly for those with fair skin (see Chapter 36). Vigilance of changes to moles suggestive of melanoma is also important.
- To educate patients to recognise other warning symptoms such as sudden unexplained weight loss, rectal bleeding or haemoptysis (see Chapter 1).
- Routine screening of stool samples for early detection of colorectal cancers.
- Future screening may include screening for ovarian cancers.

Goals of treatment

The clear and ultimate goal of treatment is cure with eradication of the cancer and where this is not possible treatment is used to reduce the tumour load, increase cancer-free survival time and relieve symptoms. The outcome for cancers varies considerably between cancer types and location and survival is quantified in terms of 5- or 10-year survival rates.

According to Cancer Research UK, the 5-year survival rate (2010–11) for the following cancers were:

	5-Year survival rate (%)
Solid tumours	
• Testicular	98%
• Breast	87%
• Prostate	85%
• Bowel	59%
• Ovary	46%
• Brain	19%

• Stomach	19%
• Oesophagus	15%
• Lung	10%
• Pancreatic	3%
Haematological tumours	
• Hodgkin's lymphoma	85%
• Leukaemias	52%

Principles of treatment

Treatment of cancer is usually by hospital specialists and is divided into surgery, chemotherapy and radiotherapy. The aim of surgery is to remove the tumour and, if the tumour is localised, this may be curative. Surgery may also be used palliatively, e.g. to remove obstructions, or even preventively, such as the removal of a second breast in women at very high risk of the recurrence of breast cancer.

Types of treatment

Current treatments include surgical removal of the tumour for cure or symptomatic relief, and chemotherapy to kill rapidly dividing cells to reduce tumour load and kill cancerous cells which may have spread to a distant site. Radiotherapy involves the use of localised high energy radiation to kill tumour cells. Biological therapy involves the use of advanced biological molecules to specifically target markers or biochemical pathways associated with cancer cells. A number of tumours and their growth are enhanced by hormones, for example, some forms of breast cancer and some forms of prostate cancers are sensitive to sex hormones, and modifying hormonal action with receptor antagonists and synthase inhibitors is used to reduce cell growth. In certain haematological cancers, and usually in conjunction with chemotherapy and whole body irradiation, stem cell transplantation of bone marrow is used curatively.

Cancer chemotherapy

In the treatment of cancers, chemotherapy may be curative, e.g. in the treatment of testicular cancer, or may be used to kill leukaemia cells before bone marrow transplantation leading to a cure. Chemotherapy may be used in addition to surgery, e.g. after the removal of a solid tumour, courses of anticancer chemotherapy may be used to prevent recurrence or suppress the growth of any metastases. It may also be used in palliation to reduce tumour size or growth and to prolong life. There are a number of chemotherapeutic agents and these are often used in specific combinations, generally involving three agents. The purpose of using combinations is to attack different pharmacological targets and so limit the development of resistance. Aside from the conventional agents mentioned above, newer approaches include the use of monoclonal antibodies, which selectively target certain cell types, e.g. rituximab targets B lymphocytes and is used in non-Hodgkin's lymphomas.

Cytotoxic anticancer chemotherapy

Chemotherapy is the use of cytotoxic drugs to kill fast growing cells and the target is generally associated with DNA structure, function and replication. This is quite a poor targeting strategy and affects rapidly dividing cells, leading to widespread side effects. Drugs used in anticancer chemotherapy generally target the synthesis of nucleotides (antimetabolites such as methotrexate and mercaptopurine), may chemically modify the DNA by alkylation (e.g. busulfan, chlorambucil, cyclophosphamide), cause fragmentation (e.g. bleomycin) or intercalation (e.g. dactinomycin), or may destroy mitotic spindle fibres (vinca alkaloids) involved in cell division (Table 32.1). Accordingly, the lack of selectivity gives rise to a wide range of side effects, including myelosuppression leading to pancytopenia, which is associated with anaemia, increased susceptibility to infections due to neutropenia and increased bleeding due to thrombocytopenia. Myelosuppression is a common occurrence with many agents and is a reason to carry out chemotherapy in cycles, because this allows the bone marrow to recover between cycles. Colony stimulating factors may be used under some circumstances to increase the white cell count and reduce the time between cycles. Prophylactic antimicrobial agents may also be required. As a result of the toxic nature of cytotoxic agents they may exhibit a range of side effects which, depending on the agent, may include:

- alopecia
- nausea and vomiting
- mouth ulcers
- renal damage
- bladder damage
- infertility
- lung damage
- cardiotoxicity
- carcinogenic effects.

Given the toxicity of cytotoxic anticancer drugs they are often used in combination to reduce the doses required. Many regimens involve three or four agents which target different stages in the cell cycle, e.g. DNA synthesis (e.g. an antimetabolite), DNA structure and replication (e.g. an alkylating agent) and cell division (e.g. a microtubule inhibitor). Regimens are often given in cycles (e.g. every 21 days) so that the body and especially the bone marrow can recover between doses. A core principle in this approach is that an initial treatment might lead to a substantial reduction in cancer cell number but be associated with side effects due to other, healthy rapidly dividing cells (e.g. bone marrow) being killed off. The body is then allowed to recover and next phase leads to another substantial reduction in cancer cell number. The ideal goal is total destruction of the cancer cell load or at least to achieve a remission.

Regimens

Some commonly used regimens include:

- CHOP (e.g. for non-Hodgkin's lymphoma)

    - cyclophosphamide
    - doxorubicin
    - vincristine
    - prednisolone

- ABVD (e.g. for Hodgkin's lymphoma)

    - doxorubicin
    - bleomycin
    - vinblastine
    - dacarbazine

Table 32.1 Summary of cytotoxic anticancer drugs

Class of chemotherapeutic drug	Examples	Mechanism of action	Comments
Antimetabolites	Folate antagonists, methotrexate	Inhibits dihydrofolate reductase to decrease thymidylate, purine nucleotide, and interfere with DNA synthesis	Folinic acid is given to reduce associated myelosuppression
	Pyrimidine analogues, mercaptopurine and thioguanine	Activated by hypoxanthine phosphoribosyltransferase to toxic metabolites	Mercaptopurine is inactivated via thiopurine S-methyltransferase and pharmacogenetic differences mean that some patients are more susceptible to its toxicity.
	Purine analogues 5-flurouracil, capecitabine, cytarabine, gemcitabine	Incorporated into DNA as false metabolites and lead to damage of the DNA	Capecitabine is given orally and metabolised to 5-flurouracil
Alkylating agents	Cyclophosphamide, busulphan	Cause chemical cross-linking of DNA leading to defective DNA replication	Widely used in combination therapy in a number of haematological malignancies and solid tumours
Platinum compounds	Cisplatin	Inhibition of DNA synthesis by cross-linking guanine residues	Associated with a high level of emesis
Anthracycline antibiotics	Doxorubicin, epirubicin and daunorubicin	Interfere with nucleotide synthesis by intercalating between DNA strands, inhibiting topoisomerase and generating free radicals	• Widely used in a variety of haematological malignancies and solid tumours • Doxorubucin is associated with cardiac toxicity
Topoisomerase inhibitors	Etoposide	Inhibition of topoisomerase II prevents ligation of DNA, leading to breaks in the DNA strand	
Microtubule inhibitors	• Vinca alkaloids: vincristine and vinblastine • Taxanes: paclitaxel and docetaxel	• Vinca alkaloids block the formation of the mitotic spindle • Taxanes stabilise spindle fibres	

- EC (e.g. for small-cell lung cancer)
  - etoposide
  - cisplatin

- FEC (e.g. for breast cancer)
  - flurouracil
  - epirubicin
  - cyclophosphamide.

Targeted cancer therapy

Newer targeted therapies have been introduced and target cell signalling. For example imatinib inhibits tyrosine kinase activities and is used in chronic myeloid leukaemia. In this condition there is a translocation between chromosomes 9 and 22, known as the Philadelphia chromosome, that results in fusion of two proteins to form BCR-Abl, a constitutively active tyrosine kinase, which may be inhibited by imatinib with relative selectivity. Some key examples are summarised in Table 32.2.

Hormone-based therapy plays a significant role in certain tumours, e.g. the oestrogen receptor antagonist tamoxifen is widely used in oestrogen receptor-positive breast cancer. It is given after surgery, with or without chemotherapy, and is effective at suppressing the growth of oestrogen-sensitive cells, including residual cells and metastases. Other approaches include the use of aromatase inhibitors, such as aminoglutethimide, which prevent the metabolism of androgens to oestrogens. Corticosteroids also have a role, although this is poorly understood. In targeting these processes, the agents kill rapidly dividing cells in the tumour but also suppress growth of 'normal' cells with high rates of division, such as

bone marrow cells producing blood cells and epithelial cells.

Chemotherapy is also used in non-systemic therapy, which has the clear advantage of limiting side effects. Example of this include the use of topical 5-flurouracil for skin cancers, bladder instillation in localised bladder tumours and intraperitoneal instillation for some peritoneal tumours.

Radiotherapy also plays a role, whether by radiation from isotopes or from X-rays. By targeting the radiation on the tumour, cancerous cells may be killed. Certain tumours are especially sensitive to irradiation (such as bladder cancers) and radiotherapy may play an important role in localised disease. Radiotherapy is also used when surgery is not possible in vital organs such as the head and neck. In addition, radiotherapy may be used after

Table 32.2 Summary of targeted anticancer drug

Class	Example	Mode of action	Comments
Monoclonal antibodies	Bevacizumab	Anti-VEGF to reduce angiogenesis and hence metastasis	Used in advanced colon or breast cancer as an adjuvant
	Rituximab	Anti-CD20, targeting leukocytes in non-Hodgkin's lymphoma	
	Trastuzumab	ErbB2 (Her-2) inhibitor to reduce EGF receptor signalling	Used in breast cancers expressing Her-2
	Cetuximab	Targets EGF receptor	Used in advanced colorectal cancers
EGF receptor tyrosine kinase inhibitors	Erlotinib and gefitinib	Targets EGF receptor kinase, often over-expressed in certain cancers	EGF receptor tyrosine kinase inhibitors used to treat lung and pancreatic cancers
Tyrosine kinase inhibitors	Imatinib	Inhibition tyrosine kinase activities associated with *abl* proto-oncogene and PDGF	• In chronic myeloid leukaemia, a translocation between chromosomes 9 and 22, known as the Philadelphia chromosome, results in fusion of two proteins to form BCR-Abl, a constitutively active tyrosine kinase, which may be inhibited by imatinib with relative selectivity • Also used in some gastrointestinal stromal tumours
	Sunitinib	Inhibition of tyrosine kinase activity associated with PDGF and VEGF receptors	Used in advanced renal cell carcinoma
Proteasome inhibitor	Bortezomib	Inhibition of intracellular proteasomes alters the regulation of intracellular proteins	Used in multiple myeloma

EGF, epidermal growth factor; PDGF, platelet-derived growth factor receptor; VEGF, vascular endothelial growth factor.

surgery, in palliation to reduce the size of tumours, to reduce obstruction of the vena cava and for relief from bony metastases. This may allow a reduction in doses of analgesics and/or stepping down the analgesic ladder.

Side effects and implications

As commented, anticancer chemotherapy is associated with widespread and significant adverse effects.

- **Bone marrow suppression:** almost all cytotoxic agents cause myelosuppression and as commented above this is a key limiting factor in tolerance to chemotherapy and why chemotherapy is carried out in cycles. The bone marrow suppression decreases leucocyte production, leading to neutropenia with decreased resistance to infection which can lead to potentially fatal neutropenic sepsis. Clearly white cell counts should be taken during chemotherapy and their recovery determines suitability for the next cycle. For prevention of infection antibiotic prophylaxis is used in some but not all regimens. In the presence of neutropenic sepsis intravenous broadspectrum antibiotics are used and colony stimulating factors such as granulocyte colony stimulating factor (GCSF) may be given to increase white cell production. Bone marrow suppression can also leads to thrombocytopenia with the potential for serious haemorrhages and platelet transfusions may be required.

- **Nausea and vomiting** (see Chapter 9): different agents have differing levels of emetogenic potential with platinum compounds being notably emetogenic. As discussed in Chapter 9, a variety of agents are available for prevention and include 5HT$_3$ receptor antagonists; dexamethasone is effective both pre- and post-chemotherapy. Chemotherapy is also associated with anticipatory nausea before treatment and lorazepam is used here.

- **Alopecia:** some but not all agents can lead to hear loss by poorly understood toxic effects on hair follicle cells. Prevention can involve cold caps to reduce scalp blood flow during chemotherapy to limit exposure.

- **Skin reactions:** as with many drugs, skin reactions are common; a specific example is hand–foot syndrome with a number of drugs, notably capecitabine. This involves reddening, swelling and pain on both the palms of the hands and soles of the feet.

- **Cardiac toxicity:** this is particularly a problem with anthracyclines, where a maximum cumulative dose only can be given. This well established event leads to damage to the myocardium and may lead to heart failure and so patients should be monitored via echocardiography.

- **Neurotoxicity:** irreversible nerve damage is commonly associated with vinca alkaloids as the main culprit and may need dose reduction. Past medication errors with vinca alkaloids being administered intrathecally by mistake have led to fatal neurotoxicity.

- **Tumour lysis syndrome:** this is associated with the release of purines from the breakdown of cancer cells which are then metabolised to uric acid. It is associated with hyperkalaemia, hyperphosphataemia, hypocalcaemia and may lead to nephrotoxicity. The xanthine oxidase inhibitor allopurinol is used to inhibit uric acid formation and rasburicase (uricase) is used to reduce uric acid levels.

- **Renal toxicity:** this is a particular problem with cisplatin and the patient should be well hydrated before treatment.

- **Extravasation:** intravenous administration can be associated with leakage of highly irritant and toxic chemicals into the surrounding tissue leading to damage. This can be prevented by administering cytotoxic chemicals via a central line and/or using high flow rates. If extravasation occurs then attempts should be made to dilute or neutralise the irritant.

- **Mucositis:** this involves painfull oral inflammation and ulceration due to damage to epithelial cells in the mouth. Patients require mouth care, e.g. to use antiseptic mouth washes such as chlorhexidine. Relief may be achieved by sucking ice cubes.

- **Diarrhoea:** damage to the rapidly dividing gastrointestinal mucosa commonly leads to diarrhoea and this can be treated with loperamide.

Practice points

- Cytotoxic anticancer chemotherapy has poor selectivity and is associated with widespread side effects.

- Appropriate use of antiemetics may reduce the associated nausea and vomiting.
- Be alert of signs of neutropenic sepsis which requires immediate treatment.

CASE STUDY

A 65-year-old woman with small-cell lung cancer has been recommended for chemotherapy with the following intravenous regimen:

Etoposide
Cisplatin

Explain the principles of cytotoxic anticancer chemotherapy.

- The key target in cytotoxic anticancer chemotherapy is to kill fast growing cells, cancerous cells in particular. The pharmacological targets are DNA and DNA synthesis and replication and the aim is to kill the tumour cells either for cure or palliatation. Combined therapy is often used to target different parts of the cell cycle and this may mean lower doses of the toxic compounds can be used.

Why is this regimen given in 21-day cycles?

- The cell killing affects 'normal' rapidly growing tissue, in particular leading to myelosuppression. Myelosuppression leads to anaemia and neutropenia (both pose significant issues for the patient) and so the use of cycles allows the body to recover.

What particular side effects would you anticipate from this regimen? How might they be prevented?

- Nausea (especially cisplatin): recommend an effective antiemetic (e.g. ondansetron, metoclopramide). May need a benzodiazepine for anticipatory nausea. Cisplatin requires intensive hydration before treatment to reduce nephrotoxicity. To manage myelosuppression the regimen is given in cycles and with monitoring of the full blood count.
- Alopecia may be limited by use cold caps for cooling the scalp.

Prior to the third cycle, her haematological measurements (which were normal at the start of therapy) were as follows:

Variable	Value	Normal range
Haemoglobin	7.6 g/dL	11.5–16.5 g/dL
White blood cell count	0.4×10^9/L	$4–11 \times 10^9$/L
Platelet count	50×10^9/L	$140–400 \times 10^9$/L

(continued)

(continued)

What do these changes indicate?

The reduction in all cells counts is pancytopenia due to myelosuppression. There is associated anaemia, the reduced white cell counts is consistent with an increased risk of infection (neutropenic sepsis) and reduced platelet count means there is an increased risk of bleeding.

What are the possible consequences for this patient?

Problems due to anaemia, increased risk of infection and increased risk of bleeding and this may mean delay of next cycle. Colony stimulating factor might be considered and if there are signs of infection, antimicrobials are required.

Online resources

www.cancerresearchuk.org/health-professional/cancer-
    statistics/statistics-by-cancer-type
Cancer Research UK (accessed September 2015).

33

The cancer patient and palliative care

Palliative care

The following section is intended as an introduction to some of the issues encountered during palliative care, particularly relating to common symptoms, the importance of regular monitoring to optimise treatment and the education of patients and carers. Specialist information should be sought from references given at the end of the chapter and local palliative care teams.

What is palliative care?

The term 'palliative' is used to describe treatment that addresses and alleviates symptoms associated with an incurable disease. Palliative care is therefore applied commonly to the treatment of terminal malignancy but may also include conditions such as the end-stages of chronic heart failure, respiratory diseases, AIDS and motor neuron disease. The aim of treatment is to improve the quality of life of both patients and carers, and includes the control of physical symptoms and attention to spiritual, emotional and social needs. A multidisciplinary palliative care team therefore comprises specialist nurses, doctors, pharmacists, counsellors, dieticians, physiotherapists, social workers and ministers of religion. The National Institute for Health and Care Excellence (NICE 2004) has issued guidance for the provision of cancer services including supportive and palliative care. The World Health Organization (WHO 1990) also includes the following recommendations as to the role of palliative care:

- Consider dying as a normal process (see Nuland 1997).
- Death should not be hastened or postponed.
- Patients should be offered the support required, enabling them to live as actively as possible until death.
- The quality of life should be enhanced and care may also provide a positive influence throughout the course of the illness.

Types of cancer pain

Pain is one of the most common and feared symptoms of cancer. However, this is not inevitable and approximately a third of patients do not suffer severe pain at any stage of their illness. When treating pain, the first step is to determine the location and likely source because this will determine the choice of treatment, e.g. pain resulting from compression by a tumour may be reduced by chemotherapy or radiotherapy to remove or reduce the size of the tumour. Some types of pain (see Chapter 30) respond to treatment with opioids, but neuropathic or bone pain may be more resistant to opioids. Bone pain is a somatic pain produced by nociceptors in the bone and tends to be localised, described as gnawing or aching, and often results from secondary tumours in the bone. Visceral pain is triggered by infiltration, compression, distension or stretching of the viscera due to the presence of a tumour, and tends to be diffuse and constant.

WHO analgesic ladder

Once the nature and likely cause of pain are assessed, the recommendation of analgesia follows the analgesic ladder, as recommended by the WHO (see Chapter 30). Analgesia is prescribed continually and not 'when required' for optimum pain management and therefore improved quality of life. Additional analgesia is prescribed for pain occurring despite continuous treatment. This is commonly described as breakthrough pain, for which 'when required' analgesia is appropriate. Adjuvants may be added to treatment at any stage and include tricyclic antidepressants, anticonvulsants and corticosteroids (see Chapter 30). Choice is dependent on the

nature of the pain, risk of drug interactions and side effect profile.

Other symptoms

Other common symptoms of advanced cancer may include fatigue, weakness, anorexia, weight loss, lack of energy, dry mouth, constipation, dyspnoea and early satiety. Symptoms may be drug related and may vary according to the nature of the tumour, e.g. cancer of the head and neck often causes dysphagia whereas dyspnoea is associated with lung, breast or other cancers affecting the thorax. The cause and treatment of common symptoms are summarised in Table 33.1.

Pharmacology

The pharmacology of analgesics is described in Chapter 30. The pharmacology of corticosteroids is summarised in Chapter 22.

Table 33.1 Examples of the causes and treatment of common symptoms encountered in palliative care

Symptom	Treatment	Comments/common causes
Anorexia	Identify and treat the cause. A short course of corticosteroids may be given or high doses of a progestogen such as megestrol acetate or medroxyprogesterone	• Possible causes include dry mouth, nausea, constipation, anxiety, dyspepsia, pain, gastric stasis, hypercalcaemia, uraemia, depression and malodorous tumours • Dietary supplements may be added but do not replace normal meals. The intake of calorific food such as cheese and full-fat milk should be encouraged • The effects of progestogens may be delayed for a few weeks and side effects such as oedema and the risk of thromboembolic disease may prevent their use. They tend only to be used if the prognosis is greater than 3 months
Anxiety	SSRIs, β blockers, benzodiazepines, e.g. lorazepam sublingually	• May be associated with depression and this may worsen pain (Chapter 25) • Benzodiazepines may be appropriate and the risk of dependence may not be relevant
Breathlessness	• Identify cause and treat as appropriate. Breathing techniques may be beneficial, particularly when dyspnoea is worsened by anxiety • Opioids may be of symptomatic benefit due to reduction of the central respiratory drive • Oxygen is required if the patient is hypoxic	Causes include anaemia, bronchospasm, fluid retention, respiratory infection, COPD, pulmonary embolism, congestive heart failure or drugs such as β blockers or aspirin (Chapter 16)
Confusion	• Identify cause • Treatment may include haloperidol or chlorpromazine if the patient is agitated or distressed	• Hyponatraemia, hypercalcaemia, uraemia, pain, constipation, infection, urine retention • Drug causes include opioids, hypnotics and antimuscarinics (Chapter 6)

Table 33.1 *(continued)*

Symptom	Treatment	Comments/common causes
Constipation	A softener and stimulant are required, e.g. regular lactulose and senna or co-danthrusate (Chapter 10). Suppositories or enemas may be required if severe	• Opioids, reduced mobility, dehydration • Laxatives should be given to all patients prescribed regular opioids
Dehydration	Small amounts of fluids may be administered regularly. Causes should be identified and treated	• Causes include diuretics, laxatives, sweating or difficulty swallowing • Dehydration may lead to deterioration of renal function and should therefore be avoided or identified and corrected promptly
Depression	Tricyclic or SSRI antidepressants (Chapter 25)	• Consider the prognosis and delayed efficacy before initiating antidepressants • Monitor for hyponatraemia as a cause of confusion and drowsiness • Antimuscarinic effects of tricyclics may be a disadvantage. Review other medications for risk of additive effects and consider problems such as dry mouth and constipation
Diarrhoea	Loperamide (Chapter 10), other opioids, rehydration	Causes include impacted faeces, bowel obstruction or infections. Drug causes include opioid withdrawal, antibiotics, iron salts, laxatives, NSAIDs and magnesium salts (Chapter 6)
Dry mouth and oral candidiasis	• Sugar-free chewing gum or sweets may help to stimulate saliva production (consider sorbitol as a cause of diarrhoea), artificial saliva, ice or unsweetened pineapple chunks and regular sips of water • Candidiasis may be present and is treated with nystatin or miconazole oral gel • Antiseptic mouth washes (e.g. chlorhexidine) may be used if patients are unable to brush their teeth	• Drug causes include opioids, drugs with antimuscarinic effects (sedating antihistamines, TCAs, hyoscine; Chapter 6) • Reduce the prescribing of antimuscarinic drugs if possible • Glycerol-based mouthwashes are best avoided because they cause drying • Broad-spectrum antibiotics and steroids (particularly inhaled) and general debilitation may cause candidiasis • Asthmatic patients treated with inhaled steroids are at increased risk of developing oral candidiasis and may benefit from using a spacer device and should be advised to rinse their mouth after inhaler use
Hiccup	Antacid with antiflatulent (simeticone), e.g. Asilone suspension or Maalox Plus, metoclopramide or chlorpromazine	• May be caused by gastric distension • Avoid antacids containing aluminium salts alone, which may cause constipation • Avoid bicarbonate salts, which may increase flatulence from carbon dioxide production
Insomnia	Benzodiazepines, e.g. temazepam	• Causes include anxiety, depression, cramps, pain, night sweats, joint stiffness, fear or discomfort • Drug causes include corticosteroids (administer dexamethasone before 6pm), caffeine, alcohol, sympathomimetics (Chapter 27) or withdrawal from benzodiazepines
Intractable cough	Consider changing posture, particularly at night, or opioids, e.g. morphine	Gastric distension

(continued)

Table 33.1 *(continued)*

Symptom	Treatment	Comments/common causes
Muscle spasm	Diazepam, baclofen or dantrolene	• Pressure or nerve irritation • The efficacy of dantrolene may be delayed by a few weeks
Nausea and vomiting	The cause should be determined and treated if appropriate. Antiemetics include domperidone, metoclopramide, haloperidol, cyclizine, levomepromazine, prochlorperazine when required (Chapter 9). Ondansetron may be used for chemotherapy-induced nausea and vomiting	• For example, gastric stasis, constipation, bowel obstruction, hypercalcaemia (stop drugs such as thiazides, which retain calcium), renal failure, raised intracranial pressure, motion sickness, severe pain, cough, severe anxiety, infection, uraemia or chemotherapy • Antimuscarinic drugs may oppose prokinetic drugs (Chapter 6) • Common cause is initial treatment with opioids but this is usually transient, resolving after a few days • Review every 24 hours • Many drugs cause nausea and vomiting (Chapter 6) • Note that extrapyramidal effects of metoclopramide are more common in children
Pruritus	Emollients (cool in the fridge) and/or oral antihistamines. Avoid heat and try cotton clothing. Obstructive jaundice may require treatment with colestyramine	Jaundice or drugs such as opioids (Chapter 36). Note that itching due to opioids is more common in children
Sedation	Reduction of opioid dose if pain is controlled. Also review other drugs causing sedation such as antihistamines (chlorphenamine), antidepressants (amitriptyline, dosulepin, trazodone) or benzodiazepines	• Tends to occur when opioid dose is increased and should be transient, resolving after a few days • Patient should not perform skilled tasks such as driving • If sedation persists, consider toxicity and review dose and factors such as deteriorating renal function
Sweating	Paracetamol or NSAIDs, or hyoscine (opioid-induced sweating)	• Malignancy, infection, anxiety, hyperthyroidism, menopause. Drug causes include antidepressants • Monitor for dehydration, e.g. diuretic doses may need to be withheld

COPD, chronic obstructive pulmonary disease; NSAIDs, non-steroidal anti-inflammatory drugs; SSRIs, selective serotonin reuptake inhibitors; TCAs, tricyclic antidepressants.

Drug choice

Treatment is given according to the analgesic ladder, as described in Chapter 30. The following section outlines analgesic choice according to the analgesic ladder, as applied to palliative care.

Step 1

Regular paracetamol is an effective first choice and is often an adequate analgesic used alone for mild pain, with or without an NSAID. This should be used regularly and may be continued at all stages of the ladder.

Step 2

Mild opioids such as codeine or dihydrocodeine may be added (see Chapter 30). Each tablet should contain the equivalent of 30 mg codeine or more and combination analgesics containing less than this dose per tablet are not recommended for cancer pain (National Prescribing Centre 2003). It should be noted that constipation is a problem even with low doses of opioid and a laxative will be required with regular treatment.

Tramadol

Tramadol is considered suitable for use at the second step of the analgesic ladder, as it has fewer opioid side effects such as constipation and respiratory depression compared with strong opioids. However, this may not be appropriate for the management of cancer pain in the absence of evidence for an advantage over weak opioids and also recommendations in the summary of product characteristics (SPC) that the maximum dose of 400 mg/day is not exceeded except in special circumstances due to the risk of convulsions at higher doses. It is also unsuitable for patients with epilepsy or those prone to seizures, e.g. patients with cerebral tumours or uraemia. It should be avoided with other drugs known to lower the convulsive threshold, such as antidepressants (see Chapter 6).

Step 3

Strong opioids

The properties of the strong opioids such as fentanyl, morphine, pethidine, oxycodone and buprenorphine are summarised in Table 33.2 and also in Table 30.1. The latest *British National Formulary* should be consulted for equivalent doses of opioids when calculating doses of strong opioids after treatment with milder agents, e.g. codeine and dihydrocodeine are approximately one-tenth the potency of morphine and the use of these opioids is considered when calculating the morphine dose. The dose is then titrated against pain because doses higher than those required to control pain lead to respiratory depression.

Despite the introduction of agents such as oxycodone, morphine remains the first-line strong opioid for moderate-to-severe pain. Strong opioids such as morphine cause euphoria and mental detachment, which may be beneficial, as well as reducing respiratory symptoms. However, bone pain and neuropathic pain are often resistant to even strong opioids, although the response is unpredictable and therefore a trial of opioids is recommended.

Where possible, it is reasonable to give drugs orally, even in advanced cancer. For patients with vomiting or difficulty swallowing, oral suspensions, patches or suppositories may be used. Alternatively syringe drivers provide a useful and continuous method of drug administration (see below).

Syringe drivers

For patients in the final stages of a terminal illness, syringe drivers can provide an extremely useful way of delivering medication. Syringe drivers provide a continuous subcutaneous infusion and therefore allow effective control of symptoms. When converting from oral morphine to a syringe driver, the more soluble opioid diamorphine is used and the equivalent doses of these opioids are tabulated in the BNF. The dose may, however, need to be increased because of worsening pain and/or increased tolerance by patients at the time that a syringe driver is initiated.

Table 33.2 A summary of some important characteristics of strong opioids in relation to palliative care	
Opioid	**Comments**
Buprenorphine	• Vomiting may be a problem and withdrawal effects may occur if added to high-dose opioid treatment, resulting from its partial agonist activity. It is therefore not often suitable for cancer pain • Patches have recently been introduced
Cyclimorph	• Cyclimorph is a combination product containing both morphine and cyclizine. This is not appropriate for chronic pain because nausea is a transient effect of opioid treatment, so ongoing treatment with cyclizine is not necessary. In addition, dose increases lead to excessive sedation due to cyclizine • Diconal is a combination product of cyclizine and dipipanone and is therefore also unsuitable in palliative care
Dextromoramide	• A short duration of action makes dextromoramide unsuitable for control of continuous pain and this is rarely used • Available as a sublingual tablet
Diamorphine	• More soluble than morphine and therefore used for infusion due to reduced volume • Activity one-quarter to one-third that of oral morphine • Injection is given by the subcutaneous route, which is easier to administer and less painful than other routes

(continued)

Table 33.2 *(continued)*	
Opioid	**Comments**
Fentanyl	• The efficacy of fentanyl is comparable with morphine and this is therefore not a suitable alternative when pain is not controlled by morphine (suspect opioid-resistant pain). The time taken for transdermal fentanyl to reach steady state also makes this preparation unsuitable for unstable pain • Patches changed at the same time every 3 days are useful for patients with dysphagia, malabsorption or poor compliance • Less constipating than morphine and more suitable in renal impairment as there are no active metabolites, although dose reduction may be required • Oral transmucosal fentanyl citrate lozenges are now available for breakthrough pain • New preparations should be started 12 hours after the last patch is removed. It should also be noted that fentanyl effects remain for up to 72 hours after removal of the patch • When starting fentanyl treatment, apply patch at the same time as the last dose of slow-release morphine. The full effect may take 36–48 hours and therefore breakthrough pain may occur and should be treated as required • When changing from morphine, withdrawal symptoms such as colic, diarrhoea, nausea, sweating and restlessness may persist for a few days, although pain may be controlled. Doses of short-acting oral morphine may be given • Adjuncts or alternative analgesia should be considered if pain is not controlled by doses >300 micrograms/hour
Hydromorphone	• To date, hydromorphine appears to demonstrate efficacy and tolerability comparable to morphine and is reserved for patients with confusion, loss of concentration, vivid dreams or hallucinations occurring with even low doses of morphine • The contents of controlled-release capsules may be sprinkled on cold soft food
Methadone	Useful in renal failure
Morphine	• Remains the first choice for the treatment of chronic cancer pain • Oral slow-release and quick-acting preparations available for good pain control, including breakthrough pain
Oxycodone	• Suppositories offer alternative routes of administration • Role in relation to morphine remains to be established as side effect profile and efficacy appear similar but may provide an alternative if symptoms such as hallucinations become problematic with morphine
Pentazocine	Avoided due to high risk of confusion and hallucinations
Pethidine	Pethidine is avoided in palliative care due to the short half-life, reduced potency compared with morphine and the accumulation of toxic metabolites during regular use

It should be noted that a misconception exists whereby patients and carers view the administration of opioids via the parenteral route to be more effective than the oral route, and an inevitable part of the treatment of advanced disease. The BNF indications for the parenteral route include patients unable to take medication by mouth, e.g. due to dysphagia or nausea and vomiting and, importantly, when patients request that they receive their medication by this route.

Important roles for pharmacists include the calculation of diamorphine dose required when converting from oral morphine and assessing the compatibility of drugs to be added to diamorphine infusions, thereby maintaining the stability of the infusion and preventing adverse effects in the patient. The infusion solution should be checked regularly for discoloration or precipitation. Examples from the BNF of drugs that may be added to diamorphine infusions include:

• cyclizine
• dexamethasone
• haloperidol
• hysoscine butylbromide
• hyoscine hydrobromide
• metoclopramide
• midazolam.

Drugs contraindicated for use in syringe drivers include chlorpromazine, prochlorperazine and diazepam due to irritation at the injection site.

Adjuncts used in the treatment of pain

Adjuncts may be added at any step of the analgesic ladder and include corticosteroids, antidepressants and anticonvulsants. Other treatment includes nerve block, relaxation therapy and the use of transcutaneous electrical nerve stimulation (TENS) machines (see Chapter 30).

Corticosteroids

Corticosteroids such as dexamethasone are particularly useful for treating pain due to nerve compression, tissue swelling or raised intracranial pressure.

Dexamethasone (doses up to 16 mg/day) is used for raised intracranial pressure, severe bone pain, nerve or soft-tissue infiltration by the tumour or oedema, and hepatic capsular pain. The last dose should be given before 6pm to avoid causing insomnia. Additional benefits include increased appetite, energy and general wellbeing. To avoid side effects, the lowest effective dose is prescribed and the course duration is as short as possible. For patients taking corticosteroids and NSAIDs, gastric protection in the form of a proton pump inhibitor is appropriate.

Neuropathic pain

Neuropathic pain (see Chapter 30) results from treatment such as radiotherapy, or from infiltration of a tumour into peripheral nerves or the central nervous system, causing compression or damage. It may be described as burning, stabbing, tingling, a constricting sensation or shooting pains. The skin may feel numb or oversensitive. Neuropathic pain is often unresponsive to opioids, the most effective being methadone, tramadol and oxycodone, and is managed by a combination of corticosteroids, tricyclic antidepressants and antiepileptic drugs such as gabapentin and pregabalin (see Chapters 24 and 25). Specialists may also consider the use of ketamine or antiarrhythmics such as flecainide, mexiletine or lidocaine.

Bone pain

Bone pain often arises from secondary tumours, which result in either increased or reduced bone density and the release of prostaglandins. NSAIDs are therefore the analgesics of choice. If an NSAID remains ineffective after 1 week, an alternative NSAID is selected (see Chapter 30). The addition of a weak opioid may be considered but is not often beneficial. Bisphosphonates or calcitonin may be used to reduce bone turnover or inhibit calcium resorption into bone, respectively. Corticosteroids are useful for treating bone pain due to anti-inflammatory properties and also by reducing oedema surrounding the tumour. Regular use of paracetamol is useful at each step of the analgesic ladder.

Colicky pain

Pain associated with the gastrointestinal tract and reported as 'colicky' pain may respond to antimuscarinic agents, such as hyoscine, which reduce intestinal transit.

Common symptoms

Table 33.1 summarises the causes of some common symptoms associated with cancer and their management.

Concurrent disease

Analgesic prescribing decisions complicated by concurrent diseases are outlined in Chapter 30. Key considerations include gastrointestinal toxicity due to NSAIDs and worsening renal function. For patients with effective pain control with NSAIDs, a proton pump inhibitor may be added for gastric protection. Misoprostol may not be suitable due to colic or diarrhoea. It should be noted, however, that respiratory depression in terminal care does not preclude the use of strong opioids and careful dose titration prevents this effect. Signs of opioid overdose include drowsiness, reduced respiratory rate and the presence of hallucinations, and pain tends to be well controlled. Opioid toxicity may be precipitated by renal impairment.

In general, the risks of initiating further treatment are compared with the likely benefits. Unnecessary treatment is withheld to prevent further complications of drug regimens, e.g. the treatment of hyperlipidaemia may not be appropriate in terminal care. Palliative care is one of the exceptions when polypharmacy is often necessary and adverse drug reactions (ADRs) are treated as they arise. Patients and carers should be as involved as possible in treatment choices and the impact on quality of life considered, e.g. the use of drugs with sedative properties may be avoided for as long as possible in patients wishing to retain the independence gained from driving.

Terminal symptoms

Terminal symptoms occur when death is likely to be within days. These include noisy breathing (death rattle), confusion, fever and severe fatigue. Symptoms should be monitored regularly and those considered to be causing distress, such as urinary retention, constipation, pain and dyspepsia, should be identified and treated. It should be noted that restlessness and agitation may occur in the presence of worsening pain but this is not always the case and care should be taken to avoid misinterpretation. Increasing doses of opioids may worsen such symptoms and dose reduction or an alternative opioid should be considered when other causes, including pain, have been excluded. Any unnecessary treatment such as antihypertensives, diuretics, antiarrhythmics and hypoglycaemics may be stopped. Artificial feeding such as via a nasogastric tube is not appropriate because it may cause distress to both the patient and the carers.

Drug interactions

See Chapter 30.

Monitoring

The impairment of renal or hepatic function may increase side effects, particularly to opioids, and requires dose reduction or less frequent dosing (see Chapter 30).

The role of the community pharmacist

The community pharmacist is an important source of support and information, particularly for carers of cancer patients who are often involved in collecting and administering medication. Pharmacists are an essential part of the palliative care team, being experts on the use and availability of medicines, e.g. pharmacists can advise on alternative preparations such as suspensions, suppositories and patches available for patients with dysphagia.

Perhaps the most important role of the pharmacist is in the education of patients and carers on the best use of medicines because this improves compliance. The needs of the patient and carers should be considered, e.g. a complicated medication regimen is of no benefit if it causes anxiety and poor compliance. Verbal and written information should be provided; an up-to-date list of medication, dosing information and indications for use of each product may help both patients and carers. Advice may need to be repeated. Regular supply of medication should be ensured and patients and carers encouraged to report new or altered symptoms for early recognition of ADRs or new symptoms. Providing a list of contacts and sources of further information is also helpful, particularly in the early stages of the disease. Pharmacist input to medication assessment and review, of a multidisciplinary palliative care team staffing palliative care clinics, is also to be encouraged because this improves pharmaceutical care for patients (Needham and Wong 1999; Austwick *et al.* 2002).

General advice for patients and carers

- Key words to consider when providing advice include education, empathy, reassurance, approachability and resourcefulness.
- Good mouth care should be encouraged to prevent problems such as infection.
- Take care not to run out of medicines.
- Pharmacists may consider producing specific information leaflets to cover the use of medicines outside the product licence.

Pain

- Patients and carers may fear the use of morphine, because it is wrongly associated with 'imminent death'. Reassurance should be given that morphine is an extremely safe and useful analgesic, which may be used for years and with little risk of psychological dependence when used for severe pain.
- Drowsiness caused by strong opioids is often transient. Skilled tasks such as driving should be avoided and prolonged drowsiness should be reported to the prescriber.
- Advice should be given as to the timing of morphine doses, e.g. regular administration of a long-acting preparation twice a day means as close to 12 hours as practical between doses,

with additional doses of an immediate-release preparation (usually morphine solution) given up to every 4 hours as required for breakthrough pain. The total amount of oral solution taken during a 24-hour period allows the prescriber to calculate the 12-hourly dose required.

- Reassurance should be given that the effectiveness of morphine will persist even if started early in the disease. It is a common misconception by patients that starting morphine treatment too early may leave them without adequate pain control when the pain worsens.
- The control of neuropathic pain may take a week or more but if the pain worsens the prescriber should be contacted. If agents such as antidepressants or anticonvulsants are used, the use of these drugs for neuropathic pain should be explained.

Opioids, NSAIDs and adjuvant counselling

See Chapter 30.

Fentanyl patches

- Patches should be changed at the same time every 3 days.
- A new patch should be applied to a different area of skin, and not applied to inflamed skin, scar tissue, or swollen or broken skin.
- Direct contact of heat such as from hot-water bottles should be avoided.
- There should be good contact between the skin and the patch, and porous adhesive tape (e.g. Micropore) may be used if necessary.
- Used patches should be folded inwards, protecting the side that contained the drug, and disposed of carefully.

Fentanyl lozenges

- For breakthrough pain with a maximum dose of 4 dose units a day.
- No more than 2 dose units for each pain episode.
- The lozenge should be sucked and moved around the mouth over about 15 minutes, dissolving any lozenge left after pain is relieved, under hot running water.

Co-danthramer

This may colour urine red.

Self-assessment

Consider whether the following statements are true or false. In the management of cancer:

1 Cyclimorph is a good choice for chronic pain.
2 Cyclizine may be added to an infusion of diamorphine though there is a risk of precipitation (see BNF).
3 NSAIDs are effective in bone pain.
4 An oral solution of morphine is sometimes used to determine the required dose of a modified-release preparation.
5 Treatment with morphine should be delayed as efficacy will reduce with time.

Practice points

- Psychosocial and spiritual support for both patient and family are important components of palliative care and may impact on the severity of symptoms.
- The progressive nature of cancer means that the symptoms and patients' needs are constantly changing. Regular review of medication is therefore essential and should identify ADRs and new symptoms and assess the continued benefit from treatment. Palliative care medicine is a balance between symptom control and avoidance of unacceptable ADRs.
- Palliative care is a specialist area though encountered commonly in the community. It is therefore important for community pharmacists to be familiar with the general principles of pain management and liaise with specialist pharmacists.

General pain control

- Pain control should follow the stepped approach recommended by the WHO (see Chapter 30).
- The WHO also recommends that analgesia be provided continually and not 'when required', although additional

(continued)

(continued)

analgesia is prescribed for use when required for breakthrough pain.

- Frequent review is required for optimum pain control.
- Consider the timing of doses, e.g. before painful changing of dressings.
- It may be useful to ask the patient to indicate the severity of each symptom on a scale of 1–10 to assess treatment outcome and the need for dose changes or further intervention. A list of drugs, including those found to be ineffective, is useful to prevent omissions and unnecessary treatment.

Opioids

- The total daily dose of morphine should be reviewed daily and the regular dose adjusted according to the number of rescue doses required. In practice, a doubling of the rescue dose may be given at night (50% increase for elderly patients) to ensure a pain-free night and prevent the patient waking for a further dose.
- There is no maximum dose for morphine and therefore the dose is titrated according to increased pain relief compared with side effects. A poor response may necessitate the introduction of adjuncts, e.g. the cause of pain should be reassessed if more than 200 mg/day of morphine is required.
- There are now many brands of morphine that are designed for either daily or twice-daily administration. When prescribing, it is good practice to indicate both the generic and brand name to avoid over- or underdosing.
- Patients sensitive to the adverse effects of one strong opioid can be changed to a similar opioid so long as toxicity has been excluded, but note that frequent changes result in poor pain management.
- Softener and stimulant laxatives (see Chapter 10) should be started when any

opioid is initiated and the dose increased according to response rather than the opioid dose. When changing from high doses of morphine, however, laxative doses should be halved as severe diarrhoea may occur.

- Note that, unlike stronger opioids, opioids for mild-to-moderate pain produce a maximum analgesic effect, which is not exceeded by further dose increases. At this stage, stronger opioids are substituted according to step 3 of the WHO analgesic ladder. Substituting for an alternative weak opioid is of no benefit.

Syringe drivers

- Check infusion solutions regularly for discoloration or precipitation and ensure the correct rate of infusion.
- Infusion solutions should not be used for longer than 24 hours to reduce the risk of infection.
- Breakthrough pain may be treated with subcutaneous (or intramuscular) injections of diamorphine (a sixth of the total 24-hour dose being given by subcutaneous infusion).
- Monitor the injection site and consider changing to an alternative site if there is pain or prominent inflammation.

References

Austwick EA, Brown LC, Goddyear KH *et al.* (2002). Pharmacist's input into a palliative care clinic. *Pharm J* 268: 404–406.

British National Formulary, latest edition. London: British Medical Association and Royal Pharmaceutical Society of Great Britain.

Dickman D, Littlewood C, Varga J (2002). *The Syringe Driver. Continuous infusions in palliative care.* Oxford: Oxford University Press.

Miles CL, Fellowes D, Goodman ML *et al.* (2006). Laxatives for the management of constipation in palliative care patients. *Cochrane Database System Rev* issue 4: CD003448.

National Institute for Health and Care Excellence (2004). *Guidance on Cancer Services. Improving supportive and palliative care for adults with cancer.* London: NICE.

Needham D, Wong I (1999). An expert panel review to evaluate the effectiveness of community pharmacist's interventions in the palliative care setting. *Pharm J* 263 (suppl): R32–R33.

Nuland SB (1997). *How We Die*. Berkshire: Vintage.

World Health Organization (1990). *Cancer Pain Relief and Palliative Care: Report of a WHO Expert Committee*. Geneva: WHO.

Online resources

www.palliativedrugs.com
Provides access to drug information on the use of drugs in palliative care, access to books such as the *Palliative Care Formulary* and a monthly newsletter (accessed July 2015).

www.who.int/cancer/palliative/en
For WHO cancer information and publications, including the International Agency for Research on Cancer (IARC) (accessed July 2015).

www.hospiceuk.org
National charity for hospice care (accessed July 2015).

www.macmillan.org.uk
For Macmillan Cancer Relief, a charity providing information and support to patients with cancer and their carers, including information on access to Macmillan nurses (accessed July 2015).

www.mariecurie.org.uk
For access to Marie Curie Cancer Care, providing access to ongoing research, education and Marie Curie Hospices across the UK (accessed July 2015).

PART I

Infections

34

Bacterial infections

Bacterial infections comprise a wide range of diseases from simple, troublesome conditions to life-threatening events. The purpose of this chapter is to give a brief overview of common infections and antibacterial agents. In some cases infections such as respiratory tract and skin infections are dealt with elsewhere (see Chapters 20, 22 and 36). The aim is to illustrate common examples and principles; more detailed sources and guidelines should be consulted for specific information relating to bacterial sensitivity to antibiotics.

Disease characteristics

Infection or invasion by foreign, pathogenic organisms may result from those living as commensals on the body or from gut flora, in addition to those present in soil, food or on other animal hosts. Pathophysiological changes may result from bacterial infection of any part of the body, often entering via a wound or mucous membranes, by contact, ingestion or opportunistic infection, e.g. of immunocompromised patients.

Risk factors for infection include reduced immunity in young, elderly, immunocompromised or malnourished individuals, those with diabetes mellitus, or prosthetic valves or joints, or after surgery, or as a result of burns. Foreign travel may also result in infection due to exposure to organisms for which immunity has not developed previously. Drugs may increase the risk of infection by immunosuppression (e.g. corticosteroids), and effects on white cell production (e.g. drugs associated with agranulocytosis such as clozapine) and broad-spectrum antibiotics by affecting the gut flora.

Clinical features of common infections (Table 34.1)

Signs and symptoms of infection may include pyrexia, sweating, tachycardia, hypotension, nausea and vomiting, pallor, local pain and inflammation or purulence. A full blood count may indicate white cells elevated to $>12 \times 10^9$/L, with neutrophilia, but reduced due to depletion in chronic infections (such as tuberculosis [TB], although monocytes may be elevated) or in septicaemia. There may also be a raised erythrocyte sedimentation rate (ESR, see Chapter 2).

Gastrointestinal infections

Infections of the gastrointestinal tract include gastroenteritis, campylobacter enteritis, invasive salmonellosis, shigellosis, typhoid fever, antibiotic-associated pseudomembranous colitis, biliary tract infection (cholangitis) and peritonitis. Specific symptoms include diarrhoea, vomiting and abdominal pain. Cholangitis presents as pain in the right upper quadrant of the

Table 34.1 Some common examples of bacteria and their related conditions

Bacterium	Associated disease
Gram-positive cocci	
• *Staphylococcus aureus*	Associated with styes, impetigo, conjunctivitis, sinusitis, food poisoning, endocarditis, meningitis, pneumonia, UTI and osteomyelitis
• *Streptococcus pyogenes*	Causes scarlet fever, acute tonsillitis, erysipelas; dangerous if it affects wounds because it may cause sepsis
• *Streptococcus pneumoniae*	Pneumonia, bronchitis, infections of the ears and sinuses, meningitis
• *Streptococcus viridans*	Endocarditis
Gram-negative cocci	
• *Neisseria gonorrhoeae*	Purulent ophthalmia or gonorrhoea
• *Neisseria meningitidis*	Cerebrospinal fever or meningococcal meningitis
Gram-positive rods	
• *Bacillus* spp. (*B. anthracis, B. cereus*)	Anthrax, food poisoning
• *Clostridium* spp. (*C. botulinum, C. tetani C. difficile*)	Dangerous anaerobes causing tissue damage, affecting wounds and leading to gangrene, food poisoning (botulism), tetanus, pseudomembranous colitis (often secondary to use of broad-spectrum antibiotics such as clindamycin)
Gram-negative rods	
• *Pseudomonas aeruginosa*	Dangerous secondary infection of wounds, pneumonia, eye infections, UTI
• *Helicobacter pylori*	Associated with peptic ulcer
• *Haemophilus influenzae*	Infantile meningitis, conjunctivitis, chronic bronchitis, infections of ear and sinuses
• *Escherichia coli*	Enterobacteria (inhabitants of intestines) causing enteritis in young infants, also pyelitis, pyelonephritis and UTIs
• *Salmonella* spp.	Enteric bacteria causing typhoid, food poisoning
• *Shigella* spp.	Enteric bacteria causing dysentery
• *Proteus* spp.	Enteric bacteria infecting the urinary tract and wounds
• *Klebsiella pneumoniae*	Enteric bacteria and cause of acute bronchopneumonia
• *Campylobacter jejunum*	Enteritis due to food poisoning. Anaerobe
• *Bacteroides fragilis*	Oropharyngeal or gastrointestinal infection. Anaerobe
• *Chlamydia trachomatis*	Trachoma, conjunctivitis and non-gonococcal urethritis
• *Legionella pneumophila*	Legionnaires' disease transmitted in water, pneumonia
Acid-fast organisms	
Mycobacterium tuberculosis	Tuberculosis (*Mycobacterium* spp. also cause leprosy)
Spirochaetes	
• *Leptospira icterohaemorrhagiae*	Weils' disease (jaundice) carried by rats
• *Borrelia vincenti*	Vincent's angina

UTI, urinary tract infection.

abdomen and may be associated with jaundice and high fever. Chronic infection of the stomach or duodenum with *Helicobacter pylori* is associated with ulceration and is dealt with in Chapter 8.

Cardiovascular infections

Endocarditis, inflammation of the lining of the heart cavity (endocardium) and valves, may result from rheumatic fever or bacterial infection by streptococci, enterococci or staphylococci. Patients with existing abnormalities of the heart such as valvular disease are at increased risk. Specific clinical features are chest pain, murmur, tachycardia and palpitations. Patients may be frightened that they are suffering a heart attack, because symptoms can be severe and rapid in onset.

Respiratory infections

Respiratory infections include bronchitis and pneumonia, which are discussed in Chapters 20 and 22.

The incidence of TB is increasing, mainly due to the spread of acquired immune deficiency syndrome (AIDS), increased homelessness and the emergence of resistant strains. An initial latent phase may be asymptomatic. Progressive pulmonary TB produces symptoms of fatigue, night sweats, weight loss, cough with haemoptysis and chest pain. Chest radiology reveals abnormalities such as pulmonary infiltration, visible cavities and fibrosis. These abnormalities may occur before the clinical symptoms. The causative organisms are *Mycobacterium tuberculosis* and *M. avium,* of which multidrug-resistant strains are common.

Central nervous system

The most common infection of the central nervous system is meningitis, or infection with inflammation of the membrane (meninges) surrounding the brain. *Neisseria meningitidis* (meningococci), *Streptococcus pneumoniae* (pneumococci), *Haemophilus influenzae* and *Listeria monocytogenes* are important causative agents of bacterial meningitis. Clinical features include photophobia, neck stiffness, headache, rash that does not blanch under pressure (the glass test), general malaise and fever. A rash is not always present. Suspected meningitis is treated with 'blind' antibiotic therapy.

Urinary tract

Bacteriuria may indicate genitourinary infection affecting the kidney (pyelonephritis), bladder (cystitis), prostate in men (prostatitis) or urethra (urethritis), collectively known as urinary tract infections (UTIs). Acute pyelonephritis is an acute kidney infection presenting with fever, chills, rigors and pains, and tenderness. Lower UTIs are more common in women due to a shorter urethra and produce symptoms of urgency, frequency and dysuria (painful urination). More serious symptoms indicating renal involvement include haematuria, lower back or loin pain, and fever with diarrhoea and vomiting.

Risk factors for developing a UTI include diabetes mellitus, pregnancy, impaired voiding and catheters. *Escherichia coli* causes most UTIs occurring in the community. UTIs acquired during a stay in hospital may include infection by staphylococci, streptococci or *Pseudomonas* or *Proteus* species. UTIs are also commonly associated with long-term urinary catheters.

Genital infections

Genital infections include gonorrhoea, uncomplicated genital chlamydial infection, non-gonococcal urethritis and non-specific genital infections, pelvic inflammatory disease and, rarely, syphilis. *Neisseria gonorrhoeae* can infect the urethra, cervix, rectum, pharynx and conjunctiva. Infection is associated with a purulent discharge and may be otherwise asymptomatic and a cause of infertility. Non-gonococcal infection may produce a thinner discharge but also requires further investigation. Pyrexia and pelvic pain require urgent referral.

Genital infections are often transmitted sexually and partners should be referred for screening even in the absence of symptoms. Recurrent requests for cystitis or thrush treatment, particularly when previous treatment has been unsuccessful, should be referred to the general practitioner (GP) or genitourinary clinic for further investigation. This is particularly important due to the risk of complications such as infertility.

Blood

Septicaemia (blood poisoning) often results from an existing infection and in susceptible patients such as elderly or immunocompromised individuals. It may be caused by any of a number of pathogens. Treatment is therefore dependent on the nature of the initial infection. Symptoms include chills, diarrhoea, fever and vomiting. Urgent treatment is required to prevent spread, leading to secondary infection of organs and ultimately life-threatening septic shock, which involves severe hypotension and may lead to multiorgan failure.

Musculoskeletal system

Prompt treatment of osteomyelitis (infection and inflammation of bone marrow) and septic arthritis is imperative to prevent bone or joint damage. Alerting symptoms of infection include red, hot and painful swelling of the affected site with difficult movement. Septic arthritis most often involves *Staphylococcus aureus* and occasionally *H. influenzae* or *N. gonorrhoeae* (gonococci). Patients with existing damage to joints, such as those with rheumatoid arthritis and patients taking corticosteroids, are at increased risk of developing septic arthritis. This may also follow osteomyelitis affecting a nearby bone. Osteomyelitis in turn may follow a fracture or bone surgery. Treatment includes high doses of antibiotics, aspiration, analgesia and support of the affected joint or limb.

Eye

Purulent conjunctivitis may indicate bacterial infection requiring antibiotic eye drops such as chloramphenicol or gentamicin. Fusidic acid is used to treat suspected staphylococcal infections. Gonococcal conjunctivitis requires both topical and systemic antibiotics.

Ear, nose and throat

Infections affecting the ear, nose and throat include dental infections, sinusitis, otitis externa, otitis media and throat infections, which are covered in Chapter 20.

Acute otitis media

Acute otitis media is dealt with in Chapter 20.

Skin

Infections of the skin produce the conditions impetigo, erysipelas (*Streptococcus pyogenes* infection of

the skin and underlying tissue of the face and scalp), cellulitis and acne (see Chapter 36).

Goals of treatment

The aims of antibacterial treatment are to:

- eradicate the infection
- prevent spread
- prevent complications such as septicaemia and secondary infection.

The appropriate antibiotic is chosen with the spectrum of activity to cover the specific infection while avoiding the development of resistance. Symptomatic treatment may include the use of analgesics such as paracetamol and/or ibuprofen.

Prophylaxis

The use of antimicrobial agents to prevent infection plays an important role in patients at risk due to concurrent disease, surgery or contact with infection. Important examples where prophylaxis is appropriate include the following:

- Patients with rheumatic fever who receive antibiotic prophylaxis until 25 years of age and for subsequent surgery and dental surgery.
- Patients who have had a splenectomy.
- Patients with sickle cell anaemia.
- Patients with a history of endocarditis and/or those with prosthetic heart valves who require antibiotic prophylaxis before dental surgery.
- Patients in contact with meningitis or TB.
- Patients undergoing surgery.

Pharmacological basis of management

The aim of pharmacological treatment is the selective destruction of pathogens without harming human cells. Possible targets are mechanisms unique to pathogens and include protein synthesis and disruption of the unique construction and presence of a cell wall.

β-Lactam antibiotics (penicillins, cephalosporins)

Penicillins: amoxicillin, ampicillin, benzylpenicillin, flucloxacillin, phenoxymethylpenicillin

Penicillins target bacterial cell wall synthesis, by inhibiting cross-linking of peptide side chains, and so are effective only against dividing organisms. Penicillins are thus bactericidal, causing lysis of the bacteria. Some penicillins are inactivated by β-lactamases secreted by resistant bacteria (see below). Benzylpenicillin is active only after parenteral administration.

Cephalosporins, e.g. cefaclor, cefalexin, cefotaxime, cefradine, cefuroxime

Cephalosporins exhibit similar pharmacology to penicillins, binding to β-lactam-binding sites and inhibiting cell wall synthesis. They show cross-reactivity with penicillins and approximately 10% of penicillin-allergic patients will also be allergic to cephalosporins.

Glycopeptides: teicoplanin, vancomycin

These also inhibit bacterial cell wall synthesis by inhibiting the growth of the peptidoglycan chain.

Antibiotics that target bacterial protein synthesis

Tetracyclines, e.g. doxycycline, minocycline, oxytetracycline, tetracycline

Tetracyclines are bacteriostatic following inhibition of protein synthesis, through interference with tRNA binding. They are broad-spectrum antibiotics taken up into bacteria by active transport. Resistance has reduced the clinical indications for tetracyclines (Table 34.2).

Aminoglycosides: amikacin, gentamicin, neomycin, tobramycin

Aminoglycosides bind irreversibly to the bacterial ribosomes, leading to an inhibition of protein synthesis. They enter the bacterial cells via an oxygen-dependent active transport process and are therefore less effective against anaerobes. The bactericidal activity of aminoglycosides is enhanced when they are used with agents that target cell wall synthesis such as penicillins and vancomycin.

Macrolides, e.g. azithromycin, clarithromycin, erythromycin

Macrolides prevent the translocation movement of the bacterial ribosome along the mRNA and so prevent protein synthesis, resulting in bacteriostatic actions. In some organisms they are bactericidal.

Quinolones, e.g. ciprofloxacin, norfloxacin, ofloxacin

These are bacterial DNA gyrase inhibitors, which inhibit the supercoiling of the bacterial DNA that is essential for DNA repair and replication. This group of agents is bactericidal.

Others

- Clindamycin inhibits protein synthesis by a similar mechanism to the macrolide antibiotics (see above).
- Chloramphenicol inhibits protein synthesis by binding to the bacterial ribosome and inhibiting the formation of peptide bonds.
- Fusidic acid is a narrow-spectrum antibiotic inhibiting predominantly protein synthesis by Gram-positive bacteria.

Sulphonamides and trimethoprim

Sulphonamides inhibit the growth of bacteria (bacteriostatic) by inhibiting the enzyme dihydropteroate synthase involved in the synthesis of folate from p-aminobenzoic acid. The availability of DNA and RNA precursors is therefore reduced. Human folate synthesis is also reduced, although it may be obtained from the diet. The presence of thymidine and purines from pus and tissue breakdown bypass the need for folic acid, thereby reducing the effectiveness of these agents in such situations.

Trimethoprim is structurally related to folate, thereby acting as a folate antagonist and inhibiting dihydrofolate reductase, which converts folate to tetrahydrofolate. Previously, trimethoprim was widely used in combination with sulfamethoxazole (co-trimoxazole), but the side effects of sulfamethoxazole

Table 34.2 Some antibiotic sensitivities

Antibiotic	Sensitivities	Comments and indications
Penicillins (phenoxymethylpenicillin)	Streptococcal (including *Streptococcus pneumoniae*), *Neisseria gonorrhoea* and *N. meningitidis* infection	• Phenoxymethylpenicillin is less active than benzylpenicillin but may be given orally for respiratory tract infections in children, streptococcal tonsillitis and as prophylaxis against streptococcal infections following rheumatic fever, and against pneumococcal infections after splenectomy or in sickle cell disease • Benzylpenicillin may be given intravenously for bacterial meningitis • See text for note on resistance
Penicillinase-resistant penicillin (flucloxacillin)	Penicillin-resistant staphylococci	Otitis externa, adjunct in pneumonia, impetigo, cellulitis, wound infections, osteomyelitis and endocarditis if infection is known or likely to be caused by staphylococci producing penicillinases
Broad-spectrum penicillins (ampicillin, amoxicillin)	Gram-positive and Gram-negative bacteria but inactivated by penicillinases secreted by common Gram-negative bacilli and *Staphylococcus aureus*	• Indicated for exacerbation of chronic bronchitis, otitis media and UTIs • See text for note on resistance • Co-amoxiclav is used for animal bites
Cephalosporins	Varying sensitivities to Gram-positive and -negative bacteria depending on generation of the cephalosporin	Septicaemia, pneumonia, meningitis, biliary tract infections, peritonitis and UTIs
Glycopeptides	Only Gram-positive bacteria	• Vancomycin and teicoplanin are used against MRSA infections • Vancomycin is effective against *Clostridium difficile*
Macrolides	Similar spectrum to penicillins. Also active against *Chlamydia, Mycoplasma, Campylobacter, Legionella* spp.	• Suitable alternative in patients who are allergic to penicillin • Respiratory infections, whooping cough, Legionnaires' disease, campylobacter enteritis • Poor activity against *Haemophilus influenzae*
Chloramphenicol	Broad-spectrum against mainly Gram-positive cocci and -negative bacteria	• It is associated with aplastic anaemia and systemic use is reserved for life-threatening infections such as *Haemophilus influenzae* • It is widely used for bacterial conjunctivitis
Tetracyclines	Gram-positive and -negative bacteria	• Resistance is a problem • *Chlamydia,* exacerbation of chronic bronchitis (*Haemophilus influenzae*), periodontal disease, acne, respiratory and genital mycoplasma infections
Quinolones	Aerobic Gram-negative bacilli, particularly *Pseudomonas aeruginosa, Haemophilus influenzae, Campylobacter* spp.	• Nalidixic acid and norfloxacin used to treat UTIs • Ciprofloxacin for respiratory infection (except pneumococcal pneumonia), UTIs, gastrointestinal infections (including typhoid), gonorrhoea and septicaemia • Ofloxacin for UTIs, lower respiratory tract infections, gonorrhoea, non-gonococcal urethritis and cervicitis • Many staphylococci are resistant to quinolones, which are therefore avoided for MRSA infections
Metronidazole	Anaerobes and protozoa	• Trichomonal vaginosis (*Gardnerella vaginalis*), giardiasis (*Giardia lamblia*), surgical and gynaecological sepsis (*Bacteroides fragilis*), pseudomembranous colitis, fungating tumours and rosacea • Resistance is common

Table 34.2 *(continued)*

Antibiotic	Sensitivities	Comments and indications
Sulphonamides and trimethoprim	*Pneumocystis jiroveci*, meticillin-resistant *Staphylococcus* spp., some Gram-negative rods	• Decreased use due to resistance and availability of less toxic alternatives • Trimethoprim is now often used alone in place of sulfamethoxazole plus trimethoprim (co-trimoxazole) • Pneumonia in AIDS patients, toxoplasmosis and nocardosis. Acute exacerbation of chronic bronchitis, acute otitis media in children and UTI if good bacteriological evidence
Aminoglycosides	Some Gram-positive and many Gram-negative	• Gentamicin is administered systemically (thus hospital use) and plays an important role in serious infections such as septicaemia, meningitis, acute pyelonephritis and endocarditis • Inactive against anaerobes and poor activity against haemolytic streptococci and *Streptococcus pneumoniae* • Synergism with agents that target cell wall synthesis such as penicillins and vancomycin • Requires therapeutic drug monitoring (Chapter 7)
Clindamycin	Gram-positive cocci, including penicillin-resistant staphylococci, many anaerobes	• Staphylococcal joint and bone infections, e.g. osteomyelitis and intra-abdominal sepsis • Limited use due to toxic side effects

AIDS, acquired immune deficiency syndrome; MRSA, meticillin-resistant *Staphylococcus aureus;* UTIs, urinary tract infections.

are pronounced and therefore trimethoprim tends to be used alone.

Metronidazole

Metronidazole was originally developed to treat amoebiasis (protozoan infection). The mechanism of action is thought to be via DNA damage due to toxic oxygen products generated from the drug by these parasites. It is also active against anaerobic bacteria, containing nitroreductases, which activate metronidazole. It is useful for the treatment of dental abscesses, fungating tumours, pseudomembranous colitis and sepsis secondary to bowel disease when anaerobic infection is suspected.

Antituberculous drugs: ethambutol, isoniazid, pyrazinamide, rifampicin

First-line agents include a combination of isoniazid, rifampicin, ethambutol (if resistance to isoniazid is likely) and pyrazinamide. Combination therapy is given in two phases to prevent resistance. The initial phase includes the use of at least three drugs for 2 months. A combination of two drugs is then given for the continuation phase lasting 4 months or longer in drug-resistant infection, meningitis or bone/joint

involvement. Intermittent regimens are recommended when compliance is a problem.

Isoniazid

Isoniazid possesses selective bacteriostatic activity against mycobacteria, with some bactericidal activity against actively dividing mycobacteria. It is actively taken up: possible inhibition of *Mycobacterium-specific* mycolic acid constituents of the cell wall is the suggested mechanism. Disruption of cell metabolism may also be involved.

Resistance occurs due to reduced penetration of the drug. Side effects include allergic skin eruptions, fever, hepatotoxicity, haematological changes, arthritis and vasculitis (see Chapter 6).

Rifampicin

Rifampicin binds to and inhibits DNA-dependent RNA polymerase in prokaryotic but not eukaryotic cells. It is also active against some Gram-positive and -negative species. Resistance occurs rapidly due to a mutation in the chromosome encoding the DNA-dependent RNA polymerase. Adverse drug reactions (ADRs) include skin eruptions, jaundice, hepatotoxicity, fever and gastrointestinal disturbances.

Ethambutol

Ethambutol inhibits the growth of mycobacteria, although resistance is common if used alone. The development of optic neuritis is dose related, with an increased risk in renal impairment. Colour blindness and reduced visual acuity may occur, so monitoring of visual symptoms is required. Additional ADRs include gastrointestinal disturbance, arthralgia, headache, dizziness and mental disturbances.

Pyrazinamide

This agent becomes tuberculostatic at acidic pH. It is effective against intracellular mycobacteria found in macrophages after phagocytosis. Pyrazinamide is most effective against rapidly dividing intracellular organisms and is most effective in the first 2 months. Unwanted effects include gout, gastrointestinal disturbances and hepatotoxicity.

Drug choice

Current guidelines can be found at the start of Section 5 of the *British National Formulary*. Local guidelines may be available from health authorities, primary care trusts or the local infectious diseases centre, and based on local sensitivities these may well differ from those in the *British National Formulary*. Table 34.2 summarises examples of the main sensitivities of some antibiotics in regular use. Factors for consideration when prescribing antibiotics include:

- the likely causative organism
- risk of pathogen resistance
- age and sex of patient
- history of drug allergy
- tolerance of gastrointestinal side effects
- renal and hepatic function
- concurrent illnesses, e.g. epilepsy (Table 34.3)
- concurrent drug treatment (Table 34.4)
- route of elimination (renal excretion of active drugs resulting in therapeutic concentrations in the urinary tract, a distinct advantage in UTIs)
- is the patient pregnant or breastfeeding?
- risk factors, e.g. immunocompromised
- is the patient taking oral contraceptives?

Common organisms causing disease in humans

Bacteria are classified according to a staining method developed by Christian Gram in the nineteenth century. Gram-positive bacteria retain a solution of dye, which can be washed away from Gram-negative bacteria due to differing cell wall structures. Further nomenclature results from additional properties including morphology, the formation of spores and movement. Acid-fast bacteria are also named according to a staining reaction. For examples of disease-causing bacteria, see Table 34.1; some sensitivities of antibacterial agents are indicated in Table 34.2.

Resistance

Antibiotic resistance is now a major global concern, with the prospect of currently available antibiotics becoming ineffective in the near future. It occurs as a result of evolution of the rapidly dividing populations of bacteria. The spread of resistance occurs by the transfer of bacteria between people and the transfer of genetic material encoding resistance properties between bacteria. Mechanisms of resistance include the following:

- Development of pumps to exclude the drug from the bacteria, e.g. resistance to quinolones.
- Impermeability of bacteria to drugs, e.g. resistance to streptomycin.
- Inactivation of the drug, e.g. production of the enzyme β-lactamase by *Staphylococcus* spp. results in the breakdown of both phenoxymethylpenicillin and benzylpenicillin. Flucloxacillin is penicillinase resistant and therefore used for treating infections caused by penicillin-resistant *Staphylococcus* spp. Alternatively, the combination of the broad-spectrum penicillin amoxicillin with clavulanic acid may be given. Clavulanic acid inhibits β-lactamase.
- Some Gram-negative bacteria have reduced permeability of the cell wall, thereby impeding penetration of hydrophilic antibiotics to the target site.
- Alternative metabolic pathways to bypass blockade, e.g. in resistance to trimethoprim.
- Alteration in the drug target so that it is no longer recognised by the drug, e.g. in resistance to erythromycin, aminoglycosides.

Table 34.3 Concurrent disease and antibiotic prescribing

Concurrent disease	Drugs to avoid or use with caution	Comments
Arrhythmias	Macrolides	Prolongation of Q–T interval
History of allergy	Penicillins (phenoxymethylpenicillin, flucloxacillin, amoxicillin, pivmecillinam)	Increased risk of penicillin hypersensitivity including urticaria, fever, joint pains, rashes, angio-oedema
Penicillin allergy	Penicillins and cephalosporins	• If possible, penicillin side effects should be differentiated from true penicillin allergy (see text) • Usually occurs within 72 hours of starting treatment • Penicillin allergy is a contraindication to using penicillins and a reason not to use cephalosporins
Asthma (see also above)	Co-trimoxazole	May cause shortness of breath or pulmonary infiltrates
Epilepsy	Quinolones	May induce convulsions
Immunocompromised	All antibiotics	Higher doses are often required, as infections may be severe
Porphyria (hereditary disorder of haem biosynthesis)	Flucloxacillin, cephalosporins, erythromycin, isoniazid, sulphonamides, chloramphenicol, co-trimoxazole, trimethoprim, nitrofurantoin, nalidixic acid, tinidazole, oxytetracycline	For complete list see *British National Formulary*
Sore throat	Broad-spectrum penicillins (ampicillin, amoxicillin)	Due to a rash with glandular fever
Psychiatric disorders	Quinolones	Discontinue if there is a psychotic reaction
Diabetes mellitus	Cephalosporins, nitrofurantoin	False-positive urinary glucose (test for reducing substances)
Myasthenia gravis	Aminoglycosides	Impairment of neuromuscular transmission
Diarrhoea	Clindamycin	Contraindicated
History of deafness	Vancomycin, gentamicin	Ototoxic

Given the global concerns over antibiotic resistance the judicious use of antibiotics is a major goal for prescribers and education of patients is essential to ensure that antibiotics are only used when essential.

Meticillin-resistant *Staphylococcus aureus*

Resistance of *Staphylococcus aureus* bacteria to the discontinued drug meticillin is known as meticillin-resistant *Staphylococcus aureus* (MRSA). MRSA has received much attention because its incidence is on the increase and is associated with significant mortality. Although the bacterium responsible for these infections may be present innocently on many individuals (e.g. colonising the nasal passages), it poses a special problem for debilitated patients in hospital. Wounds may become infected leading to infection of major organs (e.g. the lungs), which may proceed to septicaemia.

The mechanism of resistance includes the modification of bacterial penicillin-binding sites. Treatment is indicated according to the infecting strain and currently includes vancomycin and teicoplanin. In addition to treatment, carriers may require eradication of the bacterium by using topical antiseptics such as mupirocin. New antibiotics effective against MRSA are reserved for strains resistant to conventional antibiotics and as such are currently beyond the scope of this book. These agents include linezolid (an oxazolidinone) and a combination of the streptogramin antibiotics quinupristin and dalfopristin.

Table 34.4 Examples of drug interactions involving antibiotics

Drugs	Consequences	Comments
Aminoglycosides with furosemide	Increased risk of aminoglycoside toxicity	• Monitor carefully for signs of nephrotoxicity and/or ototoxicity • Bumetanide does not appear to interact
Aminoglycosides with vancomycin	Increased risk of nephrotoxicity due to both drugs	Monitor for signs of nephrotoxicity
Rifampicin with oral contraceptives	Risk of contraceptive failure and pregnancy	Additional precautions are required during treatment and for 4–8 weeks after withdrawal due to enzyme induction and accelerated metabolism of oestrogens
Quinolones (ciprofloxacin, ofloxacin) with NSAIDs and drugs lowering seizure threshold (Chapter 6)	Increased risk of seizures	• Rare and limited evidence • These drugs should not be used in combination in patients with epilepsy
Quinolones with antacids	Reduced absorption of quinolones	• Aluminium and magnesium antacids particularly may reduce serum levels to below therapeutic concentrations • Separate administration by 2–6 hours
Ciprofloxacin with theophylline	Increased serum levels of theophylline	• Dose reduction (by half) is required with ciprofloxacin, enoxacin, and possibly norfloxacin • Monitor for signs of theophylline toxicity (Chapter 7)
Metronidazole, tinidazole, the cephalosporin cefamandole with alcohol	Risk of disulfiram-like reaction	• Most antibiotics do not interact with alcohol • Avoid alcohol with the drugs listed, as reaction may be frightening, although not serious
Erythromycin with alcohol	Erythromycin may increase the plasma concentrations of alcohol	• Some reports have also shown that alcohol reduces the absorption of erythromycin ethyl succinate • Drivers should be advised of this potential interaction
Antibiotics with warfarin	Effects of warfarin may be increased	See Chapter 17
Isoniazid with phenytoin, carbamazepine	Increased levels of anticonvulsants	Isoniazid inhibits cytochrome P450
Rifampicin with corticosteroids, oestrogens, phenytoin, carbamazepine, sulphonylureas, anticoagulants	Reduced levels	Rifampicin induces cytochrome P450, therefore increasing metabolism
Macrolides with simvastatin	Increased plasma concentrations of simvastatin with increased risk of myopathy	This combination should be avoided
Macrolides with ciclosporin	Increased levels	• Reduced ciclosporin dosage is usually required (approximately 60% with erythromycin). Monitor levels • Azithromycin appears not to interact
Erythromycin, clarithromycin, with other drugs which prolong the Q–T interval (Chapter 6)	Risk of potentially life-threatening cardiac arrhythmias	Concurrent use of two or more drugs that prolong the Q–T interval should be avoided because of the risk of additive effects

Table 34.4 *(continued)*

Drugs	Consequences	Comments
Erythromycin with various drugs: alfentanil, theophylline, warfarin, atorvastatin, some benzodiazepines, nadolol, carbamazepine (may become toxic), ciclosporin, digoxin (occasionally), felodipine, omeprazole	Inhibition of metabolism and therefore increased levels	Erythromycin inhibits cytochrome P450 enzymes
Erythromycin with zafirlukast	Reduced plasma concentrations	Monitor treatment outcome with zafirlukast

NSAIDs, non-steroidal anti-inflammatory drugs.

Measures to limit resistance include the following:

- The use of short courses of antibiotics such as a 3-day course to treat uncomplicated UTI.
- A reduction in unnecessary use of antibiotics in the treatment of viral infections and other self-limiting infections.
- The avoidance of antibiotics on repeat prescriptions.
- The avoidance of inappropriate prescribing of broad-spectrum agents (see Table 34.2).
- Ensuring that patients complete courses of antibiotics, so that more resilient strains do not survive.
- In the case of TB, the use of combination therapy.

Clostridium difficile

This 'superbug' infection is also receiving interest because it is associated with significant mortality, largely in debilitated hospital patients. Once again this bacterium is present in the gastrointestinal tracts of many otherwise healthy individuals. Broad-spectrum antibiotic treatment may alter the normal gut flora, killing off many harmless bacteria that normally keep pathogenic bacteria in check and this may lead to an outgrowth of *Clostridium difficile*, resulting in pseudomembranous colitis, which may present as severe bloody diarrhoea. To confound the problem, the spores of this bacterium are resistant to heat and some disinfectants, and so the spores are widespread in hospitals and may lead to severe outbreaks.

Penicillin allergy

Reports of penicillin allergy are common and it is often difficult to distinguish between true penicillin allergy (see Chapter 21) and less serious ADRs. Penicillin allergy is a class effect and all penicillins should be avoided, and there is the possibility of cross-reactivity with cephalosporins and these are also avoided.

Concurrent conditions

Although bacterial sensitivity of the causative organisms is a prime factor in the choice of appropriate antibacterial agents, concurrent conditions should also be taken into account. Some considerations are detailed in Table 34.3.

Children less than 12 years of age should not receive tetracyclines due to deposition in the teeth, leading to discoloration.

Pregnancy

The safest antibiotics for use during pregnancy are considered to be the penicillins, erythromycin and cephalosporins. The following drugs should be avoided or used with caution:

- Ciprofloxacin and other quinolones: adverse effects on developing cartilage have been reported in animal studies, even though there is no evidence of teratogenicity in humans.
- Co-trimoxazole: this is a folate antagonist, so there is a possible teratogenic risk.
- Fusidic acid: not known to be harmful; consider risk versus benefit.
- Gentamicin: there is a risk of auditory damage to the fetus.
- Metronidazole: avoid high doses if possible but this is an important treatment of trichomoniasis and giardiasis infections.

- Nitrofurantoin may cause nausea.
- Tetracycline: there is a risk of deposition in growing bones and teeth and the resultant risk of fetal abnormalities if given during pregnancy.

Breastfeeding

Amoxicillin, erythromycin or cephalosporins are appropriate for use during breastfeeding. Penicillins may in theory produce hypersensitivity in the infant and therefore mothers should be vigilant for signs of allergy such as a rash. Tetracyclines are not recommended, although calcium should prevent the infant from absorbing the small amounts present in breast milk.

Chloramphenicol eye drops as an over-the-counter medicine

Chloramphenicol eye drops are now available as an over-the-counter (OTC) medicine and may be recommended to patients aged >2 years for the treatment of bacterial conjunctivitis for a maximum of 5 days. This move is clearly to be welcomed because it utilises the pharmacist's expertise and makes readily available an effective treatment for this condition without the need to visit a doctor. However, this raises a number of issues because it requires the pharmacist to differentiate bacterial conjunctivitis from a range of other eye conditions, some of which could be potentially serious. Therefore, the pharmacist should be cautious and seek the advice of a specialist if there are any uncertainties such contact lens wearing, eye trauma, concurrent glaucoma and pregnancy. Furthermore, if there is treatment failure after 48 hours or the condition gets worse the patient should visit their doctor.

Despite the introduction of chloramphenicol as the first OTC antibiotic, a study has indicated that its use in otherwise healthy children results only in a very modest improvement in outcome (Rose *et al.* 2005). Therefore, the use of chloramphenicol for most children offers little in the way of benefit as the infection usually resolves in a similar time frame. Simple measure such as bathing the eye in cotton wool soaked in sterile physiological (0.9%) saline may be helpful.

Drug interactions

Antibacterial agents comprise a diverse group of drugs and can be expected to exhibit a range of interactions. In particular, the macrolides are inhibitors and rifampicin an inducer of cytochrome P450 with the ability to alter the metabolism of a range of other drugs. Until recently it was assumed that broad-spectrum antibiotics could potentially affect oral contraceptives. However, this is no longer supported by the evidence and caution is no longer needed. Some important interactions are detailed in Table 34.4.

General counselling

- Antimicrobials should be taken regularly, at evenly spaced intervals, and the prescribed course should be completed to prevent recurrence and resistance. Explaining that more resistant bacteria may survive if the course is not completed, creating an increased risk of resistance to subsequent treatment, may aid compliance.
- Patients should be advised that antibacterial agents will take several days for an effect but, if the condition does not resolve by the end of the course, patients should visit their GP.
- Patients should be advised not to hoard antibacterials or allow them to be used by others.
- A key point to reinforce is that colds and most sore throats are viral in origin and will not respond to antibacterial agents (see Chapter 20).
- An important point is that taking broad-spectrum antibiotics is associated with super-infection, which may lead to candidiasis and diarrhoea. If the diarrhoea is severe (possibly accompanied by pain and pyrexia), this may indicate pseudomembranous colitis and patients should contact their GP urgently. This is particularly associated with clindamycin treatment (see Chapters 6 and 10).
- Many antibacterial agents are associated with rashes and this is particularly true of penicillin allergy. In the case of penicillin allergy, antihistamines may relieve the rash. However, as with any drug, if there is itching, angio-oedema or breathing difficulties, then medical attention should be sought immediately because this may be due to anaphylaxis (see Chapter 21).
- A prominent record of penicillin allergy should be made on all medical records and patients should also be advised to inform GPs, dentists, pharmacists and nurses.

Penicillins

- Penicillins should be taken an hour before food or on an empty stomach for improved absorption, with the exception of amoxicillin.
- Penicillins should not be taken by patients with a history of penicillin allergy.
- Side effects are mild and may include diarrhoea and indigestion.
- Flucloxacillin may rarely cause jaundice.

Cephalosporins

Report increased bruising or signs of bleeding, due to possible interference with blood-clotting factors.

Quinolones

- Separate administration of antacids, particularly aluminium- and magnesium-containing preparations, by 2–6 hours because these antacids may reduce serum levels to below therapeutic concentrations.
- Quinolones may impair performance of skilled tasks such as driving. Advice given in the *British National Formulary* suggests that these effects are enhanced by alcohol, but evidence presented in *Stockley's Drug Interactions* by Baxter (2013) suggests that quinolones do not interact with alcohol.
- Due to risk of tendon damage treatment should be withdrawn at the first sign of pain or inflammation. The affected limb should be rested until tendon symptoms have resolved. Contact the GP immediately.

Macrolides

- Macrolides may cause nausea, so should be taken with or after food.
- Macrolides and erythromycin in particular are associated with a high incidence of nausea and vomiting.

Tetracyclines

- Do not take at the same time as milk, iron or zinc supplements, calcium supplements or indigestion remedies that may hinder absorption. Separate doses by at least 2 hours.
- Swallow whole with plenty of water while sitting or standing.

- Doxycycline may cause photosensitivity, so avoid exposure to the sun or use high-factor sun cream. Avoid using sun beds and sun showers.

Metronidazole and tinidazole

- Do not take these with alcohol due to very unpleasant effects such as flushing.
- Take with or after food.
- Swallow whole and do not chew.
- Take with plenty of water.
- For treatment exceeding 10 days, consider providing advice about the increased risk of adverse effects such as peripheral neuropathy (see Monitoring below).

Trimethoprim

- Contact the GP if a rash and/or itching develop.
- If taking trimethoprim long term, report signs of bruising, bleeding, mouth ulcers or sore throat due to rare effects of this antibiotic on the blood.

Clindamycin

- Capsules should be swallowed whole with plenty of water.
- See comments above regarding diarrhoea.

Antituberculous drugs

- Soft contact lenses should not be worn during treatment with rifampicin. Gas-permeable or hard lenses are appropriate.
- The patient should report any signs of liver disease such as persistent nausea, vomiting, malaise or jaundice immediately.
- Rifampicin may colour the patient's urine orange-red.
- Isoniazid should be taken 30–60 minutes before food.
- The patient should report visual deterioration with ethambutol immediately. This may be irreversible if treatment is continued.
- The importance of compliance should be explained.
- Pyridoxine (vitamin B_6) should be taken with isoniazid to prevent peripheral neuropathy. Increased risk factors include diabetes mellitus, alcohol misuse, renal failure and malnutrition.

Eye drops and ointments

- Eye drops should be applied at least every 2 hours and then the frequency reduced as the infection is controlled.
- Treatment should be continued for 48 hours after symptoms have cleared.
- Patients should not share eye drops.
- Eye ointment may be used at night or three to four times a day if used alone.
- Remaining drops or ointment should be discarded.
- Sterile saline solution may help soothe the eyes and remove discharge.

Chloramphenicol

The introduction of chloramphenicol requires clear counselling once it is established that its use is appropriate. The following are additional counselling points:

- If there is deterioration or no improvement after 48 hours then the patient should consult a doctor.
- The course is for 5 days.
- Although contact lens wearers should consult an optometrist, patients prescribed choramphenicol should not wear their contact lenses until 24 hours after completing treatment.

Monitoring

Metronidazole

Laboratory and clinical monitoring is advised if treatment with metronidazole exceeds 10 days. This is due to an increased risk of adverse effects, particularly peripheral neuropathy, and possibly transient seizures, cholestatic hepatitis, jaundice and leukopenia. Full blood counts and liver function tests may be required (see Chapter 2).

Renal impairment

Many drugs require dose reduction, particularly in severe renal impairment. The following are some general considerations:

- Piperacillin: dose adjustment is required.
- Aminoglycosides: dose reduction and monitoring are required with even mild renal impairment.

Plasma concentrations should be monitored due to renal and ototoxicity.
- Ethambutol: dose reduction and monitoring are required.
- Isoniazid: maximum dose recommended in severe impairment is 200 mg/day.
- Sulphonamides: maintain a high fluid intake with moderate impairment due to the risk of crystalluria.
- Tetracyclines: other than doxycycline and minocycline, may exacerbate renal failure and should not be given to patients with renal disease.
- Trimethoprim: dose reduction is required in moderate renal failure. Avoid if creatinine clearance is <10 mL/minute unless plasma trimethoprim levels are monitored.

Hepatic function

Many antibiotics may cause hepatic disease see (Chapter 6) and therefore monitoring for suspected ADRs is important:

- Clindamycin: dose reduction is required.
- Co-amoxiclav: risk of cholestatic jaundice. Treatment should not normally exceed 14 days.
- Erythromycin may cause idiosyncratic hepatotoxicity.
- Flucloxacillin: a risk of cholestatic jaundice.
- Fusidic acid: impaired biliary excretion and increased risk of hepatotoxicity. A reduced dose is used if treatment is necessary.
- Isoniazid: monitor liver function tests regularly and particularly during the first 2 months of treatment.
- Metronidazole: in severe hepatic disease, the dose of metronidazole is reduced by a third and given once a day.
- Minocycline: monitor liver function tests if treatment exceeds 6 months.
- Pyrazinamide: avoid in liver disease.
- Rifampicin: monitor for toxicity.
- Tetracyclines should be avoided or used with caution in liver disease.

Over-the-counter considerations

Pharmacists are ideally placed to reassure patients and recommend symptomatic relief of infections that do not require antibiotics. Consultations about infections are particularly important in the identification of underlying disease. Patient counselling on the appropriate use of anti-infective agents and preventive measures is important, particularly in preventing drug resistance and treatment failure. General lifestyle advice (see Chapter 3) may also be appropriate.

Genitourinary infection

Recurrent UTIs or candida infections may indicate diabetes mellitus, recent antibiotic treatment or undiagnosed sexually transmitted infection (STI). Appropriate referral including the first UTI in men, pregnant women, abdominal or lower back pain, resistance to treatment and haematuria is warranted.

The following advice is important in the prevention of recurrent infection:

- The avoidance of nylon underwear (cotton is preferable).
- The importance of sexual hygiene, including urination after sexual intercourse.
- Drink plenty of water.
- Urinate frequently with double voiding (go again after 5 minutes).
- Cranberry juice has been shown to be effective at preventing bacteria adhering to bladder epithelial cells and may be helpful in the treatment of UTIs.
- Consider treating partners.

ADRs

Requests for antidiarrhoeal agents should be dealt with carefully to exclude possible antibiotic-associated colitis, e.g. the severity and duration of diarrhoea should be determined. Throat preparations containing local anaesthetics may cause hypersensitivity.

Drug interactions

For interactions between NSAIDs or antacids and antibiotics, see Table 34.4.

Products for cystitis containing sodium are inappropriate for patients with hypertension or those prescribed lithium. Alternative products containing potassium salts should not be given to patients taking angiotensin-converting enzyme inhibitors or potassium-sparing diuretics such as spironolactone or amiloride.

Practice points

- Broad-spectrum antibiotics are more likely to result in fungal infections (vaginitis or pruritus ani) or ADRs such as pseudomembranous colitis.
- Viral infections such as simple coughs and colds and viral sore throats should not be treated with antibacterials.
- Whenever possible, an accurate diagnosis and clear documentation of penicillin hypersensitivity should be made.
- Chloramphenicol eye drops are now available as an OTC medicine and patients should be identified and counselled as appropriate. If there is any doubt as to the diagnosis the patient should be referred to his or her doctor.
- In prescribing chloramphenicol, community pharmacists might consider developing links with local opticians for assistance in diagnosis.

Self-assessment

For the following questions concerning the management of bacterial infections, choose the most appropriate answers:

1 *Which one of the following antibacterial agents or groups is associated with significant drug interactions?*

   A Gentamicin
   B Amoxicillin
   C Cephalosporins
   D Erythromycin
   E Flucloxacillin

2 *Which one of the following is often a sign of acute infection?*

   A Decreased erythrocyte sedimentation rate (ESR)
   B Raised C-reactive protein (CRP) levels
   C Raised international normalised ratio (INR)
   D Raised B-type natriuretic peptide (BNP) levels
   E Decreased platelet count

3 Which one of the following best describes the mode of action of penicillins (such as amoxicillin)?

A Inhibition of DNA gyrase to prevent DNA uncoiling
B Inhibition of bacterial ribosomes to prevent protein synthesis
C Inhibition of bacterial transpeptidases to prevent cross-linking of cell walls
D Inhibition of bacterial dihydropteroate synthase
E Chelation of bacterial DNA

4 Clavulanic acid is added to amoxicillin to:

A Prevent its degradation by bacterial β-lactamases
B Limit its renal excretion
C Give it a more rigid structure
D Prevent cellular uptake
E Optimise the pH for amoxicillin to act

5 Which one of the following is contraindicated in children?

A Amoxicillin
B Tetracycline
C Ciprofloxacin
D Gentamicin
E Trimethoprim

6 What problem does the anti-tuberculosis drug rifampicin pose?

A Interacts with milk
B Powerful enzyme inducer
C Most infections are resistant to it
D Suppression of bone marrow
E Contraindicated in asthma

7 Which one of the following is an OTC licence?

A Gentamicin ear drops for otitis externa
B Trimethoprim tablets for a simple urinary tract infection
C Amoxicillin tablets for a simple chest infection
D Chloramphenicol eye drops for conjunctivitis
E Erythromycin cream for acne

8 Which of the following poses a high risk for Clostridium difficile infection?

A Vancomycin
B Metronidazole
C Tetracycline
D Trimethoprim
E Clindamycin

9 Cellulitis affects which of the following?

A Heart muscle
B Skin
C Lungs
D Liver
E Nerves

10 Which one of the following shows a significant interaction with alcohol?

A Amoxicillin
B Co-amoxiclav
C Gentamicin
D Metronidazole
E Tetracycline

CASE STUDIES

Case 1

A 60-year-old woman requests loperamide for acute diarrhoea. On further questioning you discover that she is taking clindamycin.

Do you give loperamide?

- No! Clindamycin is associated with antibiotic-associated colitis, which is potentially fatal. This is most common in middle-aged and elderly women and particularly postoperatively. The antibiotic should be stopped immediately.

Case 2

A 65-year-old man presents at the accident and emergency department complaining of a persistent productive cough with haemoptysis and general ill health. A chest X-ray reveals a lesion.

How would TB be confirmed?

- TB is becoming more prevalent. A positive Mantoux (tuberculin test) confirms TB together with the above symptoms and possibly a sputum sample culture, although the former is the quickest means of diagnosis.

What tests would be carried out before starting drug treatment?

- Liver function tests are required, because isoniazid, rifampicin and pyrazinamide are all associated with liver toxicity. Renal function would be determined because doses of ethambutol and isoniazid may need to be adjusted. Visual acuity is monitored with ethambutol because this can cause loss of acuity, colour blindness or restriction of visual fields.

Is it necessary to treat contacts?

- Yes. Chemoprophylaxis with isoniazid for 6 months is the current recommendation.

What are the possible causes of treatment failure?

- Treatment failure may result from incorrect prescribing, poor compliance or drug resistance. Taking a sample of urine, which is orange-red when taking rifampicin, may be a useful method to monitor compliance.

Case 3

A 55-year-old male patient presents with an acute exacerbation of chronic bronchitis. He has seen adverts about overuse of antibiotics and is reluctant to take them. He reports purulent green sputum.

What is the appropriate treatment?

- Amoxicillin is an appropriate first-line treatment, assuming that this patient is not allergic to penicillin. His symptoms and history indicate the use of antibiotics and he should be advised accordingly. Amoxicillin is a broad-spectrum antibiotic covering the main organisms causing community-acquired infection, such as *Streptococcus pneumoniae*, *Haemophilus influenzae* or *Staphylococcus aureus*. Erythromycin is a suitable alternative in penicillin allergy, though drug interactions should be considered. Smoking cessation advice should be reinforced if necessary.

References

Baxter (2013). *Stockley's Drug Interactions*, 11th edn. London: Pharmaceutical Press.

British National Formulary, latest edition. London: British Medical Association and Royal Pharmaceutical Society of Great Britain.

Rose PW, Harnden A, Brueggemann AB *et al*. (2005). Chloramphenicol treatment for acute infective conjunctivitis in children in primary care: a randomised double-blind placebo-controlled trial. *Lancet* 366: 37–43. pmid: 15993231.

Further reading

Denyer SP, Hodges NA, Gorman SP, Gilmore BF, eds (2011). Hugo and Russell's *Pharmaceutical Microbiology*, 8th edn. Oxford: Wiley-Blackwell.

Online resources

www.hpa.org.uk
The website of the Health Protection Agency; provides the latest information relating to infectious diseases (accessed October 2015).

35

Non-bacterial infections

The term 'parasite' describes organisms that rely on another organism or host for food and shelter without providing a positive contribution to the host. Parasitic infections therefore include bacteria, fungi, worms, viruses and protozoa. Non-bacterial infections include:

- fungal: *Candida albicans* and tinea (see Chapter 36)
- viral: herpes simplex and varicella-zoster (see Chapter 36), influenza (see Chapter 20)
- protozoan: *Plasmodium* spp. (malaria)
- helminthic: roundworms (ascariasis), thread worms (enterobiasis)
- ectoparasitic infections: head lice (*Pediculus humanus capitis*), crab lice (*Phthirus pubis*) and scabies (*Sarcoptes scabiei*).

Goals of treatment

The main aims of treatment are to:

- prevent or treat infections such as malaria
- prevent spread of lice or scabies
- prevent re-infection by implementing hygiene measures and contact tracing.

Malaria

Malaria is a potentially fatal mosquito-borne infection of red blood cells (erythrocytes) caused by the protozoan parasites *Plasmodium falciparum, P. vivax, P. ovale* and *P. malariae*. Red blood cells are destroyed by the parasites, resulting in haemolytic anaemia. Other symptoms include shivering, fever, muscle pain and sweating. The parasites live and reproduce inside the liver, being re-released into the bloodstream in a continuous cycle.

Drug treatment for prophylaxis of malaria

The choice of antimalarial agent depends largely on the destination of travel and the presence of resistance. Recommendations for effective prophylaxis are reviewed regularly and therefore the latest guidelines should be sought from organisations such as the National Pharmaceutical Association, the Health Protection Agency, Schools of Tropical Medicine, the Department of Health or the World Health Organization (see the *British National Formulary* and Online resources at the end of this chapter).

4-Aminoquinolines (chloroquine)

Chloroquine is a disease-modifying antirheumatoid drug (DMARD, see Chapter 31). In protozoal infections, chloroquine becomes concentrated in infected erythrocytes as it binds to a breakdown product of haemoglobin. It then inhibits haem polymerase, an enzyme produced by *Plasmodium* spp., which prevents the parasite from digesting haemoglobin. It is therefore effective against the erythrocytic forms *P. malariae*, *P. ovale* and *P. vivax*. It is not, however, effective against latent forms of *P. ovale* and *P. vivax*, which reside in the liver. The resistance of *P. falciparum* to chloroquine tends to result from increased efflux of the drug and/or reduced uptake.

Quinoline methanols (quinine, mefloquine)

Quinine is active against all erythrocytic forms of *Plasmodium* spp. but is mainly used to treat *P. falciparum* infections. In view of its adverse effects, it is not appropriate for prophylaxis. Quinine is an alkaloid with negative inotropic effects on the heart, a mild oxytocic effect on the uterus in pregnancy (although use is appropriate for malaria treatment) and a weak antipyretic effect. Mefloquine has no effect on hepatic forms of the parasites but is often used for prophylaxis or treatment of *P. falciparum* infection, particularly against chloroquine-resistant forms. Quinine resistance occurs after increased expression of an efflux transporter.

Drugs affecting the synthesis or utilisation of folate (pyrimethamine, proguanil)

These agents exhibit activity similar to that of sulphonamides (see Chapter 34) in that they inhibit the utilisutilisation of folate by inhibiting dihydrofolate reductase. Combinations of folate antagonists with drugs targeting folate synthesis are used to produce a synergistic action resulting from blockade of different parts of the synthetic pathway.

8-Aminoquinolones (primaquine)

Primaquine is active against the latent phase of *P. ovale* and *P. vivax* and may be used in combination with other drugs such as chloroquine. It enters the parasites in the liver and is thought to inhibit mitochondrial respiration. Active metabolites may also bind to parasitic DNA. Resistance is currently rare.

Doxycycline

Doxycycline may be used as an alternative when antimalarials are contraindicated (see Chapter 34).

Artemether with lumefantrine

This combination is a relatively recent introduction for the treatment of acute uncomplicated falciparum malaria. These drugs target the conversion by the parasites of toxic haem to haemozoin in red blood cells during active infection. This stops the re-infection cycle at the blood stage.

Drug choice

Local guidelines may be available from health authorities, primary care trusts or on the advice of the local infectious disease centre. Factors for consideration when prescribing include:

- risk of pathogen resistance
- age and sex of patient
- history of drug allergy
- concurrent disease (Table 35.1)
- is the patient pregnant or breastfeeding?
- time and destination of travel.

Patient counselling

Patients should be encouraged to consult healthcare professionals at least 2 months before foreign travel to ensure time for immunisations.

Antimalarials

- Preventive measures are extremely important, even during prophylaxis with antimalarials.
- The application of repellents containing diethyltoluamide (DEET, now called diethyl-methylbenzamide), with increasing concentration (up to 50%) or frequency of applications, offers greatest protection (Fradin and Day 2002). These products are suitable for children aged >2 months and during pregnancy and breastfeeding.
- Mosquito nets should be used at night. Nets impregnated with permethrin and vaporised insecticides are also effective.
- Protective clothing should be worn in the evening, after dusk.

Table 35.1 The effects of concurrent disease on drug choice

Concurrent disease	Drugs to avoid or use with caution	Comments
Arrhythmias	Mefloquine, quinine, artemether with lumefantrine	Prolongation of Q–T interval (Chapter 6)
Asthma and/or eczema	Pesticides and particularly those containing alcohol	Some pesticide preparations may trigger an allergic response. All pesticides should be applied in a well-ventilated room. Dimeticone or wet combing is preferred
Epilepsy	Chloroquine, mefloquine, piperazine	May induce convulsions and should therefore be avoided
Gastrointestinal disease (severe)	Chloroquine	Use with caution
Glucose-6-phosphate dehydrogenase (G6PD) deficiency	Primaquine	• G6PD activity should be assessed before starting treatment • Patients with G6PD deficiency may suffer haemolysis if given standard doses • Reduced doses are appropriate
Hepatic disease	All antimalarials with the possible exception of proguanil and atovaquone (HPA)	• Avoid in severe liver disease • Mefloquine may also be used in moderate impairment • Chloroquine and doxycycline (with caution) are additional choices in mild impairment (HPA)
Psychiatric disorders	Mefloquine	Contraindicated for patients with a history of psychiatric disorders including depression
Psoriasis	Chloroquine	May exacerbate psoriasis
Renal impairment	Proguanil (avoid or reduce dose), piperazine	• Chloroquine, mefloquine or doxycycline are appropriate for malaria prophylaxis • The dose of chloroquine may require reduction in severe impairment • Malarone should not be used for prophylaxis in patients with creatinine clearance <30 mL/minute • Piperazine should be avoided in severe renal impairment

HPA, Health Protection Agency.

- Patients may be concerned about side effects from antimalarials and should be advised of the importance of taking these drugs because malaria is life threatening, e.g. many people are worried about the psychiatric effects of mefloquine (see Chapter 6).
- Prophylaxis is recommended for 1 week before travel (2–3 weeks for mefloquine to identify psychiatric adverse drug reactions before travel), during the stay and for 4 weeks after return with the exception of Malarone, which should be stopped 1 week after leaving.
- Any illness within 1 year of travel to an area associated with risk of malaria should be reported, particularly within the first 3 months.

Helminthic and ectoparasitic infections

Pruritus is the most common feature of the presence of worms, head lice, crabs or scabies. These parasites may then be observed, e.g. head lice on the hair or worms in the faeces. Scabies are more difficult to diagnose because they burrow under the skin, but close examination will reveal 'tracks' along the skin and a magnifying glass may be used to view the mites. Suspicion of scabies is aroused if more than one patient living in the same house is affected and often the wrists are the first sites of infection.

Pharmacological basis of management

Anthelmintics: mebendazole, piperazine

Anthelmintics target the formation of intracellular microtubules in helminths (parasitic worms). They must penetrate the cuticle of the worm or be eaten by the worm. The resultant effects are paralysis, partial digestion or an immune response to the damaged cuticle. Alternatively, helminth metabolism may be targeted. This is a species-dependent effect, explaining the varied activity of some anthelmintics.

Mebendazole is a broad-spectrum agent and may take several days to expel worms by targeting intracellular organelle function such as microtubules.

Piperazine is used to treat the common roundworm (*Ascaris lumbricoides*) and threadworm (*Enterobius vermicularis*). It inhibits neuromuscular transmission in the worm, possibly by activation of γ-aminobutyric acid (GABA)-gated chloride channels in nematode muscle, leading to muscle relaxation. The paralysed worms are passed alive. Side effects include gastrointestinal disturbance and urticaria.

Malathion, carbaryl, phenothrin, permethrin, dimeticone

Malathion and carbaryl are organophosphorous inhibitors of acetylcholinesterase, and so prevent the breakdown of acetylcholine, which causes paralysis and kills the louse. The use of carbaryl is, however, restricted to prescription use when lice are resistant to other agents. Phenothrin and permethrin are pyrethroid compounds, which also produce death by paralysis after activation of sodium channels on peripheral nerves. Dimeticone is a silicone-based substance and is used as an alternative choice to insecticidal neurotoxins; it probably acts by coating the louse and disrupting its function. Dimeticone has the advantage that it does not readily cause skin irritation and resistance that develops to neurotoxins is not a problem.

Drug choice

Anthelmintics

These are combined with hygiene measures to prevent re-infection. Mebendazole is used to treat threadworms in patients aged >2 years. This is available over-the-counter but not for use during pregnancy. A fatty meal aids the absorption of mebendazole, which is given as a single dose for threadworm infection, or twice a day for 3 days to treat hookworms or roundworms, and repeated after 2 weeks. Mebendazole is the most commonly used benzimidazole; gastrointestinal disturbances are the main side effect.

Piperazine is an alternative, e.g. given to children aged from 3 months by a general practitioner (GP), as a single dose, and repeated after 14 days for threadworm infections or monthly for up to 3 months for roundworms.

Levamisole is available on a named-patient basis and is the drug of choice for the common roundworm *Ascaris lumbricoides*.

Head lice preparations

The choice of preparation depends upon previous treatment and the presence of asthma or skin sensitivity such as eczema (see Table 35.1). Dimeticone and wet combing are suitable first-line choices. Alternatively, products with an aqueous base, such as Derbac M, are preferred for people with asthma or sensitive skin, and young children. Lotions or liquid formulations are recommended rather than shampoos, mousses and cream rinses because the contact time is too short for the latter products to be effective and some preparations may be too dilute. If a previous treatment has failed, an alternative agent should be used, once the reason for treatment failure has been established, e.g. failure to apply a second application after 7 days. The presence of live head lice 7–9 days after treatment indicates the survival of eggs and therefore is not treatment failure. The same treatment should be repeated. Resistance is also becoming a problem, and this is most marked with pyrethroids but less of a problem with carbaryl (Clark 2007). Other causes of treatment failure include the following:

- Re-infection due to the lack of treatment of close contacts including parents and grandparents.
- The product not being left on the hair for sufficient time.
- The application of conditioner before the product, which should be applied to dry hair.
- Application of too low a concentration of active ingredient.

Carbaryl

It should be noted that carbaryl preparations have been restricted to prescription-only use due to the observation that carbaryl is carcinogenic in rodents. The risk to humans is reported to be theoretical, especially if use is intermittent. Carbaryl and malathion can irritate the skin and should not be used in damaged skin or where there is infection.

Crab lice

Permethrin, phenothrin and malathion are licensed for the eradication of crab lice. Aqueous preparations are applied to all parts of the body for 12 hours.

Patient counselling

Head lice preparations

Prevention

- Parents should be reassured that head lice have no preference for dirty or clean hair. Long hair may, however, be more accessible as head lice 'walk' from head to head. They do not hop, jump or fly. Long hair should therefore be braided close to the head if possible. Shaving the hair is not an effective method because lice only need 1 mm of hair to cling to. Head lice are not harmful but may cause an itchy scalp with the risk of secondary bacterial infection after chronic scratching.
- Regular checking for lice is advisable using a fine nit comb when the hair is wet, going through a small section at a time. This will help to remove lice, aid early diagnosis and prevent the spread of head lice. The excessive use of pesticides may then be prevented. The use of conditioner may help the manual removal of lice. The eggs may appear similar to dandruff but are differentiated by their ability to stick to the hair.
- The presence of lice should be confirmed before treating, because infection is not prevented by treatment. The hair may be combed over white paper to identify live lice.
- Contact tracing is important to prevent spread of the infection. This includes all close contacts such as grandparents who should be treated if infected.

Wet combing

Wet combing is useful for detection and treatment of head lice infestation and some products for this method can be prescribed. However, this is not necessarily an easy option because to fully wet comb the hair can take a significant amount of time. The *British National Formulary* recommends an interval of 4 days and a minimum of 2 weeks with hair conditioner or vegetable oil used to make combing and removal of eggs and lice easier. An appropriate comb should be used from the scalp to the ends of the hair and lice removed after each stroke. Conditioner can then be washed off. Information leaflets with detailed instructions about wet combing should be provided. Weekly wet combing is recommended for detection if head lice are present in a school or nursery (Clark 2007). Note that metal combs are not appropriate for wet combing but can be useful for removing noticeable nits.

Treatment

- Treatment is most likely to be successful if patients understand the mode of action of preparations for head lice and the life-cycle of lice. This enforces the likelihood of a second application being required after 7 days. A leaflet should be provided alongside verbal advice.
- Most products require a 12-hour application and should be applied to dry hair at night, in a well-ventilated room. The hair and scalp should be soaked in the product and then allowed to dry naturally. The hair may then be washed the following morning.
- A second application is required after 7 days, after which time any eggs not eradicated by the initial treatment may begin to hatch. This should not be confused with treatment failure or reinfestation.
- Repeat applications should be avoided within a week and for more than three consecutive weeks. The manufacturers suggest that not more than five applications of head lice preparations be used per year. The likelihood of eradication is not increased.
- It should be noted that Full Marks mousse contains alcohol and may not be suitable for patients with asthma or eczema.

Crab lice

Apply aqueous lotion to all parts of the body, including scalp, neck, ears and face, for 12 hours. A second treatment is recommended after 7 days to kill lice hatching from eggs, which may have survived the initial treatment (BNF).

Anthelmintics

- Combine with hygiene measures to break the cycle of re-infection. Hands should be washed and nails scrubbed before each meal and after each visit to the toilet. A bath immediately after rising will remove ova laid during the night. Fingernails should be kept short.
- A second dose may be required to prevent re-infection.
- Infected patients should use separate towels.
- Avoid using dirty towels in public toilets.
- All members of the same household should be treated, even if asymptomatic.

Concurrent conditions

Table 35.1 provides examples of the influence of concurrent disease on the choice of non-antibiotic anti-infective drugs.

Pregnancy

Antimalarials

Ideally, travel to areas with malaria should be avoided during pregnancy but proguanil and chloroquine may be used. Folic acid 5 mg supplementation is required with proguanil. Mefloquine is considered for areas of chloroquine resistance but the manufacturer recommends that it should be avoided. Malarone is used only if there is no alternative. Doxycycline is contraindicated.

Anthelmintics

Mebendazole should be avoided during the first trimester. The *British National Formulary* reports a lack of evidence of harm with piperazine but the manufacturer advises avoidance of use during the first trimester.

Head lice

Dimeticone or wet combing is preferred. Malathion products were used before the introduction of dimeticone.

Drug interactions

Table 35.2 summarises examples of drug interactions with antimalarial and anthelmintic drugs.

Table 35.2 Examples of drug interactions with antiparasitic agents		
Drugs	**Consequences**	**Comments**
Antimalarials with antacids or antidiarrhoeals	Reduced absorption of chloroquine and proguanil	Doses of antimalarials and antacids (particularly magnesium trisilicate or kaolin) should be separated by at least 2–3 hours
Antimalarials with warfarin	Increased effects of warfarin and other anticoagulants	• Chloroquine does not appear to interact and interactions with proguanil are rare • A baseline INR should be checked and then re-checked 1 week after taking malaria prophylaxis (HPA)
Mefloquine or quinine with drugs which prolong the Q–T interval (Chapter 6)	Increased risk of arrhythmias	• Mefloquine and quinine prolong the Q–T interval • WHO has warned that mefloquine should be used with caution with concurrent antiarrhythmics, β blockers, calcium-channel blockers, antihistamines or phenothiazines
Mefloquine or chloroquine with other drugs which lower the convulsive threshold (Chapter 6)	Increased risk of convulsions	Consider patient with increased risk (Chapter 6)

Table 35.2 *(continued)*

Drugs	Consequences	Comments
Chloroquine with cimetidine	Increased effects of chloroquine due to reduced hepatic metabolism	• Risk of increased adverse effects of chloroquine • Ranitidine may be a suitable alternative
Mebendazole with cimetidine	Increased levels of mebendazole	Monitor for adverse effects of mebendazole
Mebendazole with phenytoin or carbamazepine	Reduced levels of mebendazole	Increased doses of mebendazole may be required but not when treating infections of the gut
Mefloquine with β blockers, calcium-channel blockers, digoxin or antidepressants	Increased risk of bradycardia	Concurrent use should be avoided if possible, particularly for patients considered to be at increased risk of developing bradycardia, until more is known about these interactions
Quinine with cimetidine	Increased levels of quinine	• Monitor for adverse effects of quinine • Ranitidine is a suitable alternative

INR, international normalised ratio; HPA, Health Protection Agency; WHO, World Health Organization.

Self-assessment

Consider whether the following statements are true or false. In the management of non-bacterial infections:

1 Insecticides are a useful prophylactic treatment for recurrent head lice.
2 Doxycycline is a suitable choice for a pregnant woman travelling to an area with malaria.
3 Doxycycline is a suitable choice for a patient with epilepsy.
4 Proguanil, atovaquone, doxycycline and mefloquine do not exacerbate psoriasis.
5 Doxycycline can affect progestogen-only contraception.

Practice points

Malaria

- The latest guidelines should always be consulted when recommending malaria prophylaxis due to increased resistance and the potentially fatal nature of this disease.
- Pharmacists should be vigilant of flu-like symptoms in patients who have recently returned from abroad, particularly from regions associated with malaria.

Helminthic and ectoparasitic infections

- Contact tracing should be encouraged when eliminating head lice.
- Hygiene measures are important when recommending treatment for worms and head lice.
- Repeat applications of pesticides are generally recommended after 7–9 days for head lice.
- The mosaic approach to head lice treatment is no longer used. Current recommendations consist of using a different insecticide for a second application after treatment failure.
- A leaflet should be provided alongside verbal information, e.g. *The Prevention and Treatment of Head Lice* is available from the Department of Health (www. dh.gov.uk).
- Pharmacists should refer treatment failure and infants aged <6 months for assessment of scabies. Pharmacists may wish to refer to a general practitioner patients exceeding five applications of pesticide per year and when counselling has failed.

References

British National Formulary, latest edition. London: British Medical Association and Royal Pharmaceutical Society of Great Britain.

Clark C (2007). Head lice treatments and advice. *Pharm J* 279: 185–188.

Fradin MS, Day JF (2002). Comparative efficacy of insect repellents against mosquito bites. *N Engl J Med* 347: 13–18. pmid: 12097535.

Further reading

Marshall S (2008). Malaria: the issues and advice. *Pharm J* 280: 603–606.

Online resources

www.hpa.org.uk
The Health Protection Agency for information on infectious diseases including an informative section on malaria with answers to commons questions (accessed October 2015).

www.who.int/ith
The website for World Health Organization travel and health information (accessed October 2015).

www.travelhealthpro.org.uk
The website provides up to date travel health advice (accessed October 2015).

Dermatology

36

Dermatology

Dermatology is a relatively specialised area but the pharmacist has important roles, which include:

- identifying and treating common skin diseases or advising appropriate referral
- recognising skin conditions caused by an adverse drug reaction (ADR), including topical preparations (see *British National Formulary*, Section 13.1.3 for excipients associated with sensitisation)
- dispensing and monitoring treatment in more complicated cases
- identifying and referring serious skin diseases or serious diseases presenting with skin changes.

Dermatology encompasses common conditions such as eczema and skin infections and serious (such as skin cancers) and rare conditions, which are only likely to be dealt with by hospital specialists. In addition, ADRs may manifest as dermatological changes, which are considered in Chapter 6. This chapter concentrates on common skin conditions including eczema, psoriasis, acne, fungal infections and some cancers. In order to aid recognition of dermatological conditions the reader is referred to the many textbooks and atlases of dermatology, such as *Dermatology in Focus* by Wilkinson *et al.* (2005).

Eczema

Disease characteristics

This is a common inflammatory skin condition, which has many forms. Within dermatology, the terms 'eczema' and 'dermatitis' are both used but eczema should be used for the endogenous inflammatory conditions and dermatitis for reactive changes, e.g. to allergens. Examples of eczema/dermatitis include:

- atopic or infantile eczema
- irritant contact dermatitis
- allergic contact dermatitis
- seborrhoeic eczema: cradle cap in infants and a dry and itchy scalp in older children and adults.

In addition, rarer forms include pompholyx (vesicles on hands or feet, which may be related to heat, stress or a reaction to fungal foot infections, or may be cryptogenic), hyperkeratotic palmar eczema (typically occurring in middle age and presenting with fissured eczema on hands), asteatotic eczema (reduced lipids in the skin, drying and cracking, which give rise to a 'crazy paving' appearance) and discoid eczema (rare, discoid lesions, perhaps related to alcohol abuse).

Atopic eczema

Atopic or infantile eczema is the most common form of eczema and is associated with an inherited tendency for asthma and hayfever. It often appears in babies at around 3 months of age and, by the age of 5, almost a third of children will have been diagnosed as having atopic eczema at some stage. Fortunately, most children grow out of the condition. It is characterised by the following:

- Prominent pruritus: this is a central feature and its absence may suggest another condition.
- Itchy papules on the cheeks.
- The skin is often dry or inflamed and lichenified, especially around the flexures of the elbows and knees.
- There may be sensitivity to allergens. The dry and inflamed skin may be aggravated by cold, heat, hard water, infections and clothes (especially wool).
- The affected area is often scratched and may become infected, particularly with staphylococci or streptococci, and this may lead to a flare of eczema and, sometimes, impetigo. Viral infection with herpes simplex (eczema herpeticum) leads to painful vesicles and is a serious complication requiring immediate antiviral treatment.

Management

Guidelines for the management of eczema have been produced on behalf of the British Association of Dermatologists (and for children, by the National Institute for Health and Care Excellence or NICE 2007) and these should be consulted.

The initial treatment is regular use of emollients, which hydrate the skin and prevent drying. Emollients have a range of constituents that may include liquid and soft paraffins and cetomacrogol. The most effective are the oily emollients but these may be cosmetically less acceptable. To prevent dehydration of the skin, soap and bubble bath should be avoided, and bathing should be with emollient bath oils and use of emollient creams as a soap substitute. Other lifestyle measures include keeping the house cool (to reduce itchiness), limiting allergens such as house-dust mite (see Chapter 21) and cutting the child's nails to reduce scratching.

Pharmacological management

Topical steroids

When emollients are not sufficient, topical steroids should be considered for treatment, especially in inflamed eczema. Topical 1% hydrocortisone is the first-line agent and is the only agent suitable for infants aged <1 year. It is very effective at reducing the inflammatory response and should be used for short bursts of aggressive treatment rather than occasional 'dabbing'. Ointments give better skin penetration for the steroid than creams, although creams are less greasy and may be more acceptable to patients. Topical 1% hydrocortisone is a mild corticosteroid and is rarely associated with side effects. However, failure of treatment may lead to the short-term use of more potent corticosteroids such as hydrocortisone butyrate, betamethasone and clobetasol propionate to bring the condition under control. These are, however, more likely to be associated with side effects, especially if used for prolonged periods or excessively, and these include:

- secondary infections due to immunosuppression
- thinning of the skin
- telangiectasia (appearance of dilated arterioles in the skin due to thinning)
- acneiform lesions
- glaucoma which may be caused by application near to the eyes or on the eyelids; use with caution
- mild depigmentation
- pituitary–adrenal axis suppression
- Cushing's syndrome.

If oral steroids (e.g. prednisolone) are used in severe disease, height suppression is an important side effect in children and this should be monitored. However, it may be appropriate to use 'steroid-sparing' approaches as described below in preference.

The steroid creams may also be combined with topical antibacterial agents or antifungal agents to prevent infection. Oral antibacterial agents may also be required occasionally to bring any infections under control.

Topical calcineurin inhibitors: tacrolimus and pimecrolimus

These are a relatively new addition to therapy and have immunosuppressant actions similar to ciclosporin. They act indirectly by interfering with the induction of interleukin-2 (which is involved in cell growth and differentiation) in T lymphocytes and so dampen down the immune response. These agents are now available for use as topical agents by dermatologists for patients with moderate-to-severe disease who are unsuitable for or who do not respond to topical steroid treatment. In the case of pimecrolimus, it is recommended for use on the face and neck of children (>2 years).

Oral antihistamines

Non-sedating antihistamines may be of benefit where there is marked itching. Some practitioners might use sedating agents where scratching interferes with sleep.

Additional treatments

Ultraviolet phototherapy is used by hospital dermatologists in some patients.

Counselling

Lifestyle measures are the first step and are detailed earlier.

Emollients

- These are best applied after bathing when the skin is hydrated.
- They may sting on application.
- They should be applied liberally at least twice daily.
- They should be used even after the condition has improved.
- Paraffin-based emollients are associated with a fire hazard and patients should be advised not to smoke when using large amounts of these products, and to keep away from flames.

Topical steroids

The use of topical steroids requires clear counselling:

- They are very effective and safe in the treatment of eczema if they are used correctly.
- Steroids have different potencies and mildly potent agents such as topical hydrocortisone have few side effects. More potent steroids may be used to bring the eczema under control.

- Apply the cream or ointment thinly.
- The steroid should be applied once or twice daily as directed.
- Avoid application to the face (unless specifically prescribed). This is to limit systemic absorption, facial telangiectasia and acne.
- Avoid application to the anogenital region (unless specifically prescribed) to limit systemic absorption.
- Over-the-counter (OTC) use of hydrocortisone is appropriate only for children aged >10 years for 7 days. Longer treatment or application to the face or anogenital region requires referral to the general practitioner.
- Clobetasone cream is available over-the-counter for short-term symptomatic control of eczema and dermatitis (except seborrhoeic dermatitis) for adults and children aged >12 years.
- Avoid application to infected areas including cold sores, acne and fungal infections (in the absence of a concomitant antifungal agent).
- The preparation is applied in 'fingertip units' in adults:

  - hand: 1 unit
  - face: 2.5 units
  - arm: 3 units
  - leg: 6 units
  - foot: 2 units
  - front of trunk: 7 units
  - back of trunk: 7 units.

Contact dermatitis

This is also a common form of eczema, which is either an irritant reaction to chemicals such as detergents or an allergic reaction to chemicals such as nickel, cosmetics and creams (e.g. some constituents such as lanolin, sodium stearate). It is characterised by inflammation with dryness and chapping after exposure to the irritant or allergen. The initial management is to remove or avoid the cause, coupled with emollients, barrier creams, topical steroids or oral antihistamines as appropriate. Occupational causes should be referred for patch testing to identify the irritant.

Napkin dermatitis

This form of contact dermatitis is due to the irritant effects of ammonia from faeces and urine in the nappy region and may often coexist with fungal infection. In napkin rash that results solely from irritation, the skin folds are relatively spared, because there is less contact in these areas. Treatment should include improved hygiene, such as frequent nappy changes, leaving the nappy off for a time and washing, with the application of barrier creams (e.g. dimeticone) to prevent contact and emollients to hydrate the skin. In more severe dermatitis not responding to these measures 1% hydrocortisone cream may be prescribed for up to a week. Fungal infection should be suspected if the skin folds are affected or there are small red dots, because the fungi may spread. Accordingly, antifungal treatment with a topical imidazole, clotrimazole (see later), is appropriate, often with hydrocortisone to reduce the inflammation. Bacterial infections may present as pustules.

Seborrhoeic eczema

In infants this manifests on the scalp as cradle cap, for which there are a number of preparations, some of which include oils to soften the skin and facilitate removal.

In children and adults seborrhoeic eczema may present as a dry and flaky scalp for which corticosteroid lotions are effective. The condition may be related to a hypersensitivity to yeast infection due to *Pityrosporum* spp. and ketoconazole shampoo is effective.

Other forms

In relation to the rarer forms of eczema, pompholyx may be managed by potent topical steroids and potassium permanganate. Oral antihistamines may provide symptomatic relief and, if the condition is a reaction to a fungal infection, this should be treated with antifungal agents (see later). Hyperkeratotic palmar eczema is treated with emollients, topical steroids, keratolytics and, in severe disease, immunosuppressants. Asteatotic eczema is treated with emollients, emollient bath oils and weak topical steroids. Discoid eczema is treated with emollients and steroids.

Psoriasis

This is a reasonably common inflammatory skin condition that affects 2–3% of the population and is due to rapid epidermal transit caused by increased cell division and increased passage of keratinocytes through the epidermis. As part of the inflammatory response, there is infiltration of the dermis with lymphocytes and the epidermis with neutrophils. The release of cytokines and lymphokines stimulates keratinocyte proliferation and alters their maturation.

The most common form is plaque psoriasis, which presents as a well-demarcated, erythematous region with thick silvery scales, and is associated with pruritus. The plaques may be localised to a few areas or are extensively distributed. Less common forms include guttate psoriasis ('raindrop' lesions that may follow a streptococcal throat infection in younger patients), pustular psoriasis (a rare and serious condition, which presents as sterile pustules) and flexural psoriasis (well-demarcated erythematous regions). Decreased levels of cAMP (adenosine cyclic 3′:5′-monophosphate) are found in lesions and β blockers may exacerbate the condition. In addition, lithium may exacerbate psoriasis.

Pharmacological management

There are a number of pharmacological approaches to psoriasis that may be tried and used according to their response. A central theme of the agents used is to reduce the proliferation of dermal cells and the inflammatory response, which contribute to the condition.

Emollients

As with eczema, emollients play an important role in hydrating the skin and should be used widely.

Topical steroids

Their anti-inflammatory actions may be of benefit but they may become less effective on continued use and there may be rebound effects on withdrawal.

Topical dithranol

This is often used first line in plaque psoriasis and has antiproliferative properties by inhibiting mitotic activity. It may lead to hypersensitivity and so patch testing is sometimes used before treatment. The ability of this agent to stain skin and clothes may limit its acceptability with patients.

Topical vitamin D₃ analogues: calcipotriol, tacalcitol

Vitamin D₃ analogues act on keratinocyte vitamin D receptors, with antiproliferative actions, and reduce epidermal proliferation. They are also anti-inflammatory through their interference with the release of cytokines and suppression of both lymphocyte proliferation and neutrophil accumulation. Calcipotriol has now been formulated with betamethasone (in Dovobet) and appears to give good control of stable plaque psoriasis.

Coal tar

The keratolytic, antipruritic and anti-inflammatory actions of coal tar provide relief.

Phototherapy

Phototherapy with ultraviolet A (UVA) reduces dermal cell proliferation by interfering with DNA synthesis and reduces lymphocyte infiltration of the psoriatic epidermis. In extensive disease, the patients are treated with oral or topical methoxsalen (a psoralen) as a photosensitising agent, to enhance the effects of UVA, and this is known as PUVA (psoralen UVA). Alternatively, the patient may receive narrow-band UVB treatment, which does not require a photosensitising agent.

Oral retinoids: acitretin

Acitretin (a metabolite of etretinate) binds to nuclear retinoic acid receptors and affects gene transcription, resulting in antiproliferative actions and normal keratinocyte maturation. It should be avoided in pregnancy and in females of childbearing age; adequate contraception should be used and conception should be delayed for 3 years after stopping treatment. Acitretin may also alter the lipid profile by increasing plasma triglycerides and cholesterol, so this should be monitored along with liver function tests. Tazarotene is available as a topical retinoid.

Other treatments

Low-dose methotrexate is used by dermatologists for its cytotoxic actions, which reduce cellular turnover. Ciclosporin is also used by dermatologists for its immunosuppressant actions. In addition, etanercept and infliximab are now used by specialists in severe and refractory disease (see Chapter 31).

Counselling

Emollients and steroids

See earlier.

Dithranol

- This should be applied for 30–60 minutes and then washed off.
- It should be applied only to the lesions.
- It may stain skin and clothes.
- Patients should wash their hands thoroughly after application.

Oral acitretin

- This agent is teratogenic and should not be used during pregnancy. In females, conception should be delayed for at least 3 years after the patient has stopped taking the drug.
- Acitretin may also cause cracked and dried lips, which may be helped by the application of petroleum jelly.
- It may cause a drying of mucous membranes.
- It may cause thinning of the skin.
- The effects may be delayed for 2–4 weeks.
- The patient should not donate blood for at least 1 year after stopping treatment.
- Excessive exposure to sunlight should be avoided.

Acne

Acne vulgaris is a common condition, typically affecting teenagers, but in a few patients it may persist beyond these years. It is due to excessive sebum production in response to androgens, and results in the formation of comedones and pustules. Closed comedones are white cysts and open comedones are blackheads.

The bacterium *Propionibacterium acnes* is present in the skin and can lead to inflammatory lesions. The lipid-rich sebum favours the growth of *P. acnes*, which produces lipases that act on the sebum to release fatty acids, favouring comedone formation. The *P. acnes* also activates the complement system, leading to the release of proteases, which cause inflammation. Pustules form as part of the inflammatory lesions.

Management

In the mild form of the disease, general cleansing may provide relief. There is no evidence that altering the diet will bring about an improvement. The treatments for acne are directed against the comedones and/or the infected lesions and the following are used.

Topical agents

Topical benzoyl peroxide

Topical benzoyl peroxide is used for its keratolytic and bactericidal properties and is used in all forms of acne.

Azelaic acid

This may be used as an alternative to benzoyl peroxide and is less irritating.

Topical retinoids

If topical benzoyl peroxide fails, then topical applications of retinoids (tretinoin and isotretinoin) are used for their keratolytic actions by reducing adhesion between epidermal cells. The main adverse effect is skin irritation. Retinoids are teratogenic and are used only in patients who are not pregnant.

Topical antibiotics

The topical antibiotics erythromycin, tetracycline or clindamycin are prescribed. When used alone they are ineffective against comedones but in pustular disease they are as effective as tretinoin and benzoyl peroxide. However, resistance may develop and this may be partly overcome by combining either zinc (such as Zineryt, which is erythromycin plus zinc acetate) or benzoyl peroxide with the antibiotic. They are often used for a 10- to 12-week trial.

Systemic treatments

Oral antibiotics

In moderate-to-severe acne or when there is a poor response to topical treatments, oral antibiotics are used. Tetracycline is used first line, with oxytetracycline, minocycline, erythromycin, clindamycin or trimethoprim as alternatives. The penetration of the antibiotics into the sebaceous glands is low and so treatment can take up to 3–4 months for an effect; maximal effects may take up to 2 years. Tetracycline and erythromycin may exert additional anti-inflammatory actions, independent of their antibacterial activity.

When minocycline is used for more than 6 months the *British National Formulary* recommends that hepatotoxicity, skin pigmentation and signs of systemic lupus erythematosus are monitored every 3 months.

Oral retinoids (tretinoin and isotretinoin)

A failure of oral antibiotics or severe acne may lead to referral to a dermatologist, who may prescribe the oral retinoid isotretinoin. This inhibits sebum production by reducing the number and activity of sebaceous glands. It can be highly effective but is associated with depression. It may also alter the lipid profile by increasing plasma triglycerides and cholesterol, so this should be monitored along with liver function tests. It is teratogenic and used only in patients who are not pregnant and who should be advised to avoid conception for at least 1 month after stopping treatment.

Hormonal therapy

In females only, co-cyprindiol (oral cyproterone, a testosterone receptor antagonist, plus ethinylestradiol) may be used because it will alter the hormonal balance away from androgens.

Counselling

General counselling should include hygiene advice and emphasise the importance of not touching lesions, to reduce the spread of infection.

Benzoyl peroxide

- It may bleach hair and clothes.
- It may irritate the skin and cause dryness.
- Apply once daily in the evening to begin with, in case there is redness or peeling.
- If there is irritation, reduce the frequency or stop and consider reintroducing gradually.
- Apply to the affected area, not just the spots.

Topical retinoids

- These are a photoirritant: patients should avoid UV sun beds and may need to wear sunscreen in the sunshine.
- Topical retinoids are teratogenic and females should take adequate contraceptive measures.

Oral antibiotics

- See Chapter 34.
- Broad-spectrum antibiotics may reduce the effectiveness of combined oral contraceptives containing ethinylestradiol (by altering the gastrointestinal flora), so alternative barrier contraceptive measures should be used. This reduction in effectiveness lasts for only 3 weeks because resistance within the gastrointestinal flora develops, so additional measures need be taken only for this time.
- Patients developing severe diarrhoea while taking antibiotics (especially clindamycin) should stop taking them and consult their GP urgently.
- An improvement may take 3–4 months.

Oral isotretinoin

- This is teratogenic and females must not become pregnant during treatment and for at least 1 month after treatment.
- Patients should not donate blood during treatment and for 1 month afterwards.
- This drug may cause depression.
- Patients should not exceed the daily allowance of vitamin A and should not take supplements containing vitamin A without consulting their pharmacist or GP.
- Patients should not take other products for acne unless advised to by their GP or dermatologist.
- Isotretinoin may cause thinning of the skin: patients should not wax or epilate their skin for 5–6 months after stopping treatment. Petroleum jelly may be helpful in preventing dry and cracked lips. Dry eyes may also affect vision and hypromellose eye drops may be helpful.
- Patients should avoid strong sunlight and UV light and wear sunblock if exposed.

Co-cyprindiol

- As with other oestrogen-containing contraceptives, there is a risk of thromboembolism, which is compounded by other risk factors such as smoking and increased age (see Chapter 3).
- An improvement may take several months.
- This should be used as a contraceptive only for patients with severe acne or hirsutism because there is an increased risk of thromboembolism

compared with other hormonal contraceptives. Treatment should be stopped 3–4 months after complete resolution of symptoms.

Rosacea

Rosacea is an inflammatory condition with acneiform lesions, and telangiectasia (prominent and dilated arterioles) but without comedones. It is more common in women with fair skin, especially around the menopause. It may be precipitated by sunshine, alcohol and spicy foods. Hypertrophy of sebaceous glands around the nose may lead to an enlargement, rhinophyma, which is more common in men.

Management

The first active treatment is topical metronidazole gel (0.75%) and this may be followed by oral erythromycin or tetracycline. β blockers or clonidine may be used to help the symptoms of flushing. Sunscreen should be used to reduce the effects of the sun.

Fungal infections

The skin is a common site of fungal infection due to tinea (dermatophyte) or *Candida* spp., and is commonly encountered in primary care. Common forms are as follows.

Ringworm (tinea infections)

This may occur at different sites on the body, as shown in Table 36.1.

Pityriasis versicolor

This is a relatively common condition, which presents as hypo- or hyperpigmented macules. It is due to infection by the yeast *Pityrosporum* spp.

Candidiasis

This is a common yeast infection due to *Candida albicans* and is known as thrush. It commonly affects the skin and mucous membranes. Skin infections tend to present as moist, inflamed regions, which are less

Table 36.1 The different forms, sites and features of tinea infection

Form	Site	Features
Tinea corporis	Trunk and limbs	Discoid, erythematous scaly plaques
Tinea capitis	Scalp	Bald, scaly patches
Tinea pedis (athlete's foot)	Between the toes	May present as scaling or inflammation between the toes
Tinea unguium	Nails	Nails become yellow and crumbly
Tinea cruris	Groin	Reddened and scaly groin

well demarcated than in tinea infection, presenting with pain and itching. The infections are favoured by warm and moist skin folds, such as the groin, breasts, armpits and buttocks, especially in obese individuals (intertrigo). Mouth infections present as white patches and vaginal infections as pruritus with a creamy discharge, which is sometimes described as being like cottage cheese in appearance although it is sometimes watery. Candidiasis is favoured by the use of antibiotics and corticosteroids in diabetes mellitus, eczema and immunocompromised patients. Patients who have recurrent candidiasis should be investigated to exclude diabetes mellitus. It may also present as angular stomatitis at the corner of the mouth. Nails may be affected and become discoloured.

Management

In superficial infections, simple hygiene measures should be advocated and these may involve thorough drying after washing, not sharing towels and avoiding occlusive clothing (e.g. nylon). In athlete's foot, more frequent changes of socks and shoes may help.

Topical imidazoles: clotrimazole, miconazole, tioconazole

These act to inhibit a cytochrome P450-dependent demethylase which converts lanosterol to ergosterol, a fungal membrane lipid. This results in the accumulation of lanosterol which disrupts the membrane phospholipids. The imidazoles are fungistatic and so must be used for about 2 weeks after healing to prevent a relapse. They are widely used in superficial skin infections and are effective against both tinea and candidal infections.

Oral imidazoles and triazoles ('azoles')

The imidazole ketoconazole and the triazoles itraconazole and fluconazole are orally active and act via inhibition of cytochrome P450-dependent demethylase, as described above. The azoles are associated with hepatotoxicity. The prescribing of oral ketoconazole has been restricted because of this risk and increased monitoring of liver function is recommended during treatment (MHRA).

Polyenes: nystatin

This polyene macrolide binds to fungal ergosterol in the cell membrane. It disrupts the cells and is effective in candidiasis but not tinea.

Allylamines: terbinafine

Terbinafine inhibits the conversion of squalene to lanosterol, with the accumulation of squalene causing cell death. This fungicidal action has the advantage that shorter treatment courses are required. Terbinafine is available as a cream, spray or gel for superficial infections or orally for deeper infections, such as those affecting the nails. It is available over-the-counter for the treatment of tinea pedis, cruris and corporis. The indication varies according to the preparation.

Griseofulvin

This interferes with fungal microtubules and nucleic acid synthesis but has largely been replaced by oral terbinafine and azoles. It is suitable for tinea infections but not candidiasis, because it is ineffective against the yeast.

Topical steroids

These may be used in addition to antifungal agents to relieve the symptoms due to irritation and are especially useful in concomitant eczema.

In terms of the use of antifungal agents, topical agents are used in more superficial infections and oral agents for deeper infections. The agents are chosen according to the spectrum of activity; some recommendations are given in Table 36.2.

Failure of topical treatment or extensive infection should be treated with oral agents, such as terbinafine or itraconazole. The recommended agents and duration of the above therapies are largely derived from the *British National Formulary*.

A pulse is a twice-daily dose for 7 days followed by 21 days without the drug.

Counselling

A long course is often required and should be completed.

Imidazole creams

- For cutaneous infections, these should be applied two to three times daily and for 2 weeks after the infection has healed.
- For vaginal infections, hygiene advice should be given and sexual partners treated if they are symptomatic. Other sources of infection may include fingernails, umbilicus, gastrointestinal tract and bladder.
- Vaginal preparations (excluding nystatin pessaries) may damage latex condoms and diaphragms.
- Vaginal preparations should be administered high into the vagina and may be used during menstruation.
- They may cause a burning sensation on application.

Table 36.2 Treatment for fungal infections	
Condition	**Possible primary treatments**
Tinea corporis	• Topical imidazole, continued for 2 weeks after healing • Topical terbinafine: 1–2 weeks • Topical imidazole is first-line while terbinafine is reserved for resistance
Tinea capitis	• Oral griseofulvin: 8 weeks • Oral terbinafine: 4 weeks (unlicensed) • Oral itraconazole (unlicensed)
Tinea pedis (athlete's foot)	• Topical imidazole, continued for 2 weeks after healing • Topical terbinafine: 1 week
Tinea unguium	• Oral terbinafine: 6 weeks to 3 months, sometimes longer in toenail infections • Oral itraconazole: 3 months or 2 pulses (fingernails) or 3 pulses (toenails) • Oral griseofulvin for 6 months (fingernails) or 12 months (toenails) • In mild infection limited to 1–2 nails, local therapy with amorolfine or tioconazole may be used
Tinea cruris	• Topical imidazole, continued for 2 weeks after healing • Topical terbinafine: 1–2 weeks • Topical imidazole is first line whereas terbinafine is reserved for resistance
Pityriasis versicolor	• Selenium sulphide shampoo daily for 1 week • Topical imidazole for 10 days • Itraconazole for 1 week
Candidiasis – cutaneous	• Topical imidazole, continued for 2 weeks after healing • Topical terbinafine: 2 weeks • Topical nystatin, continued for 7 days after healing
Candidiasis – nail	Oral itraconazole: 3 months or 2 pulses (fingernails) or 3 pulses (toenails)
Vaginal candidiasis	Either clotrimazole pessaries (single dose) or cream (10% clotrimazole is available for single application); oral fluconazole (150 mg as a single dose); may also be used for candidal balanitis

Oral azoles and oral terbinafine

- These may cause gastrointestinal side effects. Itraconazole capsules (but not liquid) and ketoconazole should be taken with food.
- Patients taking oral antifungal agents should report signs of liver toxicity such as nausea, vomiting, dark urine or jaundice (see Chapters 6 and 11).

Nystatin

The cream may stain clothes yellow.

Griseofulvin

- Avoid during pregnancy.
- Males should avoid fathering children for 6 months after stopping treatment.

Other infections affecting the skin

In addition to fungal infections, the skin is also the site of a wide range of bacterial and viral infections, which vary from benign to potentially serious. Some of the infections may be related to increased susceptibility due to chronic skin conditions, e.g. impetigo (as a complication of eczema) or as a result of manifestations of viral infections with both skin and systemic symptoms. A summary of the features and management of a range of common skin infections is given in Table 36.3.

Pruritus

This is a symptom of a range of conditions and presents as itchiness. Possible causes include (Greene and Harris 2008):

- dermatological inflammatory conditions:
  - eczema
  - psoriasis
- skin infections:
  - lice/scabies
  - viral infection – chickenpox, herpes
  - fungal infection
- reactions:
  - drug reactions
  - urticaria
- psychogenic
- ageing
- manifestations of systemic changes:
  - diabetes
  - pregnancy
  - liver failure
  - renal failure
  - malignancy.

The treatment should be directed at the cause, but additional symptomatic measures include the use of crotamiton cream or lotion and oral antihistamines. Colestyramine is used in pruritus associated with liver failure, because it will bind bile salts and so reduce plasma bilirubin, which causes pruritus (see Chapter 11). Anogenital pruritus may be due to fungal infection, haemorrhoids or contact dermatitis caused by irritation from poor hygiene. It should be treated with hygiene measures, antifungal agents, emollients if due to dry skin or short-term hydrocortisone as appropriate, but topical local anaesthetics are best avoided because they may lead to hypersensitivity.

Manifestations of systemic disease

In addition to pruritus as a symptom, systemic diseases may manifest as changes in the skin. Examples of this include the following:

- Pigmentation that may be yellow in jaundice (due to increased bilirubin in liver disease), a lemon tinge in renal failure or vitiligo in Addison's disease.
- Spider naevi are dilated central arterioles with spidery arterioles feeding from them, and are present, especially above the nipple line, in liver cirrhosis, frequently due to alcohol.
- Fungal infections that recur may suggest that the patient has impaired immunity. Frequent candidiasis occurs in diabetes mellitus.

Skin cancers

The incidence of skin cancers is on the increase and they are dealt with by specialists in dermatology. However, recognition of potential skin cancers in primary care is clearly important and the pharmacist should be vigilant for changes in the skin that require referral.

Table 36.3 Additional skin infections and their treatment

Condition	Comments	Management
Impetigo	Usually a staphylococcal or occasionally streptococcal infection of the skin. Reddening with a golden crust. Contagious and may complicate eczema	• Limited infection may be treated with topical fusidic acid or mupirocin (use limited to 10 days to prevent the emergence of resistance). More extensive infections require oral flucloxacillin (or phenoxymethylpenicillin if there is streptococcal infection) or erythromycin if penicillin allergic • Antiseptic bath oils may reduce colonisation
Cellulitis	Deep streptococcal or staphylococcal infection, often following trauma. There may be a red, oedematous rash which may be accompanied by pyrexia	Phenoxymethylpenicillin plus flucloxacillin or erythromycin if penicillin allergic
Erysipelas	Superficial cellulitis of the skin, often due to *Streptococcus pyogenes*. Often affects the face or legs	Phenoxymethylpenicillin in mild infections. Flucloxacillin is added if staphylococcal infection is suspected
Herpes simplex	Painful vesicles on mucous membranes and skin due to herpes simplex virus. Tingling precedes the lesions	Analgesics provide symptomatic relief. Topical aciclovir and penciclovir reduce the length of symptoms if started at the first signs of an attack. Oral aciclovir may be less effective
Chickenpox	• Varicella infection leading to fever and vesicular rash. Usually uncomplicated in children but in adults may be complicated by pneumonia, hepatitis, encephalitis and myocarditis • Smoking increases the chances of complications of pneumonia • Chickenpox is especially severe in patients taking systemic steroids	• Antihistamines may provide symptomatic relief • Emollients may be soothing • Older remedies such as calamine lotion may be ineffective • Aciclovir is indicated for high-risk patients who develop the infection and should be started in the first 24 hours • Immunoglobulin is appropriate for pregnant contacts and those taking steroids who do not have immunity
Shingles	Reactivation of varicella-zoster virus leading to pain, with red papules that become vesicular. Shingles cannot be caught from contact with chickenpox but contact of patients with shingles may lead to chickenpox in patients who are not immune	• Aciclovir is indicated for patients aged >60 years or immunocompromised. It should be started within 72 hours of the appearance of the rash • Neuralgic pain after infection may require low doses of tricyclic antidepressants such as amitriptyline or carbamazepine, which are routinely used in older patients as a preventive measure
Warts and verrucae (plantar warts)	Warts are hyperkeratotic papules and verrucae are deep lesions on the soles. They are caused by the human papillomavirus	• Warts generally resolve but may be treated with salicylic acid, glutaraldehyde or cryotherapy with liquid nitrogen or dry ice • Verrucae may be treated with salicylic acid plasters or podophyllin/salicylic acid ointment or cryotherapy
Molluscum contagiosum (water blisters)	Drop-like papules affecting infants and children due to a virus	None indicated and reassurance is all that may be required
Hand, foot and mouth disease	Coxsackie viral infection in children with vesicles around the mouth, palms and soles	None
Scabies	Severe pruritus due to scabies mite infestation	• Malathion or permethrin as aqueous preparations as alcohol may irritate damaged skin (Chapter 35) • All members of the family should be treated • Treatment should be applied to the whole body, particularly to the web of digits and fingernails • Two applications, 1 week apart, are recommended • Crotamiton and/or sedating antihistamines may be used for pruritus

Basal cell carcinoma (rodent ulcer)

This is the most common skin cancer and presents as a colourless lump with pearly edges, but may become ulcerated and crusty in the centre and is often on the edge of the ear, temple or side of the nose. It is very slow growing and may have been present for several years. Although it is a malignant tumour, it has only very limited local invasion and is cured by surgical removal. Extensive invasion may require radiotherapy or cryotherapy. Topical 5-fluorouracil is also used. Prevention of occurrence or recurrence (which is common) should be stressed by advising sun protection measures, such as wearing a hat in the sun and using a high-factor sun block.

Solar keratosis

These are common, premalignant lesions with crusts on an erythematous base. Solar keratosis is associated with exposure to the sun and occurs more often on fair-skinned patients on the forehead, scalp, face or hands. It may be managed by cryotherapy and topical 5-fluorouracil.

Squamous cell carcinoma

This is a relatively common malignancy, often appearing on sun-damaged skin on the hand and face, especially the ear and lip. It is removed surgically but metastases may occur if it is untreated.

Malignant melanoma

This involves evolution and possibly malignant transformation in a large mole. This is more likely in larger moles and in sun-exposed skin. The following features may be seen:

Asymmetry
Border irregular
Colour irregular
Diameter >0.5 cm
Elevation irregular.

Any change in a mole requires referral for an expert opinion. In malignant melanoma, surgical excision has a good outlook in small lesions that are caught early. Chemotherapy is palliative in disease that has spread.

Drug interactions involving drugs widely used in dermatology

In drugs used in dermatology there are a wide range of potential drug interactions, generally affecting the oral azoles, and also ciclosporin and methotrexate, which are initiated only by specialists. Table 36.4 contains a summary of some important interactions.

Table 36.4 Some important drug interactions for drugs used in dermatology

Interacting drugs	Consequences	Comments
Methoxsalen with phenytoin	Phenytoin may, by enzyme induction, reduce concentrations of methoxsalen	This combination should be avoided
Acitretin with ciclosporin	An increase in ciclosporin concentration may occur	
Acitretin with methotrexate	Increased toxicity of methotrexate	BNF recommends avoiding concomitant use of acitretin and methotrexate
Isotretinoin with carbamazepine	The plasma concentration of carbamazepine may be reduced	Epileptic control should be monitored
Isotretinoin with tetracycline/minocycline	Increased risk of benign intracranial hypertension	Their concomitant use should be avoided
Methotrexate	Toxicity of methotrexate is known to be enhanced by NSAIDs and so extreme caution should be exercised, although this is less likely to occur at the lower doses used for psoriasis	Methotrexate exhibits a wide range of interactions and *Stockley's Drug Interactions* (Baxter 2013) should be consulted

Table 36.4 *(continued)*

Interacting drugs	Consequences	Comments
Ciclosporin		Ciclosporin exhibits a wide range of interactions and *Stockley's Drug Interactions* (Baxter 2013) should be consulted
Oral cyproterone plus ethinylestradiol (co-cyprindiol)	Efficacy may be reduced by broad-spectrum antibiotics and enzyme inducers. When used with minocycline there may be an enhancement of facial pigmentation	
Oral imidazoles and triazoles	• Phenytoin reduces the plasma concentrations of itraconazole and ketoconazole but fluconazole may increase the concentrations of phenytoin • Carbamazepine may reduce the plasma concentrations of itraconazole • Rifampicin reduces the plasma concentrations of itraconazole, fluconazole and ketoconazole. • Additional interactions include reduced absorption of ketoconazole and itraconazole (but not fluconazole) by antacids and H_2-receptor antagonists	• These are inhibitors of cytochrome P450 and will inhibit the metabolism of a range of drugs, increasing their plasma concentrations (Chapter 6) • Similarly, inducers of cytochrome P450 may accelerate the metabolism of the azoles, reducing their plasma concentrations • Inhibitors of cytochrome P450 may inhibit the metabolism of azoles and increase their concentrations
Antifungals (fluconazole, itraconazole, ketoconazole and miconazole) with warfarin	Increased anticoagulant effect	Includes oral and vaginal preparations of miconazole
Griseofulvin with warfarin	In some patients, griseofulvin decreases the plasma concentration of warfarin	Monitoring is recommended
Itraconazole with clarithromycin	Itraconazole levels doubled	Monitoring and possible dose reductions are recommended
Ketoconazole with omeprazole	Reduced antifungal effects	• Fluconazole is a suitable alternative for patients prescribed omeprazole • Alternative proton pump inhibitors such as lansoprazole may also interact and an alternative such as H_2-receptor antagonists is recommended
Oral terbinafine	• Plasma concentrations are decreased by concomitant rifampicin and its dose may need to be increased • Terbinafine may increase plasma levels of theophylline but this is unclear	
Amphotericin with corticosteroids	Adverse cardiac effects due to potassium loss and water and sodium retention	Electrolytes should be monitored, particularly in patients at risk (e.g. elderly people)
Oral aciclovir	• There is a report of aciclovir reducing plasma concentrations of phenytoin and sodium valproate • Aciclovir can increase plasma concentrations of theophylline, which may lead to toxicity	Monitoring may be appropriate

BNF, *British National Formulary;* NSAIDs, non-steroidal anti-inflammatory drugs.

Self-assessment

For the following questions concerning the management of skin diseases, choose the most appropriate answer:

1 *Which one of the following is a feature of atopic eczema?*

   A It is caused by a virus
   B It is caused by a fungus
   C It is characterised by dry and inflamed skin
   D It protects against asthma in later life
   E It protects against hayfever in later life

2 *Widespread impetigo is best managed by which one of the following?*

   A Retinoids (such as isotretinoin)
   B Oral terbinafine
   C Topical hydrocortisone
   D Aciclovir
   E Oral flucloxacillin

3 *Dermatophyte fungal infections can be treated by which one of the following?*

   A Retinoids (such as isotretinoin)
   B Oral terbinafine
   C Topical hydrocortisone
   D Aciclovir
   E Oral flucloxacillin

4 *The use of retinoids (such as isotretinoin) leads to which one of the following?*

   A Reduced sebum production
   B Thickening of the skin
   C Sterilisation of the skin
   D Hydration of the skin
   E Removal of dead skin

5 *The use of retinoids (such as isotretinoin) is complicated by their association with which one of the following?*

   A Significant drug interactions
   B Increased risk of infection
   C Birth defects

   D Carcinogenesis
   E Sedation

6 *Acne may be managed by which one of the following?*

   A Hydrocortisone
   B Oral antibiotics (such as tetracycline)
   C Emollients
   D Methotrexate
   E Antifungal agents (such as terbinafine)

7 *Psoriasis is best described by which one of the following?*

   A Increased epidermal transit
   B Fungal infection
   C Cancerous
   D Associated with the menopause
   E Associated with prolonged steroid usage

8 *Rosacea is often managed by which one of the following?*

   A Topical hydrocortisone
   B Retinoids (such as isotretinoin)
   C Methotrexate
   D Aciclovir tablets
   E Topical metronidazole

9 *A rodent ulcer (basal cell carcinoma) is best described as which one of the following?*

   A It is widely metastatic
   B Is usually due to a change in a mole
   C It is usually cured by minimally invasive surgery
   D They are often caused by metastasis
   E They are associated with alcohol abuse.

10 *The presence of multiple spider naevi is often a sign of:*

   A Lung disease
   B Alcoholic liver disease
   C Renal disease
   D An adverse drug reaction
   E Thrombocytopenia

CASE STUDIES

Case 1

Toddler TR is 2 years old and has scaly inflamed skin on her back and on the back of her knees. A diagnosis of atopic eczema has been made.

How might the parents manage this condition using lifestyle changes and OTC treatments?

- Simple lifestyle measures should involve regular but not excessive washing, and using emollients in place of soap. After bathing, emollient should be applied liberally and reapplied throughout the day. Keeping the house cool may help reduce the discomfort of itching. Limiting allergens in the house is controversial and may or may not help. The child's nails should be kept short to avoid scratching and a sedative oral antihistamine given at night might help her sleep and reduce scratching at night.

Might the toddler benefit from topical antihistamines?

- These are of no benefit in eczema and they may actually sensitise the skin.

What are the treatment options open to her general practitioner?

- For poorly controlled and inflamed eczema, topical corticosteroids (1% hydrocortisone preferred in infants) may be prescribed (not over-the-counter at this age) for short periods to bring the condition under control.

What other conditions will she be susceptible to?

- Atopic individuals are more susceptible to asthma and hayfever.

Toddler TR's skin condition deteriorates and becomes covered with a golden crusty coat over a red and inflamed surface. The GP decides that she has an impetigo-like infection.

What is impetigo?

- A staphylococcal or streptococcal infection of the skin leading to reddening with a golden crust, which may complicate eczema.

How would this be treated?

- In limited infection, topical fusidic acid 2% is used. If widespread, either oral flucloxacillin 125 mg four times daily or erythromycin 250 mg four times daily is appropriate. If streptococcal infection is suspected, then phenoxymethylpenicillin 125 mg four times daily may be prescribed.

Case 2

Ms GS is a 16-year-old (50 kg) girl with acne vulgaris.

What are the goals of treatment?

- Eradication of acne, which is important both cosmetically and psychologically

(continued)

(continued)

- Reduction in sebum production
- To limit the growth of the bacteria involved
- To prevent recurrence
- To prevent scarring.

What would the ladder of treatment be in her case?

- Step 1: mild acne – general cleansing.
- Step 2: topical benzoyl peroxide for its keratolytic and bactericidal actions.
- Step 3: if there is a poor response to the above, then topical tretinoin or topical antibiotics (not effective against comedones).
- Step 4: if there is a poor response to the above, then oral antibiotics.
- Step 5: if there is a poor response to the above, then oral isotretinoin.
- Any stage: co-cyprindiol may be used. Severe acne should be referred to a dermatologist.

At one stage she is prescribed tetracycline 500 mg twice daily.

How would you counsel her?

- Do not take at the same time as milk and antacids: take at least 30 minutes before food or on an empty stomach. Calcium in milk and antacids will bind tetracycline and prevent it from being absorbed.
- Complete the course.
- Avoid direct sunlight/ultraviolet light because of photosensitivity.
- An improvement may take 3–4 months.

What might be tried if there is no improvement?

- Oral erythromycin or trimethoprim might be tried.

Later her dermatologist prescribes isotretinoin orally

Suggest an appropriate dosage.

- 500 micrograms/kg daily, so her dose is 25 mg daily.

How would she be counselled?

- Isotretinoin is teratogenic and she will require a pregnancy test and must not become pregnant until at least 1 month after stopping treatment. She should use effective contraception.
- Her skin may become thin.
- She should avoid waxing or epilation, because this will strip skin.
- Her lips may become dry and petroleum jelly may help.

Case 3

An elderly man presents a prescription for metronidazole 0.75% gel 30 g for his wife. You notice from her patient medication record (PMR) that she is receiving medication for palliative care.

How do you proceed?

- Confusion can arise when prescribing topical metronidazole preparations.

- A product providing 0.75% metronidazole gel in a 30 g pack size is indicated for acne rosacea.
- It is important to check the indication because it is possible that the above prescription is for a malodorous fungating tumour.
- An appropriately licensed product should be supplied.

References

Baxter K, ed. (2013). *Stockley's Drug Interaction,* 10th edn. London: Pharmaceutical Press.

British National Formulary, latest edition. London: British Medical Association and Royal Pharmaceutical Society of Great Britain.

Greene RJ, Harris ND (2008). *Pathology and Therapeutics for Pharmacists.* London: Pharmaceutical Press.

National Institute for Health and Care Excellence (2007). *Atopic Eczema in Children.* Clinical Guideline 57. London: NICE.

Wilkinson JD, Shaw S, Orton D (2005). *Dermatology in Focus.* Edinburgh: Elsevier Churchill Livingstone.

Further reading

Brown SK, Shalita AR (1998). Acne vulgaris. *Lancet* 351: 1871–1876. pmid: 9652685.

Cunliffe W (2002). A rational approach to acne management. *Prescriber* 13: 46–67.

Hindle E (2001). Eczema: first- and second-line drug treatments. *Prescriber* 12: 49–71.

Rudikoff D, Lebwohl M (1998). Atopic dermatitis. *Lancet* 351: 1715–1721. pmid: 9734903.

Stern RS (1997). Psoriasis. *Lancet* 350: 349–353. pmid: 9251649.

Online resources

www.eczema.org
The website of the UK National Eczema Society (accessed October 2015).

www.bad.org.uk
The website of the British Association of Dermatologists providing professional guidance and patient information (accessed October 2015).

PART **K**

Endocrine disorders

37

Diabetes mellitus

Diabetes mellitus is a serious condition associated with a considerable disruption to a patient's life and potentially serious long-term consequences. In particular, diabetes mellitus is a major risk factor for cardiovascular disease, comparable to hypertension and hypercholesterolaemia. Diabetes mellitus is broadly classed as either type 1 (previously known as insulin-dependent) or type 2 (non-insulin-dependent) diabetes mellitus. Both conditions are characterised by impaired glucose metabolism. In type 1, there is an inability to produce insulin whereas in type 2 there is reduced production and/or a reduced sensitivity to its actions. Type 1 is generally associated with onset at an early age, whereas type 2, previously termed 'maturity-onset diabetes', presents later in life and is strongly associated with obesity. A small subset of type 2 diabetes is maturity-onset diabetes of the young (MODY), a genetic condition, with onset at an earlier age. It is now recognised that the incidence of type 2 diabetes mellitus is increasing, with many cases remaining undiagnosed, and it is believed that we are on the edge of a hidden epidemic. Type 2 diabetes represents 90% of patients who have diabetes.

Common clinical features of diabetes are:

- increased thirst (secondary to increased plasma osmolality)
- increased urination (due to osmotic diuresis secondary to glucose in the urine)
- glycosuria
- increased superficial infections such as genital candidiasis due to glucose in the urine
- tiredness
- weight loss in type 1
- ketoacidosis (in the form of dehydration, nausea, vomiting, thirst, weight loss, hyperventilation, ketone breath) in type 1, rarely in type 2.

Diagnosis may be secondary to complications of diabetes, such as hypertension, myocardial infarction, retinal damage, peripheral vascular disease and renal damage. Diabetes can be induced in certain conditions such as pregnancy (gestational diabetes), endocrine conditions associated with the increased production of counter-regulatory hormones (such as corticosteroids in Cushing's syndrome and growth hormone in acromegaly), diseases of the pancreas such as chronic pancreatitis, and by certain drugs (e.g. thiazides, corticosteroids).

Diagnosis is based on elevated plasma glucose levels of >7.0 mmol/L in the fasting state or 11.1 mmol/L on a random test on two occasions. An oral glucose tolerance test may also be carried out and involves measuring plasma glucose levels before and 2 hours after a challenge with a glucose-rich drink (75 g). In this test, a diagnosis is made if the fasting glucose is >7.0 mmol/L or the 2-hour glucose is >11.1 mmol/L. A fasting value of 6–7 mmol/L is consistent with impaired glucose tolerance and referred to as 'pre-diabetes'. A newer measure is based on glycated haemoglobin (HbA_{1c}) levels which reflect long-term glucose levels and a value of 48 mmol/mol is consistent with diabetes. HbA_{1c} levels are increasingly used to diagnose diabetes. Diabetes may be suggested by detection of glucose in the urine, but this is a less valuable test as individuals vary in their renal threshold (about 7–15 mmol/L) for the appearance of glycosuria.

Type 1 diabetes mellitus

This form is generally associated with onset at a young age (<40 years) but may occur at any age. It may be caused by destruction of β cells of the islets of Langerhans after certain viral infections or due to an autoimmune process. It is characterised by an inability of the β cells to produce insulin and is fatal if not treated.

Pharmacological management

Treatment is directed towards replacing the insulin in an attempt to return blood glucose to normal and preventing diabetic complications. The insulin used is now generally the human peptide derived from recombinant DNA technology, although insulin derived from porcine and bovine (rarely) pancreases is used. The insulin is given by injection (sometimes initially by slow intravenous infusion) and in the maintenance phase by subcutaneous injection. Insulin acts on insulin receptors on target tissues of the body to enable blood glucose to be controlled. This follows the insertion of glucose transporters to promote glucose uptake into muscle, liver and adipose tissue, and by stimulation of glycogen, triglyceride and fatty acid synthesis.

Insulin preparations

As insulin has a short plasma half-life, it may be complexed with various agents to retard its absorption, so prolonging its action.

Human insulin analogues

These are modified insulin peptides (insulin lispro and insulin aspart) which have a rapid onset but short duration of action and may be injected just before a meal or when necessary just after a meal. These preparations increase flexibility and are particularly useful for patients prone to pre-lunch hypoglycaemia and those who tend to eat late in the evening and may therefore be at risk of nocturnal hypoglycaemia.

Short-acting insulins

Soluble insulins have relatively short-lived effects of 6–8 hours, with peak effects at 2–5 hours. These are given approximately 15–30 minutes before meals.

Intermediate and long-acting insulins

Combination of insulin with protamine gives rise to intermediate-acting insulin (isophane insulin), binding to zinc gives intermediate-to long-acting insulin and combination with protamine plus zinc gives long-acting insulin. Crystalline insulin zinc suspensions are also long acting. Biphasic preparations contain both an intermediate-acting agent (e.g. isophane insulin) and a shorter-acting form (e.g. soluble insulin).

The aim of insulin therapy is to maintain a plasma glucose level as close to 7.5 mmol/L as possible to prevent future complications, but also to avoid hypoglycaemia. The ideal situation is to match the physiological changes in insulin profile in non-diabetic patients. One method of achieving good glycaemic control is by multiple insulin injections of differing durations of action in an attempt to mimic physiological responses. The aim is to give a long-acting agent to achieve a basal level and to add short-acting preparations in relation to a meal; this is termed 'basal bolus dosing'. The disadvantage here can be one of compliance, because patients are required to monitor blood glucose frequently and administer multiple injections per day. This can be difficult to achieve.

There are no fixed rules and regimens can be adopted to suit the individual needs of the patient. Here are some of the regimens that are commonly used:

- Twice-daily regimens: two daily injections, one 30 minutes before breakfast and one before the evening meal of short- and longer-acting insulins in combination, with two-thirds of the insulin given as the morning dose. This is the most common regimen.

- Multiple dosing regimens: a single dose of medium-acting insulin is given at bedtime and doses of short-acting insulin are given 30 minutes before each meal. This allows more flexibility with the timing of meals.

  Alternatively, a short-acting insulin mixed with intermediate-acting insulin is given before breakfast; short-acting insulin is given before the evening meal and an intermediate-acting insulin is given at bedtime.

- Single daily regimens: these are rarely used but involve one daily injection before breakfast or at bedtime of intermediate-acting insulin, with or without a short-acting insulin. They are generally for patients with type 2 diabetes who are unable to control their blood glucose with antidiabetic drugs.

Insulin requirement is increased by stress, infection, accidental or surgical trauma, puberty (effects of growth hormone) and during the latter two trimesters of pregnancy. Reduced insulin requirements may occur in coeliac disease, renal or hepatic impairment, and endocrine disorders such as untreated Addison's disease.

Insulin administration

Intravenous infusion of soluble insulin is a reliable route of administration and may be used in hospital in an acute setting, to bring the diabetes under control. The amount required to control blood glucose may give an indication of daily requirements for future treatment. In the early stages, patients may encounter what is termed a 'honeymoon period', during which time less insulin is required (due to residual β-cell function). The most conventional route is via subcutaneous injection using a disposable syringe, in which the different insulins may be mixed to achieve the desired combination. This method has largely been superseded by the introduction of more convenient injection pens and biphasic insulins.

Insulin pumps may be used that allow continuous subcutaneous administration. These are particularly useful in diabetes that is difficult to control. They have the advantage of providing a continuous infusion, which may be increased at meal times.

Complications of insulin therapy

As the role of insulin is to reduce blood glucose levels, excessive dosing in relation to food intake can lead to hypoglycaemia. Patients may become aware of this through autonomic (anxiety, sweating, trembling, tachycardia and hunger) and neuroglycaemic (confusion, drowsiness, and problems with concentration, speech and coordination) symptoms. Awareness of these symptoms is important so that action may be taken, such as intake of 10–20 g glucose in lumps or in glucose-rich drinks to prevent a hypoglycaemic coma, e.g. 10 g glucose is provided by two teaspoons of sugar, three sugar lumps, 200 mL milk, 50–55 mL Lucozade, 90 mL Coca-Cola or 15 mL Ribena original (to be diluted). If this is not sufficient, the same dose may be repeated in 10–15 minutes. Hypostop gel may be easier to administer with a reduced risk of choking, and it contains 10 g/23 g ampoule. Glucagon may be given by subcutaneous, intramuscular or intravenous injection for acute insulin-induced hypoglycaemia resulting in unconsciousness.

Strict glycaemic control and the use of human insulin may also impair hypoglycaemic awareness, and it is for this reason that some patients prefer to be maintained on porcine or bovine insulin. Hypoglycaemia is also common at night, because the evening insulin injection may have peak effects at this time, even if the patient has an evening snack (see insulin regimens).

Exercise not only reduces insulin requirements because glucose is used, but also accelerates the absorption of insulin from the subcutaneous sites. Accordingly, patients may need to reduce the dose of insulin before and after exercise and also to take a snack before exercise. In highly trained patients, multiple daily insulin injections may be the best approach to attain glycaemic control, and avoid hypoglycaemia.

Subcutaneous injection of insulin may lead to changes in the skin. At a site of repeated injections, there may be lipohypertrophy, leading to unpredictable insulin absorption. It is for this reason that patients should rotate the sites used.

Inhaled insulin

Delivery of insulin by inhalation was introduced to therapy. Although this represented an advance in delivery of insulin, it was relatively expensive and was subsequently withdrawn from the market.

Drug interactions and effects on concurrent diseases

A number of drugs may alter glucose control and hence the effects of insulin (Table 37.1). By altering glucose metabolism they will also affect control in diabetes and in some cases uncover diabetes.

Intercurrent illnesses and conditions

As commented in Chapter 1, patients with diabetes are a special group who should have a lower threshold for referral to a general practitioner (GP) during illness. In addition, during an illness there may be a loss of appetite but patients should not reduce their insulin intake. In fact, the illness itself may increase blood glucose levels. Carbohydrate 10 g (see Complications of insulin therapy above) should be taken every hour or sips every 20 minutes if nauseated. It is also important to allow

for the glucose content in rehydration solutions, e.g. Dioralyte powder contains 3.56 g glucose per sachet. Pregnancy is a major issue in patients with diabetes and requires specialist supervision.

Type 2 diabetes mellitus

The UK is facing an epidemic of type 2 diabetes and this is likely to pose substantial challenges to the health service. Type 2 diabetes is generally associated with increased insulin resistance, in which the body's tissues become less responsive to insulin, leading to increased blood glucose levels. There is also a strong family association. The β cells of the islets of Langerhans still produce insulin but there is sometimes a loss of cells or reduced glucose sensitivity. The patient may also have other associated diseases such as obesity, hypertension and hyperlipidaemia. Type 2 diabetes generally presents after the age of 40 years

Table 37.1 Examples of the effects of some important drugs on glucose control and insulin activity

Drug	Effects on diabetes	Comments
Alcohol	May mask the signs of hypoglycaemia	• Alcohol should not be consumed in excess and should be taken with food • The carbohydrate content of the drink should also be taken into account (see Counselling in text)
ACE inhibitors	These can sometimes lead to hypoglycaemia	The dose of insulin or antidiabetic drug may need to be reduced
β blockers	These may mask the awareness of hypoglycaemia by reducing the tremor and tachycardia, although sweating is not affected (as this is cholinergic)	This is most marked with propranolol. This is a reason to choose alternative agents or favour the use of β_1-adrenoceptor antagonists
Corticosteroids	These oppose the actions of insulin and cause hyperglycaemia	The dose of insulin may need to be increased
Isoniazid	Variable effects	Monitoring is appropriate
Lithium	May reduce glucose tolerance	May induce diabetes. Monitoring is appropriate
MAOIs	These may enhance the hypoglycaemic actions of insulin	Monitoring is appropriate
Oral contraceptives	Insulin requirements may be altered	
Thiazides	May increase blood glucose	This is a reason to avoid using thiazides in diabetes
Tobacco smoking	This increases the insulin requirements	Smoking substantially enhances the cardiovascular damage in diabetes

ACE, angiotensin-converting enzyme; MAOIs, monoamine oxidase inhibitors.

and may have a gradual onset, such that the patient may have the condition for several years before recognition. This includes the pre-diabetic state, where either fasting glucose and/or post-prandial glucose levels are above the normal range (see above) but below the diagnostic criteria. Pre-diabetes is associated with increased cardiovascular risk and many patients will develop diabetes. Lifestyle changes involving weight loss, exercise and dietary changes have the potential to reverse the pre-diabetic state or slow progression to diabetes.

Pharmacological basis of management

In mild or initial disease, all that may be required is dietary modification to reduce the amount of simple carbohydrates in the diet, weight loss in obesity and increased exercise to achieve control of blood glucose. The alteration of diet should limit the intake of mono- and disaccharides, increase non-starch polysaccharides, and reduce the intake of saturated fat to minimise the risk of atherosclerosis, such that fat is 30–35% of the calorific intake and carbohydrate is 50–55%. A specific dietary modification is to aim for a diet with foods with a low glycaemic index (GI). GI reflects the ability of a food to lead to a rise in plasma glucose, and high GI foods, such as sugar-rich foods, lead to a rapid rise. Lower GI foods include lentils, wholegrain breads such as granary and rye, pasta, basmati rice, porridge and bran cereals.

If dietary changes alone are insufficient after 3 months, antidiabetic drugs are used. If these fail to achieve control at maximum doses and optimal combinations insulin injections may be required. Indeed, type 2 diabetes should be viewed as a progressive disease.

Biguanides: metformin

The action of metformin is unclear but may involve AMP-kinase activation. There are several proposed mechanisms of action, including:

- increased glucose uptake into muscle
- reduced uptake of glucose from the gastrointestinal tract
- reduced output of glucose from the liver.

Obviously these proposed mechanisms will lead to either reduced entry of glucose into the blood or increased utilisation.

Sulphonylureas, e.g. glibenclamide, gliclazide, glimepiride, glipizide, tolbutamide

The sulphonylureas rely on the fact that the β cells can still produce insulin. These drugs act to increase insulin secretion. Pharmacologically, they are inhibitors of adenosine triphosphate (ATP)-sensitive potassium (K_{ATP}) channels. Subtypes of K_{ATP} channels are present on many cell types such as β cells, smooth muscle cells, cardiac muscle cells and neuronal cells. In β cells, they regulate insulin release. When glucose is present, the production of ATP and the reduction in adenosine diphosphate (ADP) inactivate these channels, leading to cellular depolarisation, which results in calcium influx and insulin secretion. When glucose is low, ATP levels fall and ADP rises, channels open, with membrane hyperpolarisation, and this decreases insulin release. Sulphonylureas bind to a receptor associated with these channels, resulting in channel closure, which leads to insulin release.

Meglitinide analogues: nateglinide, repaglinide

These also act on β cells but at a site distinct from the sulphonylurea receptor, causing closure of the K_{ATP} channels, leading to depolarisation and insulin release. They have a rapid rate of onset and are given at mealtimes to stimulate postprandial insulin secretion, which is relatively short-lived. Their effects may be enhanced by patients having a meal and they are referred to as prandial glucose regulators, which may be regarded as producing a more physiological rise in insulin than that produced by sulphonylureas.

Thiazolidinediones (glitazones): pioglitazone

These are 'insulin sensitisers' which work by enhancing glucose utilisation in tissues, and so reduce insulin resistance. They activate the γ nuclear peroxisome proliferator-activated receptors (PPAR-γ), which alter gene expression and result in insulin-like effects. These include reduced hepatic glucose output, increased glucose transporters (GLUT) in skeletal muscle with increased peripheral glucose utilisation, and the promotion of fatty acid uptake into adipose cells.

One of the original members of the family, rosiglitazone, was withdrawn in 2010 due to increased cardiovascular events.

Modulation of incretins: exenatide, sitagliptin, liraglutide

Incretins are endogenous hormones (e.g. glucagon-like peptide-1, GLP-1) that regulate the endocrine function of the pancreas. Exenatide is an incretin mimetic that acts on β-cells of the islets of Langerhans to stimulate the release of insulin; it also acts to reduce glucagon release. Sitagliptin is a dipeptidyl peptidase-4 (DPP-4) inhibitor, which means that it inhibits the breakdown of incretins, thus enhancing their action, which promotes insulin secretion and suppresses glucagon release.

A new addition to the family is liraglutide, a long-acting GLP-1 receptor agonist, which is given once daily by subcutaneous injection. Its use is also associated with weight loss and so may have promise in the management of obesity.

Glucosidase inhibitors: acarbose

Acarbose competitively inhibits the α-glucosidases, which metabolise oligosaccharides to monosaccharides in the small intestines. This reduces the production of glucose in the gastrointestinal tract, thereby preventing sharp rises in blood glucose after a meal. The subsequent increased presence of carbohydrates in the gastrointestinal tract may lead to flatulence and osmotic diarrhoea as side effects.

Drug choice

The first-line drug in type 2 diabetes is metformin as this is considered to have the best evidence for improved outcomes. One consideration is renal function and metformin should be avoided if eGFR is <30 mL/minute per 1.73m². If monotherapy with metformin is inadequate, an additional antidiabetic drug is added, such as a sulphonylurea, pioglitazone or an incretin-based drug. A reason to choose pioglitazone or an incretin-based drug over metformin would be if hypoglycaemia were a problem with the sulphonylurea. Additionally, sulphonylureas are associated with weight gain and this may influence drug choice.

Other considerations are detailed in Table 37.2.

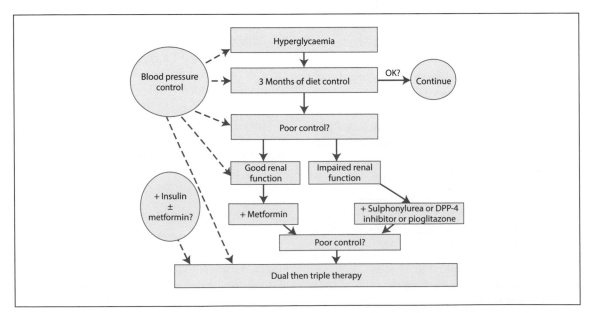

Figure 37.1 Current approaches to the management of type 2 diabetes, incorporating National Institute for Health and Care Excellence guidelines (NICE 2015).

Table 37.2 The effects of concurrent conditions on drug choice in type 2 diabetes mellitus

Condition	Effect on drug choice	Comments
Renal impairment	Avoid metformin. Tolbutamide or gliclazide is preferred	The shorter-acting sulphonylureas should be used at a reduced dose
Heart failure	Avoid metformin in severe heart failure. Avoid pioglitazone in heart failure	
Liver disease	Avoid metformin. Avoid pioglitazone	Risk of lactic acidosis
Hyperlipidaemia	Glitazones may cause modest reductions in triglycerides and increases in HDL	Fibrates may also be chosen to manage hyperlipidaemia (Chapter 13)
Porphyria	Sulphonylureas should be avoided	
Pregnancy	Insulin therapy is generally used in place of oral antidiabetic drugs	

HDL, high-density lipoprotein.

Concerns over fracture risk and glitazones

There is recent evidence that glitazones may impair bone formation and this has been identified as a risk factor for bone fractures (Meier *et al.* 2008).

Drug interactions

In addition to the effects of drugs on glucose control described above, Table 37.3 gives some important interactions with antidiabetic agents.

Complications of antidiabetic drug therapy

The main complication of treatment with the sulphonylureas and, to a lesser extent, meglitinide analogues is hypoglycaemia because they stimulate insulin release. This is most problematic at high doses or in the case of sulphonylureas with long half-lives. Incidents of hypoglycaemia may be managed by sugary drinks (see above) and may require a change in the drug used. The glitazones and metformin are far less likely to cause hypoglycaemia.

The insulin-stimulating effects of sulphonylureas and insulin-sensitising effects of glitazones may lead to weight gain, whereas metformin leads to weight loss.

Monitoring

In view of hepatotoxicity to the prototypical glitazone troglitazone, liver function tests should be carried out in patients receiving pioglitazone before and during treatment.

Diabetic complications and their prevention

Diabetic complications have serious consequences for both morbidity and mortality. The complications are macrovascular, microvascular and neuropathy.

Macrovascular complications

Diabetes is associated with a substantial increase in the risk of cardiovascular mortality through ischaemic heart disease and stroke. Furthermore, the risk is substantially enhanced by other cardiovascular risks such as hypertension, hyperlipidaemia, obesity and smoking. Cardiovascular disease occurs prematurely in patients with diabetes, even if they have had good control, and accounts for 70% of deaths in these patients. Strict regulation of blood pressure is essential in diabetes: the British Hypertension Society recommends a target of <140/80 mmHg. Evidence from trials indicates that lowering blood pressure in itself is important and reduces both macrovascular and microvascular complications. Trials with antihypertensive drugs have also focused on specific agents in patients with diabetes. In this respect, Losartan Intervention for Endpoint Reduction in Hypertension (LIFE) trial (2002) has reported that the angiotensin receptor antagonist losartan is more effective than atenolol at reducing morbidity and mortality

Table 37.3 Examples of some important interactions with antidiabetic drugs

Drugs	Consequences	Comments
Acarbose with insulin/sulphonylureas	Acarbose may enhance the hypoglycaemic effects of these drugs	Dose reduction of insulin or sulphonylurea may be needed
Chlorpropamide with alcohol	Facial flushing	This does not occur with other sulphonylureas
Glipizide with colestyramine	The absorption of glipizide may be delayed	Glipizide should be taken 1–2 hours before colestyramine
Sulphonylureas with fibrates	Enhanced effects of the sulphonylureas	This may be an advantage in poor glucose control or dose reduction of the sulphonylurea may be needed
Tolbutamide/glibenclamide with rifampicin	Rifampicin may increase the metabolism of these agents	The dose of the sulphonylurea may need to be increased
Sulphonylureas with sulphonamides	Enhanced hypoglycaemic effects	This applies to some but not all sulphonamides
Repaglinide with erythromycin, fluconazole, itraconazole, ketoconazole, phenytoin or rifampicin	These drugs may alter the actions of repaglinide	The manufacturer contraindicates these combinations
Metformin/sulphonylureas with cimetidine	Cimetidine has been reported to increase the activity of sulphonylureas (especially glipizide). Cimetidine may inhibit the renal excretion of metformin	Patients may be advised of the possibility of hypoglycaemia while taking cimetidine and a sulphonylurea. A dose reduction with metformin may be appropriate. Ranitidine does not appear to interact with these antidiabetic drugs

in hypertensive patients who have diabetes and/or left ventricular hypertrophy. The Heart Outcomes Prevention Evaluation (HOPE) trial (2000) found that treatment of patients with a high risk for cardiovascular disease with the angiotensin-converting enzyme (ACE) inhibitor ramipril reduced the complications associated with diabetes and also the development of diabetes. Accordingly, ACE inhibitors are often first-choice antihypertensives in patients with diabetes. The Heart Protection Study Collaborative Group (2002) has demonstrated, in patients with diabetes, that simvastatin protects against cardiovascular events, irrespective of their cholesterol levels.

Microvascular complications

Pathological changes in the microcirculation lead to nephropathy and retinopathy. The mechanism of damage is thought to be due to hyperglycaemia leading to glycation of structural proteins and the toxic effects of free radicals and glycation end-products. Accordingly, there is good evidence that good glycaemic control may limit these complications.

Diabetic nephropathy is a long-term consequence of diabetes and may result in end-stage renal failure. In the early stages of diabetes, there is hyperfiltration in the glomeruli. There are subsequent changes in the basement membranes, including glycation, and these lead to microalbuminuria, a marker of renal deterioration. This may be followed by hypertension and proteinuria. Microvascular damage in the retinal circulation may lead to retinopathy, which is associated with angiogenesis, haemorrhages and detachment of the retina. Retinopathy is a major cause of blindness.

All patients with type 1 diabetes who have microalbuminuria should receive an ACE inhibitor, regardless of whether they have hypertension. NICE guidance (2002) on renal disease in type 2 diabetes indicated that diabetic nephropathy is likely in patients who have albumin in the urine and/or increased plasma creatinine levels, accompanied by retinopathy. In these patients, glycaemic control should aim to achieve levels of glycated haemoglobin (HbA_{1c}) <6.5–7.5%, blood pressure should be <135/75 mmHg and an ACE inhibitor should be given for renal and cardiovascular protection. The CALM study group (2000) demonstrated, in type 2 diabetes, that the angiotensin II receptor antagonist candesartan was as effective as lisinopril at controlling both blood pressure and microalbuminuria. Furthermore, the combination of candesartan and lisinopril was even more effective. The sartan irbesartan has also been shown to be effective at reducing the incidence of diabetic nephropathy and is licensed for use in type 2 diabetes. This may be an alternative to ACE inhibitors when they are not tolerated, e.g. due to their associated cough.

The Diabetes Control and Complications Trial (DCCT 1993) reported that, in type 1 diabetes, intensive insulin therapy to maintain blood glucose as close to normal as possible delayed the onset and progression of nephropathy, retinopathy and neuropathy. Evidence from the UK Prospective Diabetes Study (UKPDS) (1998a, 1998b) indicated that intensive glycaemic control in type 2 diabetes lowers the risk of microvascular but not macrovascular complications. Furthermore, in overweight individuals metformin was more effective than sulphonylureas in reducing diabetic complications.

Peripheral vascular disease

The vascular damage associated with diabetes is a major risk factor for the development of peripheral vascular disease, leading to ischaemia, and is a major reason for limb amputation.

Neuropathy

Damage to nerves occurs through glycation and the production of polyols. This may lead to impaired nervous conduction and is referred to as neuropathy. The neuropathy may be peripheral, leading to loss of peripheral sensation and ulceration, or autonomic, which may lead to postural hypotension and impotence.

Monitoring

Monitoring of glycaemic control is important in the management of diabetes but is especially important in patients who use insulin and alter their dose according to the level of control. Monitoring is best achieved by measuring blood glucose levels using a reagent stick and simple meter, so that the levels of control may be assessed and the dose of insulin or antidiabetic drugs

adjusted accordingly. Long-term monitoring of control is by measuring the levels of HbA_{1c} in the blood. This gives a measure of the long-term control (previous 2–3 months): a value of 48 mmol/mol or less is associated with reduced diabetic complications. In addition, blood pressure, cholesterol, renal and visual function are routinely monitored.

Over-the-counter considerations

Many medicines, including many over-the-counter (OTC) preparations for coughs and colds, contain sugar and patients should be made aware of this in relation to their daily intake. Sugar-free alternatives are available but may be more expensive and often contain sorbitol, which may cause diarrhoea.

Corn plasters that contain salicylic acid should not be used in patients with diabetes, because patients with diabetic neuropathy may have less sensation in the feet and the corrosive effects of corn-plasters may go unnoticed, leading to ulceration. All foot problems affecting patients with diabetes warrant prompt referral.

Decongestants should be used with caution in patients with diabetes because the β-adrenoceptor agonist activity may alter glucose control via anti-insulin affects.

Dietary supplements

Insulin therapy or antidiabetic drugs are the only appropriate treatments for diabetes. However, a number of dietary supplements, in addition to a balanced diet, may play some role in the management of diabetes. Examples of these include aloe vera, which has been shown to exert hypoglycaemic actions and may have a potential role as an adjunct to conventional treatment; carnitine may increase glucose utilisation. Other herbal preparations with potential hypoglycaemic activity include burdock, celery, dandelion, eucalyptus, garlic, ginger, ispaghula, juniper, marshmallow, nettle and sage. Studies on animal models of diabetes suggest that evening primrose oil may be of benefit in neuropathy. Hyperglycaemic effects are associated with hydrocotyle, liquorice and rosemary. For a more detailed discussion of this topic, the reader is referred to *Dietary Supplements* by Mason (2007).

Counselling

Diabetes mellitus is a lifelong condition and patients will receive a range of counselling from doctors, specialist nurses and dieticians. Patients may also be directed to organisations such as Diabetes UK for further information and advice. The key to counselling is to ensure good glycaemic control, which is associated with the prevention of diabetic complications. In addition, practical advice that may be given includes the following.

Diabetes in general

- Give advice about the regimen.
- The patient should be made aware of the signs of hypo- and hyperglycaemia and how to respond to them.
- Patients with diabetes should inform the DVLA (Driver and Vehicle Licensing Agency) of their condition.
- Patients should be warned to avoid hypoglycaemia while driving.
- Patients prescribed insulin and those at risk of hypoglycaemia should carry glucose tablets or similar at all times.
- In addition to dietary advice, special diabetic foods are expensive and of little value.
- It is a misconception that natural fruit juice, honey and reduced-sugar products are low in sugar.
- Patients with diabetes represent a risk group (see Chapter 1) and the importance of consulting their GP should be emphasised.
- Patients with diabetes should consult their GP if they experience problems with their feet, including fungal infections.
- Patients with type 1 and type 2 diabetes (treated with drugs) are exempt from prescription charges.
- Lifestyle advice to reduce cardiovascular risk, including cessation of smoking, should be emphasised.
- Alcohol should be consumed only in moderation and it may mask the signs of hypoglycaemia.
- Alcoholic drinks will also contribute towards the carbohydrate load.
- Low-dose aspirin should be considered for patients with a significant risk of cardiovascular disease.
- Exercise improves insulin sensitivity and reduces cardiovascular risk.
- Advice should be sought before becoming pregnant.

- A MedicAlert chain or card should be carried if possible to alert doctors that the patient is prescribed insulin. A service is available whereby patients register their insulin regimen and a number is available for emergency doctors to contact if needed.

Type 1 diabetes

- Patients should be advised to maintain adequate supplies of insulin.
- Patients should not stop taking insulin.
- Give advice about injection technique.
- Insulins should be stored in a refrigerator but not frozen.
- Different injection sites should be used, although the rate of absorption may differ between sites.
- The dispensed container of insulin should be shown to the patient for confirmation that it is expected by the patient.
- The size of the pen needle should be checked carefully when prescribing and dispensing due to the increasing variety of sizes, which reflect different injection techniques.
- Sugary food may be eaten but preferably as part of a meal.
- Needles should be disposed of correctly.

Type 2 diabetes

- Metformin should be taken with or after food.
- Diarrhoea is a common side effect with metformin and acarbose.
- Nateglinide and repaglinide should be taken just before meals.

Self-assessment

For the following questions concerning the management of diabetes, choose the most appropriate answer:

1 *Which one of the following is not a clinical feature of type II diabetes?*

   A Increased susceptibility to fungal infections
   B Glycosuria
   C Racing heart rate
   D Thirst
   E Increased urination

2 *Which one of the following does NICE recommend as first-line drug treatment for type 2 diabetes in an otherwise healthy patient?*

A Acarbose

B Metformin

C Pioglitazone

D An incretin mimetic (such as exenatide)

E Insulin

3 *Which one of the following best describes the mode of action of a sulphonylurea?*

A Inhibition of ATP-sensitive potassium channels

B Insulin sensitisation

C Hyperpolarisation of pancreatic β-cells

D Increases in cAMP

E Activation of tyrosine kinases

4 *Which one of the following is a common side effect of sulphonylureas?*

A Renal failure

B Impotence

C Hypertension

D Weight gain

E Neutropenia

5 *Which one of the following is a contraindication to using metformin?*

A Asthma

B Moderate renal impairment

C Gout

D Hypertension

E Childbearing age

6 *An incretin mimetic (such as exenatide) is likely to cause which one of the following?*

A Increased insulin release

B Decreased insulin breakdown

C Enhanced activation of PPAR-γ receptors

D Increased glucagon release

E Direct activation of insulin receptors

Practice points

- Diabetes is a major risk factor for cardiovascular disease, so a healthy lifestyle (including avoidance of obesity and cessation of smoking) is essential.
- Blood pressure should be adequately controlled and ACE inhibitors are effective at reducing diabetic nephropathy.
- The risk of developing type 2 diabetes may be reduced by a lifelong healthy diet, weight control and exercise.
- Type 2 diabetes continues to be underdiagnosed.
- Good glycaemic control may prevent future complications.

CASE STUDY

A 60-year-old woman reported a raging thirst, and recurrent fungal infections. A simple 'pin-prick' blood test revealed a random blood glucose of 16.0 mmol/L [<11.1 mmol/L]. The following day her significant fasting clinical biochemistry was:

Plasma creatinine	250 µmol/L [<150 µmol/L]
Total cholesterol	6.5 mmol/L [(<5.2 mmol/L]
Triglycerides	3.0 mmol/L [0.6–1.7 mmol/L]
Glucose (fasting)	13 mmol/L [<7.0 mmol/L]

and a physical examination revealed a weight of 80 kg, height of 1.60 m and blood pressure of 160/95 mmHg.

A diagnosis of type 2 diabetes mellitus was made. The initial plan was dietary modifications with reduced intake of total calories, fat and simple carbohydrates. Her blood pressure was reviewed

(continued)

(continued)

the following week and was 165/98 mmHg and she was initially prescribed bendroflumethiazide (2.5 mg o.m.) but the pharmacist was unhappy with this and recommended that ramipril (1.25 mg o.d. increased up to 5 mg o.d.) was prescribed instead.

What are the goals of treatment for this woman?

- Control blood glucose such that HbA_{1c} is ideally below 48 mmol/mol
- Reduce cardiovascular risk
- Control blood pressure to <130 mmHg and <80 mmHg
- Reduce cholesterol levels
- Preserve renal function
- Reduce risk of other diabetic complications such as neuropathy, retinopathy

What was the rationale for the intervention made by the pharmacist?

Bendroflumethiazide would be less effective in renal impairment and might worsen diabetes and alter lipid profile. ACE inhibitors are renoprotective and so favoured in patients with diabetes.

Despite these initial measures, at the 3 months review her blood pressure was 150/90 mmHg and she had marked proteinuria and the following additions were made to her prescription:

Metformin 500 mg (o.d.) but on the advice of the pharmacist this was changed to gliclazide 40 mg (o.d.) being increased up to 160 mg (b.d.)
Atorvastatin 10 mg (o.d.) being increased over 4 weeks to 80 mg (o.d.)
Amlodipine 10 mg (o.d.)
Aspirin 75 mg (o.d.)

Comment on the choice of gliclazide over metformin in this case.

- Metformin is contraindicated in light of her renal impairment.

What was the rationale for each addition?

- Diet failed to control glucose and gliclazide was added to control this.
- Atorvastatin was added to reduce cholesterol and reduce cardiovascular risk. Amlodipine was added to bring blood pressure to target. Aspirin was added as an antiplatelet drug to reduce risk of cardiovascular events.
- Atorvastatin was chosen as it is less likely than simvastatin to interact with amlodipine.

How would you counsel the patient with respect to the new additions?

- Gliclazide: she should be warned of the risk of hypoglycaemia and how to recognise and avoid it. If she misses a meal, she should not take the sulphonylurea.
- She should monitor blood glucose regularly.
- Atorvastatin may cause gastrointestinal upsets to start with and she should report any muscle pain to her general practitioner.
- With aspirin she should be alert for dyspepsia.

At a subsequent review one year later she had significant oedema and her significant clinical biochemistry was:

Plasma creatinine	450 µmol/L [<150 µmol/L]
Total cholesterol	4.5 mmol/L [<5.2 mmol/L]
Triglycerides	2.0 mmol/L [0.6 – 1.7 mmol/L]
Glucose (fasting)	6 mmol/L [<7.0 mmol/L]

The following changes were made to her prescription:

Reduce ramipril to 2.5 mg (o.d.)
Add furosemide 250 mg (o.d.)

Comment on these changes.

- Evidence of renal impairment worsening, which could be related to diabetic nephropathy or an adverse effect of the ACE inhibitor. Either the dose of ramipril should be reduced or it should be stopped.
- Furosemide was added due to the oliguria and will reduce the oedema secondary to renal failure.

References

CALM study group (2000). Randomised controlled trial of dual blockade of the renin–angiotensin system in patients with hypertension, microalbuminuria, and non-insulin dependent diabetes: the Candesartan And Lisinopril Microalbuminuria (CALM) study. *BMJ* 321: 1440–1444.

DCCT (Diabetes Control and Complications Trial Research Group) (1993). The effect of intensive treatment of diabetes on the development and progression of long-term complications in insulin-dependent diabetes mellitus. *N Engl J Med* 329: 977–986.

Heart Protection Study Collaborative Group (2002). MRC/BHF Heart Protection Study of cholesterol lowering with simvastatin in 20 536 high-risk individuals: randomised placebo-controlled trial. *Lancet* 360: 7–22.

HOPE (Heart Outcomes Prevention Evaluation) study investigators (2000). Effects of an angiotensin-converting-enzyme inhibitor, ramipril, on cardiovascular events in high-risk patients. *N Engl J Med* 342: 145–153.

LIFE (Losartan Intervention for Endpoint Reduction in Hypertension) study investigators (2002). Cardiovascular morbidity and mortality in patients with diabetes in the Losartan Intervention for Endpoint Reduction in Hypertension study (LIFE): a randomised trial against atenolol. *Lancet* 359: 1004–1010.

Mason P (2007). *Dietary Supplements,* 3rd edn. London: Pharmaceutical Press.

Meier C, Kraenzlin ME, Bodmer M *et al*. (2008). Use of thiazolidinediones and fracture risk. *Arch Intern Med* 168: 820–825. pmid: 18443256.

National Institute for Health and Care Excellence (2015). *Type 2 diabetes in adults: management.* London: NICE.

Nissen SE, Wolski K (2007). Effect of rosiglitazone on the risk of myocardial infarction and death from cardiovascular causes. *N Engl J Med* 356: 2457–2473. pmid: 17517853.

UKPDS (UK Prospective Diabetes Study) Group (1998a). Intensive blood-glucose control with sulphonylurea or insulin compared with conventional treatment and the risk of complications in patients with type 2 diabetes (UKPDS 33). *Lancet* 352: 837–853.

UKPDS Group (1998b). Effects of intensive blood-glucose control with metformin on the complications in overweight patients with type 2 diabetes (UKPDS 34). *Lancet* 352: 854–865.

Online resource

www.diabetes.org.uk
The website of Diabetes UK, the current name of the British Diabetic Association, which provides both patient and professional information (accessed October 2015).

38

Thyroid disorders

The thyroid gland releases predominantly thyroxine (T_4), but also triiodothyronine (T_3), which is the more active hormone; indeed, T_4 may undergo peripheral conversion to T_3. Both of these hormones play important roles in the regulation of cellular metabolism and growth, while also influencing activity of the sympathetic nervous system. Clinically there may be excessive activity (hyperthyroidism) or underactivity (hypothyroidism), both of which have widespread pathophysiological effects.

Hyperthyroidism

This is also known as thyrotoxicosis and is generally characterised by elevated levels of T_3 and T_4. The most common form is Graves' disease, which is due to antibodies against the thyroid-stimulating hormone (TSH) receptor, responsible for stimulating the release of T_3 and T_4. The antibodies activate the receptor and lead to the increased production of thyroid hormone, and there is usually an increase in the size of the thyroid gland (goitre). Other less common causes include toxic multinodular goitre, toxic adenoma and iatrogenic causes. In the last case, drugs that have a high iodine content such as amiodarone and radiological contrast agents may lead to increased thyroid activity; lithium may rarely cause hyperthyroidism.

Clinical features

Hyperthyroidism is especially common in women and occurs most often between the ages of 20 and 40 years. There may be widespread changes, which include:

- weight loss
- increased appetite
- diarrhoea
- nervousness and irritability
- fatigue
- tremor
- increased sweating
- heat intolerance
- pruritus
- exophthalmos (bulging eyes, seen in Graves' disease only)
- eyelid retraction
- goitre
- cardiac arrhythmias, including palpitations and atrial fibrillation
- angina
- precipitation of heart failure

- shortness of breath on exertion
- nausea and vomiting in pregnancy
- palmar erythema.

Many of these symptoms may be attributable to the increased action of catecholamines.

Diagnosis

In addition to the above symptoms, biochemistry will reveal increased levels of thyroid hormones but undetectable levels of TSH. This latter finding is due to increased levels of thyroid hormone causing negative-feedback inhibition of TSH release from the pituitary gland. Thyroid function tests may be complicated by concurrent drug treatment, including the use of amiodarone, aspirin, β blockers, carbamazepine, corticosteroids, heparin, oestrogens, phenytoin, rifampicin and radiological contrast agents. In this respect, the enzyme inducers carbamazepine, phenytoin and rifampicin may accelerate the metabolism of T_4 and T_3, leading to reduced levels. Corticosteroids may inhibit TSH release, lowering T_4 and T_3. By contrast, heparin may give a rapid but short-lived increase in T_4 and radiological contrast agents may elevate T_4 due to their high iodine content.

Given the non-specific nature of some of the symptoms, thyroid function is often routinely measured in patients presenting with a range of symptoms, e.g. palpitations in young adults.

Goals of treatment

These are to achieve a euthyroid state (normal levels of thyroid hormones), and to provide symptomatic relief from the increased sympathetic activity.

Management

To achieve euthyroidism the choice is from the use of antithyroid drugs (thionamides), radioactive iodine to irradiate and destroy part of the thyroid gland, and a partial or subtotal thyroidectomy.

Pharmacological basis of management

Thionamides: carbimazole and propylthiouracil

These decrease the production of thyroid hormones by inhibiting the iodination of thyroglobulin, which occurs via inhibition of thyroperoxidase. The thyroid hormones have long plasma half-lives, so inhibiting their synthesis will take several weeks for an effect to occur. Thionamides may also suppress the immune response, but whether this contributes to their action in hyperthyroidism is unclear.

β blockers: atenolol, nadolol, propranolol

These are dealt with extensively in Chapter 12. In the context of hyperthyroidism, they will reduce the actions of catecholamines at β-adrenoceptors, which are augmented in this condition, and will provide relief from symptoms such as tremor, anxiety and palpitations. Non-selective β blockers (e.g. propranolol) are required to relieve the tremor. It should also be noted that hyperthyroidism accelerates the metabolism of propranolol.

Treatment (Figure 38.1)

Thionamides are indicated for the first episode of Graves' disease with a view to achieving a remission. It is also used in subsequent episodes of Graves' disease, in more elderly patients and those with toxic nodular hyperthyroidism, to achieve euthyroidism before surgery or with radioactive iodine for a definitive cure. In the case of drug-induced hyperthyroidism, the causative drug should be stopped and a β blocker used to control the symptoms.

Carbimazole is the thionamide of choice, with once-daily administration. It is initially given at higher doses, known as reducing doses, to achieve a euthyroid state, which takes about 1–2 months to achieve. During this time, unless contraindicated (asthma, chronic obstructive pulmonary disease, uncontrolled heart failure), a β blocker is given to control symptoms. Once the euthyroid state is achieved, maintenance therapy with the thionamide at a lower dose may be used, typically for 18 months, and the β blocker withdrawn gradually. Alternatively, a high dose of carbimazole may be maintained to suppress thyroid activity completely and combined with replacement T_4, and this is known as the blocking–replacement regimen. This has the advantage of avoiding hypothyroidism, which may be induced by antithyroid drugs, and a reduced requirement for monitoring of thyroid function. Block-and-replace regimens might be most appropriate for patients in whom it is difficult to achieve

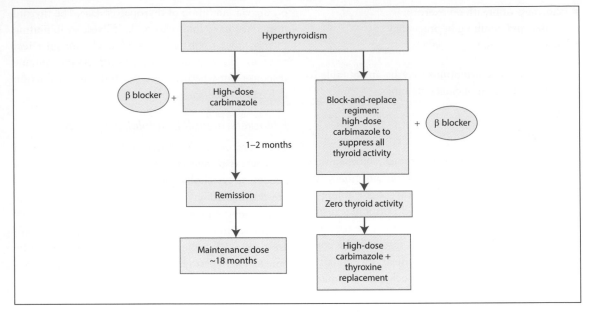

Figure 38.1 Approaches to the management of hyperthyroidism.

a euthyroid state on antithyroid drugs alone. Despite the use of antithyroid drugs, the relapse rate is around 50% on discontinuation of treatment, although it is unclear whether blocking–replacement regimens have a higher success rate.

Other considerations

Pregnancy and breastfeeding

Carbimazole may cause hypothyroidism in the fetus but is generally considered safe in pregnancy under specialist care, with the lowest effective dose used, and this may be stopped before birth. Propylthiouracil is sometimes preferred because carbimazole may induce fetal aplasia cutis (a localised absence of skin at birth). A blocking–replacement regimen is contraindicated in pregnancy, because the antithyroid drugs more readily cross the placenta than T_4 and this may lead to fetal hypothyroidism.

Carbimazole at doses of <20 mg is considered safe during lactation, because the amounts in the milk are low. Once again, propylthiouracil is sometimes preferred because it enters the breast milk to a lesser extent.

Asthma

Hyperthyroidism may sometimes lead to a worsening of asthma. β_2 agonists should be used with caution as bronchodilators because they may be expected to have enhanced systemic actions in uncontrolled hyperthyroidism. Indeed, the symptoms of toxicity with β_2 agonists may also be confused with those of hyperthyroidism. As commented above, asthma is a contraindication to using β blockers in the management of hyperthyroidism. In patients who cannot receive a β blocker, calcium-channel blockers such as diltiazem may be useful in controlling tachycardia.

Monitoring

No specific monitoring, except thyroid function, is required for treatment with thionamides. However, carbimazole and propylthiouracil may both cause agranulocytosis leading to leukopenia. If patients report with sore throats, mouth ulcers, bruising or non-specific illness, a full blood count should be carried out and the drug withdrawn if there is leukopenia. Although an alternative thionamide may be used as a replacement, there is a high degree of cross-reactivity between agents.

Drug interactions

Drug interactions with antithyroid drugs are limited and detailed in Table 38.1.

Table 38.1 Some important drug interactions with antithyroid drugs

Drugs	Consequences	Comments
Corticosteroids with carbimazole	Increased elimination of prednisolone	The dose of prednisolone may need to be increased
Digoxin with carbimazole	Carbimazole may reduce the plasma levels of digoxin. Patients with hyperthyroidism may be resistant to the actions of digoxin, such that digoxin may be less effective in atrial fibrillation in patients with hyperthyroidism	Higher doses of digoxin may be required initially and then reduced as thyroid levels fall
Theophylline with thionamides	Theophylline levels may rise in patients treated with thionamides for hyperthyroidism	Monitoring may be required and the dose of theophylline may need to be reduced
Warfarin with thionamides	The actions of warfarin may be decreased	The dose of warfarin may need to be increased

Counselling

Lifestyle advice may be helpful in relieving symptoms such as heat intolerance. Caffeine consumption should be reduced, because this may exacerbate symptoms. Ophthalmopathy in Graves' disease, presenting as photophobia and grittiness, may be relieved by sunglasses and artificial tears. Drug-specific counselling points are detailed:

- If carbimazole or propylthiouracil is taken without a β blocker, it will take several weeks for an improvement in symptoms to be noticed.
- If a β blocker is used, it is worth explaining its role to the patient, and that it is not being used for hypertension or angina, which may be indicated on the patient information leaflets. General counselling for β blockers is found in Chapter 12.
- Both carbimazole and propylthiouracil may cause agranulocytosis, leading to leukopenia. Patients should report urgently to their general practitioner (GP) with sore throats, mouth ulcers, bruising or non-specific illness.
- Both carbimazole and propylthiouracil may cause mild gastrointestinal disturbances and urticarial rashes. Pruritus may be managed with antihistamines and treatment continued. If this fails, an alternative agent may be tried because cross-sensitivity may not occur.
- Patients should be advised to report symptoms of hypothyroidism, which may indicate overtreatment.

Hypothyroidism

This is simply failure of the thyroid gland to produce sufficient thyroid hormone, leading to reduced circulating levels. The most common form (90%) is Hashimoto's thyroiditis, which is an autoimmune destruction of the thyroid gland. Hypothyroidism may also be induced by antithyroid drug treatment with thionamides, lithium, amiodarone and also radioactive iodine.

Clinical features

As with hyperthyroidism, there is an increased incidence of hypothyroidism in women and this increases with age. There are widespread changes in hypothyroidism, which include:

- tiredness
- weight gain
- hypothermia
- cold intolerance
- hoarseness
- bradycardia (rarely angina and heart failure)
- mental slowness
- delayed reflexes
- depression
- anaemia
- dry skin and hair
- goitre
- oedema, leading to puffiness around the eyes
- constipation.

Diagnosis

Hypothyroidism is identified on a thyroid function test, which reveals elevated TSH and reduced T_4 levels. In addition there may be macrocytosis and hypercholesterolaemia. In secondary failure due to pituitary or hypothalamic disease, TSH levels will be reduced. Other causes should be considered before starting treatment.

Goals of treatment

These are to achieve a euthyroid state.

Management

Restoring thyroid hormone levels is achieved by administration of levothyroxine (T_4). In young patients the starting dose is usually 50–100 micrograms/day, which may be increased after 6 weeks by 25–50 micrograms, and thereafter until maintenance levels are achieved. The dose required is the one that leads to correct TSH levels. In elderly patients, and those with ischaemic heart disease, the starting dose used is 25 micrograms, which is increased every 3–4 weeks by 25 micrograms, until TSH levels are normalised. The reason to exercise caution in patients with ischaemic heart disease is that T_4 may lead to worsening or uncovering of angina (there is also an increased risk of myocardial infarction and death) by increasing the metabolic rate and sympathetic activity. In patients who experience angina, a β blocker may be prescribed. If the TSH levels are suppressed by overtreatment, there is a significant risk of atrial fibrillation. Once established, T_4 therapy will need to be used lifelong.

Diabetes mellitus

An increased dose of antidiabetic agents, including insulin, may be required.

Pregnancy

T_4 treatment is continued during pregnancy but the dose may need to be increased to normalise TSH levels.

Drug interactions

Some important interactions with T_4 are detailed in Table 38.2. The interactions relate to altering the effects of T_4 or interacting drugs.

Counselling

Aside from guidance on the regimen, a key counselling point should be to advise patients to consult their GP if angina develops or pre-existing angina deteriorates. Additional points:

- It is difficult to distinguish between the strengths of T_4 tablets, because they are all small and white. Patients should make sure that they take tablets of the correct strength.
- If a dose is missed, the missed dose may be taken the next day with the next dose (as T_4 has a long half-life of 7 days).
- Patients should be encouraged to report symptoms of overtreatment, particularly when treatment is initiated. These include diarrhoea, nervousness, rapid pulse, insomnia, tremors or anginal pain. These symptoms may necessitate a reduced dose or the omission of a dose for 1–2 days before restarting at a lower dose.

Over-the-counter medicines in patients with thyroid disorders

Topical or oral sympathomimetic drugs should be avoided in patients with hyperthyroidism, due to the enhancement of catecholamines. Pharmacists can help to remind patients of the need for prompt referral when presenting with signs of infection on being prescribed antithyroid medication. Pharmacists may also help to identify patients presenting with symptoms suggestive of thyroid disorder and encourage referral for further investigation, e.g. the common request for over-the-counter (OTC) products for fatigue and/or slimming advice may prompt further questioning to identify the possibility of an underlying thyroid disorder.

Herbal medicines in patients with thyroid disorders

Kelp is used as herbal treatment for thyroid disorders. However, it has a high iodine content that may lead to hyper- or hypothyroidism, and it should be avoided. Preparations of ephedra should be avoided due to the ephedrine content. Shepherd's purse also has the potential to cause hypothyroidism and should

Table 38.2 Drugs interacting with levothyroxine

Drug	Consequences	Comments
Amiodarone	Reduced effects of levothyroxine	Contraindicated by manufacturers. The *British National Formulary* indicates that, if amiodarone causes hyperthyroidism, amiodarone should be withdrawn and antithyroid drugs may be required. If hypothyroidism is induced then replacement therapy may be needed
Antiepileptic drugs (carbamazepine and phenytoin)	These enzyme inducers have been reported to lower thyroid hormone levels occasionally	Monitoring may be appropriate
Colestyramine	This may reduce the absorption of levothyroxine	Their use should be separated by 4–6 hours
Ferrous sulphate	This may reduce the absorption of levothyroxine	Their doses should be separated by 2 hours
Digoxin	Hypothyroid patients are relatively more sensitive to digoxin	The dose of digoxin may need to be reduced as levothyroxine treatment is established
Sertraline	The effects of levothyroxine have been reported to be reduced	The dose of levothyroxine may need to be increased
Lofepramine		Its use with levothyroxine is contraindicated by the manufacturers
Theophylline	Reduced effects of theophylline	The dose of theophylline may need to be increased
Tricyclic antidepressants	Levothyroxine may accelerate the responses to imipramine and amitriptyline	The manufacturers of lofepramine contraindicate its use with levothyroxine
Warfarin	Increased anticoagulant effects of warfarin	The dose of warfarin may need to be reduced

therefore be avoided by patients prescribed thyroid treatment.

Other supplements

Many multivitamin and mineral preparation contain approximately 50–100% of the recommended daily intake of iodine. This is generally provided in the diet, with the possible exception of the vegan diet. Toxicity is rare at these doses but patients prescribed thyroid treatment should be careful to avoid excess doses, which may interfere with their treatment.

Practice points

- Both hyperthyroidism and hypothyroidism may present with relatively non-specific symptoms.
- Both may be readily diagnosed by thyroid function tests.
- Both may be managed by drugs; β blockers provide symptomatic relief in hyperthyroidism.
- Be alert for neutropenia in patients taking carbimazole and propylthiouracil.

Self-assessment

For the following questions concerning the management of thyroid disorders, choose the most appropriate answer:

1 *In the treatment of hyperthyroidism, which one of the following might provide some symptomatic relief in a patient who also has asthma?*

A   An antihistamine

B   Levothyroxine

C   A rate-limiting calcium-channel inhibitor (such as verapamil)

D   A β blocker (such as propranolol)

E   A muscarinic receptor antagonist (such as atropine)

2 *Which one of the following best describes the actions of an antithyroid drug such as carbimazole?*

A   It is also used to control seizures

B   It desensitises over time

C   It initially causes hypotension

D   It causes immediate relief

E   It takes several weeks for a full effect

3 *In the treatment of hypothyroidism, which one of the following is the best approach?*

A   Use of carbimazole as part of a block-and-replace regimen

B   Use of a TSH analogue

C   Use of levothyroxine

D   Iodine tablets

E   β blockers (such a propranolol)

CASE STUDY

A 35-year-old woman with a history of mild asthma developed anxiety, palpitations, rapid pulse and feelings of panic not long after a fall down a full flight of stairs. She put the symptoms down to the fall. Her symptoms worsened until she lost 10 kg (1.5 stone) in a week, developed a tremor, had broken vessels in the eye and the back of the knee, and a pulse of 150 beats/minute, at which time she visited her general practitioner. She was hyperthyroid and was prescribed propranolol and carbimazole. The pharmacist picked up a history of asthma and she was changed to atenolol. She developed a rash on her hands and feet but continued treatment for 2 years, at which point treatment was withdrawn.

- In this case it is possible that the initial palpitations and tachycardia may, in part, have been due to overuse of a β_2-adrenoceptor agonist or its increased sensitivity in hyperthyroidism. The pharmacist was correct to question the use of propranolol and atenolol was appropriate only if symptomatic control was considered absolutely essential because β_1-adrenoceptor antagonists may still lead to bronchospasm in patients with asthma. The rash would have been viewed as an acceptable side effect of carbimazole.

References

British National Formulary, latest edition. London: British Medical Association and Royal Pharmaceutical Society of Great Britain.

Online resource

www.btf-thyroid.org
The website of the British Thyroid Foundation providing professional and patient advice (accessed September 2015).

Feedback on self-assessments

Chapter 3

1 False: this is the recommendation for general health. Long sessions of 45–60 minutes are recommended to prevent obesity.
2 True: although it should be noted that this interaction may not be clinically significant with all calcium-channel blockers.
3 True: warfarin is a vitamin K antagonist and its actions may be reduced by foods rich in vitamin K.
4 True: there is a risk of symptoms of depression, including suicidal thoughts and behaviour in patients taking varenicline to help them stop smoking.

Chapter 4

1 False: they contain pharmacologically active components and may therefore produce adverse effects, particularly in concentrated form as supplements.
2 False: not many products currently have a traditional herbal registration (THR) number as this system is still in its infancy. However, these products should be supplied in preference to those without as more become available.
3 False: all serious adverse reactions to herbal preparations should be reported.
4 False: those with cardioactive activity or which alter clotting should be discontinued before surgery (see Table 4.1).
5 True.

Chapter 8

1 E: Infection with *H. pylori* is consistent with a positive ^{13}C-urea breath test.

2 D: proton pump inhibitors increase the risk of food poisoning in more vulnerable patients.
3 C: a penicillin (amoxicillin), a macrolide (clarithromycin) and a proton pump inhibitor is an example of 'Triple Therapy'.
4 D: NSAIDs reduce the production of cytoprotective prostanoids and this can increase acid secretion and reduce protection of the stomach.
5 D: misprostol is contraindicated in females of childbearing age as it may cause uterine contractions, potentially leading to an abortion in pregnancy.

Chapter 10

1 C: opioids commonly lead to constipation.
2 C: 5-amino salicylates are commonly used in inflammatory bowel disease.

Chapter 11

1 B: alkaline phosphatase along with γ-glutamyl transferase is elevated in cholestasis.
2 A: INR increases in chronic liver damage as the production of coagulation factors in impaired.
3 A: NSAIDs are fluid retaining and will exacerbate ascites.

Chapter 12

1 A: non-steroidal anti-inflammatory drugs are fluid retaining and may worsen hypertension.
2 D: hypertension is a major risk factor stroke and a compelling reason to treat hypertension.
3 A: only angiotensin-converting enzyme (ACE) inhibitors (and calcium-channel inhibitors) are

recommended as first-line antihypertensives in other healthy patients in the UK.

4 E: thiazide may worsen gout owing to impaired excretion of uric acid.

5 A: rate-limiting calcium channel antagonist plus β-adrenoceptor antagonist represents a serious drug interaction owing to the risk of asystole.

Chapter 13

1 A: HMG-CoA reductase is inhibited by statins.
2 A: atorvastatin has a long half-life and can be taken at any time of the day.
3 C: grapefruit juice should be avoided with statins as it can lead to increased plasma concentrations and adverse effects.

Chapter 14

1 E: orlistat inhibits pancreatic lipases to reduce the breakdown of lipids.
2 A: orlistat is associated with oily diarrhoea as fat is not absorbed and passes out in the faeces in an oily form

Chapter 15

1 C: the reduced heart rate increased diastole and so promotes coronary blood flow.
2 C: ST-depression on the ECG is consistent with angina.
3 C: nitrates act via guanylyl cyclase to increase cGMP.
4 E: nitrates do not reduce cardiovascular risk

Chapter 16

1 B: B-type natriuretic levels are increased in CHF.
2 B: peripheral oedema is associated with right sided failure.
3 A: rate-limiting calcium-channel inhibitors depress cardiac contractility and can worsen CHF.

4 C: renal function should be measured to determine dose and monitor for changes associated with ACE inhibitor-associated renal impairment.
5 E: angioedema is a rare but significant adverse effect of ACE inhibitors.
6 E: renal artery stenosis is a reason to avoid ACE inhibitors because of the risk of renal underperfusion and severe hypotension.
7 E: loop diuretics are commonly associated with reductions in plasma potassium.
8 A: initial reductions in cardiac output may lead to an initial worsening of symptoms.
9 C: COPD may be exacerbated by β blockers and they are used with caution.
10 C: second-line drugs after ACE inhibitors and β blockers are the aldosterone-receptor antagonists.

Chapter 17

1 B: warfarin is a vitamin K antagonist.
2 A: the effects of warfarin are delayed by 2–3 days as it impacts in the synthesis of new coagulation factors.
3 D: atrial fibrillation is a significant risk for thrombus formation leading to thromboembolic stroke.
4 E: digoxin is the only option with no appreciable interactions with warfarin.
5 C: induction of metabolism can reduce plasma concentrations leading to therapeutic failure.
6 D: low-molecular-weight heparins do not require monitoring of their effects on coagulation.
7 C: the activated partial thromboplastin time (APTT) will increase.
8 B: atrial fibrillation is a significant risk for thrombus formation leading to thromboembolic stroke.

Chapter 18

1 C: the mean corpuscular volume is in the normal range and so the anaemia is normocytic.
2 B: the reduction in oxygen carriage is associated with tiredness and breathlessness.
3 C: iron sulphate will help to build up iron stores.

Chapter 19

1 False: they are increased.
2 True: due to reduced production of EPO.
3 False: phosphate binders are used to reduce intake of phosphate from the diet.
4 True: this limits further renal damage.
5 True: ACE inhibitors have a major role in the prevention of diabetic nephropathy.

Chapter 20

1 True: simple analgesia plays a major role. Antibiotics are rarely indicated as most infections are viral.
2 False: prolonged use often leads to rebound secretion.
3 True: be alert for this in patients taking drugs associated with causing neutropenia.
4 True: requires urgent referral to exclude serious lung disease.
5 True: a common first-line drug.

Chapter 22

1 C: β blockers can cause bronchospasm and so are contraindicated in asthma.
2 A: NSAIDs can cause bronchospasm, thought to be due to increased availability of arachidonic acid for the lipoxygenase pathway.
3 D: long-acting β-adrenoceptor agonists are used at Step 3 of the stepped care and should be used in addition to steroids.
4 E: action is delayed by a few days as protein synthesis is altered.
5 E: their effectives are limited.
6 A: blocked by leukotriene receptor antagonists.
7 D: $β_2$-adrenceptors are coupled to adenylyl cyclase and a rise in cAMP.
8 B: smoking is the overwhelming cause of COPD.
9 B: bronchodilators ($β_2$-adrenceptor agonists and muscarinic receptor antagonists) are the mainstay of therapy.
10 B: COPD may lead to right-side heart failure (cor pulmonale).

Chapter 23

1 C: they activate a range of 5-HT_1 receptor subtypes.
2 B: vasoconstriction of cerebral vessels reduces the symptoms of migraine.
3 D: the antiepileptic drug is now recommended for prophylaxis.

Chapter 24

1 C: temporary loss of attention is a characteristic feature of absences.
2 C: carbamazepine induces hepatic metabolism, leading to a range of interactions.
3 A: lamotrigine has a good safety record in pregnancy.
4 D: saturation of metabolism leads to zero order kinetics with phenytoin, such that plasma concentrations can increase dramatically.

Chapter 25

1 D: nausea caused by increased levels of 5-HT is a common and early side effect of selective serotonin reuptake inhibitors (SSRIs).
2 D: beneficial effects are delayed.
3 D: SSRIs and tricyclic antidepressant (TCAs) are equally effective but SSRIs have fewer side effects and are considered safer as TCAs can lead to fatal overdoses.
4 C: SSRIs are considered safer in cardiovascular disease.
5 D: CBT is recommended in mild depression in which drug treatment is of questionable value.
6 D: St John's wort is a powerful inducer of drug metabolism, leading to a range of interactions.
7 A: lithium has a narrow therapeutic window and plasma levels are greatly influenced by renal function and also electrolyte balance.
8 D: the mode of action is unclear but it is known to affect intracellular signalling by interfering with IP_3 levels.

Chapter 26

1 C: the SSRI sertraline is used in anxiety; diazepam is only used if essential.
2 A: fluvoxamine

Chapter 27

1 True: diuretics may be associated with insomnia indirectly if diuresis occurs at night.
2 False: temazepam is a short-acting benzodiazepine and therefore suitable for short-term treatment of insomnia, having reduced hangover effects compared with longer-acting drugs.
3 True: excess caffeine and alcohol consumption and eating a large meal late at night are all associated with insomnia.
4 False: promethazine is an antihistamine available over-the-counter but should be used only occasionally due to the risk of adverse effects, e.g. antimuscarinic effects, and also reduced effectiveness after a few days of treatment.
5 True: establishing the pattern of insomnia is important so that an appropriate referral can be made and the underlying cause treated.

Chapter 28

1 D: clozapine is associated with agranulocytosis leading to neutropenia.
2 B: antipsychotic drugs are all dopamine-receptor antagonists.

Chapter 29

1 C: blockade of dopamine receptors is a key cause of drug-induced Parkinson's disease.
2 D: levodopa is metabolised to dopamine.
3 E: peripheral conversion of levodopa to dopamine leads to side effects and these are reduced by DOPA decarboxylase inhibitors.
4 B: effectiveness is finite.

Chapter 30

1 False: aspirin is generally avoided now due to gastric side effects and its use being prohibited in children.
2 True: it is devoid of anti-inflammatory actions.
3 True: a common side effect and laxatives are co-prescribed when they are used long term.

4 False: it is widely used in neuropathic pain.
5 False: it is appropriate for chronic neuropathic pain.

Chapter 31

1 True.
2 False: this is a safe and effective combination for pain relief.
3 False: it is used in rheumatoid arthritis.
4 True: risk of an interaction leading to methotrexate toxicity.
5 False: it is used by specialists when two other disease-modifying antirheumatoid drugs (DMARDs) have failed to control the condition.

Chapter 33

1 False: combined preparations of antiemetic and opioid are not recommended because opioid-induced nausea usually resolves after 4–5 days and therefore long-term use of the antiemetic is not necessary.
2 True.
3 True as this may be associated with the release of prostaglandins.
4 True: a 24-hour dose is calculated and divided by two for modified-release preparations given twice a day.
5 False: this is a common misconception and patients should be encouraged to discuss their concerns about morphine.

Chapter 34

1 D: macrolides are associated with inhibition of hepatic cytochrome P450 isoforms, leading to a range of interactions.
2 B: CRP levels rise in reponse to infections.
3 C: penicillins inhibit bacterial transpeptidases to prevent cross-linking of cell walls.
4 A: clavulanic acid inhibits β-lactamases.
5 B: because of discoloration of teeth.
6 B: rifampicin is associated induction of hepatic cytochrome P450 isoforms, leading to a range of interactions.

7 D: chloramphenicol is an OTC medicine for conjunctivitis.
8 E: clindamycin poses a risk for *C. difficile* infection.
9 B: cellulitis involves infection of the skin, often after a puncture wound.
10 D: through inhibition of aldehyde dehydrogenase.

Chapter 35

1 False: they should be used only during an infestation.
2 False: it is unsuitable for use in pregnancy.
3 True.
4 True: chloroquine exacerbates psoriasis.
5 False: combined oral contraception may be affected due to reduced enterohepatic circulation of the oestrogen ethinylestradiol.

Chapter 36

1 C: these are characteristic of eczema.
2 E: widespread infection should be treated with oral flucloxacillin.
3 B: oral terbinafine is appropriate.
4 A: the sebum is reduced by 90% which is beneficial in acne.

5 C: retinoids are highly teratogenic.
6 B: they have a key role.
7 A: the increased turnover of cells leads to the symptoms.
8 E: metronidazole has a key role.
9 C: surgical removal has a very high cure rate.
10 B: spider naevi are associated with alcoholic liver disease.

Chapter 37

1 C: the others are key symptoms.
2 B: evidence supports use of metformin as first-line treatment except where there is renal impairment.
3 A: inhibition of ATP-sensitive potassium channels leads to cellular depolarisation and insulin secretion.
4 D: weight gain caused by increased insulin secretion.
5 B: moderate renal impairment increases the risk of lactic acidosis.
6 A: acting as GLP-1 receptor agonists.

Chapter 38

1 C: β blockers are contraindicated due to asthma and so a rate-limiting calcium-channel inhibitor may be used to control heart rate.
2 E: the response is delayed.
3 C: this replaces the thyroid hormones.

Appendix 1

Formulary of some important classes of drugs, commonly used examples, mechanisms of action and uses

Class	Examples	Actions	Common uses
Gastrointestinal			
Proton pump inhibitors (PPIs)	Omeprazole,[a] lansoprazole, rabeprazole	Irreversible proton pump inhibition	Acid suppression – peptic ulceration, GORD, prophylaxis against NSAID-induced damage
Histamine H_2-receptor antagonists	Ranitidine[a]	Antagonism of histamine H_2-receptor	Acid suppression – peptic ulceration, GORD, dyspepsia
Cytoprotective prostaglandin analogue	Misoprostol	Analogue of PGE_1, reduces H^+ secretion and stimulates bicarbonate and mucus secretion	Prophylaxis against NSAID-induced damage
Triple therapy for *Helicobacter pylori* eradication	PPI plus two from amoxicillin, clarithromycin and metronidazole	Acid suppression and *H. pylori* eradication	*H. pylori* eradication in peptic ulceration
Prokinetic drugs	Metoclopramide	Increase gastric emptying	Bloating and nausea
Laxative	Lactulose,[a] senna,[a] ispaghula[a]	Lactulose: osmotic. Senna: stimulant. Ispaghula: bulk	Constipation, constipation due to drugs, IBS. Lactulose: also in liver failure to prevent encephalopathy
Antidiarrhoeal agents	Loperamide[a]	Opioid: reduces colonic motility via presynaptic inhibition	Diarrhoea
Antispasmodic agents	Mebeverine[a]	Phosphodiesterase inhibitor?	IBS
Cardiovascular			
Cardiac glycosides	Digoxin	Inhibition of Na^+/K^+ ATPase	AF, positive inotrope in CHF
Class I antiarrhythmics	Lidocaine	Inhibition of Na^+ channels	Ventricular tachycardia
Class II antiarrhythmics	β blockers (including sotalol)	Antagonism of β-adrenoceptors	Paroxysmal AF
Class III antiarrhythmics	Amiodarone, sotalol	Blockade of K^+ channels leading to action potential prolongation	AF

Class	Examples	Actions	Common uses
Class IV antiarrhythmics	Verapamil	Blockade of Ca^{2+} channels	Supraventricular tachycardia
Thiazide diuretics and thiazide-like	Bendroflumethiazide, indapamide, chlorthalidone	Inhibition of Na^+/Cl^- transporter in DCT	Hypertension, mild CHF (especially elderly people)
Loop diuretics	Furosemide, bumetanide	Inhibition of $Na^+/K^+/Cl^-$ transporter in loop of Henle; vasodilatation	CHF and LVF, renal failure
Potassium-sparing diuretics	Amiloride	Inhibition of aldosterone-sensitive Na^+ channels in DCT	Weak diuresis, especially in combination with K^+-losing diuretics (thiazides and loops)
Potassium-sparing diuretic, aldosterone antagonist	Spironolactone	Aldosterone receptor antagonist	Weak diuresis, especially in combination with K^+-losing diuretics (thiazides and loops), CHF and liver failure (ascites); Conn's syndrome
β blockers (non-selective)	Propranolol	Antagonism of β-adrenoceptors	Angina, post-MI, anxiety, migraine prophylaxis, hyperthyroidism
$β_1$ blockers	Atenolol, metoprolol, bisoprolol	Antagonism of $β_1$-adrenoceptors	Angina, post-MI; stable CHF (with caution)
ACE inhibitors	Captopril, enalapril, ramipril, lisinopril, perindopril	Inhibition of ACE, reducing synthesis of angiotensin II	Hypertension, post-MI, CHF, diabetic nephropathy
Angiotensin (AT_1) receptor antagonist (sartans)	Losartan, candesartan, valsartan	Antagonism of AT_1-receptors	Hypertension, CHF diabetic nephropathy?
Calcium-channel blockers	Verapamil, amlodipine, nifedipine, diltiazem	Inhibition of VSM Ca^{2+} channels and cardiac Ca^{2+} channels (diltiazem, verapamil)	Hypertension, angina. Diltiazem and verapamil: antiarrhythmic
Nitrates	Glyceryl trinitrate,[a] isosorbide mononitrate[a]	Act via nitric oxide to increase cGMP	Angina, CHF
K^+ channel activators	Nicorandil	Activation of ATP-sensitive K^+ channels and release of nitric oxide	Angina
α blockers	Prazosin, doxazosin, indoramin	Antagonism of α-adrenoceptors	Resistant hypertension, prostatic hypertrophy
Centrally acting antihypertensives	Clonidine, moxonidine, α-methyldopa	• Clonidine: central $α_2$-adrenoceptors • Moxonidine: central imidazoline receptors	Resistant hypertension
HMG-CoA reductase inhibitors (statins)	Simvastatin,[a] pravastatin, atorvastatin, fluvastatin	HMG-CoA reductase inhibition in cholesterol synthesis	Reduction of cholesterol in hypercholesterolaemia and in patients with a high CV risk
Fibrates	Bezafibrate, gemifibrozil	Activates α-peroxisome proliferator-activated receptors (PPAR-α)	Hypercholesterolaemia and hypertriglyceridaemia
Bile binding agents	Colestyramine	Binds bile in gastrointestinal tract	Hypercholesterolaemia

(continued)

(continued)

Class	Examples	Actions	Common uses
Fibrinolytics	Streptokinase, alteplase	Activates plasminogen to form plasmin	• Clot busting in MI, PE • Alteplase is used in ischaemic stroke
Antiplatelet drugs	Low-dose aspirin,[a] clopidogrel	Aspirin: inhibition of platelet COX. Clopidogrel: ADP ($P2Y_{12}$) receptor antagonist	Prevention of MI and CVA. Prophylaxis for CVA in low-risk patients with AF
Injectable anticoagulants	Low-molecular-weight heparins (dalteparin, enoxaparin, tinzaparin), unfractionated heparin	Activates antithrombin III	Immediate anticoagulation
Oral anticoagulants	Warfarin	Vitamin K antagonist	Prophylaxis against thrombosis, e.g. DVT, PE, CVA in AF, thrombosis on mechanical heart valves
Respiratory			
β_2 agonists	Salbutamol, terbutaline	Activation of β_2-adrenoceptors	Relief in asthma, COPD
β_2 agonists, long acting	Salmeterol, formoterol	Long-lasting activation of β_2-adrenoceptors	Long-term control in asthma, COPD
Corticosteroids	Beclometasone, budesonide	Anti-inflammatory	Prevention in asthma; 15% of COPD patients also benefit. Nasal use in hayfever[a]
Muscarinic antagonists	Ipratropium, tiotropium	Blockade of vagal bronchoconstriction	Relief in asthma, COPD
Cromones	Sodium cromoglicate	Unclear – may stabilise mast cells/sensory nerves	Prevention in asthma. Nasal and ocular use in hayfevera
Xanthines	Theophylline	Phosphodiesterase inhibition, adenosine receptor antagonist	Relief in asthma
Leukotriene receptor antagonist	Montelukast, zafirlukast	Leukotriene receptor antagonist	Prevention in asthma; NSAID-induced bronchospasm
Antihistamines	Loratadine,[a] chlorphenamine,[a] cetirizine[a]	Antagonism of H_1-receptors	Allergy, older sedating agents (diphenhydramine, chlorphenamine, promethazine) for insomnia
Central nervous system			
Benzodiazepines	Diazepam, temazepam	Enhancement of GABA at GABA-A receptors	Anxiety, insomnia. Short-term only
Z-drugs	Zopiclone, zolpidem	Enhancement of GABA at GABA-A receptors	Insomnia
Antipsychotics	Haloperidol, chlorpromazine, fluphenazine	Dopamine (D_2)-receptor antagonists	Schizophrenia
Atypical antipsychotics	Clozapine, olanzapine, risperidone	Dopamine and 5HT receptor antagonists	Schizophrenia

Class	Examples	Actions	Common uses
Antimanic drugs	Lithium	Uncertain	Bipolar affective disorder
Tricyclic antidepressants (TCAs)	Amitriptyline, lofepramine, dosulepin	Inhibition of noradrenaline (norepinephrine) and 5HT reuptake	Depression. Amitriptyline: neuropathic pain; prophylaxis in migraine, IBS
Serotonin selective reuptake inhibitors (SSRIs)	Fluoxetine, paroxetine, citalopram, sertraline	Inhibition of 5HT reuptake	Depression, anxiety, panic disorder
Monoamine oxidase inhibitors (MAOIs)	Phenelzine, moclobemide	Inhibition of MAO enzymes (moclobemide is reversible) and catecholamine metabolism	Resistant depression
Other antidepressants	Venlafaxine, reboxetine, mirtazapine	Reboxetine: noradrenaline reuptake inhibitor. Venlafaxine: serotonin–noradrenaline reuptake inhibitor. Mirtazapine α_2-antagonist and $5HT_2$ and $5HT_3$ antagonist	Depression. Venlafaxine also for anxiety
Antiobesity	Orlistat[a]	Orlistat: pancreatic lipase inhibitor	Obesity
Antiemetics	Promethazine, cyclizine,[a] hyoscine,[a] metoclopramide, ondansetron	Promethazine and cyclizine: H_1-receptor antagonists. Hyoscine: M-receptor antagonist. Metoclopramide: dopamine D_2-receptor antagonist. Ondansetron: $5HT_3$-receptor antagonist	Promethazine, hyoscine and cyclizine: motion sickness. Metoclopramide: emesis due to anticancer drugs. Ondansetron: emesis due to anticancer drugs; postoperative nausea and vomiting
Non-opioid analgesics	Paracetamol,[a] NSAIDs (ibuprofen,[a] diclofenac, naproxen, mefenamic acid)	COX inhibition. Paracetamol may inhibit the putative COX-3?	Pain, antipyretic and NSAIDs in inflammation
COX-2 inhibitors	'Coxibs' (celecoxib), etodolac and meloxicam	Inhibition of COX-2	Inflammation
Opioid analgesics	Morphine, tramadol, codeine,[a] dihydrocodeine[a]	Opioid receptors	Pain
Opioid antagonist	Naloxone	Opioid receptor antagonist	Reversal of opioids
Antimigraine (triptans)	Sumatriptan,[a] naratriptan	$5HT_{1D}$-receptor agonists	Treatment of a migraine attack
Antimigraine, prophylaxis	Pizotifen	$5HT_2$-receptor antagonist	Prevention of migraine
Antiepileptic drugs	Sodium valproate, carbamazepine, phenytoin	Valproate: potentiation of GABA. Carbamazepine and phenytoin: use-dependent inhibition of Na^+ channels, inhibiting propagation of excitation	Forms of epilepsy: all for tonic–clonic and partial seizures; valproate for absences and myoclonic seizures. Carbamazepine is also used in neuropathic pain and for bipolar affective disorder
Newer antiepileptic drugs	Lamotrigine, gabapentin	Lamotrigine: blockade of Na^+ channels and decreased release of glutamate. Gabapentin: unknown	Certain forms of epilepsy (gabapentin in combination), neuropathic pain

(continued)

(continued)

Class	Examples	Actions	Common uses
Anti-Parkinsonian drugs	Levodopa with carbidopa, ropinirole, rotigotine, procyclidine, selegiline	Levodopa: conversion to dopamine. Ropinirole, rotigotine: dopamine D_2 agonists. Procyclidine: muscarinic antagonist. Selegiline: MAO-B inhibitor	Parkinson's disease
Alzheimer's disease	Donepezil, galantamine, rivastigmine	Acetylcholine esterase inhibitors	Alzheimer's disease
Antimicrobial agents			
Penicillin	Amoxicillin, phenoxymethyl-penicillin, flucloxacillin	Inhibition of cross-linking of peptide side chains	Phenoxymethylpenicillin: tonsillitis. Flucloxacillin: impetigo, cellulitis. Amoxicillin: chest infections, otitis media, UTIs
Cephalosporins	Cefalexin, cefotaxime, cefaclor	Binding to β-lactam-binding sites and inhibiting cell wall synthesis	Septicaemia, pneumonia, meningitis, biliary tract infections, peritonitis, and UTIs
Tetracylines	Tetracycline, doxycycline	Inhibition of protein synthesis, through interfering with RNA binding	*Chlamydia* infection, exacerbation of chronic bronchitis *(Haemophilus influenzae)*, periodontal disease, acne, respiratory and genital mycoplasma infections. Doxycycline in malaria prophylaxis
Macrolides	Erythromycin, clarithromycin	Prevent the translocation movement of the bacterial ribosome along the mRNA and prevent protein synthesis	Suitable alternative in patients who are allergic to penicillin. Respiratory infections, whooping cough, Legionnaires' disease, campylobacter enteritis
Aminoglycosides	Gentamicin	Irreversibly bind to the bacterial ribosomes leading to an inhibition of protein synthesis	Gentamicin is used in various infections such as septicaemia, meningitis, acute pyelonephritis and endocarditis
Sulphonamides and trimethoprim	Trimethoprim	Inhibition of folate synthesis and reduces the precursors of DNA and RNA	Pneumonia in AIDS patients, toxoplasmosis and nocardiosis. Acute exacerbation of chronic bronchitis, otitis media and UTIs
Antituberculous	Rifampicin, isoniazid, pyrazinamide, ethambutol	Isoniazid and rifampicin most effective versus continually growing bacteria. Rifampicin versus intermittently dividing bacteria. Pyrazinamide versus rapidly dividing intracellular organisms, hence most effective in first 2 months	Tuberculosis
Quinolones	Ciprofloxacin, ofloxacin	Inhibition of bacterial DNA gyrase	*Pseudomonas aeruginosa, Haemophilus influenzae, Campylobacter* spp.

Class	Examples	Actions	Common uses
Others	Metronidazole	DNA damage due to toxic oxygen products	Trichomonal vaginosis, giardiasis, pseudomembranous colitis, tumours and rosacea
	Chloramphenicol[a]	Binds to bacterial ribosomes and inhibits protein synthesis	Eye drops used in bacterial conjunctivitis
Antiviral	Aciclovir,[a] famciclovir, zanamivir	Aciclovir: inhibition of herpesvirus DNA polymerase. Zanamivir: a neuramidase inhibitor which prevents the entry and release of the viral particles from the host cells	Aciclovir: herpes simplex and herpes varicella. Zanamivir: influenza
Imidazoles	Clotrimazole[a]	Inhibition of cytochrome P450-dependent demethylase which converts lanosterol to ergosterol; accumulation of lanosterol disrupts fungal membrane	Fungal infections
Triazoles	Itraconazole, fluconazole[a]	As for imidazoles	Fungal infections
Other antifungal agents	Griseofulvin, terbinafine,[a] amphotericin	Terbinafine inhibits the conversion of squalene to lanosterol, with the accumulation of squalene causing cell death. Griseofulvin: interferes with fungal microtubules and nucleic acid synthesis	Griseofulvin: suitable for tinea infections but not candidiasis
Endocrine			
Sulphonylureas	Glibenclamide, tolbutamide, gliclazide, glipizide, glimepiride	Inhibition of ATP-sensitive K^+ channels, leading to insulin release	Type 2 diabetes
Biguanides	Metformin	Activation of AMP kinase? This may increase glucose uptake and reduce glucose production by the liver. It may also suppress lipid synthesis and promote fatty acid oxidation	Type 2 diabetes
Thiazolidinediones	Pioglitazone	'Insulin sensitisers', which work by enhancing glucose utilisation in tissues, and so reduce insulin resistance. They activate the nuclear peroxisome proliferator-activated receptors γ (PPAR-γ)	Type 2 diabetes
Antithyroid	Carbimazole	Decreases the production of thyroid hormones by inhibiting the iodination of thyroglobulin	Hyperthyroidism

(continued)

(continued)

Class	Examples	Actions	Common uses
Corticosteroids	Prednisolone, hydrocortisone,[a] dexamethasone	A range of immunosuppressant actions, including production of lipocortin, which inhibits phospholipase A_2	Anti-inflammatory. Topical hydrocortisone for eczema. Dexamethasone for nerve compression in palliative care
Others			
Topical vitamin D_3 analogues	Calcipotriol	Acts on keratinocyte vitamin D receptors, and has antiproliferative actions and reduces epidermal proliferation	Psoriasis
Oral retinoids	Acitretin, tretinoin and isotretinoin	Binds to nuclear retinoic acid receptors and affects gene transcription, resulting in antiproliferative actions and normal keratinocyte maturation	Acitretin: psoriasis. Tretinoin and isotretinoin: acne
Folate antagonist	Methotrexate	Inhibits dihydrofolate reductase	Anticancer chemotherapy; immunosuppressant for psoriasis, asthma, Crohn's disease
Immunosuppressants	Azathioprine, ciclosporin	Azathioprine: inhibits nucleic acid synthesis and prevents lymphocyte production. Ciclosporin: prevents activation of T lymphocytes	Immunosuppression including prevention of transplant rejection
5-Aminosalicylates	Mesalazine, sulfasalazine	Yield 5-aminosalicylic acid, leading to inhibition of leukotriene and prostanoid formation, scavenging free radicals, and decreasing neutrophil chemotaxis	Ulcerative colitis, Crohn's disease

[a]Certain preparations of these drugs are available over-the-counter for certain indications.

5HT, 5-hydroxytryptamine; AIDS, acquired immune deficiency syndrome; AF, atrial fibrillation; AMP, adenosine monophosphate; ATP, adenosine triphosphate; cGMP, guanosine cyclic 3′:5′-monophosphate; CHF, chronic heart failure; CoA, coenzyme A; COPD, chronic obstructive pulmonary disease; COX, cyclo-oxygenase; CV, cerebrovascular; CVA, cerebrovascular accident; DCT, distal convoluted tubule; DVT, deep venous thrombosis; GABA, γ-aminobutyric acid; GORD, gastro-oesophageal reflux disease; HMG, hydroxymethylglutaryl; IBS, irritable bowel syndrome; LVF, left ventricular failure; MI, myocardial infarction; NSAID, non-steroidal anti-inflammatory drug; PE, pulmonary embolism; PGE_1, prostaglandin E_1; UTIs, urinary tract infections; VSM, vascular smooth muscle.

Appendix 2

Some important clinical measurements and therapeutic drug monitoring

Table A2.1 Biochemical measurements

Biochemical parameter	Reference ranges	Comments
Sodium (Na⁺)	135–145 mmol/L >155–160 mmol/L confusion and coma <120 mmol/L weakness and confusion	Sodium controls the volume of extracellular fluid. Sodium is involved in neuronal action potentials and is therefore important for excitable tissues
Potassium (K⁺)	3.5–5.3 mmol/L >6.5 mmol/L or <2.5 mmol/L are medical emergencies	• Potassium levels determine membrane potential and influence the functioning of excitable tissues such as muscles and neurons • Hypokalaemia increases toxicity with digoxin therapy
Calcium (Ca²⁺)	2.25–2.6 mmol/L >3.50 mmol/L danger of cardiac arrest <1.6 mmol/L tetany (muscle spasm/twitching)	Calcitonin and parathyroid hormones maintain calcium blood plasma levels. As well as its role as a component of bone and teeth, calcium is essential for many metabolic processes, including nerve function, muscle contraction and blood clotting
Magnesium (Mg²⁺)	0.7–1.2 mmol/L	Magnesium is found in bones and is essential for the functioning of nerves and muscles. It is also a cofactor for many enzymes
Creatinine (plasma)	60–120 micromoles/L	When calculating creatinine clearance as an indication of renal function, creatinine levels are adjusted according to age, weight and sex
Creatinine clearance	97–140 mL/minute males 85–125 mL/minute females	Used to estimate GFR
eGFR	>90 mL/minute per 1.73 m²	Used to indicate renal function
Urea	2.0–6.5 mmol/L	May be elevated in renal disease or high protein intake
Uric acid	0.15–0.47 mmol/L	• Elevated by thiazide diuretics • Excess may present as gouty arthritis due to deposits of uric acid crystals in joints
Bicarbonate (HCO₃₋)	22–29 mmol/L	• Important for acid–base balance • Reflects renal and metabolic function
HbA₁c	<48 mmol/mol	• Glycated haemoglobin • Measured to assess the glycaemic control over the previous 2 months by patients with diabetes
Cholesterol	Ideal <5.0 mmol/L	A risk factor for cardiovascular disease. Should be considered as the ratio of LDL:HDL (ideally <3)

(continued)

Table A2.1 *(continued)*

Biochemical parameter	Reference ranges	Comments
Triglycerides	<2.1 mmol/L males	A mild risk factor for cardiovascular disease.
	<1.7 mmol/L females	Associated with obesity and alcohol abuse

(e) GFR, (estimated) glomerular filtration rate; HDL, high-density lipoprotein; LDL, low-density lipoprotein.

Table A2.2 Summary of liver function tests

Parameter	Reference range (check local ranges)	Comment
Aspartate transaminase (AST)	<50 iu/L	Elevated in acute hepatocyte damage but considered to be a non-specific parameter
Alanine transaminase (ALT)	<45 iu/L	Elevated following hepatocyte damage and tends to indicate acute damage
Alkaline phosphatase (ALP)	39–117 iu/L	Indicator of cholestasis but non-specific as it is also found in bone, placenta and intestine. Consider also the level of GGT as levels of ALP may be increased in other types of liver disease
γ-Glutamyl transferase (transpeptidase) (GGT)	Up to 70 iu/L (males) Up to 40 iu/L (females)	Often used in the diagnosis of cholestasis but may also be elevated in acute or chronic hepatitis, alcoholism and in patients taking inducers such as anticonvulsants
Unconjugated (free) bilirubin	5–17 micromoles/L (>35 micromoles/L produces jaundice)	Increased levels indicate impaired liver function
Prothrombin time	10–14 s	Prolonged when clotting factor synthesis is reduced, e.g. chronic hepatitis and/or malabsorption of vitamins, warfarin treatment
INR	1–1.2	Ratio of prothrombin time compared with a control
Albumin	30–48 g/L	Reduced levels are associated with reduced synthetic activity of the liver

INR, international normalised ratio.

Table A2.3 Haematological parameters

Haematological parameter	Reference value(s)	Comments
White blood cells (leukocytes: WBC)	$4–11 \times 10^9$/L	Increased levels (leukocytosis) during infection or malignancy
Neutrophils	$2.5–7.5 \times 10^9$/L	Reduced levels (leukopenia) due to drugs (Chapter 6), viral infections, chronic infections or hypersensitivity reaction
Lymphocytes	$1.5–3.5 \times 10^9$/L	
Monocytes	$0.2–0.8 \times 10^9$/L	
Eosinophils	$0.04–0.4 \times 10^9$/L	
Basophils	$0.01–0.1 \times 10^9$/L	

Table A2.3 *(continued)*

Haematological parameter	Reference value(s)	Comments
Erythrocyte sedimentation rate (ESR)	• 0–9 mm/hour male • 0–20 mm/hour female	Elevated with increasing age, during pregnancy, chronic infection, dysproteinaemias, cancer and inflammatory diseases (e.g. giant cell arteritis, rheumatoid arthritis)
Serum ferritin	• 15–300 micrograms/L male • 15–200 micrograms/L female	A measure of iron stores
Haemoglobin (Hb) (Chapter 18)	• 13.5–17.5 g/dL male • 11.5–15.5 g/dL female	Symptoms of anaemia appear at levels <9–10 g/dL
Platelets	$140–400 \times 10^9$/L	Low due to infections, drug-induced thrombocytopenia (Chapter 18), bone marrow hypoplasia, uraemia, liver disease, severe megaloblastic anaemia and alcohol abuse
Mean corpuscular volume (MCV)	76–95 fL	• Raised in vitamin B_{12} or folate deficiency, excess alcohol consumption or liver disease • Reduced in iron-deficient anaemia or chronic blood loss or thalassaemia • May be normal during acute blood loss or anaemia of chronic disease (e.g. renal anaemia)
Red blood cells (RBCs, erythrocytes)	• $4.5–6.5 \times 10^{12}$/L male • $3.8–5.8 \times 10^{12}$/L female	
Haematocrit (Hct) or packed cell volume (PCV)	• 37–54 % male • 35–47% female	PCV of anticoagulated blood The Hct gives a crude indication of red cell volume but the RBC and MCV reveal more specific details
Mean corpuscular haemoglobin (MCH)	27–33 pg	• Consider with other red cell parameters • Raised in vitamin B_{12} or folate deficiency • Lowered due to chronic blood loss, iron deficiency, thalassaemia or megaloblastic anaemia
Vitamin B_{12}	211–911 ng/L	• Deficiency may result in macrocytic anaemia (Chapter 18) • Vitamin B_{12} deficiency may be due to low dietary intake (vegans)
Folate (serum)	2.9–18 micrograms/L	• Deficiency may result in macrocytic anaemia (Chapter 18) • Folate deficiency may be due to malabsorption or drug causes (Chapter 18)

Table A2.4 Some important examples in therapeutic drug monitoring

Drug	Concentration range	Comments
Digoxin	0.8–2.0 micrograms/L	• The risk of toxicity is increased in renal impairment • Sample >6 hours after the dose • Toxicity may present as visual disturbances, arrhythmias, vomiting, gastrointestinal disturbances, confusion • Patients should be counselled to ensure that their pulse does not drop <60 beats/minute
Theophylline	10–20 mg/L	• Risk of toxicity is increased by drug interactions • Smoking reduces plasma concentrations • Toxicity may present as nausea, vomiting, arrhythmias, convulsions

(continued)

Table A2.4 *(continued)*		
Drug	**Concentration range**	**Comments**
Lithium	0.4–1 mmol/L	• Plasma levels influenced by renal function • Patients should be hydrated and not greatly alter sodium intake • Sample 12 hours after dose • A failure of treatment might be due to subtherapeutic levels • Toxicity may present as tremor, visual disturbances, gastrointestinal disturbances, weakness, CNS disturbances
Phenytoin	10–20 mg/L	• Zero order kinetics (Chapter 7) mean that therapeutic concentrations are difficult to achieve. Patients vary considerably. Therapeutic drug monitoring guides the dosage • Toxicity may present as nystagmus, nausea, vomiting, CNS disturbances • Low therapeutic levels may lead to failure to control seizures

CNS, central nervous system.

Index